Personal Property
of
Dolores L. Hilaga RN, B.S.N

Critical Care

Certification Preparation and Review

Publishing Director: David Culverwell
Executive Editor: Richard A. Weimer
Production Editor/Text Designer: Donna M. Griffin
Art Director/Cover Designer: Don Sellers, AMI
Assistant Art Director: Bernard Vervin
Illustrators: Joe Vitek and Bruce Bolinger
Manufacturing Director: John Komsa, Jr.

Typesetting by: Carver Photocomposition, Inc., Arlington, VA
Typefaces: Palatino (text) and Optima (display)
Printed by: Fairfield Graphics, Fairfield, PA
Index by: Leah Kramer

Critical Care

Certification Preparation and Review

Dot E. Langfitt, RN, MN, CCRN

President
CRIT-ED
Columbia, South Carolina

Consultant
CRIT-MORE
Columbia, South Carolina

Formerly

Clinical Specialist in Critical Care
Richland Memorial Hospital
Columbia, South Carolina

Robert J. Brady Co.
A Prentice-Hall Publishing and Communications Company
Bowie, Maryland 20715

Critical Care: Certification Preparation and Review

Library of Congress Cataloging in Publication Data

Langfitt, Dot E.
  Critical care.

  Bibliography: p.
  Includes Index.
  1. Intensive care nursing—Handbooks, manuals, etc.
I. Title.
RT120.I5L36 1984 616'.025'024613 83-15451
ISBN 0-89303-245-X

Prentice-Hall International, Inc., London
Prentice-Hall Canada, Inc., Scarborough, Ontario
Prentice-Hall of Australia, Pty., Ltd., Sydney
Prentice-Hall of India Private Limited, New Delhi
Prentice-Hall of Japan, Inc., Tokyo
Prentice-Hall of Southeast Asia Pte. Ltd., Singapore
Whitehall Books, Limited, Petone, New Zealand
Editora Prentice-Hall Do Brasil LTDA., Rio de Janeiro

Printed in the United States of America

84 85 86 87 88 89 90 91 92 93 94 10 9 8 7 6 5 4 3 2 1

Contents

Dedicated with love to my husband William and sons, William III, Timothy Robert, and David Scott,

and to all critical care nurses who foster better patient care and increased professionalism through voluntarily obtaining critical care certification.

Acknowledgements

Many people have played significant roles in helping me write this book. I would like to thank Rick Weimer, Executive Editor, for his support, patience, and guidance throughout the months of writing and rewriting.

Donna Griffin, Production Editor, has been unfailing in her efforts to help me through the "publishing process" and has continually been available (and used) at all hours of the day and night to answer questions, clarify points, and, most importantly, to provide the encouragement needed in this undertaking. She was always positive that we would complete the project, even when I was ready to give up.

Bernard Vervin, Assistant Art Director, provided much needed support so that my ideas for pictures could actually become pictures, and Joe Vitek proved Bernard correct by drawing the illustrations so necessary for this book.

My husband and three sons gave willingly of their time and energy to put my written words into the word processor and played pivotal roles in correcting printouts and reading galleys for many months.

Dr. Larry Nelson provided help by re-inforcing the value of this undertaking and by helping me cope with many major problems that threatened to divert my resolve to write this book.

Many colleagues reviewed sections of the book for accuracy and completeness. Included in this group are Drs. Rod McMillin, William Brannon, William Keane, Richard Helman and Kay McFarland, and Eric Hoffman, Pharm. D., Mrs. Triphy Barber, RN, PhD, along with Mrs. Anne Hale, RN.

Miss Betty Branham spent many hours after work and during holidays typing the first version of this book before the word processor use became feasible.

A special thanks goes to Mr. Ed Watson, a board certified respiratory therapist who provided the pulmonary formulae and the sample calculations for the appendix.

Many others helped through continuous support and encouragement in this endeavor. Only the lack of space precludes naming everyone—but to many, many people, I express a sincere heartfelt thank you.

Introduction

Purpose of the Text

The critical care nurse is responsible for providing safe, competent, and comprehensive care to the patient experiencing a life-threatening disruption of the normal hemodynamic mechanisms of one or more body systems.

Certification by the American Association for Critical Care Nurses establishes your knowledge base of the pulmonary, cardiovascular, neurologic, renal, endocrine (metabolic), gastrointestinal, hematologic, shock, and psychosocial areas.

Certification is initially granted *only* by successful completion of the certification examination. The revised *Core Curriculum* is an outline of the basic information necessary for certification. This textbook has been written to *supplement* the revised edition of the *Core Curriculum* by filling in the outline.

This textbook is designed to provide concise, succinct knowledge needed to prepare you to complete the critical care certification exam successfully. This textbook will provide critical care nurses who do not have access to formal courses with a home study course designed to help them prepare for the critical care certification examination and/or to supplement their knowledge of critical care nursing. No course or text can guarantee successful completion of the certification examination; but, the more knowledge you have, the better your chances. We cannot assume that all readers share a common level of educational preparation or clinical practice. Consequently, basic anatomy, physiology, pathophysiology, and nursing care are all concisely and thoroughly presented. This text will assist the critical care nurse in developing an in-depth knowledge base for each of the body systems relevant to critical care. It will help the critical care nurse to correlate the pathophysiology of specific disease entities within each body system and to identify and anticipate interactions between the body systems. This text will also help to identify appropriate nursing interventions in each disease entity and help to determine a logical sequence of steps in performing complete and accurate assessments of each body system.

This book will provide the critical care nurse with a readily available reference source.

Design of the Text

Each body system is presented in a separate section. Within each section, there are a series of chapters following similar formats. The first chapter in each body system is on anatomy. The anatomy chapters include only that which is needed for critical care nursing. The second chapter in each body system explains the physiology of the specific body system. The *emphasis* is on enhancing the knowledge of anatomy and physiology needed by the critical care nurse to provide a scientific base for applying the nursing process in administering patient care. The third chapter of each section varies according to the body system involved. Some third chapters present norms, whereas others cover specific disease entities.

A special section pertaining to the assessment of each of the eight body systems involved in critical care is included. This section (Section 10) provides a consolidated ready reference to this vital process of assessments.

Each chapter is preceded by explicitly stated learning objectives. This makes it possible to screen the material and quickly select specific subject matter. Simply glance down the list of objectives and find the items you need to review. The more expert practitioner may not need the material that reviews nursing care. The entry-level critical care nurse may wish to study all the material. Whatever your specific needs are, use the objectives to guide you through the book.

There are two appendices. The first appendix contains formulae for select body systems. The second appendix contains the normal and abnormal laboratory values for each body system. A bibliography appears at the end of each section. Certain especially helpful resources are designated by asterisks.

A companion workbook, *Critical Care: Certification Practice Exams,* is available to provide you with experience in taking this type of test.

So now let us start the course that will help you to prepare to become a CCRN.

Photo Credits

The following figures are used with permission from *Atlas of Endocrine Diseases,* Jerzy Kosowicz, The Charles Press Publishers, Inc., Bowie, MD, 1978: Figures 31-4 and 31-5; Figures 32-5 and 32-6; and Figures 33-4 and 33-5.

I

The Pulmonary System

— 1

Anatomy of the Pulmonary System

Learning Objectives

By the end of this chapter, the nurse will be able to:

1. Identify the boundaries of the thoracic cage.
2. Explain the basic phases of inspiration and expiration.
3. Define the pleura and explain its function.
4. List the gross anatomic components of the lung and its structural arrangement.
5. Trace the flow of air in the respiratory tree from the nose to the alveolus.
6. List the three types of alveolar cells and their function.
7. Discuss the function of pulmonary surfactant.
8. Explain the mucociliary escalator and its importance.
9. Trace the pulmonary circulation of the lung parenchyma.
10. Explain the gas exchange at the capillary-alveolar membrane.
11. Explain the pressure system in the lungs and identify three factors that will alter the pressure.
12. Differentiate between the three neural regulators of ventilation.
13. Explain the central chemical control of ventilation.
14. Describe the physiology of the peripheral control of ventilation.
15. Explain the physical and functional differences between the cough, sneeze, and Hering-Breuer reflex.
16. Identify five factors that would modify control of ventilation.

Most textbooks approach the study of the pulmonary anatomy by starting with the most visible feature—the nose. This text does it differently. The text reviews the thoracic cage first and moves in from there to the major components: the pleura, the pleural space, and the lung, with its seg- ments, lobes, and attachments. The passageways through which air enters the thoracic cage from the nose and travels to the alveoli, where gas exchange occurs, are reviewed. Pulmonary circulation and neurogenic and chemical respiratory centers and controls are then examined.

Anatomical Components

THE THORACIC CAGE

The thoracic cage (Figure 1-1) is the bony frame of the chest. The sternum makes up the anterior portion of the thoracic cage. The sternum is actually three connected flat bones—the manubrium, the body, and the xiphoid process (Figure 1-2). Seven pairs of ribs attach to the sternum and are called the "true ribs." The remaining five ribs form the anterior bony portion of the thoracic cage. Each is attached to the rib above it by intercostal muscles.

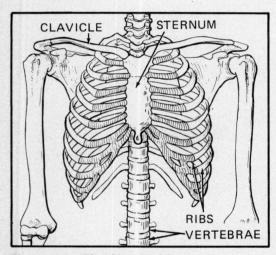

Figure 1-1.   The thoracic cage.

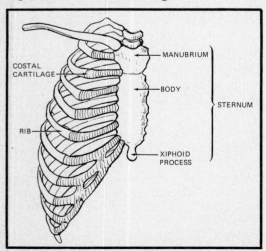

Figure 1-2.   The sternum.

The posterior thoracic cage is formed by the vertebrae and each of the twelve pairs of ribs that are attached to the vertebrae. Since the ribs are C-shaped, they serve as the bony protective side borders of the thoracic cage.

The thorax is shaped like an inverted cone with the apex about 2½ centimeters above the clavicles. The clavicles and first rib form the protective barrier of the superior portion of the thoracic cage. The diaphragm is the inferior portion of the thoracic cage (Figure 1-3). It is a muscle that contracts and flattens to enlarge the thoracic cage. When the diaphragm relaxes, it becomes dome-shaped and decreases the space in the thoracic cage.

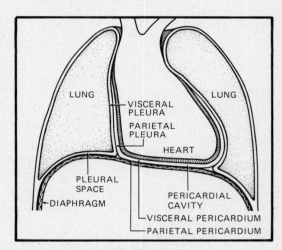

Figure 1-3.   The diaphragm.

Each of the 12 pairs of ribs has cartilage and muscle attached to it. The intercostal muscles are composed of two layers: the internal and external intercostals. Any change in the musculature of the chest alters normal thoracic pressures and affects ventilation.

The diaphragm is the major force in normal breathing. On inspiration, the diaphragm contracts (Figure 1-4), which lengthens the chest cavity, while the external intercostal muscles contract to raise the ribs, thus enlarging the diameter of the chest. Expiration is simply the act of ceasing to inhale (in the normal healthy state). It is a passive act accomplished by the relaxation

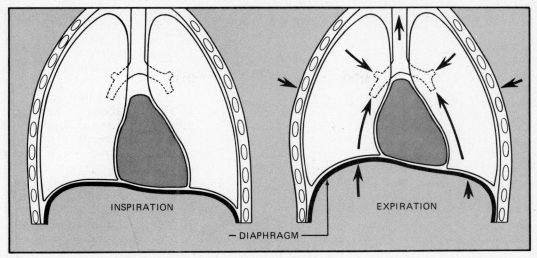

Figure 1-4.   The diaphragm on inspiration and expiration.

of the diaphragm and the relaxation of the external intercostal muscles. The lungs have a normal tendency for elastic recoil, so relaxation of the musculature provides the major mechanism for the passive act of exhalation.

The internal intercostal muscles, which pull the ribs down and inward, play a role in forceful expiration, coughing, and sneezing. The intercostal muscles are used mostly during stressful states and exertional activities. The intercostal muscles may facilitate a smooth transition from inspiration to expiration.

In cases of pulmonary distress and/or disease, accessory muscles may be used to help inspiration. These accessory muscles include the scalene, sternocleidomastoid, trapezius, and pectoralis muscles.

THE MEDIASTINUM

The lung parenchyma and the mediastinum are contained within the bony thoracic cage. The mediastinum is a space midline in the chest and contains the heart, great vessels, trachea, major bronchi, esophagus, thymus gland, lymphatics, and various nerves.

THE PLEURA

Each lung lies free in its own pleural cavity

except at its single point of attachment, *the hilum* (Figure 1-5). The pleural covering of each lung is composed of two layers. The visceral layer is contiguous with the lung and does not have pain nerve fibers. The parietal layer is the outer pleural layer that lines the inside of the thoracic cage. The parietal layer of the pleura contains pain nerve fibers.

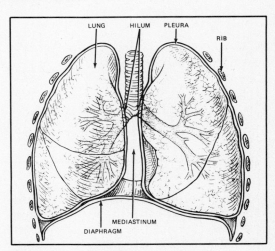

Figure 1-5.   The hilum.

The two layers are separated by a small amount of fluid. This fluid allows the two pleurae to slide easily over each other. If the

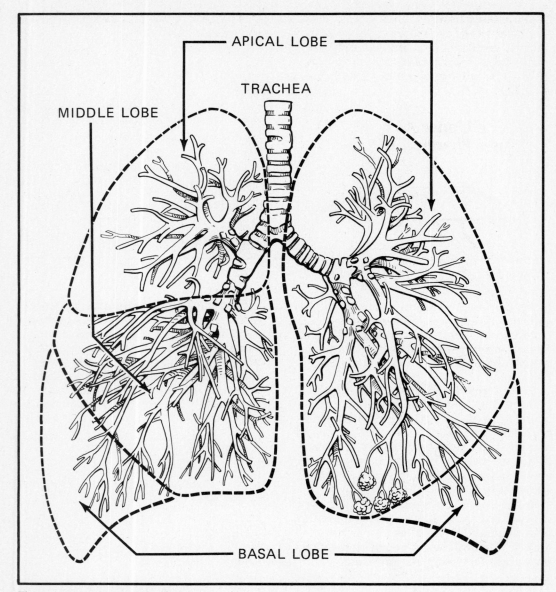

APICAL LOBE

TRACHEA

MIDDLE LOBE

BASAL LOBE

Figure 1-6.   Lobes of the lungs.

pleurae become inflamed, the minute amount of fluid between the pleural layers no longer allows free sliding movement during inhalation and exhalation. This restriction of movement and irritation of the parietal pleura account for pleuritic pain.

The diaphragm is the inferior border for each pleural space. The chest wall is the lateral border, and the mediastinum is the medial border for each pleural space.

Gross Anatomy of the Lung

Each lung is composed of divisions or segments of the bronchial tree and the lung parenchyma. There are 10 segments in the right lung and eight in the left lung. These 18 bronchial segments are grouped into lobes. Three lobes form the right lung, and two lobes form the left lung (Figure 1-6). Each lobe of the lung is separated from the adjacent lobe by fissures. The left lung also has an upper and lower division of its superior lobe, separated by a fissure. This fissure is called the lingula. The lingula is equal to or smaller than the middle lobe of the right lung.

The Upper Airway
(Nose, Pharynx, Larynx)

The upper airway consists of the nose and pharynx. The larynx is included as part of the upper airway, but it functions in part as

a transitional structure between the upper and lower airways.

THE NOSE

The first part of the upper airway (Figure 1-7) is the nose. Air normally enters the respiratory system through the nose. The nose has skeletal rigidity, which maintains patency during inspiration.

The first two-thirds of the nose is cartilaginous, and the last one-third is bony. The cartilaginous septum, straight at birth,

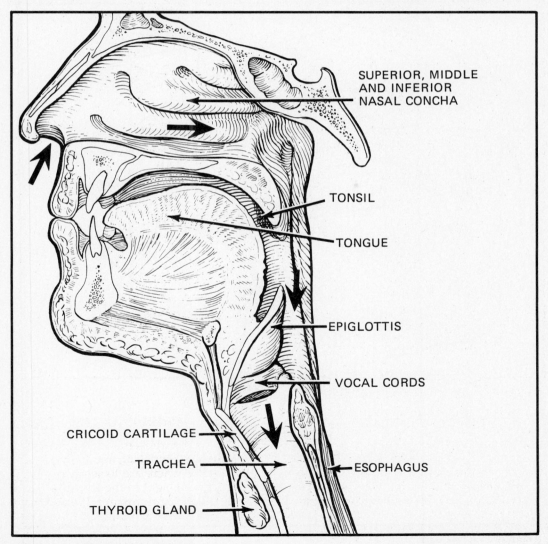

SUPERIOR, MIDDLE AND INFERIOR NASAL CONCHA

TONSIL

TONGUE

EPIGLOTTIS

VOCAL CORDS

CRICOID CARTILAGE

TRACHEA

ESOPHAGUS

THYROID GLAND

Figure 1-7.   The upper airway.

frequently becomes deviated during life for many reasons. Unless the deviation is severe enough to obstruct air flow, no medical treatment is necessary. The nasal septum divides the nose into two fossae, with the lateral border known as the alae. The opening between the alae and the nasal septum is known as the nostril or the naris (*pl.* nares). The nose has a small inlet and a large outlet. Anatomically, this feature allows inspired air to have maximum contact with the upper airway mucosa. By "sniffing" through the nose, we direct inhaled air toward the superior turbinates, where the olfactory area is located.

THE PHARYNX

The main function of the pharynx is to collect incoming air from the mouth and nose and project it downward to the trachea. Anatomically, the pharynx is subdivided into the nasopharynx, the oropharynx, and the laryngopharynx (Figure 1-8). The nasopharynx is the space behind the oral and nasal cavities and above the soft palate. It

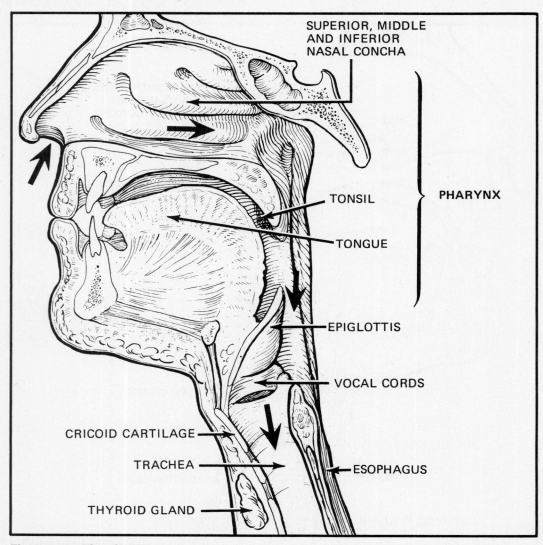

Figure 1-8.   The pharynx.

contains the orifices of the eustachian tubes. The eustachian tubes maintain proper air pressure in the middle ear, for normal tympanic membrane function. The pharyngeal tonsils (adenoids) are located in the superior nasopharynx. This lymphatic tissue is an important defense mechanism of the pulmonary system.

The oropharynx is that portion of the pharynx from the soft palate to the base of the tongue. It receives air from the mouth and nose, and food from the mouth. The faucial "tonsils" are located at the ante-

riolateral borders of the oropharynx.

The laryngopharynx is the lower portion of the pharynx, located from the base of the tongue to the opening of the esophagus. The laryngopharynx contains muscles within its wall called pharyngeal constrictors. These muscles aid in the mechanism of swallowing.

THE LARYNX

The larynx is the upper portion of the trachea and connects the upper and lower airways (Figure 1-9). It lies in the anterior

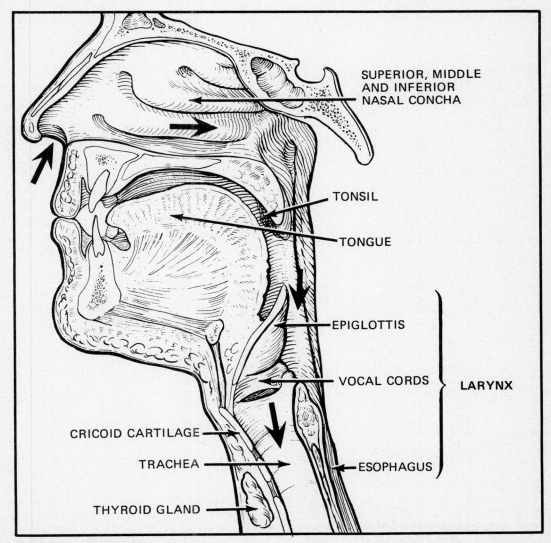

Figure 1-9. The larynx.

portion of the neck, extending from C-4 through C-6. The larynx protects the lower airway against foreign material, aids in speech, and is an essential part of the mechanism of coughing.

The glottis is the opening into the larynx. The epiglottis, a flexible cartilage attached to the thyroid cartilage, primarily functions to prevent entry of foreign material into the airway by covering the glottis when a person swallows.

The larynx is composed of cartilage, connected by membranes, and muscle. One cartilage is a complete ring and is called the cricoid cartilage. It is located just below the thyroid cartilage. The vocal cords lie inside the thyroid cartilage.

In the adult, the thyroid cartilage (Figure 1-10), housing the vocal cords, is the narrowest part of the air passage of the larynx. As muscles in the larynx contract, the vocal cords change shape and vibrate. This vibrating of the vocal cords produces sound.

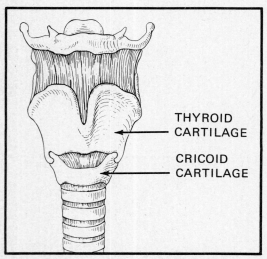

THYROID CARTILAGE

CRICOID CARTILAGE

Figure 1-10.   The thyroid-cricoid cartilages.

In children, the cricoid cartilage (Figure 1-10) is the narrowest part of the laryngeal airway. Therefore, children do *not* need a cuffed endotracheal tube. The cricothyroid membrane is an avascular structure that connects the thyroid cartilage and cricoid cartilage. It is through this membrane that an airway may be established in an emergency. The posterior wall of the larynx and the vocal cords will not be injured.

The Lower Airway

The lower airway consists of two divisions, the tracheobronchial tree and the lung parenchyma.

THE TRACHEOBRONCHIAL TREE

This is simply a system of conducting tubes to allow air to reach the alveoli. The large airways in the tracheobronchial tree are called bronchi. The small airways are called bronchioles.

The trachea is the portion of the airway that extends from approximately C-6 to the point of bifurcation of the right and left main-stem bronchi (Figure 1-11), which is called the *carina*. The trachea is composed of C-shaped cartilaginous rings.

The C-shaped cartilaginous rings have a posterior muscle that is membranous and friable. On inspiration, this muscle relaxes and the diameter of the trachea increases. On exhalation, this muscle contracts and the diameter of the trachea decreases. Occasionally, the muscle relaxes and then bows in on exhalation, decreasing the effectiveness of the mucociliary stream in clearing secretions from the lungs. This is seen in Figure 1-11.

The carina is the bifurcation of the trachea into the right main-stem bronchus and the left main-stem bronchus. The right main-stem bronchus is almost straight, whereas the left main-stem bronchus angles more acutely to the left (Figure 1-12). The right is also wider in diameter than the left, and foreign matter tends to lodge in the right side.

During endotracheal intubation, the position of the endotracheal tube must be checked frequently by auscultation and chest x-ray to insure proper ventilation to both lungs. This is because there is frequent

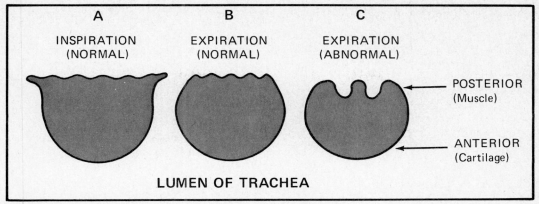

Figure 1-11. Movement of posterior muscles of the trachea.

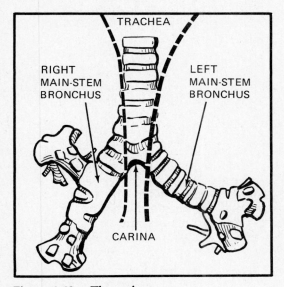

Figure 1-12. The carina.

slippage of the endotracheal tube into the right main-stem bronchus, preventing ventilation of the left lung.

If aspiration occurs, it is more likely to occur on the right side for the same reasons.

There are 22 divisions of the right and left main-stem bronchi that occur before the terminal respiratory bronchioles are reached. These divisions are cartilaginous, whereas the respiratory bronchioles are small tubes with no cartilage. Only smooth muscle *surrounds* the respiratory epithelium. Contraction of this smooth muscle results in *bronchospasms*.

The respiratory bronchioles branch directly into alveolar ducts, which give rise to the alveoli, the bulk of lung parenchyma. There are about 40 square meters or more of alveoli. This is possible only because many alveoli and alveolar ducts have common walls, termed septa. These septa play an important role in elastic recoil. The septal wall is composed of smooth muscle. It is thought that this smooth muscle contracts to narrow the alveolar duct lumen.

Alveolar sacs are the ends of the "respiratory tree" (Figure 1-13). These sacs are dead-end structures in that inhaled ambient air can go no farther. The sacs are found in groups numbering 15–20 alveoli per sac. Alveolar sacs share a common wall with adjacent sacs.

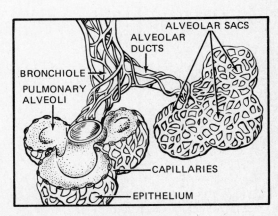

Figure 1-13. Alveolar sacs.

LUNG PARENCHYMA

The lung parenchyma (lung tissues) consist of primary lobules, which are the functioning units of the lung. Lobules are comprised of alveolar ducts and sacs. "The 200 to 600 million alveoli in the normal lung have an average total surface area of 40 to 100 square meters (M^2) [approximately the size of a football field]. The surface area is directly related to body length and decreases by about 5% per decade."[1]

Epithelium lines the entire lung parenchyma. The alveolar epithelium is lined with a fluid. The origin of the fluid is unknown. It is believed that this fluid mixes with the mucous blanket and helps to protect the parenchyma. How this is achieved is pure speculation at this time.

Since alveoli are the terminal components of the airway, gas exchange occurs over this area.

Alveolar Airways

Alveolar sacs are lined with epithelium. The alveolar epithelium is composed of three types of cells. Type I cells are characterized by cytoplasmic extensions and are the cells that make up most of the lung. Type II alveolar cells are found where one extension meets (interfaces with) another. Type II cells are active metabolic cells that contain organelles to synthesize surfactant. Type III alveolar cells are phagocytes that arise from bone marrow or maybe from Type II cells.

Pulmonary Surfactant

Alveolar epithelium is lined with a fluid that contains a phospholipid protein. This fluid is called surfactant. It functions to reduce surface tension in the alveoli. The phospholipid is insoluble but highly permeable to all gases. Normal alveolar func-

tion is dependent upon this surfactant. Two pathologic states that are complicated by insufficient or absent surfactant are (1) hyaline membrane disease in the neonate, and (2) adult respiratory distress syndrome. The pulmonary surfactant contains large amounts of dipalmitoyl lecithin, a phospholipid that decreases the surface tension of the fluid lining the alveoli. This surfactant functions by forming a thin (monomolecular) layer at the interface of the air and fluid in the alveoli. Normally, an interface of air and fluid produces surface tension that forces collapse of the small alveoli. Surfactant *decreases* the surface tension in the alveoli by preventing the development of the air-fluid interface.

The pulmonary surfactant serves two other, but related, functions in the lungs. First, the surfactant rapidly changes in individual alveoli, depending upon the given surface tensions. There is an instability of the alveoli in which the smaller alveoli have a greater pressure and tend to collapse. The pulmonary surfactant counters this instability.

Second, the absence of pulmonary surfactant alters the surface tension of the alveoli. Without surfactant in the proper amount, there is a filtration of fluid from the alveolar wall capillaries into the alveoli with the all-too-frequent picture of severe pulmonary edema or adult respiratory distress syndrome (ARDS).

The Mucociliary Escalator (Mucous Blanket)

An important portion of the respiratory system, the mucociliary escalator (Figure 1-14) should be considered at this point. The mucociliary escalator is the *primary* protective mechanism for the entire respiratory system.

The entire respiratory tree is lined with varying types of epithelium. Cells within the epithelium produce different types of mucus (watery and thick). This mucus is in immediate contact with the airway lumen. The mucous lining is called the *mucous blanket*. The mucous blanket is lined with

---

[1]Wilson RF (ed): Pulmonary physiology, Sect. F. Critical Care Manual: Principles and Techniques of Critical Care, Vol. 1. Kalamazoo, MI: The Upjohn Co., p. 10, 1977

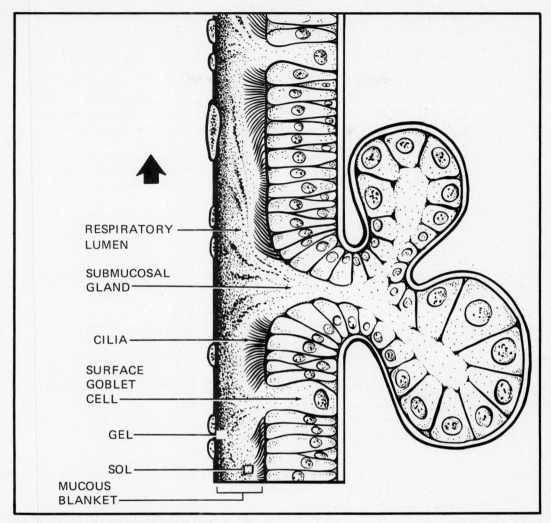

RESPIRATORY
LUMEN

SUBMUCOSAL
GLAND

CILIA

SURFACE
GOBLET
CELL

GEL

SOL

MUCOUS
BLANKET

Figure 1-14.   The mucociliary escalator.

cilia, which are fine, hairlike filaments projecting into the airway lumen.

Various mechanisms will move this mucous blanket lining of the airway lumen to the pharynx (where it will be swallowed), to the larynx (where coughing will expel it), and to the hairs in the nose (where it will be expelled by blowing and sneezing). Cilia lining the larger airways will help to move this mucous blanket up the respiratory tree to be expelled by the cilia's continuous undulating movement, which may be referred to as the *escalator*.

Linings of the Upper Airway

The first one-third of the nose is lined with nonciliated, squamous epithelium. The remaining two-thirds of the nose is lined with ciliated, pseudostratified epithelium. Coarse particles larger than four microns are entrapped by nasal hairs. The nasopharynx is lined with ciliated, pseudostratified epithelium. The laryngeal mucosa is stratified, squamous epithelium above the vocal cords and pseudostratified, columnar epithelium below. The entire upper airway is lined with a mucous membrane. This membrane is essential for accomplishing the functions of the upper airway. The ciliated portions of mucosa in the upper airway filter pollutants and irritants. Fine particles from one to four microns come in contact with the respiratory mucosa and become trapped; these are eventually carried to the pharynx by the mucociliary escalator and are finally swallowed.

The mucous membrane of the upper airway moisturizes and warms the inspired air because of the vast blood supply in the mucosa and the thick layer of mucus present from secretions of both serous glands and goblet cells. Serous glands in the mucosa secrete a watery mucus. Goblet cells in the epithelium secrete a thick, tenacious mucus. These secretions add up to 1,000 milliliters of water per day to inspired ambient air.

One cannot overstress the importance of the functions of the upper airway to warm, humidify, and filter the respiratory passageways. These functions are essential to protect the alveoli so that they may function to their fullest capacity and be guarded against erosion and hemorrhage from dry air.

Coughing and Sneezing

Coughing and sneezing help "empty" the mucociliary escalator. The sneeze reflex is a reaction to irritation in the nose, and the cough reflex is a reaction to irritation in the upper airway distal to the nose. Both processes are complex mechanisms that require the integration of increased intrathoracic pressure, complete and tight closure of the epiglottis and vocal cords, and stong contraction of the abdominal musculature, diaphragm, and intercostal muscles.

Gas Exchange Pathways

The alveoli are the areas in which gas exchange actually occurs. Consider that oxygen has been inhaled and has traveled through all the conducting tubes and is now in the alveolus. The oxygen must diffuse across the alveolar epithelium, the basement membrane, and move across the

small interstitial space. The oxygen is now halfway there! It continues the diffusion process through the capillary membrane, the plasma fluid, and the erythrocyte membrane. The capillary endothelium is very sensitive and is easily damaged by endotoxins, oxygen, or other noxious substances. At this point, the capillary is so small that the erythrocytes are lined up in single column moving through the capillary. As the erythrocyte continues its route through the capillary, the oxygen diffuses rapidly through the erythrocyte membrane and attaches to the hemoglobin molecule of the erythrocyte. While the oxygen has been diffusing in this manner, carbon dioxide molecules have been diffusing in the opposite direction across the alveolar capillary membrane. *But carbon dioxide diffuses 20 times faster than oxygen.*

Pulmonary Circulation of the Lung Parenchyma

As with all tissues in the body, the lung tissue *itself* must receive oxygenated blood and dispose of its own waste products. The lungs' arterial system follows the bronchial tree, bifurcating at each bronchial division and following close to the bronchus or its subdivisions. As the bronchioles become smaller and divide still again (remember there are 22 divisions from trachea to respiratory bronchioles), some arteries fail to bifurcate. This problem is simply solved by other nearby arteries that send out branches from their stem. Freshly oxygenated blood enters the *central* part (Figure 1-15) of the alveolar tissue (lobule).

Venous blood flows through the capillaries and venules to the periphery of the alveolus and then re-enters the venous circulation to be directed back to the right atrium.

Pulmonary Circulation of the Alveolar System

The total volume and rate of pulmonary blood circulation is about five liters per minute. Blood flow is greatest to the dependent

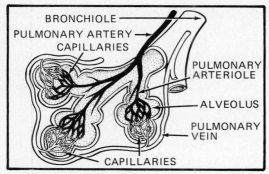

Figure 1-15.   Entrance of freshly oxygenated blood of the lung parenchyma.

portions of the lung, due simply to gravity. Thus, in an erect person, the apex of the lung will have the least circulating blood volume. When the person is lying down, the anterior lung surfaces will have the least circulating blood volume.

The erythrocyte completes the pulmonary circulation very rapidly (0.75 seconds at rest). This rapid circulation helps maintain adequate perfusion. "The total volume of blood in the pulmonary arteries, veins, and capillaries is about 500 to 750 ml in the average adult male or about 10% to 15% of the total blood volume."[2] Thus the pulmonary circulation functions as a reservoir in times of increased need of cardiac output.

[2]Wilson RF (ed): Pulmonary physiology, Sect. F. Critical Care Manual: Principles and Techniques of Critical Care, Vol. 1. Kalamazoo, MI: The Upjohn Co., p. 24, 1977

Control of Ventilation

Three major factors control ventilation. They are neural control, central chemical control, and peripheral chemical control.

NEURAL CONTROL

The respiratory center is in the medullary portion of the brain stem. Neurons initiate impulses that result in inspiration.

An increase in the rate of impulses results in an increase in respiratory rate. An increase in the amplitude (strength) of impulses increases the tidal volume.

Normally, chemical factors keep the inspiratory and the expiratory centers in balance, providing normal ventilation patterns. A spirometer pattern for normal ventilation is shown in Figure 1-16.

The inspiratory center is in the dorsal aspect of the medulla oblongata, in close association to the vagus nerve and the glossopharyngeal nerves. There appears to be an inherent automaticity in the electrical impulse release for inspiration. The apneustic center (located in the pons) acts to *prevent* the interruption of these inspiratory impulses.

If the apneustic center takes control over the normally balanced ventilation pattern, apneustic breathing patterns would be established. Apneustic breathing consists of slight pauses following some expirations in an otherwise normal breathing pattern. An apneustic spirometer pattern is shown in Figure 1-17. This and other abnormal

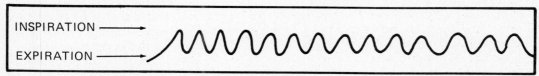

Figure 1-16.   Spirometer pattern of normal ventilation.

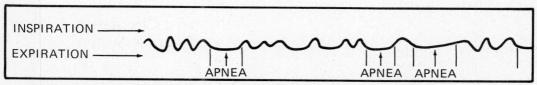

Figure 1-17.   Spirometer pattern of apnuestic breathing.

spirometer patterns are discussed in the neurologic section of this text.

Expiration control is in the pneumotaxic center located in the upper pons. The neurons located there transmit impulses to limit inspiration. When the pneumotaxic center takes control over ventilation, there is irregular, deep, and shallow breathing with randomly spaced pauses of apnea of varying length. The pneumotaxic spirometer pattern is shown in Figure 1-18. This is sometimes termed ataxic breathing.

If all three neural centers (the medullary center, the apneustic center, and the pneumotaxic center) become nonfunctional, respiration ceases.

There are four other common patterns of respiration seen in critical care areas.

Central neurogenic hyperventilation is regular, deep, and rapid respirations without periods of apnea. Neurogenic dysfunction produces this pattern. A central neurogenic hyperventilation spirometer pattern is shown in Figure 1-19.

Cheyne-Stokes is a pattern in which respirations start from apnea, reach a maximum in depth and rate, and then fade back to apnea (a crescendo-decrescendo pattern). A Cheyne-Stokes spirometer pattern is shown in Figure 1-20.

Kussmaul breathing is regular, but faster *and* deeper than normal (most often seen in diabetic ketoacidotic coma). Breathing is usually labored. A Kussmaul spirometer pattern is shown in Figure 1-21.

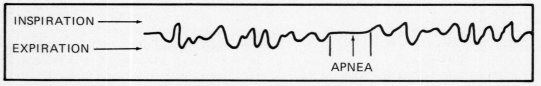

Figure 1-18.   Spirometer pattern of pneumotaxic (ataxic) breathing.

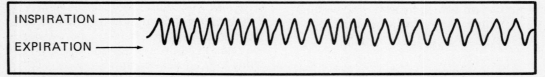

Figure 1-19.   Spirometer pattern of central neurogenic hyperventilation.

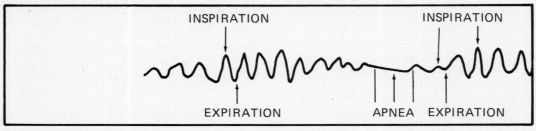

Figure 1-20.   Spirometer pattern of Cheyne-Stokes breathing.

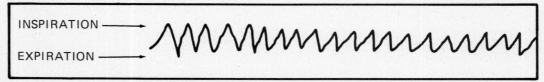

Figure 1-21.   Spirometer pattern of Kussmaul breathing.

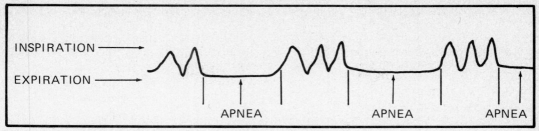

Figure 1-22.   Spirometer pattern of Biot (cluster) breathing.

Biot respirations are faster and deeper than normal with irregular, abrupt periods of apnea. Each breath is equal (as contrasted to Cheyne-Stokes). A spirometer pattern of Biot breathing is shown in Figure 1-22.

In addition to these respiratory patterns, there are five basic terms used frequently:

1. *Eupnea* is normal respiratory rate and rhythm.
2. *Tachypnea* is an increased respiratory rate, greater than 24, but normal depth of respiration.
3. *Hyperpnea* is an increased depth of respiration at a normal respiratory rate.
4. *Bradypnea* is a decreased respiratory rate with normal respiratory depth.
5. *Apnea* is the absence of breathing.

CENTRAL CHEMICAL CONTROL

Cerebrospinal fluid (CSF) pH is the primary control of respiratory center stimulation. A change in the CSF hydrogen ion concentration occurs very quickly in relation to arterial P_{CO_2}. The change in the CSF hydrogen ion concentration will result in the appropriate change in stimulation of the neural respiratory center. A rise in CSF hydrogen ion concentration (acidosis) increases stimulation to respiratory centers. A drop in CSF hydrogen ion concentration (alkalosis) decreases stimulation to neural respiratory centers.

Subsequently, arterial P_{CO_2} is the normal neurochemical control of the respiratory cycle because of its effect on the CSF pH. Usually, a rise in CSF hydrogen ion concentration (acidosis) will first increase respiratory depth and then increase respiratory rate.

PERIPHERAL CHEMICAL CONTROL

Chemoreceptors are located at the bifurcation of the internal and external carotid arteries (carotid bodies) and at the aortic arch (aortic body). These highly vascular, neural bodies are stimulated by *any* decrease in oxygen supply (e.g., decreased blood flow, decreased hemoglobin, increased pH, increased P_{CO_2}). Stimulation of the carotid and/or the aortic bodies will increase cerebral cortex activity, cause tachycardia, cause hypertension, increase respiratory rate and tidal volume, increase pulmonary resistance, increase bronchial smooth muscle tone, and increase adrenal gland secretions.

HERING-BREUER (STRETCH) REFLEX

The walls of the pulmonary bronchi and bronchioles have stretch receptors that interact with the vagus nerve when they become overstretched. This seems to be a feedback mechanism to prevent overinflation of the lungs. It functions like the pneumotaxic center in limiting the extent of inspiration and, therefore, protects the lungs from hyperinflation.

Modifying Factors

Certain drugs may depress the respiratory center. The mechanisms of depression are related to decreased alveolar ventilation or central respiratory center block. Decreased alveolar ventilation is characterized by shallow respirations and a respiratory rate of less than 12 breaths per minute. Normally, an increase in P_{CO_2} results in an increase in respirations. Drugs which depress the respiratory center block this normal, protective mechanism.

Chronic respiratory disease will modify the normal respiratory patterns. As the chronic disease progresses, a change in the respiratory drive occurs. Instead of an increase in P_{CO_2} initiating the respiratory drive, a decrease in P_{O_2} levels initiates ventilation. High flow oxygen therapy may result in apnea. Neurologic diseases such as myasthenia gravis, Guillain-Barré, amyotrophic lateral sclerosis (ALS), and such will impinge upon respiratory functions.

Neoplastic diseases may impinge on respiratory centers in the brain, resulting eventually in death. Very rarely, a neoplasm of the cervical spinal cord occurs and alters respiratory function.

— 2

Physiology of the Respiratory System

Learning Objectives

By the end of this chapter, the nurse will be able to:

1. List the four phases of the respiratory process.
2. Identify three intrathoracic and three extrathoracic causes of decreased lung compliance.
3. Explain the relationship of surfactant to lung pressures.
4. Differentiate between the three types of air flow in the lung passages.
5. Define eight lung volumes.
6. Distinguish between anatomic and physiologic dead space.
7. Explain Dalton's law and Graham's law.
8. Discuss shunting as a result of air obstruction and blood obstruction.
9. Compare the oxygen-carrying content of blood and plasma.
10. Explain the oxyhemoglobin dissociation curve.
11. List three transport systems for carbon dioxide.
12. Explain the chloride shift.
13. Define the *Haldane effect*.

Basic to any discussion of pulmonary physiology is a *clear* understanding of the terms *ventilation* and *respiration*. These terms are often used interchangeably; that is, incorrectly. Ventilation refers to the process of moving air from the atmosphere into the alveoli and moving carbon dioxide from the alveoli back into the atmosphere. Ventilation is a pattern of breathing, of inhaling and exhaling. Respiration refers to the *exchange* of oxygen and carbon dioxide. The terms are *not* synonymous and are *not* interchangeable.

Lung Functions

There are four major functions of the lungs:

1. The main function is the exchange of gases to oxygenate the blood. The main gases exchanged are carbon dioxide and oxygen. The functional re-

serve of the lung is eight times the amount needed to perform normal activities.

2. The lungs are a reservoir storing one to two liters of blood that is available for increasing cardiac output.

3. The lungs filter out bacteria and microaggregates. These microemboli are phagocytized by macrophage cells of the lung (Type III cells).

4. The lungs may function as an endocrine organ, altering certain compounds that pass through its system. Most cancers of the lung have endocrine functions producing insulin, antidiuretic hormone (ADH), and cortisol.

Respiratory Processes

The process of respiration has four phases. Phase one is pulmonary ventilation, which is the movement of ambient (normal room) air into and out of the lungs. Phase two is the diffusion of oxygen and carbon dioxide in the alveoli. This is often referred to as *external respiration*. Phase three is the transport of oxygen to the cells and carbon dioxide away from the cells. This is referred to as *internal respiration*. Phase four is the regulation of ventilation.

Mechanical Process of Phase One (Pulmonary Ventilation)

Normal atmospheric (barometric) pressure at sea level is 760 mm Hg. For the average, healthy person at rest, the intrapleural pressure is slightly subatmospheric or about 755 mm Hg. If the pressures were equal, there would be no flow of air.

As the mechanics of inspiration begin, the thoracic cage increases in size. This size increase produces a negative intrapleural *inspiratory* pressure, as compared to atmospheric pressure, resulting in air flowing into the lungs. If one considers atmospheric pressure to be zero (0), then resting intrapleural pressure is −5 and inspiratory intrapleural pressure is −10.

It is possible under extreme physical exertion, especially for athletes, to reduce the intrapleural inspiratory pressure to as low as −50 to −80. The intrapleural expiratory pressure does not exist in terms of negative pressures. As inspiratory muscle activity ends, the normal elastic recoil of the lung tissue and muscles decreases the size of the thoracic cage. Gas flows out of the lungs and back into the atmosphere. The repetition of this process establishes the breathing pattern and pulmonary ventilation.

The kinetic theory of gases helps to explain the movement of air in both inhalation and exhalation. This theory states that when a gas fills a space (like the lungs), there are many gas particles, *but* these particles do *not* form a solid mass. Within the space the gas fills, the molecules are in a state of continuous random movement. This results in the particles colliding with each other and the container walls. This perpetuates the random movement. Gas particles exert a pressure upon the walls of the container (in this case, the lungs) because of their continual colliding with each other and the container walls.

Lung Pressures

The low pressure system that exists in the right heart pumps blood into the pulmonary arterial system where there is also a very low pressure (resistance), compared to the high pressure system of the left heart and the systemic circulatory system.

This low pressure system in the lungs allows the capillaries to distend easily to accommodate increased volumes from the systemic circulatory system in times of distress and/or exertion. This distensibility helps regulate resistance to blood flow through the pulmonary system.

In the normal lung, free of disease, the mean pulmonary artery systolic pressure is 10–25 mm Hg. The mean diastolic pressure is 5–15 mm Hg. The wedge pressue is 0–10 mm Hg and the mean pulmonary venous pressure is 4–6 mm Hg. The mean pressure gradient is about 10 mm Hg.

Compliance

Compliance is a measurement of the expansibility of the lungs and the thorax. If the lungs were removed from the confines of the bony thorax, their expansion would be almost doubled. Compliance is expressed as the volume change in the lungs for each unit of pressure change in the intra-alveolar pressure. The respiratory symbol for volume is "V" and the symbol for pressure or partial pressure is "P". Greater compliance means there is a larger volume change in the lung for each pressure change. Reduced compliance means there is less volume change in the lung for each pressure change. In other words, the more pressure needed to change the volume in the lung, the *less* the compliance. The increase of intra-alveolar pressure is measured in centimeters of water (cm of H_2O).

INTRATHORACIC CAUSES (OBSTRUCTIVE)

Any disease that stiffens the lungs will decrease compliance. Diseases that increase the congestion in the lungs result in an increase in the distance oxygen (O_2) molecules must travel to exchange places with carbon dioxide (CO_2) molecules. This makes it more difficult for gas molecules to penetrate this congestion. Some diseases that decrease compliance are listed in Table 2-1.

Table 2-1.   Some intrathoracic causes of decreased compliance.

Atelectasis
Pneumonia
Pleural effusion
Empyema and lung abcesses
Bronchospasms
Pulmonary edema
Bronchitis
Asthma
Emphysema
Adult respiratory distress syndrome (ARDS)
Closed tension pneumothorax

Space-occupying neoplasms decrease lung compliance. The area the neoplasm occupies becomes stiff and noncompliant. Gas molecules cannot penetrate a solid mass.

Flail chest decreases the lung compliance in the area of the flail segment. Every time the patient inhales, the flail segment is pulled in toward the lung, instead of expanding outward. Simultaneously, every time the patient exhales, the flail segment expands outward, decreasing the effective ventilation of that portion of the lung.

EXTRATHORACIC CAUSES (RESTRICTIVE)

Any condition that limits the ability of the bony thorax to expand will decrease lung compliance. Table 2-2 lists some of the extrathoracic causes of decreased lung compliance.

Table 2-2.   Some extrathoracic causes of decreased compliance.

Flail chest
Barrel chest
Pectus excavatum (funnel chest)
Pectus carinatum (pigeon chest)
Kyphosis
Scoliosis
Kyphoscoliosis

Pregnancy (as it reaches term) displaces abdominal contents upward and prevents the diaphragm from contracting (descending) fully, thus decreasing the extent of chest wall expansion.

Morbid obesity and abdominal distention present the same deterrent on the diaphragm. Obesity presents one other problem in lung compliance. If the patient is morbidly obese, the sheer weight of excess fat on the upper torso strains the intercostal muscles in attempting to lift the massive weight. The muscles cannot function efficiently and lung compliance is decreased.

Postoperative binders and/or chest splints are seen much less frequently now that their adverse effect on lung compliance is well-recognized. Both binders and splints (or the patient in pain splinting by decreased rate and volume of each breath) decrease the ability of the bony thorax to expand over a very wide area. Lung compliance is then decreased over a large segment of the thorax.

TYPES OF COMPLIANCE

There are two types of compliance—static and dynamic.

1. *Static compliance* (C_{st}) is the change in lung volume per unit airway pressure change when the lungs are *motionless*. Static compliance can only be measured when there is *no* flow of gases, that is, at the end of inspiration or expiration. Static compliance is normally about 100 ml of pressure per centimeter of water pressure. If and only if there were no airway diseases, static compliance measurements would be a reliable index of lung compliance. Airway disease alters the rate of gas flow from the mouth to the alveoli. Airway disease results in inaccurate static compliance values, leading one to believe that the lungs are less compliant than in actuality.

2. *Dynamic compliance* (C_{dyn}). If airway disease is present, most of the resistance to air flow will be in the medium size bronchi. The massive number of airways account for the lack of decreased resistance to air flow through them, but this massive number also makes the small airways capable of developing rather extensive disease before static compliance measurement reveals the disease.

Dynamic compliance is tested by using air flow and having the patient breathe in a series of from 10 to 120 breaths per minute. Variations in the results indicate "silent" airway resistance and airway disease at a much earlier stage. Normal dynamic compliance is about 50 ml/cm H_2O. Comparing the C_{st} and the C_{dyn} gives an indication of airway resistance.

Airway resistance results from friction caused by gas molecules trying to flow in one direction and that flow being impeded by the walls of the airway or some other obstruction. This impediment changes the

ratio of alveolar pressure against the rate of air flow.

Airway resistance is increased by the collection of secretions, artificial airways, endotracheal tubes, bronchospasms, laryngeal or tracheal strictures, edema, emphysema, or space-occupying lesions.

Elasticity (Recoil Tendency)

In Chapter 1, it was mentioned that the alveolar sacs are separated by septa. These septa are a major factor in the elastic recoil of the interstitial parenchyma. The thorax and pleura and the lung parenchyma have opposing elastic forces. The interstitial parenchymal tissues are elastic fibers always trying to collapse the lungs. The fluid lining the alveoli is also trying to collapse the lung parenchyma. The thoracic cage and pleura are trying to expand the lungs.

There is a specific volume below which the elastic forces overcome other factors and the alveolus will collapse. This is known as the critical volume. As long as the volume remains above this critical volume a state of equilibrium is maintained between the surface-acting substances. This balance is between surface tension trying to collapse the alveolus and the expanding pressures of inhalation keeping the alveolus open.

As long as the thoracic cage and pleura are patent, these elastic forces tend to balance each other. If the integrity of the pleura is compromised, the parenchymal forces become greater, and the lung collapses. Life is dependent upon re-expansion of the lung within reasonable time frames.

Increased elastic resistance and dyspnea are usually seen in cardiac disease. (The thoracic cage and pleura are patent.)

Air Flow

There are three basic types of air flow within the lung airways.

1. Turbulent air flow—When a person inhales, and especially sniffs, air flows into the turbinates. Turbulent air flow looks like Figure 2-1.

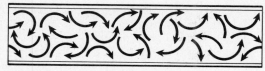

Figure 2-1.   Turbulent air flow.

2. Transitional air flow—As inspired air flows down the respiratory tree, it branches into smaller and smaller tubes. This transitional air flow looks like Figure 2-2. Transitional flow oc-

curs in large-to-medium airways at points of bifurcation and/or narrowing.

3. Laminar air flow—This is essentially flow occurring in thin, flat, continuous sheets. The outermost layer of air has minimal contact with the air passage walls, providing slight filtering in the small peripheral airways. Laminar air flow looks like Figure 2-3.

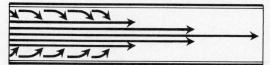

Figure 2-3.   Laminar air flow.

Lung Volumes

The total lung capacity (TLC) is the maximum amount of gas that the lungs can hold. This total lung capacity is composed of four discrete lung volumes. These volumes can be measured by spirometry. It is important to know these volumes and their abbreviations (Figure 2-4).

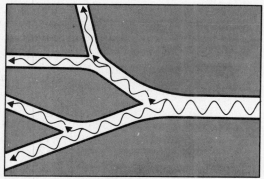

Figure 2-2.   Transitional air flow.

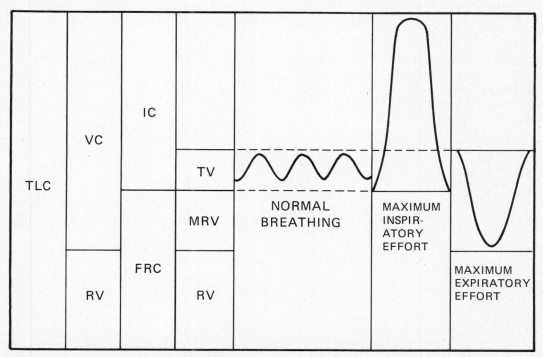

Figure 2-4.   Lung volumes and capacities.

1. Inspiratory reserve volume (IRV) is the amount of extra (reserve) gas that can be inhaled at the end of a normal inspiration. It is not usually used in normal breathing at rest. (Normal can be up to 3,000 ml.)
2. Tidal volume (V_T) is the amount of gas that is exhaled during normal breathing. (Normal is about 500 ml in a young adult.)
3. Expiratory reserve volume (ERV) is the amount of gas that can be exhaled after a normal expiration. It is not used in normal breathing patterns. It does provide a reserve means of increasing tidal volume (V_T). (Normal ERV is about 1,100 ml.)
4. Residual volume (RV) is the amount of gas that *always* remains in the lungs. This is of real interest to the pathologist who must decide if a baby was born dead. If one breath is inhaled, there will be a residual volume of gas in the lungs. No residual volume would indicate a stillborn infant. (If there is residual volume, the lung tissue floats in water.)

There are four potential lung volumes called lung capacities. Total lung capacity has already been defined. This TLC can be calculated by combining two or more of the lung volumes just listed.

1. The TLC = IRV + V_T + ERV + RV (Normal is about 5,800 ml.)
2. Vital capacity (VC) is the amount of gas that can be *forcefully* exhaled after a maximum inspiration. VC = V_T + IRV + ERV (Normal is about 4,500 ml.)
3. The inspiratory capacity (IC) is the amount of gas that can be inhaled after a normal exhalation. IC = V_T + IRV (Normal is about 3,500 ml.)
4. The functional residual capacity (FRC) is also called the resting lung volume. It is the amount of air left in the lungs after normal expiration. FRC = ERV + RV (Normal is about 2,300 ml.)

It is important to know these values and that they are averages and will differ according to body size, weight, and age.

Very early in a critical illness, these respiratory volumes and capacities can be used to prevent respiratory deterioration. Throughout the patients' illness, monitoring the effectiveness of treatment modalities is by measuring these components. Vital capacity, inspiratory force, and tidal volume are the most frequently measured parameters of respiratory muscle function.

Measuring the flow of gas being exhaled and the time of exhaling helps distinguish between restrictive and obstructive lung diseases (Chapter 6). Forced vital capacity (FVC) measures the vital capacity that the patient can forcibly exhale. The FVC is important because it reveals the maximum volume of air the patient will have under stress for ventilation.

FEV_t is the forced expiratory volume over a specific time interval. Normally FEV_1 or $FEV_{1\%}$ rather than FEV_t is seen. The patient inhales as much as possible, holds his or her breath briefly, and then exhales as forcibly as possible. The recording machine actually records three measurements of interest. One is the FVC. One is the amount of gas exhaled in one second, FEV_1. One is the maximum mid-expiratory flow rate. Some experts say this maximum mid-expiratory flow rate is the most accurate indication of airway resistance. $FEV_{1\%}$ is just a comparison of the FVC and the FEV_1. Obstructive lung diseases decrease the FEV_1 and $FEV_{1\%}$. In restrictive lung diseases, the FVC will be decreased, but the FEV_1 and $FEV_{1\%}$ will be normal.

Mechanical Process of Phase Two (Diffusion of the Alveoli)

This phase is often called *external respiration*. Up to this point, no oxygen has reached the erythrocyte to be transported throughout the body. All the mechanics of getting the oxygen from the atmosphere into the alveolus so that oxygen can be consumed have been discussed. Some very important laws affect the exchange of oxygen and carbon dioxide and some very important measurements are made in relation to the diffusion process.

DEAD SPACE

Not all the oxygen inhaled reaches the alveoli. In fact, none of the oxygen from the nose and mouth and the pathway down to, but not including, the alveoli participates in exchanging with carbon dioxide. This area is called *anatomic dead space*. It is difficult to measure but is estimated to be 150 ml (or 1 ml/pound of ideal body weight). If the tidal volume (V_T) is about 500 ml in normal breathing, approximately 350 ml of each inhalation will reach the alveolar areas. And, of course, each time one exhales, a similar volume of gas remains in the airway passages. Volume of dead space is abbreviated V_D. It can be calculated by the following formula (where $\dot{V}_E$ is minute ventilation):

$$V_D = \frac{(P_{A_{CO_2}} - P_{E_{CO_2}})}{P_{A_{CO_2}}} \times \dot{V}_E$$

A sample computation of this formula is found in Appendix I.

The amount of inhaled air that is not anatomic dead space but that also does *not* participate in gas exchange is called *physiologic dead space*. Physiologic dead space is more helpful in assessing effective pulmonary ventilation than anatomic dead space. It can be calculated by the Bohr equation:

$$\frac{V_D}{V_T} = \frac{P_{A_{CO_2}} - P_{E_{CO_2}}}{P_{A_{CO_2}}}$$

A sample calculation of the Bohr equation can be found in Appendix I.

The amount of inhaled air that reaches the alveoli *and* takes part in gas exchange is termed *alveolar ventilation*. It is abbreviated V_A. Note that the "A" is a capital "A". This is important because the capital "A" stands for alveolar. (Note: The lowercase "a" stands for arterial.) V_A can be measured by Pa_{CO_2} (arterial carbon dioxide pressure) which is inversely related to V_A. The formula for this is:

$$Pa_{CO_2} = \frac{V_{CO_2}}{V_A} \times P_B$$

The V_A can be calculated by using any of the following three formulae.

1. $V_A = V_T - V_D$

2. $\dot{V}_A = \dfrac{\dot{V}_{E_{CO_2}} \times 0.863}{P_{A_{CO_2}}}$

3. $\dot{V}_A = \dfrac{\dot{V}_{E_{CO_2}}}{F_{A_{CO_2}}\%} \times 100 \times F$

Calculation of these three formulae is presented in Appendix I.

Now one can assess the patient's minute ventilation—the volume of air that is moving through the patient's respiratory system every minute. (Any time that a measurement involves a unit of time it is abbreviated as a letter with a dot over it. So minute ventilation is $\dot{V}_E$.) The $\dot{V}_E$ stands for the expired volume of a gas per time unit. The formula for minute ventilation is:

$$\dot{V}_E = V_D \times V_A$$

Minute ventilation equals volume of dead space per minute plus the volume of air participating in gas exchange per minute. The dead space is both anatomic and physiologic dead space.

Usually, a rate or a single breath measurement is done.

The patient can breathe normally and the nurse or respiratory technician can measure the amount exhaled with a small spirometer. If desired, just one breath can be measured (the amount inhaled usually equals the amount exhaled). This single measurement will identify the patient's V_T. Or, in addition, one can count the respiratory rate for one minute and calculate how much air the patient is moving. Almost always, a measurement and/or a rate is included in minute ventilation figures. Now that presents a problem.

Physiologic dead space is that amount of the available 350 ml of gas that does *not* become involved in oxygen and carbon dioxide exchange. But physiologic dead space cannot be directly measured because it depends upon the carbon dioxide which diffuses 20 times more rapidly than oxygen in the alveolus. If the person is in a fairly stable state, the *arterial* carbon dioxide is inversely related to alveolar ventilation. *Arterial* carbon dioxide can be measured, and it will indicate if the amount of alveolar ventilation is adequate for the body's demands. Arterial carbon dioxide is abbreviated Pa_{CO_2}. Pa_{CO_2} stands for the partial pressure of carbon dioxide in the *arterial* blood.

If the V_A is elevated and the Pa_{CO_2} is low, hyperventilation is present. If the V_A is low and the Pa_{CO_2} is high, hypoventilation is present (and very likely the patient may have some degree of COPD). If the V_A is normal, and the Pa_{CO_2} is normal, alveolar ventilation is adequate for the body's metabolic demands.

The entire purpose of the second phase of respiration is the diffusion of oxygen into the erythrocyte and the diffusion of carbon dioxide out of the erythrocyte. There are three major components of the diffusion of gases.

1. Partial pressure of individual gases (Dalton's law).

Every gas has a pressure determined by its molecular weight. Atmospheric pressure (P_B) at sea level is equal to the *sum* of all gases that compose atmosphere; mainly, oxygen, nitrogen, carbon dioxide, and a few others in minute amounts. Atmospheric gas contains some water vapor that adds to the total gas tensions. The only thing that affects the water pressure is temperature. At body temperature (37°C), the water pressure is equal to 47 mm Hg. Dalton's law says that the total pressure is equal to the sum of the individual gas pressures, as if they occupied the same space—corrected for water pressure. So each gas has its own pressure or tension (P) and is present in a certain concentration (C) or fractional concentration (F).

Using Dalton's law of partial pressures, one can calculate the pressure of any desired gas. Since the kinetic theory states that gas molecules are always moving randomly, one can correctly conclude that there is always a pressure gradient in every body compartment. The presence of a pressure gradient means that not all (or any) gases in any compartment of the body are

going be in a state of equilibrium. When gas molecules are moving freely among themselves, the process is called *diffusion*. With inspiration, there will be a greater concentration of oxygen in the alveolus than carbon dioxide gas. This constitutes a concentration gradient and diffusion will occur to move all the gases toward a balance. At first, the diffusion will be rapid, and this adds to the pressure gradient.

In summary, all gases have individual pressures, move freely, and always toward a state of equilibrium, that is, always from an area of high pressure or concentration towards an area of lower pressure or concentration.

On inspiration, oxygen concentration or pressure is greater in the alveolus compared to the oxygen concentration in the area of the erythrocyte. At exactly the same time, the carbon dioxide concentration is greater in the erythrocyte, so it diffuses toward the low concentration area of the alveolus, and carbon dioxide does this *20 times faster* than oxygen.

2. Diffusion through the respiratory membrane.

In addition to the pressure and concentration gradients, a few other factors affect the ability and speed of gas molecules to diffuse through membranes. With the massive number of alveoli and their sharing of common walls, the actual area of space across which gases have to diffuse is very thin. In some electron micrographs, this thickness has been measured to be as thin as 0.2–0.5 microns. In reality, the alveoli and the capillaries are so small and so thin that they look like a single sheet of blood, but they are instead made up of six layers. (These six layers receiving incoming air are the alveolus, alveolar membrane, interstitial space, capillary membrane, plasma, and the erythrocyte membrane. For exhaled carbon dioxide, the layers are the same, but in reverse order.) These six layers are collectively called the *respiratory membrane*. If it becomes thickened (e.g., pulmonary edema), the diffusion of gases will slow.

Another factor affecting diffusion through the respiratory membrane is the amount of membrane surface area available. If a lobe of the lung is filled with pus, that portion of the respiratory membrane is not available for diffusion and diffusion will be slowed or stopped completely. In emphysema, when tiny alveoli collapse and disintegrate (or coalesce) to form larger alveoli, the amount of surface area of the respiratory membrane decreases and diffusion slows. Many other such examples could be listed.

The solubility of gases will affect the speed of diffusion. This is Henry's law. It states that the volume of a gas dissolved in a liquid is proportional to its partial pressure. The structure of some gas molecules is such that they dissolve more easily in some fluid such as water or plasma than in others.

Graham's law states that in the gas phase, the rate of diffusion of gas is inversely proportional to the molecular weight of that gas. This simply means that the lighter the weight of a gas, the slower it will diffuse; and the heavier the gas, the faster it will diffuse.

3. Diffusion of gas in relation to composition.

The specific composition of the alveolar, arterial, and venous compartments will directly affect the diffusibility of gases. The compartments concerned are shown in Table 2-3.

Shunting is the final segment in phase two of respiratory ventilation that needs our attention and understanding. A shunt exists when blood bypasses the alveolus without participating in gas exchange.

When alveolar ventilation was discussed, it was defined as that part of the V_T that was not dead space and that *did* participate in gas exchange. Of the normal 500 ml inspiration, about 150 ml would be anatomic dead space. It is estimated that an equal amount would be physiologic dead space. So approximately 200 ml are available for gas exchange.

Normally, about 2% of the blood flowing through the lungs does not come into contact with inspired air for gas exchange (shunt). This is due to the anatomic arrangement of the circulatory system of the lungs.

Any shunting that occurs (outside of the normal 2%) may be classified as one of three types:

1. **Physiologic Shunt:** There is an obstruction of inspired air. The air cannot pass through the respiratory membrane to diffuse into the erythrocyte. This is termed a *physiologic shunt* (Figure 2-5) and results in no increase in physiologic dead space. Ac-

Table 2-3.   Composition of gases in the alveolar, arterial, venous, and atmospheric components.

Alveolar	Arterial	Venous	Atmospheric
$P_{H_2O} = 47$	$P_{H_2O} = 47$	$P_{H_2O} = 47$	$P_{H_2O} = 47$
$PA_{CO_2} = 40$	$Pa_{CO_2} = 40$	$PV_{CO_2} = 46$	$PI_{CO_2} = 0$
$PA_{O_2} = 100\text{--}110$	$Pa_{O_2} = 92$	$PV_{O_2} = 40$	$PI_{O_2} = 150$
$PA_{N_2} = 563$	$Pa_{N_2} = 563$	$PV_{N_2} = 563$	$PI_{N_2} = 563$
			760 mm Hg

Remember the respiratory abbreviations?

P = pressure or partial pressure
A = alveolar
a = arterial
V = venous
I = inspired

H_2O = water
O_2 = oxygen
CO_2 = carbon dioxide
N_2 = nitrogen

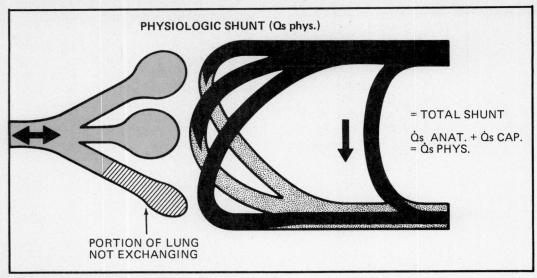

Figure 2-5.   Physiologic shunt.

cumulated secretions, atelectasis, pulmonary edema, neoplasms, and foreign objects caught in the throat are only a few of many causes of obstruction.

2. **Anatomic Shunt:** It may be that there is adequate ventilation in the alveolus, but blood perfusion is absent or markedly decreased and does not have the chance to participate in gas exchange (Figure 2-6). Normal pulmonary anatomy accounts for 2–5% of anatomic shunts due to anomalies in the pulmonary vasculature, which chan-

nel unoxygenated blood into the left atrium through thesbian, pleural, and bronchial veins. Pathological conditions causing anatomic shunts include states of pulmonary embolisms, thrombi, neoplasms, and similar conditions.

3. **Right-to-Left Shunt:** It may be that there is a true right-to-left shunt (Figure 2-7) such as in intracardiac septal defects. This would allow some venous blood to move directly from the right heart to the left heart, completely bypassing the lungs.

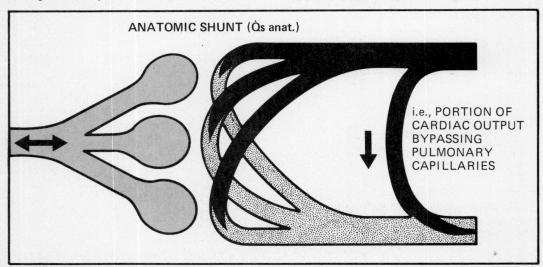

Figure 2-6.   Anatomic shunt.

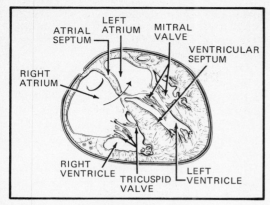

Figure 2-7.   Right-to-left shunt.

These three types of shunts may significantly alter the ventilation/perfusion rate of normal respiratory patterns and cause a mismatching. This ventilation/perfusion is abbreviated $\dot{V}/\dot{Q}$ in respiratory parlance. The "V" stands for ventilation and the "Q" stands for the quantity of blood for perfusion. $\dot{V}/\dot{Q}$ is always a ratio relationship.

The ultimate result of shunting is to decrease driving pressures of gases (which alters diffusion) and to increase the A-a oxygen gradient (which is the difference between alveolar and arterial oxygen tensions). These factors allow one to calculate the intrapulmonary shunt volume. Both of these factors are indicators of how well the lungs are meeting the oxygen needs of the body tissues. The topic of driving pressures is covered in phase three of the respiratory process. A-a oxygen gradient relates to hypoxia and will be discussed in Chapter 5, under respiratory failure.

Mechanical Process of Phase Three (Transport of Gases)

Once oxygen has penetrated the erythrocyte membrane, it will be carried through the systemic circulatory system to all body tissues.

Oxygen is transported in only two possible forms in the body. It is either dissolved in plasma or combined with hemoglobin. Very limited amounts of oxygen are dissolved in plasma. The amount is determined by Henry's law, that is, the amount dissolved is proportional to the partial pressure. This amounts to 0.003 ml O_2/100 ml of blood. This means that about 3% of the total body oxygen is in the dissolved state. When arterial blood gases are performed, the value for P_{O_2} measures the dissolved oxygen.

The remaining 97% of oxygen being transported through the system's circulation is in combination with hemoglobin (Hgb) within the erythrocyte. If the hemoglobin were chemically pure, a gram could combine with 1.39 ml of oxygen. Usually, the body hemoglobin is not pure. There is an estimated 2–4% of impurities such as methemoglobin and sulfhemoglobin. So, a more practical estimate would be that each gram of hemoglobin can combine with 1.34 ml of oxygen.

The transport of oxygen to body tissues is influenced most by cardiac output, by hemoglobin concentration, and by oxygen-hemoglobin binding and releasing factors.

Cardiac output is usually 4–6 liters per minute. As the cardiac output varies, the quantity of blood being oxygenated in the lungs will be altered. With normal, healthy lungs, a somewhat decreased cardiac output will not greatly alter oxygen content. The dynamics of the gas pressures allow for rapid oxygen equilibration between the alveolus and the erythrocyte. A markedly decreased cardiac output will alter the oxygen content—but what blood is available will have its maximum amount of oxygen. If hemoglobin is abnormally low, the cardiac output will increase to help compensate and to maintain adequate oxygen content. The amount of oxygen transported per minute is determined *basically* by the cardiac output, even though other factors will contribute some effect.

Oxygen capacity (Ca_{O_2}) is the maximum potential amount of oxygen that blood can carry. It is expressed as milliliters of oxygen per 100 milliliters of blood. In oxygen capacity, the dissolved oxygen in plasma is virtually ignored since it is so small an amount. It is not ignored in other instances.

Oxygen capacity = Hgb × 1.34 (ml of O_2)

Remember, only *pure* Hgb can be combined with 1.39 ml of oxygen. (Note: Hb and Hgb both are used as abbreviations for hemoglobin.)

Oxygen content = Hgb × 1.34 (oxygen capacity) + Pa_{O_2} × 0.003 (dissolved O_2).

Oxygen content is equal to the actual amount of oxygen in both the plasma and the erythrocytes.

Oxygen saturation (Sa_{O_2}) is the ratio comparing the actual amount of oxygen that could be carried with the amount actually carried. It is expressed as a percentage.

$$Sa_{O_2} = \frac{O_2 \text{ content}}{O_2 \text{ capacity}} \times 100(\%)$$

Hemoglobin is like a magnet and has a natural affinity for oxygen. Once the oxygen diffuses through the erythrocyte membrane, it readily attaches to a site on the hemoglobin molecule. Under ideal conditions, 100 ml of blood will have enough hemoglobin to carry 20 ml of oxygen. (Patient Hgb = 15 gm%) If this amount of oxygen is in fact present, the hemoglobin is said to be 100% saturated. Hemoglobin cannot be oversaturated. One hundred percent is the maximum—under human physiologic conditions. However, it may not always be 100% saturated. This is important when one remembers that hemoglobin is the major factor that determines how much *total* oxygen will be carried in the blood. Oxygen that is attached to hemoglobin (oxyhemoglobin) is not dissolved. Therefore, it does *not* directly exert a gas pressure.

Oxygen transportation is expressed as milliliters of oxygen/minute. To express this, the cardiac output must be considered and a factor of 10 is used to convert the oxygen content.

O_2 transport = O_2 content × 10 × cardiac output (in liters per minute)

Oxygen content and oxygen transport are a more reliable index of hypoxemia than the Pa_{O_2} alone. The oxygen content and transport include consideration of the Hgb level and the cardiac output. The Pa_{O_2} simply reflects the oxygen content dissolved in the plasma. Considering both the oxygen content and the cardiac output helps prevent an underestimation of the presence and severity of hypoxemia.

Oxygen-hemoglobin binding/releasing factors effect the oxygenation of blood even in the presence of marked disease. The effects of these factors are seen on the oxyhemoglobin dissociation curve (Figure 2-8). It is an S-shape curve. The relationship is not linear.

Physiologically, the mechanisms for oxygen-binding and oxygen-releasing factors are astonishing. If one is interested in *deeply* understanding these mechanisms, the reader is referred to the many medical texts available. For critical care nursing, at its best, one needs to understand what the curve shape indicates, what factors "shift" the curve to the right and to the left, what the results of this "shift" are, and what appropriate interventions will return the "shift" toward normal position.

Without much imagination, one can see that the oxyhemoglobin dissociation curve looks like an escalator. So let us look at it as if we were riding down one—starting from the upper right-hand side of the curve all the way to the bottom left corner.

The amount of oxygen *dissolved* in solution (plasma) provides the "driving pressure" that forces oxygen to combine with hemoglobin. This dissolved oxygen is directly proportional to its partial pressure and is termed the *arterial oxygen tension*. This driving pressure of dissolved oxygen exists until the alveolar (PA_{O_2}) and the arterial (Pa_{O_2}) pressures are almost equal and the pressure gradient no longer exists. All the oxygen pressure gradient between the alveolus and the erythrocyte is now almost in equilibrium. This is the point of the normal curve in the upper right of Figure 2-8. At this point in the normal healthy person, the oxygen tension is 95–97 mm Hg and the saturation of hemoglobin with oxygen (Sa_{O_2}) is about 97%.

With the curve indicating a move from the lungs into the systemic circulation, there is a steep down-slope portion to the curve. The hemoglobin saturation and the oxygen pressure are dropping. This is be-

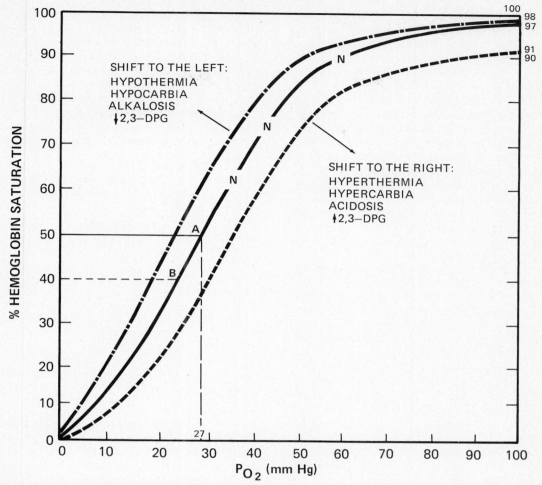

Figure 2-8. Oxyhemoglobin dissociation curve. (N = normal curve; A = hemoglobin 50% saturated with O_2; B = hemoglobin bound tightly with O_2, refusing to release the O_2 to the tissues, leading to hypoxia.)

cause the hemoglobin is readily giving oxygen out into the tissue capillaries. Another way of saying this is that in the lungs, because of high oxygen gas pressure, hemoglobin has an affinity for oxygen and absorbs as much as possible. Each hemoglobin molecule has four and *only* four sites to which an oxygen molecule can attach, but as the hemoglobin in the blood moves through the body, the arterial oxygen tension drops. With this drop, hemoglobin loses its affinity for oxygen and readily releases it into the tissues. But there is a slowing down point. When *hemoglobin saturation drops to 50%*, the hemoglobin begins to give up its oxygen

much less readily. On Figure 2-8, the normal is the point marked P_{50}. At P_{50}, the partial pressure of oxygen is about 27 mm Hg. As the curve slope becomes less steep (where the oxygen content is about 40 ml/l), the blood will soon re-enter the lungs to become reoxygenated.

The normal curve can be "shifted" to the right or to the left by specific factors. A shift in either direction indicates a change from the normal hemoglobin saturation and oxygen tension.

A shift to the right will occur in acidosis, hypercarbia (increased carbon dioxide), and a fever. As one can tell from the change from the normal slope to the slope of a right shift in Figure 2-8, the arterial oxygen tension and hemoglobin saturation are less than the normal curve (upper right starting point). This means that there is *less* oxygen content of the blood; *but* it also means that in the down slope portion of the curve, the hemoglobin will *more* readily give oxygen up to the tissues. Consequently, although there may be less oxygen in the blood, it is more readily given to the tissues, preventing hypoxia. Physiologically, this is an advantage only within certain limits. If the shift is not returned toward normal, eventually the decreased oxygen content will not prevent tissue hypoxia. If the oxygen is not there, it simply does not matter how easily hemoglobin gives it up.

A shift of the curve to the left occurs in alkalosis, hypocarbia, and hypothermia. Looking at Figure 2-8, note that the arterial oxygen tension and hemoglobin saturation are only very slightly changed from the normal curve (top right-hand corner, left shift curve line). The normal curve is an oxygen tension of 95–97 mm Hg, and the saturation of hemoglobin with oxygen is about 97%. There is just not much more oxygen that can be added. So a shift to the left does not actually help supply any extra oxygen to the tissues. In fact, the opposite occurs. With a shift to the left, hemoglobin binds oxygen much more tightly and releases less oxygen to the tissues.

2,3-Diphosphoglycerate is commonly referred to as 2,3-DPG. It is an important organic phosphate that also shifts the normal curve to the right and left. 2,3-DPG is a phosphate-type enzyme that is present in the erythrocyte. An increase of 2,3-DPG in the hemoglobin of the erythrocyte shifts the curve to the right and facilitates release of oxygen in the tissues. A decrease of 2,3-DPG in the hemoglobin of the erythrocyte shifts the curve to the left and hinders the release of oxygen into the tissues.

Transport of Carbon Dioxide

As long as life processes are functioning, carbon dioxide is formed as a waste by-product. It is produced in large quantities (average—2 pounds/day), and the body must continually rid itself of this waste product. This is transported in the blood in five different states: (a) dissolved in plasma, (b) as bicarbonate ion, (c) as carbonic acid, (d) in combination with hemoglobin, and (e) an extremely small amount as the carbonate ion. Let us look at the ways of ridding the body of carbon dioxide individually, even though all five processes are being used concurrently in the body.

1. The Dissolved State: Much like oxygen, only a very small amount of carbon dioxide is transported in the dissolved state. It constitutes about 7% of the total quantity of carbon dioxide. The presence of carbon dioxide in a dissolved state creates a pressure gradient or driving force and is measured as carbon dioxide tension or P_{CO_2}. Since carbon dioxide is a gas in solution, it follows Henry's law. The pressure gradient that develops from the dissolved CO_2 at the tissue level continues until the blood reaches the pulmonary capillaries. Since no CO_2 is normally inhaled, the pressure gradient is almost completely one-sided—pushing carbon dioxide from the capillary into the alveolus to be exhaled.

2 & 3. Bicarbonate Ion and Carbonic Anhydrase: The dissolved carbon dioxide in the blood reacts with water to form carbonic acid. The amount dissolved in the plasma takes several seconds to complete the reaction and form the carbonic acid. The amount of carbon dioxide that diffuses into the erythrocyte comes into contact with carbonic anhydrase, an enzyme that is a strong catalyst enabling dissolved carbon dioxide to convert to carbonic acid rapidly. The actual rate of the reaction is about 5,000 times faster than in the plasma portion. About 70% of the body's carbon dioxide waste is handled in this manner. Therefore, this is the most important method the body has for transporting carbon dioxide to the lungs for exhalation; but the process is not complete yet. As soon as carbonic acid is formed, it immediately breaks down into hydrogen ions and bicarbonate ions. This breakdown process is called *dissociation*. The hydrogen ions combine with hemoglobin (which has been giving up oxygen).

The bicarbonate ions diffuse into the plasma, and chloride ions diffuse into the red blood cells to maintain homeostasis. The bicarbonate ion movement results in the chloride ions being able to move into the erythrocyte. This is called the *chloride shift*. Since this is the body's *most important* way of transporting carbon dioxide, it is important to review these steps by looking at the chemical reactions.

Carbon dioxide enters the erythrocyte and does the following:

a. Combines with hemoglobin:

$$CO_2 + Hgb \rightarrow Hgb \cdot CO_2$$

(The dot between Hgb and CO_2 indicates a loose bonding.)

b. Combines with water:

$$CO_2 + H_2O \quad CA \quad H_2CO_3$$
(carbon dioxide $\rightleftharpoons$ (carbonic
and water)   acid)

(CA indicates carbonic anhydrase.)

c. The carbonic acid of step b dissociates (breaks down).

H_2CO_3

$$\rightarrow HCO_3^- \quad + \quad H^+$$
(bicarbonate   (hydrogen
ion)   ion)

d. HCO_3^- leaves the erythrocyte and enters the plasma allowing the Cl^- to enter the erythrocyte (the chloride shift).

e. The H^+ from step c binds with hemoglobin

$$H^+ + Hgb^- \rightarrow HHgb$$

Here are the formulae again without interrupting your thinking.

$CO_2 + Hgb \rightarrow Hgb \cdot CO_2$ and also
$CO_2 + H_2O \rightleftharpoons H_2CO_3$

$\rightarrow HCO_3^- + H^+$
$+$
Hgb^-

$HHgb$

erythrocyte
membrane

plasma   enters plasma and
             allows Cl^- to enter
             erythrocyte

4. In combination with hemoglobin: A small amount of the dissolved carbon dioxide enters the erythrocyte and binds loosely with hemoglobin.

$$CO_2 + Hgb \rightarrow Hgb \cdot CO_2$$

This type of compound formation is termed *carbaminohemoglobin* and these compounds are referred to as carbamino groups. A small amount of dissolved carbon dioxide will combine loosely with protein molecules in the plasma. A total of something close to 23% of total body carbon dioxide will be transported in this way.

5. The Carbonate Ion: The carbonate ion, $CO_3^=$, carries so little carbon dioxide that this transport method can be completely ignored.

Just one more concept must be explored as having a significant effect upon carbon dioxide transport. This is called the *Haldane effect*. Consider that hemoglobin picks up oxygen in the pulmonary capillaries. In order to do this, carbon dioxide *must* be released from the hemoglobin and subsequently is exhaled. Oxygen then attaches to the hemoglobin. By the time the hemoglobin reaches the body tissue capillaries, its oxygen is displaced by the metabolic waste product carbon dioxide. This is, of course, an oversimplification. But hemoglobin cannot hold or bind equal amounts of oxygen and carbon dioxide at the same time. "Therefore, in the tissue capillaries the Haldane effect causes increased pickup of carbon dioxide because of oxygen removal from the hemoglobin, and in the lungs it causes increased release of carbon dioxide because of oxygen pickup by the hemoglobin."[1]

Mechanical Process of Phase Four (Regulation of Ventilation)

The chemical balance or composition of the blood is probably responsible for alterations in the respiratory center of activity. It is now believed that there is a chemosensitive area in the medulla. This area is just behind the inspiratory neuron area. It is sensitive to changes in the hydrogen ion concentration and in the blood carbon dioxide levels. It is thought that this area responds to these general changes by increasing activity in the inspiratory neurons— first by increasing the depth of inspiration, and then the rate of inspiration. *Blood carbon dioxide has a much stronger effect in exciting the inspiratory centers than hydrogen ions have.*

Hydrogen ions cross the blood-brain barrier and the blood cerebrospinal fluid barrier very poorly, whereas carbon dioxide

---

[1]Guyton AC: Textbook of Medical Physiology, 6th ed. Philadelphia: W. B. Saunders, p. 513, 1981

passes through these barriers rapidly. Once the carbon dioxide is in the cerebrospinal fluid, it reacts immediately with water and forms hydrogen and bicarbonate ions. ($CO_2 + H_2O \rightleftharpoons H_2CO_3 \rightleftharpoons H^+ + HCO_3^-$). The increase in hydrogen ions makes the cerebrospinal fluid more acidic. This stimulates the inspiratory centers almost immediately because there are very few protein buffers free in the cerebrospinal fluid to absorb the hydrogen ions.

The effect of a decrease in blood carbon dioxide on respiration will achieve a peak reaction within a minute or so of the change in the carbon dioxide. If the blood carbon dioxide remains decreased, hydrogen ions begin to have a more potent effect on respiration. It simply takes longer for hydrogen ions to move across barrier membranes, but as they accumulate, their effect is increased. Both blood pH (normal range 7.35–7.45) and blood P_{CO_2} (normal range 35–45 mm Hg) exert continuous control on respirations; but the P_{CO_2} *is the main control for minute-to-minute changes in pulmonary ventilation.*

The aortic body and carotid bodies contain neurons that are sensitive to changes in blood composition. These bodies all contribute to the control of pulmonary ventilation. They were discusssed in Chapter 1.

3

Acid-Base Physiology and Arterial Blood Gases

Learning Objectives

By the end of this chapter, the nurse will be able to:

1. Define the terms: acid, base, pH, acidosis, acidemia, alkalosis, and alkalemia.
2. List three defense mechanisms for acid-base imbalances.
3. Explain the following buffer systems:
   a. Bicarbonate buffer system
   b. Phosphate buffer system
   c. Protein buffer system
4. Identify the normal range values in adult arterial blood at sea level for: pH, P_{O_2}, P_{CO_2}, S_{O_2}, HCO_3^-, base excess.
5. Identify the parameters for respiratory acidosis and alkalosis.
6. Identify the parameters for metabolic (nonrespiratory) acidosis and metabolic (nonrespiratory) alkalosis.
7. Name two synonyms for respiratory acidosis.
8. Name two synonyms for respiratory alkalosis.
9. Interpret abnormal values in arterial blood gases (ABGs).
10. Differentiate between compensation and correction of abnormal acid-base states.
11. Explain the mechanism of compensation for:
    a. Respiratory acidosis
    b. Respiratory alkalosis
    c. Metabolic (nonrespiratory) acidosis
    d. Metabolic (nonrespiratory) alkalosis
12. List an intervention used to correct:
    a. Respiratory acidosis
    b. Respiratory alkalosis
    c. Metabolic (nonrespiratory) acidosis
    d. Metabolic (nonrespiratory) alkalosis
13. List four etiologies of respiratory acidosis and four etiologies of respiratory alkalosis.
14. Explain "unmeasurable anions" and "anion gap."
15. List four etiologies of metabolic acidosis that have an increase in unmeasurable anions.
16. List four etiologies of metabolic acidosis that have *no* increase in unmeasurable anions.

Life processes continue only as long as the acid-base state in our bodies is kept within a very narrow range. An acid state that is not corrected will eventually result in a coma and then death. A base state that is not corrected will eventually result in convulsion or tetany and then death.

Acid-Base Physiology

Since acid-base physiology is so vital to our survival, there is a need to review some terminology.

An acid is a chemical substance that dissociates (breaks down) into ions. Ions have an electrical charge, positive or negative. The positive ion is called a *cation*. The negative ion is called an *anion*. That is easy to remember if we look at the first three letters of the word anion: ani- relates to "a negative ion." Hydrogen is a cation. It has a positive charge; and it is special in all the things that it can do, so it is given the name *proton*. Now an acid can be defined a little more specifically. An acid is a substance that dissociates and gives up a proton (H^+) to the solution. The electrical charge placed as a superscript, e.g., H^+, Cl^-, indicates that the substance is an ion.

A base is a substance that can and will accept a proton (H^+) while in solution. Water is the most common and abundant base in the body.

The pH represents the hydrogen ion concentration. The hydrogen ion concentration indicates the intensity with which the hydrogen ion will react with bases in solution. The pH was determined by Henderson and Hasselbalch. pH is an expression of the hydrogen ion concentration as a negative logarithm.

Acid-Base Balance

Two types of acids are formed in the body. They are classified as volatile acids or nonvolatile (fixed) acids. These acids are formed by the metabolism of food and by anaerobic glycolysis. There is an extremely important difference between volatile and nonvolatile acids.

VOLATILE ACIDS

Carbonic acid is the major volatile acid in the body. It is made by the combination of carbon dioxide and water:

$$CO_2 + H_2O \rightleftharpoons H_2CO_3$$

The double direction arrow indicates that the reaction readily moves in either direction. Volatile acids are those acids that can form a gas *and*, that because of an open system, can be eliminated in its gas form. All volatile acids can, therefore, be eliminated by the lungs. The two main sources of volatile acids are the body's metabolism of glucose and fat.

$$\text{glucose} \xrightarrow{+O_2} H^+ + HCO_3^-$$
$$\text{fat} \xrightarrow{} H^+ + HCO_3^-$$

Remember now that $H^+ + HCO_3^- = H_2CO_3$ (carbonic acid) *and* that carbonic acid breaks down into carbon dioxide and water.

$$H_2CO_3 \rightleftharpoons CO_2 + H_2O$$

The lungs eliminate about 24,000 mEq of volatile acids per day.

NONVOLATILE (FIXED) ACIDS

Acids that cannot be converted into gas form for elimination are termed nonvolatile acids. Fortunately, the daily production of nonvolatile acids is very small. Nonvolatile acids are excreted mainly by the kidneys in the urine, and some in the stool. Nonvolatile acid sources are anaerobic glycolysis, amino acid metabolism, and phosphoprotein/phospholipid metabolism.

$$\text{glucose} \xrightarrow{\text{anaerobic}} H^+ + \text{lactate}$$

$$\text{amino acid} \xrightarrow{+O_2} H^+ + \text{sulfate}$$
$$\text{(e.g., cystine)}$$
$$\text{phosphoproteins} \xrightarrow{+O_2} H^+ + \text{phosphate}$$

The kidneys excrete these fixed acids, which total about 50 mEq/day. Disease can also produce nonvolatile acids, such as butyric acid, in diabetic ketoacidosis.

Acid-Base Disturbance

When there is any disruption in the acid-base balance of the arterial blood toward acidosis, the body has three main defense mechanisms. The three mechanisms are buffering, increasing alveolar ventilation, and increasing hydrogen ion elimination along with increasing bicarbonate reabsorption. These three defense mechanisms "kick-in" in the order listed. Let us take a quick look over all three as they would enter the battle to maintain acid-base balance, and then look at just how each mechanism functions. (Body defense of the alkalotic state is explained under altering acid-base abnormalities.)

1. *Buffering:* This response starts immediately in reaction to an acid-base disturbance in an attempt to prevent changes in hydrogen ion concentration. All of the body's fluids have acid-base buffer systems, so this response begins within a fraction of a second.
2. *Increasing alveolar ventilation:* This defense mechanism will begin in 1–15 minutes. As hydrogen ion concentration builds up suddenly, the lungs attempt to control the hydrogen ion concentration by "blowing off" more carbon dioxide.
3. *Increasing hydrogen ion elimination along with increasing bicarbonate ion reabsorption:* The kidneys provide the stongest defense against acid-base disturbances. Unfortunately, it takes from several hours to several days for the kidneys to rebalance the hydrogen ion concentration.

Each of these three defense mechanisms needs to be examined to see how they function independently.

BUFFERING

Essentially there are three buffering systems: the bicarbonate buffer system, the phosphate buffer system, and the protein buffer system. All three are important buffers, but they function under different conditions. Chemical buffers have the ability to yield or combine with hydrogen ions.

The **bicarbonate buffer system** is by far the most important system because the end products of the chemical buffer are regulated by both the kidneys and the lungs. The chemical reaction in this system is reversible and occurs extremely rapidly due to the catalyst carbonic anhydrase (CA). The general reaction is:

$$H^+ + HCO_3^- \overset{CA}{\rightleftharpoons} H_2CO_3 \overset{CA}{\rightleftharpoons} CO_2 + H_2O$$

(Hydrogen ion plus bicarbonate ion yields carbonic acid which yields carbon dioxide and water, and vice versa.)

If the buffering moves toward the left, bicarbonate ion is the end product. Bicarbonate ion is regulated by the kidneys. If the buffering moves toward the right, the end product is carbon dioxide. Carbon dioxide is regulated by the lungs. Since one end product is regulated by the kidneys and the other end product is regulated by the lungs, and because buffering must occur by the lungs or the kidneys, this system is especially important. It means that the pH can be shifted up or down by either or both the renal system and the respiratory system. With so many possible controls, even though this is a weak chemical reaction, it is a *very important and easily manipulated system.*

The **phosphate buffer system** is similar to the bicarbonate system in function. The phosphate system buffers best at a slightly different pH than bicarbonate. It buffers mainly in the tubular fluids of the kidney. This system buffers strong acids (e.g., hydrochloric) and strong bases (e.g., sodium hydroxide) into weak acids and bases that will have little effect upon the blood pH.

The **protein buffer system** is the most inexhaustable buffering system in the body. All the plasma proteins buffer and so do all of the intracellular proteins, including hemoglobin. The majority of the proteins are intracellular. Carbon dioxide diffuses readily, and bicarbonate ion diffuses slowly into the cells. Proteins will buffer carbon dioxide quickly and bicarbonate ion over a period of several hours. The extreme importance of the system is that it helps to buffer the extracellular fluids through the diffusion of carbon dioxide and bicarbonate ion. The supply of protein is infinite.

INCREASED ALVEOLAR VENTILATION

Assuming that buffering has not rectified an acid-base disturbance within 1–15 minutes, the respiratory system will enter the battle. Alveolar hyperventilation increases the rate at which the body "blows off" carbon dioxide. Acid-base balance and ABGs are important in *early* identification and intervention to alter potentially fatal changes in the patient's status.

Increased alveolar ventilation alters the relationship between pH, P_{CO_2}, and bicarbonate ion. The Henderson-Hasselbalch equation is an expression of the relationship between pH, P_{CO_2}, and bicarbonate ion. This equation can be understood more readily by breaking it into parts: Henderson first, and then, Hasselbalch.

Henderson states:

1. An acid (HB) dissociates (breaks down) into a proton (H^+) and a base (B^-).
2. The acid dissociates at a specific rate.
3. The acid dissociates in relation to a constant characteristic for each reaction. For example, carbonic acid (H_2CO_3) dissociates into a proton (H^+) and a base (HCO_3^-). H_2CO_3 dissociates at a specific rate—no faster, no slower. H_2CO_3 dissociates in relation to a constant characteristic—equilibrium. It will continue to dissociate until equilibrium is reached. Then it stops.
4. When the acid releases the proton, H^+, the H^+ and the base will be bound together at a specific rate until equilibrium (the constant characteristic) is reached.
5. Now, put all four of the principles first mentioned together. Henderson is saying that in an acid-base reaction, equilibrium will be maintained, that is, the acid will dissociate at a rate equal to the proton binding to the

base. Look at that as a written equation:

$$\frac{\text{Rate of reaction}_1}{\text{Rate of reaction}_2} = \frac{\text{(acid)}}{\text{(proton) (base)}}$$

or

$$\frac{r_1}{r_2} = \frac{\text{(HB)}}{\text{(H}^+)\text{(B}^-)}$$

Henderson and others did not stop there. They discovered some more interesting facts, which are summarized as follows:

6. The ratio of proton (H^+) release (r_1) by the acid to the ratio of proton (H^+) bonding (r_2) to the base is constant (K).

In symbols:

$$\frac{r_1}{r_2} = K$$

Then Henderson came up with a final equation based on the first ones. Henderson's final equation in symbols is:

$$(H^+) = K \frac{(H^+)}{(B^-)}$$

This says that the proton-binding of a solution is equal to the strength of the bases plus the ratio of the concentrations of its bases to the bonded acids.

Using all of these principles, normal hydrogen ion concentration of blood was calculated to be 0.0000001 to 0.00000001 moles/liter of blood. (That equals 10^{-7} moles/liter.) It is difficult to comprehend such tiny numbers.

In the early twentieth century, Sorenson eliminated all these zeros by redefining the hydrogen ion concentration in 10^{-7} moles/liter as *seven puissance hydrogen*. (The term puissance was simply a French word expressing logarithm in a specific way.)

Then Hasselbalch came along and simplified all of this by referring to the hydrogen ion concentration simply as pH. In equation form then, pH $= \log \frac{1}{H^+}$.

Hasselbalch also determined that $pK = \log \frac{1}{K}$. (Remember K is the *constant* ratio of the release of protons from acids to the bonding of protons to bases.)

The final version of Henderson and Hasselbalch's combined equations is:

$$pH = pK + \log \frac{base}{acid}$$

This means that the behavior of hydrogen ion in a solution is equal to its chemical energy or potential. This potential is dependent upon (or results from) the activity of the substance.

Blood has a major acid (carbonic acid) and a major base (bicarbonate ion). The pK, dissociation reaction constant, has been calculated to be 6.10 in blood. The ratio of bicarbonate to carbonic acid in the blood is 20:1. The log of 20 is 1.30. These figures in the Henderson-Hasselbalch equation equal:

$$pH = pK + \log \frac{HCO_3^-}{H_2CO_3} = \underset{(pK)}{6.10} + \underset{\underset{of\ 20)}{(log}}{1.30}$$
$$= 7.4$$
$$pH = 7.4$$

The pH expresses the driving pressure of the acid-base balance.

The pH is a negative logarithm; so the smaller the value of the pH, the greater the concentration of hydrogen ions and the more acidic the solution. Conversely, the larger the value of the pH, the smaller the concentration of hydrogen ions and the less acidic the solution.

Alveolar ventilation attempts to balance acid-base disturbances by altering the relationship of pH, P_{CO_2}, and HCO_3^-. This relationship and its alterations are expressed by the Henderson-Hasselbalch equation. The extremely *important ratio* to remember is that of *bicarbonate to carbonic acid in the blood, which is 20:1*. This gives the logarithm of 20, which 1.30.

Increased Hydrogen Ion Elimination Along with Increased Bicarbonate Ion Reabsorption

This is the final mechanism that the body can utilize to alter acid-base disturbances.

This defense mechanism involves both the lungs and the kidneys. This puzzle fits together quite nicely if we once again combine Henderson-Hasselbalch with this third defense mechanism. Then we can say:

$$pH = \frac{HCO_3^-}{Pa_{CO_2}} = \frac{Kidney\ function}{Lung\ function}$$

The kidney function of acid-base disturbances will join the battle within a few hours of the disturbance. However, it is a slow acting defense mechanism and may take several days to rebalance the acids and bases.

The kidneys are able to excrete some hydrogen ions in relation to excretion of nonvolatile acids. This is a very small additional percentage of hydrogen ion elimination (since the lungs excrete most of hydrogen ions). At the same time, however, the kidneys will reabsorb bicarbonate ion (in the proximal tubule) to equal the excessive number of hydrogen ions. As this reabsorption proceeds, carbon dioxide and water are formed (remember the formula? $H^+ + HCO_3^- \rightleftharpoons H_2CO_3 \rightleftharpoons CO_2 + H_2O$).

If this reabsorption is not adequate to restore acid-base balance, then sodium ions and hydrogen ions will trade places (maintaining electrical neutrality). The sodium bicarbonate then returns from the kidney tubules to the plasma.

If this defense does not re-establish acid-base balance, the kidneys will conserve still more bicarbonate. The kidneys do this by substituting ammonium ions (NH_4^+) for bicarbonate ions, again on a one for one basis, to maintain electrical neutrality.

Assuming the acid-base disturbance continues, and all of the possible bicarbonate ions have been retained, hydrogen ions will reach the distal tubules and combine with phosphates. These phosphates, with the added hydrogen ions, will then be excreted in the urine.

Alterations in potassium and in extracellular fluid volume are final efforts of the kidney to restore acid-base balance.

Arterial Blood Gases

A single arterial blood gas sample gives a

Table 3-1. Normal adult blood gas values at sea level.

| | Arterial | | Mixed Venous |
	Range	Midpoint	
pH	7.35–7.45	7.40	7.36–7.41
P_{O_2}	80–100 mm Hg	93	35–40 mm Hg
P_{CO_2}	35–45 mm Hg	40	41–51 mm Hg
HCO_3^-	22–26 mEq/l	24	22–26 mEq/l
S_{O_2}	95–100%	97%	70–75%
Base excess	−2 to +2	0	+2

starting point for treating and assessing the patient. However, by far more important than any sampling is the *trend* of movement in serial arterial blood gases.

There are six values of importance in interpreting arterial blood gases. Each of these values has a range (Table 3-1). In addition to the range is a specific midpoint value. Nurses need to learn both the ranges and the midpoint value of at least arterial blood, and preferably, both arterial and mixed venous values.

In the rest of this chapter, reference will be to the arterial blood gas values, which are used more as guidelines in critical care than mixed venous samples. Remember, from now on (unless otherwise stated), all references are to **arterial blood gas values at sea level**.

Acidosis is an acid-base disturbance with acids being predominant in quantity.

Acidemia is a state in which the arterial blood pH is below the normal minimum of 7.35 (because of an increase in hydrogen ions).

Alkalosis is an acid-base disturbance in which acids are insufficient in quantity or base is excessive. Acid insufficiency is more commonly a cause than is base excess.

Alkalemia is a state in which the arterial blood pH is above the normal maximum of 7.45 (because of a decrease in hydrogen ions).

Altering Acid-Base Abnormalities

There are only two ways in which the pH may be returned toward the normal 7.40 in

acid-base disturbances. Compensation or correction will return the pH toward normal.

Compensation occurs when the body itself responds to the acid-base abnormality. The system not primarily affected will compensate. If the disturbance is respiratory acidosis, the kidneys will respond to shift the pH toward normal. Remember from earlier in this chapter, the kidney is slow to respond, but the response (compensatory mechanism) is strong.

Since the lungs are responsible for the state of respiratory acidosis, the kidneys will try to compensate by excreting more acid in the urine and increasing reabsorption of the bicarbonate ion. These two concurrent actions will move the pH nearly back to the normal value of 7.40.

If respiratory alkalosis is the acid-base disturbance, the kidneys (system not primarily affected) will try to compensate. The kidneys will increase the amount of bicarbonate excreted.

If metabolic (nonrespiratory) acidosis is the acid-base disturbance, the kidneys are the system primarily affected. For the body to compensate and return the pH toward normal, the respiratory system (not primarily affected) will come into action. The respiratory system is stimulated, and there is an increase in alveolar ventilation. This hyperventilation "blows off" carbon dioxide, an acid waste product of metabolic processes. This is an effective and rapid way to decrease arterial carbon dioxide (Pa_{CO_2}) levels. As opposed to the slow kidneys, the respiratory system can compensate in metabolic acidosis in just a few hours.

If metabolic (nonrespiratory) alkalosis is

the acid-base abnormality, the respiratory system (not primarily affected) will try to compensate. The respiratory system will be inhibited by the metabolic alkalosis, and the patient will hypoventilate. This retains carbon dioxide to shift the pH toward normal. However, the body cannot fully compensate for metabolic alkalosis. The hypoventilation necessary for compensation causes a decrease in the arterial oxygen (Pa_{O_2}) levels. When the oxygen level becomes too low, the respiratory system will respond to the decreased oxygen by increasing ventilation. Although this compensation effort is rapid, it is not a complete compensation.

Many authorities agree that the most significant fact about compensation as a defense mechanism in acid-base disturbance is that the body *never* overcompensates. Compensation will return the body pH to near normal (7.40), but it will *never* "overshoot the mark."

Correction is the other way in which the pH may be returned toward its normal value (7.40). Correction is the return of the system primarily affected toward normal by an outside source, that is, ventilation and medication. Nurses, doctors, and respiratory technicians do something to correct an imbalance. Unfortunately, they are not as finely tuned as the compensation process; and therefore, they do overcorrect the acid-base balance on occasion.

If the primary acid-base disturbance is respiratory acidosis, it is corrected by increasing ventilation. The increase will enable more carbon dioxide (acid) to be "blown off." For the patient on a respirator, the respiratory rate is increased to decrease the P_{CO_2} and maintain effective ventilation, or the tidal volume is increased.

If the primary acid-base disturbance is respiratory alkalosis, it is corrected by decreasing the respiratory rate or by increasing carbon dioxide inhalation. (The hyperventilating patient is told to breathe into a paper bag. Each time the patient inhales, he or she breathes back some of the carbon dioxide previously exhaled.)

If the patient is on a respirator, decreasing the respiratory rate or decreasing the tidal volume, or adding additional tubing (dead space) will correct the imbalance.

If the primary acid-base disturbance is metabolic (nonrespiratory) acidosis, treatment with intravenous sodium bicarbonate will correct the disturbance. (It may well overcorrect the acid-base imbalance.) If given judiciously, bicarbonate will begin to return the pH toward normal, while the underlying cause of the imbalance is treated. Base excess values help the doctor determine the amount of bicarbonate needed.

If the primary acid-base disturbance is metabolic (nonrespiratory) alkalosis, the imbalance is corrected by giving the patient acetazolamide (Diamox®) or potassium chloride (KCl). These drugs force the kidneys to excrete potassium or chloride instead of hydrogen ions. This correction is used to return the pH toward normal, while the actual cause of the imbalance is being treated.

Respiratory Disturbances

A look at the respiratory parameter will help determine some of the clinical conditions that may precipitate a respiratory acid-base imbalance. It is known that the Pa_{CO_2} (arterial carbon dioxide level) represents our measurement of the effective alveolar ventilation. From the Pa_{CO_2}, the presence of respiratory acidosis or alkalosis can be determined.

RESPIRATORY ACIDOSIS

If the Pa_{CO_2} is elevated (normal 40 mm Hg) and the pH decreased, respiratory acidosis is present and indicates hypoventilation. Hypoventilation may be of an acute or chronic nature. Regardless, the clinical cause must be determined and treated. Pathologic conditions usually cause respiratory acidosis.

All obstructive lung diseases (most commonly asthma, bronchitis, and emphysema) result in a degree of hypoventilation. Since obstructive lung diseases tend to be progressive and chronic, one can anticipate elevated Pa_{CO_2} values in the arterial blood gas studies. Eventually, the Pa_{CO_2} will become ineffective as a means of stimulating ventilation, and the P_{O_2} will become the driving force for inspiration.

Any clinical condition that depresses the respiratory center in the medulla oblongata may precipitate hypoventilation and result in respiratory acidosis. These conditions include head trauma, oversedation, and general anesthesia, as the leading causes. More rarely, neoplasms in the medulla oblongata or nearby areas with increasing intracranial mass, size, and, therefore, pressure may cause a respiratory acidosis.

Neuromuscular disease including myasthenia gravis, Guillain-Barré, multiple sclerosis, amyotrophic lateral sclerosis (ALS, also known as Lou Gerhig's disease), and trauma to the cervical spinal cord may cause hypoventilation and the resulting respiratory acidosis.

If the patient is on a respirator, inappropriate mechanical ventilation may cause respiratory acidosis. These causes could include too low a respiratory rate, too low a tidal volume (V_T), or too much dead space in the tubing.

RESPIRATORY ALKALOSIS

If the Pa_{CO_2} is decreased (normal 40 mm Hg) and the pH is increased, respiratory alkalosis is present and this indicates hyperventilation.

Restrictive lung diseases are the common pathologic causes of respiratory alkalosis.

Excluding these pathologic etiologies, most causes of respiratory alkalosis are anxiety, nervousness, agitation, hyperventilation on a respirator, and excessive "ambu-bagging" during a cardiopulmonary arrest.

Two conditions often cause a "temporary" respiratory alkalosis. During the third trimester of pregnancy, when the diaphragm cannot descend fully, alkalosis may occur intermittently (usually during periods of physical exertion). The second "temporary" alkalosis occurs with a change to a higher altitude. The oxygen content is lower, and the oxygen saturation is lower. Because of this lower oxygen content, the respiratory centers are stimulated, and a person may hyperventilate until physiologic adjustment to the high altitude occurs.

Metabolic (Nonrespiratory, Renal) Disturbances

The bicarbonate ion (HCO_3^-) and base excess are the parameters of the arterial blood gases used to identify nonrespiratory imbalances.

Base excess is an easy guide to use in identifying metabolic acidosis versus alkalosis. Base excess is the amount of base above the normal level, after adjusting the level for hemoglobin. The normal midpoint value is zero. If the base excess is above $+2$, there is an excess of metabolic base in the body fluids. Therefore, a metabolic alkalosis exists. If the base excess is below -2, there is not enough metabolic base in the body fluids. Therefore, a metabolic acidosis exists.

METABOLIC ALKALOSIS ($HCO_3^- \uparrow$; POSITIVE BASE EXCESS)

Any condition that increases metabolic processes beyond the ability of the body to eliminate or neutralize the waste products results in an increase in bicarbonate ions. Nonrespiratory alkalosis is less common than nonrespiratory acidosis, except in the surgical patient with nasogastric suctioning. Metabolic alkalosis is a condition with an excess base. The three most common causes are diuretic therapy, excessive vomiting of stomach contents, and excessive ingestion of alkaline drugs. Less commonly, treatment with corticosteroids (especially mega-dose therapy), hyperaldosteronism, and, rarely, Cushing's syndrome result in nonrespiratory alkalosis.

These conditions result in a loss of hydrogen ions (diuretics), chloride ions (vomiting), and potassium ions (hyperaldosteronism) through the kidneys. The effect of these three conditions is to enhance bicarbonate ion (HCO_3^-) reabsorption in the kidneys, which forces excretion of the hydrogen, chloride, and potassium ions in the urine.

Excessive ingestion of alkaline drugs usually occurs in patients with gastritis; they ingest antacids and soda bicarbonate to quiet their stomachs.

The remaining major cause of non-respiratory alkalosis is excessive loss of gastric acids. This can be from excessive vomiting or nasogastric (N/G) suctioning. Since nasogastric suctioning is a common and often lengthy treatment in critical care units, patients with nasogastric tubes should be monitored closely for acid-base disturbances. Corrective therapy is far easier in the early stages of the disorder, before electrolyte imbalances become markedly abnormal.

METABOLIC ACIDOSIS (HCO$_3$ ↓ ; NEGATIVE BASE EXCESS)

Metabolic (nonrespiratory, renal) acidosis occurs in the body when there is an increase of any metabolic acid, except carbon dioxide. Although carbon dioxide is an acid end-product of body metabolism, it is excreted by the lungs. Therefore, it is classified as a respiratory acidosis when elevated.

Nonrespiratory acidosis may occur with an excess loss of body alkali (bicarbonate ion) in diabetes mellitus, in uremia, with certain medications, with retention of hydrogen ions, and in prolonged vomiting and diarrhea of small intestine fluids.

Nonrespiratory acidosis is classified into two major groups—those with an increase in unmeasurable anions, and those with no increase in unmeasurable anions. Understanding which causes of nonrespiratory acidosis result from an increase in unmeasurable anions and which result from no increase in unmeasurable anions helps to alert us to possible problems for which the patient needs monitoring.

To calculate unmeasurable anions, add the serum chloride and the bicarbonate ion values. Then, subtract this sum from the serum sodium level. If the difference is greater than 15 mEq/l, there is an increase in unmeasurable anions. This is called an *anion gap*.

Common etiologies of nonrespiratory acidosis with an increase in unmeasurable anions include (the specific anion is in parentheses): diabetes mellitus (ketone bodies), uremia (phosphates and sulfates), lactic acidosis (lactate), aspirin poisonings (salicylate), methyl poisoning (formic acid), ethylene glycol poisoning (oxalic acid and formic acid), and paraldehyde.

There are several common etiologies of nonrespiratory acidosis with no increase in unmeasurable anions. Diarrhea is probably the most common cause. Large amounts of bicarbonate ion are in the intestines and are "washed out" in cases of diarrhea. The more severe the diarrhea, the greater the likelihood of nonrespiratory acidosis.

Drug therapy using acetazolamide (Diamox®) to induce diuresis blocks renal reabsorption of the bicarbonate ion. Ammonium chloride will also block bicarbonate ion reabsorption when overused.

A general guide for the possible development of nonrespiratory acidosis with no increase in unmeasurable anion is the presence of any drainage tube (except a Foley catheter) below the umbilicus. This includes drainage of pancreatic juices, ureterosigmoidostomies, and any others drainage tubes in use.

A final major category is uremia. With severe renal failure, the kidneys cannot excrete the normal acids formed daily by the body. As the acids build up, uremia develops; and with the uremia is an increase in unmeasurable anions.

Nonrespiratory acidosis is the most difficult acid-base disturbance to correct. The high hydrogen ion concentration stimulates the body to attempt compensation by increasing both the depth and the rate of respiration. Compensation is not usually enough by itself. However, the electrolytes are often quite abnormal and complicate the correcting of acid-base disturbance.

Interpreting Normal Arterial Blood Gases

The identity of basic acid-base disturbances can be determined by following a step-by-step procedure of analyzing arterial blood gases (ABGs).

There is a "cardinal rule" *to be memorized* and *applied every time* a set of ABGs are interpreted. If the pH and the P$_{CO_2}$ move in opposite directions, the primary cause of acid-base disturbance is respiratory. If the pH and the P_{CO_2} move in the same direction, the primary cause is metabolic (nonrespiratory). If mnemonics help, use the word *same* as a key. The word *same* indicates the direction of the pH and P_{CO_2} movement, and the word *same* has an "m" for metabolic (or nonrespiratory) cause.

Step 1: Look at the pH.

If it is 7.40, it is normal.

If it is between 7.35 and 7.39, *consider* it compensated acidosis.

If it is between 7.41 and 7.45, *consider* it compensated alkalosis.

Only a pH of 7.40 is perfectly normal. Any deviation from that value is compensated or uncompensated acidosis (if pH value is down) or alkalosis (if pH value is up). Step 1 identifies the presence of an acidosis or alkalosis. Most authorities feel that the mitochondria in cells are unable to function if the pH falls below 6.9 to 7.2.

Step 2: Look the P_{CO_2}. P_{CO_2} is used since many hospitals report the arterial carbon dioxide under this title. It is actually Pa_{CO_2}. We have dropped the "a" since we did state that we were looking at arterial blood gases. There are two stages in this step:

(a) If the P_{CO_2} is 40, it is normal.

If it is between 35 and 39, *consider* it compensated.

If the value is below 35, *consider* it uncompensated.

If the value is between 41 and 45, *consider* it compensated.

If the value is above 45, *consider* it uncompensated.

(b) If the P_{CO_2} moves in the *same* direction as the pH, the primary cause is metabolic.

If the P_{CO_2} moves in the opposite direction of the pH, the primary cause is respiratory.

Only a P_{CO_2} of 40 is perfectly normal. Any deviation between 35 and 39 or 41 and 45 indicates an abnormal state; *but* the abnormal state is not extreme. A value of less than 35 or more than 45 indicates that the body defense mechanisms are not functioning adequately.

When we look at only the pH and P_{CO_2} for any set of blood gases, respiratory or metabolic acidosis or alkalosis can be determined. (There is a movement toward referring to the oldest term *metabolic* as *nonrespiratory*, and an even more current movement toward referring to the term *nonrespiratory* as *renal*.) Depending upon which text you read, think of these three terms—metabolic, nonrespiratory, and renal—as being synonyms.

Step 3: Look at the bicarbonate ion (HCO_3^-) value.

If it is 24, *consider* it normal.

If it is between 22 and 24, *consider* it compensated.

If it is less than 22, *consider* it uncompensated.

If it is between 24 and 26, *consider* it compensated.

If it is greater than 26, *consider* it uncompensated. (Step 2 is the real key. Step 3 confirms step 2 or identifies a secondary imbalance.)

Step 4: Look at the S_{O_2}.

S_{O_2} indicates the percent oxygen saturation.

The normal is 95–99%.

Generally, if the S_{O_2} is at least 93% and the remaining ABG values are within a compensated range, the patient's oxygenation status is at least adequate. Most times, this patient needs only to be monitored. If the S_{O_2} falls lower, the patient will need treatment to prevent the occurrence of respiratory failure and tissue hypoxia (Chapter 5).

Step 5: Determine base excess.

If it is between a -2 and a $+2$, consider it normal. (Zero is the midpoint.)

Base excess is a reflection of a nonrespiratory acid-base disorder since it is altered only by the nonvolatile acids. It is used to determine the amount of bicarbonate the patient needs to buffer the nonvolatile acids.

Step 6: Look for mixed imbalances.

Many times, arterial blood gases will reveal a condition in which the pH, the P_{CO_2}, and the HCO_3^- will be outside compensated ranges. This indicates that both respiratory and nonrespiratory causes are present. Here is an actual set of values:

pH = 7.52, P_{CO_2} = 60, HCO_3^- = 52, S_{O_2} = 50

This is mixed. The pH indicates alkalosis (it moved up). The pH and P_{CO_2} moved in the same direction, indicating that a nonrespiratory disturbance is the *primary* disorder. Both the P_{CO_2} and the HCO_3^- are abnormally high. The HCO_3^- is 28 points above midpoint in its range of values. The P_{CO_2} is 20 points above midpoint in its range of values. Look at the P_{CO_2}. It is a measure of acid (CO_2). The acid is increased, so a condition of acidemia exists (along with, but less than, the arterial blood alkalemia). Since the acid product is CO_2, it must be respiratory. (Remember, the lungs control CO_2 and the kidneys, HCO_3^-.) So respiratory acidosis is present. The final label would be metabolic alkalosis and respiratory acidosis, both uncompensated. Do not become caught in the trap of thinking that the pH indicates alkalemia, so acidemia cannot exist. Use the pH and P_{CO_2} to identify the primary condition—*not* the only condition.

Once the primary condition is identified, then identify any additional abnormal condition. These are only *general* guidelines. The most important factors in labeling the patient are his or her *trend* of movement in serial ABGs, followed by the patient's condition, current respiratory treatment, drug therapies, and diagnosis.

The steps of interpreting arterial blood gases can be condensed into three general statements.

1. If only the pH and one other parameter are abnormal, an uncompensated single disorder exists.
2. If the pH is normal, but *both* the P_{CO_2} and HCO_3^- are abnormal, a compensated single disorder exists.
3. If the pH, P_{CO_2}, and the HCO_3^- are all abnormal, a single uncompensated or a mixed disorder exists.

These general rules are not a substitute for the clinical picture of the patient. The combination of an acidosis and an alkalosis is tolerated better by the body than the combination of two acidoses or two alkaloses. The combination of two acidoses or two alkaloses tend to block compensation for each other. The result is severe acid-base and electrolyte disturbances. The combination of an acidosis and an alkalosis tend toward a more normal pH since they have opposite effects on the carbonic acid/bicarbonate ion ratio. These *guidelines* for acid-base imbalance are summarized in Table 3-2.

Compensated or uncompensated cannot actually be identified in a single arterial blood gas sample. Generalizations about compensated and uncompensated are just that—generalizations. A single ABG sample cannot be definitive.

Synonyms: Respiratory acidosis (pH ↓, P_{CO_2} ↑) is also known as arterial hypercap-

Table 3-2.   Summary of parameter values in arterial blood gases.

	Uncompensated	Compensated	Value	Compensated	Uncompensated
pH	7.34	7.35–7.39 (acid)	7.40	7.41–7.45 (alkaline)	>7.45
P_{CO_2}	<35	35–39	40	41–45	>45
HCO_3^- Base excess	<22 < −3 (or more neg.)	22–23 −1 to −2	24 0	25–26 +1 to +2	>26 > +3 (or more positive)

nia (elevated P_{CO_2} in the arterial blood) and alveolar hypoventilation (decreased oxygen available for diffusion in the alveolus).

Respiratory alkalosis (pH $\uparrow$, $P_{CO_2} \downarrow$) is also known as arterial hypocapnia (decreased P_{CO_2} in the arterial blood) and alveolar hyperventilation (too rapid a respiratory rate).

One needs to know these synonyms and be able to use them interchangeably without becoming confused.

Interpreting Abnormal Arterial Blood Gases

Here are two sample blood gases to interpret using the first three steps of the procedure for interpreting ABGs.

1. pH = 7.50, P_{CO_2} = 28, HCO_3^- = 22, S_{O_2} = 90%

   Step 1: The pH is increased, so the acid-base state is alkalosis.

   Step 2: The P_{CO_2} is decreased. It has moved in the opposite direction of the pH, so the *primary* disturbance is respiratory.

   Step 3: The HCO_3^- is at the minimum compensated range point. Therefore, a metabolic disorder is *not* complicating the primary disturbance.

FINAL INTERPRETATION:
Respiratory alkalosis

2. pH = 7.25, P_{CO_2} = 28, HCO_3^- = 12, S_{O_2} = 50%

   Step 1: The pH is decreased, so acid-base state is acidosis.

   Step 2: The P_{CO_2} is decreased and outside the range of compensation. The P_{CO_2} has moved in the same direction as the pH. The same direction means a primary metabolic (or nonrespiratory) imbalance.

   Step 3: The HCO_3^- is decreased and has moved outside the normal range. Thus, there may be a secondary disturbance that is respiratory, or the patient may have endstage metabolic acidosis with an inability to compensate. Only *serial* blood gases would be definitive. All values are outside the ranges of compensation.

FINAL INTERPRETATION:
Mixed metabolic acidosis and possible respiratory acidosis, uncompensated

With practice, interpreting arterial blood gases will become easy and fast. On two of these three samples identified, the conditions are uncompensated. For textbook learning, this helps us. In clinical practice, the *trend* of movement toward normal indicates compensating processes are functioning. It is far safer for any patient to look at the *trend* in serial sample gases and not make a judgment on only one sample.

— 4

Oxygen Therapy and Ventilators

Learning Objectives

By the end of this chapter, the nurse will be able to:

1. Define the objectives of oxygen therapy.
2. Differentiate between high flow and low flow gas systems.
3. List advantages and disadvantages of oxygen therapy administered by a catheter, cannula, simple mask, ventimask, venturimask, non-rebreathing mask, and partial rebreathing mask.
4. Explain the difference among pressure-cycled, time-cycled, flow-cycled, and volume-cycled ventilators.
5. List two universal reasons for placing a patient on a ventilator.
6. State the objectives of ventilator therapy.
7. Discuss the complications of ventilator therapy.
8. Distinguish between IPPB, CPAP, and PEEP.
9. List four complications of oxygen therapy.

Oxygen is a colorless, odorless, tasteless gas that comprises approximately 21% of our atmosphere. Oxygen itself is not combustible; nor is it an explosive. One should be careful around oxygen because it supports combustion. By itself, oxygen cannot initiate a flame. However, in the presence of a spark or flame, oxygen will support the burning of the flame to such an extent that the intensity and speed of the flame may well cause catastrophic results.

Oxygen therapy is indicated only when tissue hypoxia is present. Tissue hypoxia is present when the available oxygen is insufficient to meet the metabolic needs of the body. (Hypoxia is considered in detail in Chapter 5, *Respiratory Failure and Adult Respiratory Distress Syndrome*).

Gas Flow Systems

There are two types of gas flow systems through which a patient's oxygen needs can be met: a low flow system or a high flow system. A low flow system is one in which the device supplying the gas flow is *not* able to meet the patient's inspiratory needs by itself. Ambient (room) air must be used with the low flow system device to meet these inspiratory needs. Low flow systems can deliver oxygen concentrations in a range from about 21% to 90%.

A high flow system is one in which the device supplying the gas flow *is* able to meet all of the patient's inspiratory needs. High flow systems can deliver oxygen concentration in a range from 24% to 100%. The concentration of oxygen being delivered DOES NOT determine if the system is a high flow or low flow system.

Unfortunately, high flow and low flow are frequently used to mean the high and low concentrations of oxygen. Since using the terms interchangeably is not correct, misunderstanding can be avoided by referring specifically to high or low flow systems and high or low concentrations of oxygen.

Oxygen Administration

Oxygen is a potent drug. Used appropriately, it saves lives. Used inappropriately, it has serious or even potentially fatal side effects.

Oxygen may be administered by many devices. The patient's clinical condition and oxygen needs will determine the route of administration. There are advantages and disadvantages with each method. There are two cardinal rules in oxygen therapy.

1. *Without* a patent airway, oxygen therapy is useless.
2. Administer the *lowest effective concentration of oxygen for the shortest possible duration!*

How many hours a patient may safely receive a specified concentration of oxygen has not been clearly determined. It has been proven, however, that definite physiologic changes occur in pulmonary tissues of patients on 100% oxygen continuously for 24 hours. FI_{O_2} means the fraction (or concentration) of inspired oxygen. Forty percent oxygen appears to be safe for several days.

Devices for Administering Oxygen

Nasal catheters (Figure 4-1a, b) are difficult to insert; the nasal passages must be patent (no deviated septum); nasopharyngeal trauma is common; and gastric distention occurs if the catheter is not positioned in

exactly the right spot. The catheters must be changed every 8 hours, alternating between nostrils. Because of the trauma to nasal mucosa, it becomes difficult to insert the catheters, and it is painful for the patient. They are sometimes used with restless patients. The nasal catheter has generally been replaced with the nasal cannula.

Nasal cannulas, also called nasal prongs (Figure 4-1c), are in common use in most hospitals. An oxygen concentration of 30–40% will be achieved with a flow rate of 4–6 l/min. If the flow rate is increased to 8–10 l/min, the patient may complain of a frontal headache or irritation of the nasal passages (close to the bridge of the nose) or both. Since a flow rate greater than 6 l/min will not substantially change the oxygen concentration, there seems little justification for using flow rates greater than 6 l/min. Although some studies dispute this, it is thought that a patient will receive more oxygen with the nasal prongs if he or she is a nose breather rather than a mouth breather. Oxygen therapy by nasal cannula is a low flow system since the patient breathes in ambient air through both the mouth and nasal passages around the prongs (assuming patent nasal passages). The most common disadvantages are: irritation to the nares (vaseline or plain xylocaine gel at the nasal entry may help), crimping of the tubing when the patient turns, the frontal headache already mentioned, and the patient feeling that the

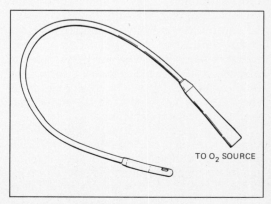

TO O₂ SOURCE

Figure 4-1a. Nasal catheter.

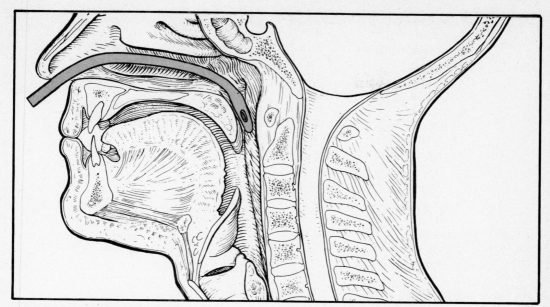

Figure 4-1b.   Nasal cannula.

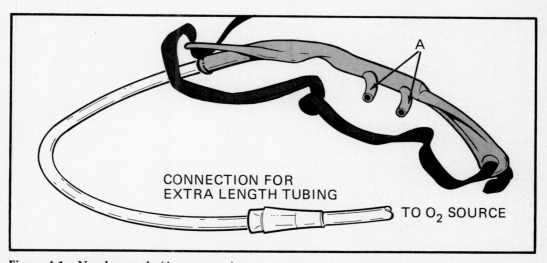

CONNECTION FOR
EXTRA LENGTH TUBING

TO O$_2$ SOURCE

A

Figure 4-1c. Nasal cannula (A = prongs).

prongs decrease his or her breathing. Emotional support may alleviate this feeling and the associated fears.

Simple masks (Figure 4-2a) are lightweight, usually plastic, fairly comfortable, and disposable. They do not have a reservoir bag. They are used for short-term or intermittent therapy. With a flow rate of 6–10 l/min, oxygen concentrations of 35–60% may be achieved. Flow rates must be at least 6 l/min to prevent carbon dioxide buildup. Simple masks have generally been replaced by the Ventimask and Venturimask.

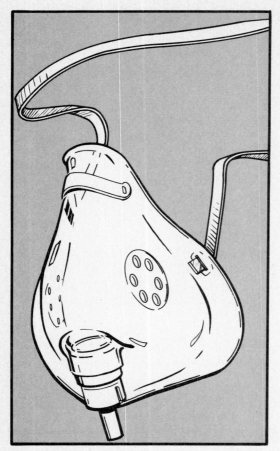

Figure 4-2a. Simple mask.

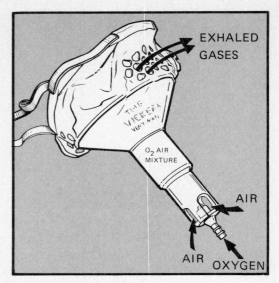

Figure 4-2b.   Ventimask.

The Ventimask (Figure 4-2b) is a low flow system. Sufficient air is entrained through holes in a valve connected to the mask to mix with the oxygen being delivered to meet the patient's inspiratory needs. The oxygen concentration is controlled by varying size cones (valves) attached to the mask. Concentrations can be 24%, 28%, 35%, and 40%. During exhalation, carbon dioxide escapes through multiple side ports in the mask.

The Venturimask (Figure 4-3) is often used instead of the Ventimask. The Venturimask is a high flow system. Oxygen concentrations of 24%, 28%, 35%, 40%, and 50% can be achieved. The major disadvantages of these masks (and all masks) are the elastic strap, which may cut into the skin

just above the ears; moisture, which collects in the mask; and the need to remove the mask to eat, vomit, or be suctioned.

Pressure from the strap may be relieved with cotton balls or folded tissues placed between the strap and the ear. The moisture is removed by frequent drying of the mask and the patient's face. NEVER apply talc (or talcum powder) to the mask or the patient's face to "absorb" moisture. Inhaled particles of talc irritate the lungs and may cause abcess formation and/or adhesions. While the mask is off for eating, nasal prongs may be used.

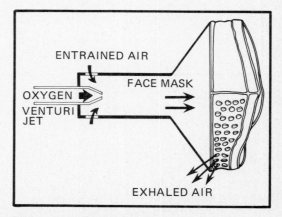

Figure 4-3.   Venturimask.

Oxygen masks should always have a flow rate set at a minimum of 6 l/min. If the flow rate is less than 6 l/min, carbon dioxide in the exhaled air may not be forced from the system. If this is the case, the patient is being treated with a rebreathing mask, which will elevate the P_{CO_2}. (COPD patients will be treated by cannulas or prongs, not a mask.)

Non-rebreathing masks (Figure 4-4a) are often used if the patient needs a high concentration of oxygen (90–100%). A reservoir bag is attached to the mask by a valve. The valve forces carbon dioxide laden air out of vents in the mask. The valve opens for inspiration so that oxygen travels from the reservoir bag into the patient's airway. This is a very good system for high oxygen concentrations for short periods of time PROVIDING there are no leaks in the system and the bag remains inflated.

Partial rebreathing masks (Figure 4-4b) are used to increase the concentration of inspired oxygen. The principle is that the last third of inspired air (V_T) remains in the upper airway passages, trachea, and bron-

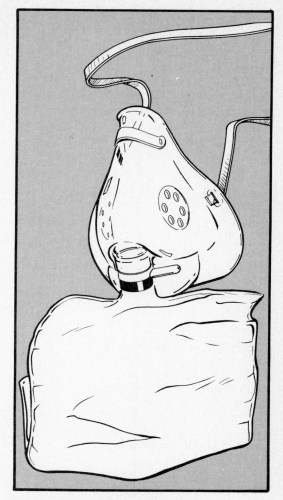

Figure 4-4b.   Partial rebreathing mask.

chi. Therefore, this oxygen-rich air is in the anatomic dead space and does not participate in gas exchange. As the patient exhales, this one-third of the tidal volume (V_T) enters the reservoir bag, and the remaining exhaled air is vented to the room air. When the patient rebreathes, the new oxygen is inhaled along with this one-third V_T which is still oxygen-rich. In this way, oxygen concentration is increased. Partial rebreathing masks can deliver oxygen concentrations of 35–60%. The disadvantage is the possibility of carbon dioxide retention if the gas flow is not high enough to prevent collapse of the bag.

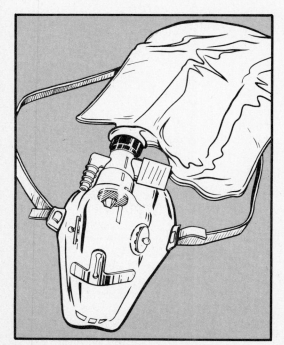

Figure 4-4a.   Non-rebreathing mask.

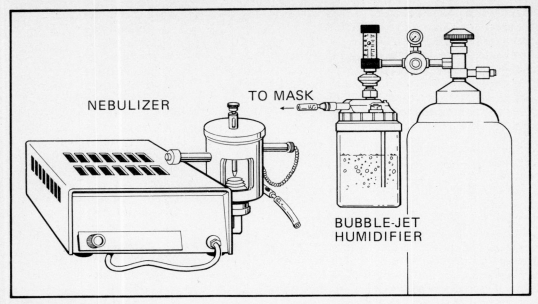

Figure 4-5. Nebulizer.

Nebulizers (Figure 4-5) are used for conditions that produce excessive mucus. The nebulizer will add sufficient water in the form of an aerosol or mist to prevent drying of the mucous secretions. Secretions must be kept moist to enable the mucociliary escalator to remove them. If the patient cannot expel the secretions, suctioning must be used. Even suctioning will not remove dried secretions. These ultimately cause obstruction to air flow in the respiratory passages.

Humidification may lead to water overload if the aerosoled water particles are 1–2 microns in size. Water particles of 2–5 microns tend to stay in the pharynx, trachea, and bronchi where they will attach to mucus. Most often, nebulizers also warm the aerosoled water. The flow rate with a nebulizer is extremely important to insure an adequate oxygen concentration since some oxygen is used in the nebulizing process and is not available in gas form for the patient.

T-pieces on intubated or tracheostomy patients need to have heating nebulizers attached. Since oxygen inspired through an endotracheal tube or a tracheostomy bypasses the normal paths of humidification and warming of the respiratory system, dried secretions are a problem. The problem is solved by using a heated nebulizer. Oxygen concentrations of 25–75% are obtained with a flow rate of 6–12 l/min. If a tracheal mask is used instead of a T-piece, oxygen concentrations of 35–75% are obtained with the same flow rate. Water overload may become a problem, so frequent assessment of lung sounds are essential.

IPPB stands for intermittent positive pressure breathing. This respiratory treatment is usually administrated by a Bird positive pressure ventilator that is pressure cycled. When the patient initiates inspiration, the Bird immediately begins to deliver a preset pressure of oxygen. Even if the patient ceases inspiratory effort, the Bird will continue the positive pressure. When the preset pressure is achieved, the Bird stops and the patient passively exhales, still under positive pressure. The amount of volume delivered is determined by the pressure that is set and achieved in the patients' airways. The volume is variable and depends upon the airway pressure. Oxygen concentrations of 21%–100% are deliverable. Medications such as saline, to moisten secretions, or Bronkosol®, to dilate bronchioles, are administered as a mist during inspiration. Although controversial, alcohol may be administered as a mist in severe pulmonary edema. Theoretically, alcohol has an antifoaming property which enhances the efficiency of pulmonary surfactant and/or helps to force fluid from the alveoli back into the venous system.

IPPB is often used to help expand alveoli. After surgery, it is used to prevent respiratory complications. It is used to treat atelectasis, to promote excretion of secretions, and to improve ventilation.

Disadvantages of IPPB treatment are listed in Table 4-1.

Table 4-1.   Some disadvantages of IPPB.

Pneumothorax
Hemoptysis
Frank bleeding after instituting IPPB
Increased pressure after carotid
  endarterectomy (48 hours)
Increased pressures after thoracic resection
  causing bronchial leakage

Although IPPB seems to decrease the work of breathing and improves oxygenation, its value is controversial. Contraindications to IPPB therapy are: (a) a pneumothorax that does not have a patent, functioning chest tube, (b) hemoptysis (secondary to coughing), (c) frank pulmonary bleeding, (d) subcutaneous emphysema of unknown origin, and (e) gastric or upper intestinal surgery with a significant ileus.

Oxygen tents are still occasionally used. They are dangerous because of the large reservoir of increased oxygen concentration within the tent. This, plus the difficulty of maintaining a specific oxygen concentration, has led to their replacement by masks and ventilators in most hospitals. Oxygen tents are still useful for the pediatric patient.

Hyperbaric oxygen chambers are found in some centers. In these chambers, oxygen is administered under high atmospheric pressures. These chambers were originally for deep sea divers who surfaced too quickly and developed the "bends" (severe disturbances in respiratory and nervous systems due to rapid changes in atmospheric pressures). The chambers are still used in treating decompression sickness (the "bends") and are also used in treating gas gangrene, radiation therapy, burns, and some carbon monoxide poisonings. The patient and staff are slowly acclimated to the increased pressures and must also be slowly deacclimated. Convulsions are a complication due to the hyperbaric chamber pressures, not the oxygen therapy per se. The slightest spark may cause massive fire and explosion. The time involved to reach therapeutic pressures which will force more oxygen into the patient's system limits the use of these chambers.

Types of Ventilators (Respirators)

There are two types of ventilators: negative external pressure and positive pressure ventilators.

Negative external ventilators are those which exert a pressure less than room air pressure against the thorax. The most widely known type is the iron lung. Since the prevention of polio, the iron lung is rarely seen, except in the hospital basement. The cuirass ventilator is occasionally seen. It is a chest ventilator that applies subambient pressure to the thorax as did the iron lung. Since the cuirass is much smaller (covering only the chest), it is used mainly in home treatment of patients with neuromuscular dysfunction. Use of the cuirass ventilator is a long-term situation. The cuirass does not require an artificial airway; so, other than skin care, it is not difficult for home use. It does reduce patient activities, and negative pressure on the abdomen causes venous pooling which results in decreased cardiac output.

Positive pressure ventilators are almost always seen in critical care areas. The Ohio, MA-1, MA-2, Bear, and such are all positive pressure ventilators. These ventilators are classified according to (a) what factor initiates inspiration and (b) what factor causes cessation of inspiration.

Initiation of inspiration is either assisted or controlled. In assisted inspiration, the patient makes an inspiratory effort which triggers the ventilator to deliver a preset volume. Minimal patient effort triggers the ventilator. In controlled inspirations, the ventilator initiates all inspirations. Conscious patients may need sedation to prevent them from "fighting" the ventilator.

Ventilators are also classified according to the factor responsible for cessation of inspiration. These factors are volume, pressure, time, and flow.

Pressure-cycled ventilators are not commonly used now. Inspiration starts and continues until a preset pressure is obtained. Major disadvantages exist with this system. Volume of inspired air varies with resistance in the airways. Concentration of inspired oxygen (FI_{O_2}) is variable in relation to pulmonary compliance and resistance in the airways. These factors also alter alveolar ventilation. If a leak develops in the system, a continuous inspiration flow is possible since the preset pressure would not be reached.

Time-cycled ventilators and flow-cycled ventilators are controlled by either time or flow and are not commonly used anymore.

Volume-cycled ventilators (Figure 4-6) are currently the most commonly used ventilators in critical care units. Inspiration is either controlled or assisted. Once initiated, inspiration continues until a preset volume (V_T) is achieved; then the inspiratory force stops and the patient passively exhales. *All* positive pressure ventilators decrease venous return to the heart. Consequently, a decrease in cardiac output resulting in hypotension may develop when a patient is put on a ventilator. This potential problem must be carefully and continuously monitored.

Volume-cycled ventilators are pressure limited. They can deliver from 21% to 100% oxygen. In spite of changing airway pressure or lung compliance, the preset volume (tidal volume) will be delivered with each inspiration. The MA-1, MA-2, Ohio, and Bear (Bournes-Bear-1) are types of volume cycled ventilators.

The ventilators have certain common characteristics and functions, although control knobs may be located in different areas or built in. A bellows type system pumps oxygen through a humidifier to

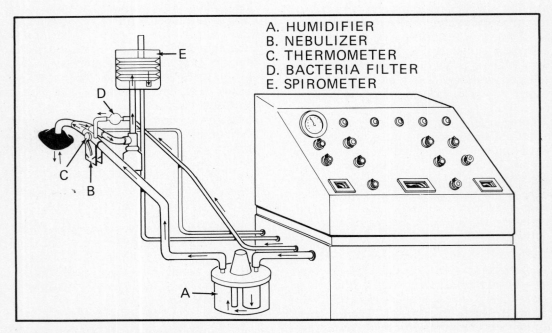

A. HUMIDIFIER
B. NEBULIZER
C. THERMOMETER
D. BACTERIA FILTER
E. SPIROMETER

Figure 4-6.   Volume cycle ventilator.

warm and moisturize the oxygen before it is delivered to the patient through an endotracheal tube, a tracheostomy, or sometimes a mask. Controls on the ventilator must be set to determine the FI_{O_2}, the respiratory rate, the tidal volume, sighs (if they are used), pressure and flow rate, and the ventilatory control.

Ventilatory control may be control, assist-control, assist, and intermittent mandatory ventilation, more commonly called IMV. In the control mode, the ventilator initiates *all* inspirations. The patient has no control. In the assist-control mode, a preset number of inspirations is established. However, if the patient wishes to breathe faster, the ventilator will respond. If the patient ceases to breathe adequately (a sufficient number of times per minute), the ventilator will take control and initiate inspiration. In the assist mode, the patient initiates all inspirations. In IMV, the patient may breathe faster than the preset rate, *and* the breathing may be of any depth. When the IMV breath is initiated, it is at the preset tidal volume.

IMV is sometimes used to help wean a patient off a ventilator by decreasing the number of IMVs per minute by one or two a day. This helps the patient develop respiratory strength.

PEEP

PEEP is positive end-expiratory pressure, and it prevents alveoli from collapsing at the end of inspiration. If the alveoli collapse, greater inspiratory pressure is needed to re-open them. PEEP is measured in centimeters of water. Figure 4-7 shows the effect of PEEP.

Continuous Positive Airway Pressure

Continuous positive airway pressure (CPAP) is used with a *spontaneously* breathing patient. The patient *may* be on a ventilator—BUT the ventilator is not forcing the patient to breathe. In instances of weaning, the number of *mandatory* breaths from the machine will be *zero*; but the patient is breathing *spontaneously* through the ventilator (or the CPAP machine) and is, therefore, exhaling against continuous positive airway pressures. This is often used in weaning PEEP-dependent patients because the positive pressure improves arterial oxygen tensions. This allows the oxygen concentration (FI_{O_2}) to be lower.

Goals of Ventilators

The goal of respiratory therapy by ventilators is to provide adequate and efficient ventilation while decreasing the work of breathing. A decrease in the work of breathing results in a decreased strain on the respiratory system and subsequently, a decreased strain on the cardiac system. Ventilators are used to *support* ventilation while the underlying disease process is treated. By and of themselves, ventilators are not curative treatments—merely supportive.

Indications for the Use of a Ventilator

There are two universal indicators for using ventilators. They are (1) alveolar hypoven-

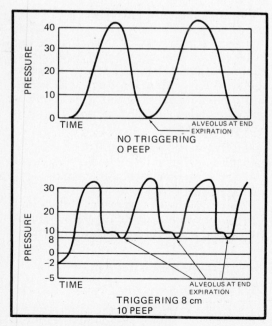

Figure 4-7.   Effects of PEEP.

tilation and (2) some hypoxic states. Alveolar hypoventilation includes apnea, impending respiratory failure, and respiratory failure.

1. Technically, apnea is the absence of ventilation. However, irregular respiratory patterns or extemely weak respirations may be clinically treated as apnea. If the cause of the apnea is treatable, ventilatory support is warranted. Such cases might include head injuries (with brain activity), postcardiopulmonary arrest, attempted suicides, Pickwickian syndrome, multiple trauma, postoperative patients, and such.

2. Impending respiratory failure is clinically seen by serial blood gases. The patient increases his or her breathing efforts (which stress the body systems), but his or her blood gases indicate an increasing Pa_{CO_2} and a decreasing pH (respiratory acidosis). The patient is usually restless, becomes agitated, tachypneic, diaphoretic, and develops some mucous membrane cyanosis.

3. Respiratory failure is inadequate ventilation. If hypercarbia is present with acidemia, the failure is acute and indicates an approaching severe cardiopulmonary imbalance. In these cases, the alveolar-arterial oxygen difference is usually greater than 350 mm Hg and the pH is less than 7.25. (Alveolar-arterial oxygen is discussed in Chapter 5.)

4. Hypoxic states may be of multiple etiologies. These could include obstructive lung diseases, restrictive lung diseases, neuromuscular diseases, infectious diseases, multiple trauma, and upper airway obstructions. Adult respiratory distress syndrome (ARDS) is one of the most common causes of hypoxic states.

Artificial Airways

In order to use a ventilator, the patient must have an artificial airway: either an endotracheal tube or a tracheostomy (Figure 4-8).

ENDOTRACHEAL TUBES

Endotracheal tubes may be inserted through the nose (nasotracheal) or the mouth (orotracheal). Only trained and experienced persons should intubate a patient. Immediately after intubation, auscultation of peripheral chest fields is essential to ascertain that both lungs are being ventilated. Chest x-ray is important and needed as soon as possible to determine that the tip of the endotracheal tube is about one inch (two to three centimeters) above the carina.

The advantage of nasotracheal intubation is that it allows the patient to eat and drink, and mouth care is simplified for the nurse. The disadvantages are the possibility of tissue necrosis, nosebleed, rupture of nasal polyps (with or without plugging the tube), and submucosal dissection. Increased mucus production as a result of the irritant properties of the tube increases the patient's susceptibility to infection. Stabilization of the tube is difficult if the patient is diaphoretic.

The advantages of orotracheal intubation are direct visualization and rapid intubation. Some feel that orotracheal tubes are easier to stabilize than nasotracheal tubes. Oral tubes should be moved to the opposite side of the mouth at least every 24 hours and preferably every 8 hours. Precautions relating to nasal intubation apply also to oral intubation.

Disadvantages of oral intubation include increased drying of oral mucosa, increased mucus production, increased gagging, and increased susceptibility to infection.

Complications of intubation (regardless of route) are laryngeal trauma, intubation of the right main-stem bronchus, and infection.

Cuffs of Endotracheal Tubes

Most endotracheal tubes have inflatable cuffs. The cuff provides a closed system with a seal and prevents aspiration of fluids into the lungs. Soft, low pressure (<25 cm

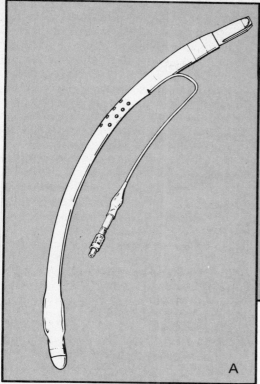

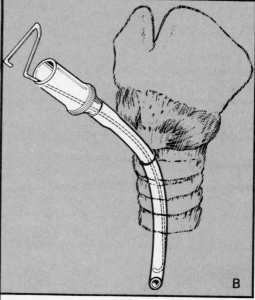

Figure 4-8.   (A) Endotracheal tube and (B) tracheostomy tube in place.

water pressure, 20 mm Hg pressure) cuffs are preferred. Cuff leaks are associated with increased mortality. Soft cuffs minimize tracheal necrosis and fistula development. Pressure is distributed over a large area, and only sufficient pressure to provide a seal is necessary.

Policies vary from hospital to hospital regarding the deflation of cuffs. Precautions to prevent aspiration are necessary when the cuff is deflated. Cuff pressure should be checked every 4–8 hours, regardless of policies on inflation-deflation and minimal leak procedure. Children do *not* need an inflated cuff.

TRACHEOSTOMY

Tracheostomy, the formation of an opening into the trachea, may be performed instead of oral or nasal intubation (or as a replacement) if ventilatory support may be longterm. Tracheostomies bypass upper airway obstruction, decrease dead space, may help prevent aspiration, and may decrease the possibilities of necrosis and/or tracheoesophageal fistula formation. Tracheostomy tubes are uncuffed for children but cuffed for adults needing ventilatory support. Hospitals *vary in the policies relating to changing tracheostomy tubes. Regardless* of policy, if a tube is to be changed, a patent airway must be maintained. An endotracheal tube on standby or a bag-valve-mask may be needed to maintain a patent airway, especially in the "fresh" tracheostomy patient. In emergencies, a hemostat will keep the tracheostomy site open. A sterile tracheostomy tube of the same size as is in the patient, should be taped to the head of the bed—for as long as the patient is dependent upon a tracheostomy.

Complications of Endotracheal Tubes and Tracheostomies

The major complication of endotracheal tubes and tracheostomies is obstruction.

Obstruction is usually caused by dried secretions. The patient appears to be in *acute* respiratory distress. Mucus production is increased by the "foreign body." As long as either tubes or tracheostomies are patent, the patient cannot talk. Endotracheal tubes become displaced rather easily. This can lead to carinal rupture, ventilation of only one lung, tension pneumothorax, and atelectasis.

Signs of tube misplacement into a bronchus include diminished or absent lung sounds on the contralateral side, little if any chest excursion on the contralateral side, expiratory wheezing, and sometimes uncontrollable coughing.

Pneumothorax may occur in the lung that has become intubated. This is one of the most serious complications of ventilatory support. The only treatment is a chest tube to "bleed out" the air of the pneumothorax. Without adequate treatment, pneumothorax can be rapidly fatal.

A tracheostomy tube that ends bluntly at the same point as an inflated cuff will cause acute airway obstruction (if the cuff ruptures) due to herniation. Very few such tracheostomy tubes are now used.

If a tracheostomy tube fluctuates with the patient's pulse, suspect that the tube is rubbing against the innominate artery. Notify the physician immediately. Erosion of the artery usually results in exsanguination. The tracheostomy tube may become misplaced, causing subcutaneous and/or mediastinal emphysema or pneumothorax. Progressively deteriorating blood gases, poor air movement throughout lung fields, and/or difficulty in suctioning the patient should alert one to a possible shift in the tracheostomy tube.

Tracheal dilatation, ischemia, and necrosis may occur because tracheostomy tubes and endotracheal tubes are round, whereas the trachea is oval. If ischemia and necrosis progress, a tracheoesophageal (TE) fistula may occur. If suspected, this can be easily tested by instilling methylene blue or cranberry juice into the mouth. If it is suctioned from the endotracheal tube or tracheostomy, a TE fistula has developed. (This may

be minimized by the use of low pressure cuffs.)

Infection is always a major concern. The longer an endotracheal tube or tracheostomy tube is in place, the greater the danger. Cultures of sputum should be routine and prn (as necessary) with fever. As soon as identification of the infecting microorganism is made, appropriate antibiotic therapy is started. Proper, frequent, and correct oral hygiene is of paramount importance, both for the patient's comfort and as an aid to prevention of infection.

Weaning from Endotracheal and Tracheostomy Tubes

Weaning from tracheostomy tubes will depend upon the patient's vital signs, arterial blood gases, physiological state, and psychological readiness. If the intermittent mechanical ventilation (IMV) has been gradually reduced and the patient has tolerated this well, as evidenced by adequate arterial blood gases, a trial extubation is warranted.

If all of these parameters look good and the patient has an endotracheal tube, the tube and then the oropharynx should be suctioned, the cuff deflated, and the tube pulled out smoothly and rapidly at the peak of inspiration. Close clinical monitoring is required and arterial blood gases are often ordered in 20 minutes, 1 hour, 2 hours, and 4 hours postextubation. Supplemental oxygen by mask is usually supplied postextubation.

Patients often complain of sore throat and hoarseness. Supportive explanations that both of these conditions are temporary will often alleviate the patients' concern. Nursing interventions of mouth care and warm water gargling may help relieve the soreness.

If the patient has had a tracheostomy for a prolonged period, the tracheostomy tube may have a T-piece attached, may be covered with a tracheal button, or may be replaced with a fenestrated tracheostomy tube. As the patient adjusts to these, he or she becomes more psychologically prepared for removal of the tube. Monitoring of the patient after tracheostomy tube removal is the same as for postextubation. The tracheostomy site is normally covered with a *loose*, sterile gauze pad (4 × 4) and supplemental oxygen is supplied by mask or cannula. The incision should close within a week.

Complications of Ventilator Support

Hypotension may occur secondary to decreased cardiac output when a patient is put on a ventilator and/or when ventilator adjustments are increased. All positive pressure ventilators exert a continuous positive pressure which decreases venous return to the heart. This decreases cardiac output. The decreased cardiac output may result in a decreased urine output and cardiac dysrhythmias. Cardiac monitoring is essential. Hypotension may be caused by hypovolemia, and intravenous fluids may correct the problem. Vasopressors are indicated if the pulmonary capillary wedge pressure (PCWP) is increased and the cardiac output is decreased.

Infection is a most common complication of mechanical ventilation. Strict adherence to sterile technique, ventilator tubing changes every 8–24 hours, and sputum culture every 24 hours will help to prevent and detect infection. As soon as a culture identifies an infecting organism, specific antibiotic therapy is started. Broad-spectrum antibiotics are *not* used prophylactically since many organisms are resistant to them. The excessive use of broad-spectrum antibiotics may allow opportunistic organisms to invade the patient's system. Chest physiotherapy and pulmonary hygiene procedures are vital nursing interventions in preventing infection.

Atelectasis often occurs with mechanical ventilation. The use of the "sigh" control to administer deep inspirations (up to one and one-half to two times the normal tidal volume) helps to open alveoli. Bronchial hygiene is extremely important to prevent further complications once atelectasis has developed. Atelectasis leads to alveolar hypoventilation. This is the most common medical complication associated with increased mortality.

Pneumothorax is not unusual when PEEP is used with mechanical ventilation. The only treatment is to insert a chest tube to "bleed out" the air in the pleural space. Without adequate treatment, pneumothorax can be rapidly fatal.

Positive water balance is a major concern. Since endotracheal tubes and tracheostomies bypass the nose, mouth, and upper airways, artificial humidification must be supplied to prevent drying of small airways and the lung parenchyma. Yet, such humidification may overhydrate the patient. Weight gain and decreasing efficiency of ventilatory parameters (i.e., compliance, increased A-a gradient, decreased vital capacity, and increased dead space/tidal volume ratio) are signs of possible overhydration. The end result is pulmonary edema, which may occur very rapidly.

FIGHTING THE VENTILATOR

The patient may fight the ventilator in two ways: by being "out of sync" or by "breathing around." The "out of sync" or "out of phase" patient is trying to exhale while the ventilator is in its inspiratory phase. This markedly decreases alveolar ventilation, since the intrathoracic pressure increases. This patient is in a very dangerous state bordering on irreversible pulmonary/cardiovascular stress changes that may be fatal.

Treatment of "Out of Sync" State

The drug of choice to treat a *well-oxygenated, acid-base balanced, and well-ventilated* patient "out of sync" with the ventilator is morphine sulfate. Morphine sulfate will increase the venous capacitance—but intravenous fluids can balance any hemodynamic changes. Assuming that the ventilator system is functioning properly and that the patient is well-suctioned, large doses of intravenous morphine sulfate may be given.

Shapiro states that doses as high as 80 mg intravenously to start and up to 20 mg intravenously every hour for maintenance in *adults* have been used without untoward side effects.[1] Problems generally associated with the cardiovascular system when using morphine sulfate are due to the respiratory effects; but these effects are on spontaneously breathing patients! If the ventilator is keeping the patient well-oxygenated, the cardiovascular dysfunctions do not occur. Morphine sulfate has excellent euphoric properties and its effects are completely reversible with naloxone hydrochloride (Narcan®).

Tranquilizers are often used, and diazepam (Valium®) is the most common. However, its effects are not reversible and its respiratory depressant properties are not consistant in every patient.

Paralyzers such as pancuronium bromide (Pavulon®) are used very frequently in some hospitals. It can be reversed by neostigmine bromide (Prostigmin®) and by edrophonium chloride (Tensilon®). The greatest disadvantage to Pavulon is that a conscious patient experiences the **terrifying** sensation of **TOTAL** paralysis. Unfortunately, since the patient cannot express discomfort or fear, he or she may receive no sedation or analgesics—even if desperately needed. A golden rule would be Pavulon with sedation or no Pavulon!

Breathing Around

The patient who is "breathing around" the ventilator is *not* in distress because the patient is trying to inhale while the ventilator is in the exhale mode. This patient needs close watching in case a change is made from "breathing around" to being "out of sync." Then the patient would need immediate treatment.

Complications of Oxygen Therapy

Atelectasis is one of the most common complications of oxygen therapy. That may seem strange when oxygen is also a treatment for atelectasis. However, the more pure and concentrated the oxygen the patient receives, the more inert gases (e.g., nitrogen) are exhaled from the body. The lungs need certain amounts of inert gases for the surfactant to function optimally. As the inert gases are washed out, atelectasis develops. This form of atelectasis is termed *miliary atelectasis*.

Less common a complication of oxygen therapy today than in the past is retrolental fibroplasia in babies. High concentrations of arterial oxygen cause vasoconstriction of blood vessels in the retina. This vasoconstriction results in fibrotic development. Today, most babies are kept at oxygen concentrations of 40% or less to avoid this problem.

Oxygen therapy in COPD patients can be fatal very quickly unless the concentration of oxygen is very low and is delivered by a low flow system at 1–2 l/min. COPD patients placed on a ventilator are usually very difficult to wean because of the oxygen-induced hypoventilation.

Oxygen therapy may cause circulatory difficulties (even without ventilators and their positive pressure). Hypoxia has three major effects upon circulation: vasoconstriction, a release of catecholamines, and sympathetic nervous system stimulation. The release of catecholamines increases the colloid osmotic pressure in the plasma volume in relation to the Donnan effect.[2] As the colloid osmotic pressure increases in the plasma, some plasma volume moves into the interstitial spaces. Oxygen therapy is started, and there may be a vasodilatation which will result in a hypovolemic state. This should be monitored by a central line and intravenous fluids used as necessary.

Oxygen toxicity may range from mild to severe and/or fatal, as a complication of oxygen therapy. The pathophysiology of oxygen toxicity is the same whether the toxicity is due to high oxygen concentrations or prolonged periods of therapy. The lung parenchyma becomes damaged and ede-

[1]Shapiro BA, Harrison RA, Trout CA: Clinical Application of Respiratory Care. Chicago: Year Book Medical Publishers, Inc., p. 325, 1977

[2]Guyton AC: Textbook of Medical Physiology, 6th ed. Philadelphia: W. B. Saunders, p. 366, 1981

matous. The damage is due to micro-alveolar hemorrhage and hyperplasia of alveolar cells. This results in a hyaline membrane formation.

Theoretically, oxygen toxicity is related to the fraction (concentration) of inspired oxygen (FI_{O_2}) *and* the pressure of inspired oxygen (PI_{O_2}) in addition to the length of time of therapy. Early signs and symptoms of oxygen toxicity are vague, generalized, and may be attributed to other causes. Late signs of oxygen toxicity are all those symptoms associated with severe respiratory distress. The two most significant symptoms that alert us to oxygen toxicity are decreased compliance and an associated increasing alveolar-arterial oxygen ($A-aO_2$) gradient.

5

Respiratory Failure and Adult Respiratory Distress Syndrome (ARDS)

Learning Objectives

By the end of this chapter, the nurse will be able to:

1. Define respiratory failure.
2. Distinguish between hypoxemia and hypoxia.
3. List the three major classifications of respiratory failure.
4. Explain the difference between dead space and a shunt.
5. Define the $A - aDO_2$ and explain its significance.
6. List symptoms of respiratory failure in the early, middle, and late stages.
7. Identify three important nursing interventions in the respiratory failure patient.
8. List some complications of respiratory failure that affect other body systems, and their importance.
9. Define adult respiratory distress syndrome (ARDS).
10. Explain the pathophysiology of ARDS in each of the four phases.

Respiratory Failure

Respiratory failure is any condition in which the oxygen content of the blood is insufficient to meet the tissue demands for oxygen secondary to decreased lung function. In other words, tissue hypoxia is present. Tissue hypoxia is usually preceded by arterial hypoxemia (low oxygen content in the arterial blood).

CLASSIFICATION OF RESPIRATORY FAILURE

Respiratory failure can be classified accord-

ing to the underlying abnormality. There are three major classifications: inadequate alveolar ventilation, decreased diffusion across the respiratory membrane, and decreased oxygen transport to the tissues. Respiratory failure may also be classified as chronic or acute. The emphysema patient will at some point develop chronic respiratory failure. The burn patient, with previously normal lungs, may develop acute respiratory failure. Of course, the chronic obstructive pulmonary disease (COPD) patient may change from a chronic respiratory failure to an acute respiratory failure, with the addition of some form of stress on his or her body.

63

1. *Inadequate alveolar ventilation*: This may be caused by many factors. A low inspired oxygen content due to increased airway resistance, such as in asthma and bronchitis, is one factor. Increased tissue resistance causes inadequate alveolar ventilation. Some of these causes are listed in Table 5-1.

Table 5-1.   Inadequate alveolar ventilation.

Lack of or decreased pulmonary surfactant
Abnormally high Pa_{CO_2} (>45 mm Hg)
Depression or damage to cerebral respiratory
    center (stroke, head injury, CNS depressant
    drugs)
Neuromuscular defects
    Myasthenia gravis
    Guillain-Barré syndrome
    Tetanus
Spinal cord injuries to cervical 1–5 vertebrae
Asthma
Bronchitis
Emphysema
Restrictive lung diseases
Morbid obesity (Pickwickian syndrome)

Paralysis of respiratory muscles (cord transection, neuromuscular disease, and drugs) is another factor. A common cause of inadequate alveolar ventilation is deformity of the thoracic cage, such as kyphosis, scoliosis, and pectus excavatum.

In primary alveolar hypoventilation, if the lungs are normal, the alveolar-arterial oxygen gradient will be normal and the patient's Pa_{CO_2} will be elevated.

2. *Decreased diffusion across the respiratory membrane*: This may result in respiratory failure. Removal of a portion of the membrane (e.g., lobectomy) certainly decreases the available area for diffusion of gases and may well contribute to low arterial oxygen content. Less dramatic is any factor that alters the alveoli to prevent oxygen from reaching them. Conditions like atelectasis, emphysema, pneumonia, pulmonary edema, and such would be included.

An increase in the thickness of the respiratory membrane is termed *alveolocapillary block*. Pulmonary edema is the most frequent acute cause. However, most of the occupational pulmonary diseases cause this alveolocapillary block. In these instances, it is chronic and may be called interstitial fibrosis.

Mismatching of ventilation and perfusion results in a decreased diffusion across the respiratory membrane. This is the most common cause of arterial hypoxemia. Normally 2% of the blood passing through the lungs does not become oxygenated. If the perfect state existed, every alveolus would be ventilated (V) and every alveolus would be totally perfused (Q). There would then exist a minute ratio of $\dot{V}/\dot{Q}$ equal to 1; but the *normal* 2% of unoxygenated blood makes the $\dot{V}/\dot{Q}$ equal to 0.8. As stated in Chapter 2, "$\dot{V}$" means ventilation per minute, and "$\dot{Q}$" means perfusion (or quantity of blood) per minute. In normal, healthy lungs, the $\dot{V}/\dot{Q}$ ratio is 0.8. This is called the respiratory exchange ratio or, more commonly, respiratory quotient. The $\dot{V}/\dot{Q}$ is an index of oxygen transport in the lungs, that is, the difference between inspired tension and arterial tension per minute.

If the $\dot{V}/\dot{Q}$ is less than 0.8, there is a *decrease* of minute ventilation ($\dot{V}$) to perfusion ($\dot{Q}$), creating a physiologic shunt. When hypoxemia or low oxygen content of the blood is present, the respiratory quotient is less than 0.8. This state is often present in atelectasis, pneumonia, and such conditions.

If the $\dot{V}/\dot{Q}$ is greater than 0.8, there is normal ventilation but a decrease in perfusion. Alveoli are receiving oxygen, but the alveoli are not perfused with blood. This increases physiologic dead space and wastes ventilation. Pulmonary embolus and shock are the two main disease processes that have a respiratory quotient greater than 0.8.

3. *Decreased oxygen transport to the tissues*: This includes conditions such as anemia, hypovolemia, decreased cardiac output, carbon monoxide poisoning (which uses the Hgb), vasoconstriction, hypotension, occlusions by thrombi, and tissue ischemia. If oxygen is transported to the tissues, the oxyhemoglobin dissociation curve must allow release of the oxygen, or tissue hypoxia will still exist.

ALVEOLAR-ARTERIAL GRADIENT

The difference between alveolar and arterial oxygen tension demonstrates the efficiency of gas exchange in the lungs. The term *alveolar-arterial oxygen difference* is abbreviated in two ways: $P_{A-a}O_2$ or $A-aDO_2$. These are interchangeable. The difference is always a positive number. In young adults, the $A-aDO_2$ is usually 10 mm Hg or less on room air. As one ages, the value increases. It also increases if the fraction of inspired oxygen (FI_{O_2}) is greater than room air.

A large $A-aDO_2$ gradient normally indicates that pulmonary dysfunction is the cause of respiratory failure, as opposed to anemia. There are two conditions which cause an increase in the $A-aDO_2$: (1) a ventilation-perfusion mismatching ($\dot{V}/\dot{Q}$), that is, shunting, and (2) diffusion abnormalities. These are the two major causes of respiratory failure. (A sample calculation of the $A-aDO_2$ is found in Appendix I.)

The higher the $A-aDO_2$ value, the greater the respiratory failure. Patients who are on ventilators have little chance of successful weaning from the ventilator until their $A-aDO_2$ is less than 350 mm Hg.

PATHOPHYSIOLOGY OF RESPIRATORY FAILURE

Hypoxemia (low oxygen content of the blood) develops as the first step in respiratory failure. Hypoxemia may develop from inadequate alveolar ventilation, decreased diffusion across the respiratory membrane, and $\dot{V}/\dot{Q}$ mismatching. Hypoxia from these three conditions causes hypoxemia. Along with hypoxemia, hypercapnia (increased Pa_{CO_2}) develops if the cause of the hypoxemia is hypoventilation or circulatory dysfunction. The hypercapnia depresses cellular and tissue function. This, in turn, causes cerebral depression, hypotension, and circulatory failure.

Untreated hypoxia leads to hypoxemia. Hypoxia stimulates the sympathetic nervous system, causing peripheral vasoconstriction and tachycardia. If hypercapnia exists with the hypoxia, acidosis will develop.

The progression from hypoxia to hypoxemia (with or without hypercapnia) may be chronic or acute. Arterial blood gases will tell if the hypoxia is chronic or acute. If chronic, body compensatory mechanisms will maintain the pH above or close to 7.35. If the hypoxia is acute, the body's compensatory mechanisms will *not* have had time to respond, and the pH will be less than 7.34.

Two types of respiratory failure exist. One is hypoxic failure, such as in ARDS. In this case, the arterial blood gases demonstrate only a decrease in the Pa_{O_2}, or there may be hypoxic/hypercapnic respiratory failure. In these cases, arterial blood gases reveal an increase in Pa_{CO_2}, a decrease in Pa_{O_2}, and a decrease in pH. This is commonly found in overdoses.

CLINICAL PRESENTATION (SIGNS AND SYMPTOMS)

Unless respiratory failure is caused by an acute upper airway obstruction, the signs and symptoms are vague and insidious. Restlessness is often the first sign. It is often accompanied by anxiety and apprehension. Tachycardia and an increase in blood pressure followed shortly by hypotension are early signs of hypoxia. Headache is an early sign of hypoxia, followed shortly by signs of hypercarbia: confusion, disorientation, and lethargy.

As hypoxia progresses, air hunger is evidenced by an increase in respiratory rate and a variable tidal volume. The skin is usually cool and dry in the early stages of hypoxia, but may become warm and diaphoretic, depending upon the autonomic nervous system response.

Late stages of hypoxia are characterized by decreasing levels of consciousness from lethargy and obtundation to coma and death. Central cyanosis is present when there is a desaturation of at least 5 gm Hgb/100 ml blood. The skin is cool, moist, and ashen. If the hypoxia has progressed to this point, the patient will probably die. Many signs and symptoms are present from the start of respiratory failure. Looked at individually, they appear innocuous.

Seen within the framework of possible respiratory failure, they almost "scream" hypoxia.

DIAGNOSIS OF RESPIRATORY FAILURE

Serial arterial blood gases revealing a Pa_{O_2} below 50 mm Hg and/or a Pa_{CO_2} above 50 mm Hg are very significant. Acidosis indicates an acute and extreme state.

X-ray of the chest may be helpful if the underlying pathology can be demonstrated (that is, pneumothorax, effusion, etc.).

The patient's history, clinical appearance, and arterial blood gases are the most reliable sources for diagnosing respiratory failure.

NURSING INTERVENTIONS

The most important nursing intervention is to maintain a patent airway. Suctioning, humidification, postural drainage (if possible), and chest physiotherapy (clapping) are all effective ways of maintaining a patent airway. Chest physiotherapy (CPT) is limited only by the patient's cardiovascular status, unless a head injury is also present.

Emotional support of the "air hungry" patient and the intubated patient cannot be overstressed. This includes explanations of equipment, therapy, estimated duration of therapy, and sedation. Emotional support of the patient includes emotional support of the patient's family.

Close observation of the patient's response to therapy and close following of serial arterial blood gases will provide clues to significant changes needing new or different respiratory care orders.

COMPLICATIONS OF RESPIRATORY FAILURE

Complications of respiratory failure affect every organ system. The respiratory system itself is prone to infection, oxygen toxicity, atelectasis, and progression of failure to ARDS.

The cardiac system responds to the respiratory failure with compensatory mechanisms of tachycardia, right ventricular hypertrophy, decreased cardiac output, and cardiac myopathies due to hypotension, acidosis, alkalosis, and thrombus formation.

The renal system may respond with acute renal failure, acid-base disturbances, and electrolyte imbalances.

The neurological system responds to the lack of oxygen with evident changes in cerebral activity, nerve conduction, and muscle responses.

Emotionally, the patient may respond with every response possible from fear and anxiety to anger and rebellion.

The patient in respiratory failure is a complex, taxing challenge to the critical care nurse.

Adult Respiratory Distress Syndrome (ARDS)

Historically, the Vietnam War educated the medical world about ARDS. Because the wounded were air-transported to medical treatment centers far faster than in any other war, a pulmonary condition, ARDS, was seen very frequently. Physicians were able to observe and treat the pulmonary condition. Much of the knowledge of the course and treatment of ARDS in civilian hospitals is due to the knowledge learned in treating the wounded Vietnam veterans.

ARDS may be called by many names. Some names relate to geography, such as Da Nang lung. Other names relate to etiology of the pulmonary state (shock lung or septic lung) or to the characteristics of the lung parenchyma in ARDS (stiff lung or traumatic wet lung).

DEFINITION OF ARDS

One hundred medical centers will define ARDS in one hundred different ways. In this text, ARDS is defined as an acute respiratory failure, secondary to injury at the alveolar capillary membrane, with leakage of proteinaceous fluid into the lung interstitium and alveoli, causing hypoxia, decreased lung compliance, and a fall in lung volume.

PATHOPHYSIOLOGY OF ARDS

An initial insult to the lung disrupts the alveolar-capillary membrane. This results in an increased permeability of both the capillary endothelium and the alveolar epithelium. This progressively enlarges intercellular spaces, and interstitial edema develops because of the increased permeability. This increased permeability of the alveolar membrane is the key factor in the vicious cycle of ARDS.

Interstitial edema makes oxygen diffusion decrease, and the edema will cause some alveoli to be functionless. The proteins (especially fibrinogen) in the fluids that have leaked into the alveoli may inactivate pulmonary surfactant. Without surfactant, more alveoli collapse. A rise in intrapulmonary pressure occurs with the edema, further reducing ventilatory efficiency. This reduction makes it difficult, if not impossible, to maintain adequate arterial oxygen tension. Figure 5-1 depicts the vicious cycle of ARDS.

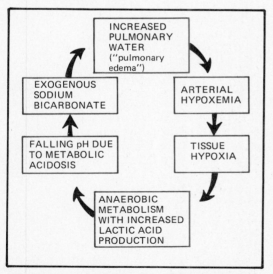

Figure 5-1.   Cycle of adult respiratory distress syndrome (ARDS).

As the alveoli collapse, the capillaries hemorrhage and collapse. This reduces blood flow to the lungs. These physiologic events lead to reduced functional residual capacity (FRC), reduced compliance, and increased pulmonary shunting. If the phys-iologic events are not reversed, the capillary hemorrhages will eventually result in no blood flow to the lungs.

CLINICAL PRESENTATION OF ARDS (SIGNS AND SYMPTOMS)

Often ARDS patients have no previous lung disease and frequently no direct pulmonary injury. The patient is often dyspneic, tachypneic, hypoxic, hypotensive, and may be cyanotic. There are four phases of ARDS that have been identified.

Phase 1 is characterized by altered tissue perfusion. The lungs are often clear. Chest x-ray will be normal, or it may show *slight* congestion. The patient may start to hyperventilate. Arterial blood gases will show normal or slightly decreased P_{O_2}, and the P_{CO_2} will average 30–40 mm Hg.

Phase 2 is subclinical respiratory distress. Chest x-ray may still be normal. The patient will hyperventilate. Hypocarbia (hypocapnia) develops due to the increased respiratory rate and decreased lung compliance. Hypoxia is evidenced by arterial blood gases; *but* usually, increasing concentrations of oxygen have no beneficial results. There is evidence of $\dot{V}\dot{Q}$ (ventilation per minute and perfusion per minute) abnormality. The mismatching of $\dot{V}\dot{Q}$ is normally toward pulmonary shunting. This indicates a respiratory quotient of less than 0.8. The P_{CO_2} is usually 25–30 mm Hg.

Phase 3 is established respiratory distress which is clinically apparent. The patient seems suddenly very ill. Continued hyperventilation has decreased the P_{CO_2} to 20–35 mm Hg, and the P_{O_2} has dropped to a range of 50–60 mm Hg. Pulmonary shunting ranges from 20% to 40%. Now, the chest x-ray shows an increasing pulmonary edema.

Phase 4 is severe respiratory failure characterized by severe hypoxia. The functioning pulmonary capillaries are markedly reduced, as shown by a continually rising P_{CO_2}. Metabolic acidosis has developed. There is evidence of a physiologic shunt approaching 50–60%, which is incompatible with life. Chest x-ray at this stage shows a complete "white out" of the lung. There is a markedly decreased functional residual capacity (FRC).

PROBABLE CAUSES OF ARDS

High on a list of precipitating causes of ARDS are vasoactive substances and enzymes from injured, ischemic, infected, or necrotic tissue. Some of the vasoactive substances are serotonins, histamines, and catecholamines. Steroid enzymes are released in reaction to the body stress.

Fat embolism from long bone fractures usually occurs 24–72 hours after the injury. Cerebral and respiratory dysfunction are clues to a possible embolism. A fat embolism carries many platelets with it; and as a consequence, microaggregates develop in the lung, resulting in pulmonary dysfunction that may be sufficient to produce ARDS.

Patients requiring massive blood transfusions are at a very high risk of developing ARDS. The longer the blood is stored, the greater the increase in particles, that is, clumping of white blood cells (WBC), red blood cells (RBC), platelets, and fibrin. Disseminated intravascular coagulation (DIC) occurs often.

Any form of trauma—intrathoracic, extrathoracic, or multiple trauma may lead to shock. Smoke inhalation is trauma to the lungs.

Aspiration, especially of gastric juices, and ingestion of many drugs traumatize the lungs. If the assault is sufficient, ARDS develops.

The *common* factor in ALL cases of ARDS is some shock or trauma sufficient to prevent the normal functioning of the lungs due to an alteration in the permeability of the alveolar-capillary membrane.

DIAGNOSIS OF ADULT RESPIRATORY DISTRESS SYNDROME (ARDS)

A medical history identifying any precipitating factor and the physical appearance of marked respiratory distress are flashing lights pointing to ARDS. On the other hand, an insignificant history and a physical exam revealing only tachypnea accompanied by flaring nostrils, grunting respirations, and perhaps cyanosis may indicate ARDS.

Chest x-ray in phases one and two may be normal or show slight diffuse congestion. By phase three and definitely by phase four, the diagnosis should have been made and treatment initiated. Radiographic proof is nice, but waiting for that proof will probably be fatal to the patient.

Arterial blood gases (serial) and the clinical picture are by far the most useful diagnostic tools to use. Special pulmonary tests for decreased lung compliance, decreased FRC, as well as other lung volumes, shunting, and an increasing $A - aDO_2$ gradient will confirm the clinical diagnosis which may have been originally only a "gut feeling."

NURSING INTERVENTIONS IN ADULT RESPIRATORY DISTRESS SYNDROME

Usually the ARDS patient will be placed on a ventilator to support alveolar ventilation. Suctioning is an essential step in the patient's care. While the patient is on the ventilator, the usual treatments include high tidal volumes, a low respiratory rate, and PEEP. Theoretically, PEEP will keep alveoli open at end expiration, increasing oxygenation and the FRC.

Many, if not most, patients with ARDS will have a central catheter for monitoring fluid balance and central venous pressure. Cardiac output and cardiac function are also monitored.

Infection must be prevented. If infection is present, vigorous chest physiotherapy and suctioning are necessary to prevent bronchopneumonia. Once identification of the infecting organism is made, antibiotic therapy is started.

Corticosteroid treatment is in use in some areas; but it is controversial since steroids stress the body and the patient's response has been variable.

Nutritional support is often overlooked. Good nutrition prevents progressive weakness of respiratory muscles. Good nutrition also helps the body's immunological state in fighting infection.

Psychological support of the patient and the patient's family will relieve some of the stress and release more energy for the patient to "fight" the ARDS state.

COMPLICATIONS OF ADULT RESPIRATORY DISTRESS SYNDROME (ARDS)

Infection is a frequent complication of ARDS.

As the ARDS progresses, cardiac dysrhythmias, neurolgical deterioration (sensorium), renal failure, and stress ulcers develop. The mortality rate in ARDS is extremely high.

6

Chronic Obstructive Pulmonary Disease, Restrictive Pulmonary Disease, and Status Asthmaticus

Learning Objectives

By the end of this chapter, the nurse will be able to:

1. Define asthma, bronchitis, and emphysema.
2. Identify the pathophysiology of asthma, bronchitis, and emphysema.
3. Compare and contrast the symptoms of bronchitis and emphysema.
4. List five major causes of chronic obstructive pulmonary disease (COPD).
5. Explain alpha$_1$ anti-trypsin deficiencies and the result of type one and type two deficiencies.
6. Explain why COPD patients often have polycythemia.
7. Name the two most common organisms cultured from the sputum of COPD patients.
8. List and explain nine nursing interventions in the treatment of COPD.
9. Define restrictive lung disease, and list the three categories of classification.
10. Explain the difference between compression and absorption atelectasis.
11. Identify factors in central nervous system depression which lead to hypoxemia.
12. Explain the effect of neuromuscular disease upon respiration.
13. Define status asthmaticus.
14. Explain the pathophysiology of status asthmaticus.
15. Identify the *immediate* treatment of a patient in status asthmaticus.
16. List the two most common complications of status asthmaticus.

Chronic Obstructive Pulmonary Disease

Chronic obstructive pulmonary disease (COPD) is actually a triad of diseases which is increasingly prevalent in our society. The triad of COPD is characterized by an ob-struction of air flow within the lungs. Asthma, bronchitis, and emphysema are the three major obstructive diseases. Bronchiectasis has the symptoms of COPD; but, in actuality, it is an infectious pulmonary disease, not a COPD. COLD means chronic obstructive lung disease, and CAO means chronic airway obstruction; they are used synonymously with COPD.

DEFINITIONS

Asthma is a condition of *episodic* bronchospasm, and between periods of bronchospasm, pulmonary function is normal or near normal in the early stages of the disease. In cases of advanced asthmatic conditions, pulmonary function is not normal. Status asthmaticus is a special circumstance that will be discussed later in this chapter.

Bronchitis is the most easily diagnosed COPD in life due to *sputum production*, cough, and wheezing. Acute bronchitis is infectious—the result of breathing in toxins. Chronic bronchitis is more difficult to diagnose. The accepted American Lung Association definition of chronic bronchitis is *a condition manifested by a productive cough present almost every day for three consecutive months out of the year for two consecutive years.*

Emphysema results in an actual destruction of pulmonary tissue by the breakdown of the alveolar wall. Lungs become hyperinflated due to a decreased elasticity. Unless a biopsy is performed, it is difficult to *definitively* diagnose during life. It is often diagnosed by autopsy. The main **symptom** is an increase in the work of breathing. In eupnea (normal breathing) 63% of the work of breathing is in overcoming the elastic resistance of the lungs and chest wall. This percent is greatly increased in emphysema.

Emphysema and bronchitis occur together 85% of the time. Before the 1930–1940s, these diseases were predominantly found in white males. Now, they are increasingly diagnosed in white females and nonwhite males. Emphysema and bronchitis together form the syndrome COPD. Since 1960, COPD has been the most rapidly increasing cause of disability in the United States. This corresponds with an increase in smoking popularity at the end of World War II.

PATHOPHYSIOLOGY OF ASTHMA

Asthma is an episodic, but generalized airway obstruction resulting from a toxin, an allergen, a pollutant, and/or a psychogenic stimulus. This airway obstruction is caused by a response to the stimulus of contraction of smooth muscle *and* increased secretion of abnormally tenacious mucus in the bronchioles. This increased contraction of the trachea and increased mucus production narrows air passages, trapping air in the terminal respiratory bronchioles (Figure 6-1). This results in dyspnea and wheezing, both inspiratory and expiratory, with the expiratory phase being prolonged as the patient tries to exhale the trapped air. In some patients, asthma is an allergic response to specific allergens. In other patients, it is simply intermittent in early stages and tends to become recurrent and paroxysmal in later stages.

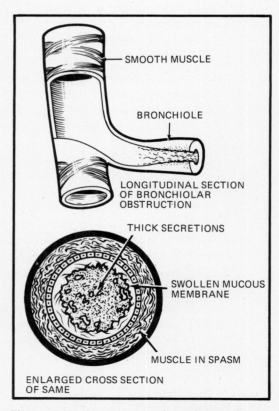

Figure 6-1. Appearance of respiratory bronchioles in asthma. (Bronchiole obstruction on expiration by muscle spasm, swelling of mucosa, and thick secretions.)

There are four stages or grades of asthma, and arterial blood gases are predictable indices of the severity of the disease process. Grade four is the most critical.

Grade One: Pa_{O_2} normal; Pa_{CO_2} normal
Grade Two: Pa_{O_2} reduced; Pa_{CO_2} reduced
Grade Three: Pa_{O_2} reduced; Pa_{CO_2} normal
Grade Four: Pa_{O_2} reduced; Pa_{CO_2} elevated

PATHOPHYSIOLOGY OF BRONCHITIS

Bronchitis is an inflammation usually caused by *Hemophilus influenzae* or *pneumococcus* that penetrates the bronchial wall. The inflammatory response results in hypertrophy and hyperplasia of the bronchial glands and goblet cells. These glands and goblet cells produce an overabundance of mucus. With repeated attacks of bronchitis, an overgrowth (metaplasia) of bronchial and bronchiolar epithelium will eventually occur. This metaplasia causes a loss of cilia and excessive mucus production. Frequent attacks cause distortion and scarring of the bronchial wall, decreasing the size of the airway lumen (Figure 6-2). The excessive mucus production in the bronchi causes the chronic or recurrent productive cough. Since the airway lumen is decreased, some secretions are trapped in the alveoli and smaller air passages.

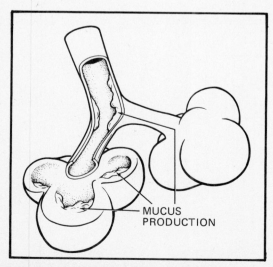

MUCUS PRODUCTION

Figure 6-2.   Airway lumen in bronchitis.

PATHOPHYSIOLOGY OF EMPHYSEMA

Emphysema is simply an enlargement of the air spaces distal to the terminal non-respiratory bronchiole, with destruction of alveolar walls. There are usually blebs and bullae in the lungs (Figure 6-3). A bleb is an air-filled space in the visceral pleura. Bullae are air-filled spaces in the parenchyma greater than one centimeter in diameter. This results in overinflation of alveoli. Lungs lose their "elastic recoil" property. There is decreased blood content due to blebs and bullae.

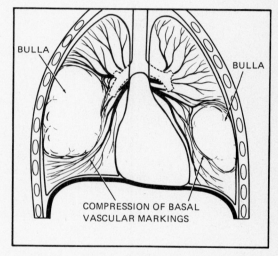

BULLA

BULLA

COMPRESSION OF BASAL VASCULAR MARKINGS

Figure 6-3.   Giant bullae of end-stage emphysema.

ETIOLOGY OF COPD

There are five major causes of COPD:

1. *Cigarette smoking* is the leading cause. Smoking effectively:
   a. Stops ciliary action so the lungs cannot clear themselves
   b. Prevents surfactant production, which results in areas of micro-atelectasis
   c. Increases the production of digestive substances, with resulting loss of elasticity and eventual breakdown in the alveolar capillary wall

2. *Pollution*—Fumes from the auto are the worst pollutant because of insufficient combustion of sulfur and nitrates. Smog, regardless of its cause, increases bronchospasm.

3. *Pesticides*—Exposure results in actual destruction of pulmonary tissue; however, one needs a fairly heavy, long-term exposure.

4. *Industrial exposure*—Sufficient exposure to cotton dust eventually causes brown lung. Coal dust causes black lung.

5. *Hereditary causes*

   a. *Propensity*—This is a state where the whole family coughs a lot. There may be some slight smoking, but *all* of the family has COPD.

   b. *Alpha$_1$ anti-trypsin deficiencies*

      (1) Trypsin is a proteolytic enzyme which dissolves small thrombi and microaggregates. If trypsin increases sufficiently, it will actually dissolve blood vessel walls, alveolar membrane, and cell walls. Anti-trypsin controls the body's trypsin level. About 0.1% of the population has no alpha$_1$ anti-trypsin factor. (Papain, found in all meat tenderizers, is almost the same as trypsin.)

      (2) There are two types of alpha$_1$ anti-trypsin deficiencies. *Type one* are the homozygous deficiencies. Homozygous deficient people have less than 10% of the normal alpha$_1$ anti-trypsin level. These people develop COPD in their early 20s, are very sick in their mid 30s, and die by their mid 40s. *Type two* are the heterozygous deficiencies. Heterozygous deficient people have less than 60% of the normal alpha$_1$ anti-trypsin levels. This may be the group of people that has a propensity for COPD.

Other causes of COPD include repeated respiratory infections, which result in greater susceptibility to pulmonary disease. As one ages, there is a high incidence of COPD among smokers; but aging, itself, is not a cause of COPD. Patients who have cystic fibrosis are classified as having COPD.

CLINICAL PRESENTATION (SIGNS AND SYMPTOMS)

In Table 6-1, a comparison is made between the major symptoms of bronchitis and emphysema.

Table 6-1.   Comparison between bronchitis and emphysema.*

Symptoms	Bronchitis	Emphysema
Nickname	Blue Bloaters	Pink Puffers
Cough	4+	no
S.O.B.	2+	4+
CO_2 retention	due to 2+ relative shunt	0 (till end stage disease)
Arterial hypoxemia	due to 2+ relative shunt	0 (till end stage disease)
Weight loss	no	yes
CHF	yes	no
Cyanosis	yes	no
VC	unchanged	unchanged
FEV$_1$	decreased	decreased
TLC	normal	increased
FRC	normal or increased	increased
RV	normal or increased	increased
With bronchodilator being given	improvement	no change

*Compiled from a masters of nursing respiratory course.

DIAGNOSIS OF COPD

A patient's history of exertional dyspnea, smoking, frequent upper respiratory infections (URI), chronic productive cough, and a family history of COPD is very suggestive of COPD in this patient.

Physical examination showing decreased chest excursion, adventitious lung sounds, cyanosis, jugular venous distension (JVD), and symptoms of cor pulmonale may be present.

Chest x-ray is of little value in diagnosing; however, if it is hyperlucent and the diaphragm is depressed, it suggests COPD.

Patients with COPD often have polycythemia: The bone marrow produces more RBC's to carry oxygen in an oxygen-deprived body.

Sputum cultures are of value to determine secondary bacterial infection. *Streptococcus pneumoniae* and *Hemophilus influenzae* are the most often found microorganisms.

NURSING INTERVENTIONS AND TREATMENT OF COPD

1. *Bronchodilators* are not effective in emphysema. They only relieve bronchospasms of asthma and bronchitis.
   a. Alpha-beta stimulators (e.g., isoproterenol hydrochloride—Isuprel®; ephedrine sulfate—Ephedrine®; and Epinephrine®) for relief of bronchial smooth muscle spasms
   b. Beta stimulators (e.g., metaproterenol sulfate—Alupent® or Metaprel®; terbutaline sulfate—Brethine®) (Propranolol hydrochloride—Inderal® are *not* used since these cause bronchospasm.)
   c. Theophyllines (e.g., Aminophylline®, Dyphylline®, Dilor®, Cyclic Aminophylline®)

   If *severe* bronchospasm is present, use Aminophylline® as a continuous drip. Nebulizing metaproterenol sulfate—Alupent® or Metaprel®—may also be used.
2. *Antibiotics* are used to control progression of the disease. An interesting

note: If a patient is admitted with COPD and with a P_{CO_2} above 50 or a P_{O_2} below 50, then there is a 90% chance that the patient will be dead within 5 years.

3. *Physical therapy and teaching* include postural drainage, abdominal breathing exercises to increase vital capacity (VC) and decrease functional residual capacity (FRC) by exhaling with pursed lips, and blow bottles for exhaling against pressure.

4. *Hydration* in an adequate volume is important to keeping secretions moist. At almost all costs, AVOID antihistamines. IPPB and ultrasonic treatments add moisture to the bronchial tree.

5. *Nourishment* is very important, especially in emphysema. However, there is not enough room in the stomach for a regular meal without compromising breathing space. Consequently, the patient should eat six or eight times daily.

6. *Corticosteroids* used systemically help in cutting down secretions and reduce the inflammatory reaction in the lung. However, glucose intolerance may develop, and resistance to infections is decreased.

   Beclomethasone dipropionate—Beclovent® or Vanceril®—is a steroid completely destroyed in the liver. It is very effective in asthma and moderately effective in chronic bronchitis. The mouth and posterior pharynx receive most of the dose. The mouth must be rinsed with water or mouth wash to prevent candidiasis.

7. *Exercise* almost to the tolerance level every day is important. Exercise will not hurt the lungs. Some patients with COPD cannot inhale enough oxygen on room air to exercise. Oxygen is available in tanks and liquids for home use.

8. *Psychotherapy* is one of the most needed interventions in COPD. These patients require a lot of encouragement and support since they suffer frequent

episodes of the sensation of suffocating and their disease process is not curable.

9. *Patient and family education* in bronchial hygiene, conservation of energy, and all of these treatment modalities is essential.

COMPLICATIONS OF COPD

Once COPD develops, it is progressive. The rate of progression may be controlled, but the patient *cannot* be cured. The most common complications are pneumonia, respiratory failure, spontaneous pneumothorax, cor pulmonale, pulmonary embolism, and peptic ulcer with or without hemorrhage. If there is even a slight question if a patient has COPD, do NOT give sleeping medicine! The respiratory centers are relatively insensitive to oxygen stimuli. If the patient is chronically hypoxic and is given oxygen in high concentrations, the patient will quit breathing and may die. If the patient quits breathing, take off the oxygen and ambu-bag the patient until help arrives.

Restrictive Lung Diseases

A restrictive lung disease is any abnormal pulmonary condition which decreases the total lung capacity and the vital capacity. These diseases are seen in critical care areas and may cause hypoxia and hypoxemia requiring treatment. Restrictive lung disease can be classified into three categories: (1) atelectasis, (2) central nervous system depression, and (3) muscular disease.

1. Atelectasis

Atelectasis is the collapse of lung tissue. Collapse occurs throughout lung fields in no discernible pattern and is termed *patchy* or *miliary* atelectasis. As the lung tissue collapses, it involves contigous areas of the lung and will eventually involve entire lobes or segments. When atelectasis has reached this point, it can be seen on x-ray. Segmental atelectasis may be caused by compression or absorption.

Compression: This may be the result of surgery with thoracotomy and is considered a part of the operative procedure. Other conditions which cause compression atelectasis include pneumothorax, pleural effusion, and space-occupying lesions.

Absorption: This is a common form of acute lung collapse. Retained secretions are almost always the cause of absorption atelectasis. Secretions have a high sugar and protein content. These retained secretions provide an excellent media for bacteria. Much of the retained secretions will be in small bronchioles. Therefore, suctioning is *less* efficient than positioning and chest physiotherapy for clearing secretions. Atelectasis needs vigorous treatment since it interrupts blood and lymphatic flow, both of which play vital roles in the body defense mechanisms.

When segments of the lung collapse, there is an immediate decrease in total lung capacity. How serious this is depends upon the size of the collapse. There is a normal hyperinflation of surrounding lung tissue. The total amount of blood passing by the collapsed lung drops remarkably—but *NOT* completely. This results in a true physiologic shunt, that is, a nonventilated, perfused lung. This shunt results in an arterial hypoxemia. Hypoxemia due to a true shunt does *not* respond well to oxygen therapy. This shunt puts a compensatory drain on the cardiovascular system. It is common to see tachycardia, tachypnea, and mild hypertension accompany absorption type atelectasis.

2. Central Nervous System Depression

Central nervous system depression by drugs or disease usually decreases total lung capacity by producing: (1) an absence of periodic deep breathing (sighs), (2) a decrease in the ventilatory drive, and (3) a decrease in central nervous system response to ventilatory stimuli. If not treated, central nervous system depression that is significant to cause these three factors will result in hypoxemia, hypercarbia, acidemia, atelectasis, cardiovascular collapse, and death.

Immediate and intensive respiratory therapy is started to prevent central nervous system depression from extending to hypoxemia and the related states. Respiratory therapy must be continued as long as there is central nervous system depression.

3. Neuromuscular Diseases

Any disease which temporarily or permanently compromises the respiratory system will cause an initial decrease in total lung capacity. It is essential to maintain optimum ventilation during the disease process. The neuromuscular diseases include tetanus, muscle-wasting disease (muscular dystrophy, congenital myotonia), myoneural junction disease (myasthenia gravis), motor nerve disease (Guillain-Barré syndrome), Landry's ascending paralysis, tickbite paralysis (porphyria), and spinal cord disease (multiple sclerosis, quadriplegia, paraplegia, and some amyotrophic lateral sclerosis).

CAUTION: Usually, in a healthy person, a preoperative vital capacity will not be comprised IMMEDIATELY postoperatively; BUT it will be comprised *sometime* during the first 24 hours post surgery. Monitor the patient closely.

TREATMENT OF RESTRICTIVE LUNG DISEASES

Treatment is directed toward the underlying disease process (or cause) that results in the restrictive lung disease. Simultaneously, intensive respiratory therapy will help prevent lung compromise.

Status Asthmaticus

This is a severe continuing attack of asthma that fails to respond to sympathomimetic drugs.

PATHOPHYSIOLOGY OF STATUS ASTHMATICUS

Initially, the same pathologic changes in asthma occur in status asthmaticus. However, as the attack continues unabated, the bronchial walls hypertrophy causing a bronchiolar obstruction. This obstruction reduces alveolar ventilation and severe atelectasis occurs.

ETIOLOGY AND CLINICAL PRESENTATION OF STATUS ASTHMATICUS

The three most common causes of status asthmaticus are (1) exposure to allergens, (2) noncompliance with the medication regimen, and (3) respiratory infections. Emotional factors play a *major* role in initiating status asthmaticus. Environments which become unusually hot, cold, and/or dusty often trigger status asthmaticus because of the effect of inspired air on the lungs.

Patients in status asthmaticus are physically exhausted from the work of breathing. They are extremely dyspneic. Their respiratory pattern is hyperpneic, which may result in the development of a dehydrated state. Inspiratory and expiratory wheezing is present, with a prolonged expiratory phase.

DIAGNOSIS OF STATUS ASTHMATICUS

All of the symptoms of asthma may be present. In addition, the history may reveal noncompliance with the medical regimen. Symptoms of URI may be present. Dyspnea, cough, wheezing, and an inability to sleep are common complaints.

Physical examination revealing tachypnea, tachycardia, use of accessory respiratory muscles, dyspnea, pallor, cyanosis, and abnormal breath sounds will help confirm status asthmaticus.

Arterial blood gases usually reveal a decreased Pa_{O_2}, and an increased Pa_{CO_2} with respiratory failure. If the status asthmaticus has reached this point, the patient is critically ill and may require respirator assistance.

Chest x-ray will probably not be helpful. It may be normal or translucent.

NURSING INTERVENTIONS IN STATUS ASTHMATICUS

The nursing interventions for status asthmaticus are the same as those for COPD. The objective is to support ventilation and respirations to prevent respiratory failure and pneumothorax. Because of the extreme life-threatening aspects of status asthmaticus, continuous intravenous theophyllines, usually aminophylline, in addition to aggresive respiratory therapies is usually instituted.

Bronchodilators, antibiotics, physical therapy, hydration, nourishment, corticosteroid use, exercise, psychotherapy, and patient and family education were discussed earlier in this chapter under COPD and are applicable to status asthmaticus.

7

Pulmonary Embolism and Chest Trauma

Learning Objectives

By the end of this chapter, the nurse will be able to:

1. Define pulmonary embolism.
2. Explain the pathophysiology of pulmonary embolism.
3. List six precipitating factors in pulmonary embolism.
4. Identify five signs of massive pulmonary embolism.
5. Name the treatment of choice in pulmonary embolism.
6. Explain why continuous I.V. therapy is better than bolus therapy every 4–6 hours in treating pulmonary embolism.
7. Define streptokinase and urokinase and state their use.
8. List six nursing interventions for patients at high risk of pulmonary embolism.
9. Classify chest trauma into three categories and explain each.
10. Identify appropriate treatment and cautions for fractures of rib 1, rib 2, ribs 3–8, ribs 9–12.
11. Define flail chest and explain its treatment.
12. Distinguish between simple closed pneumothorax, tension pneumothorax, and hemothorax.
13. Explain the difference between a cardiac contusion and a cardiac tamponade.
14. State symptoms and treatment for cardiac contusion and tamponade.
15. Discuss diaphragmatic rupture in terms of physiology, symptoms, and treatment.
16. Discuss esophageal rupture in terms of symptoms and treatment.

Pulmonary Embolism

A thrombus, which has developed in the deep veins of the lower extremities, breaks loose from its attachment and travels through the venous circulation into the pulmonary circulation where it will partially or completely occlude a pulmonary artery. A massive pulmonary embolism is one where more than 50% of the pulmonary artery bed is occluded. In this discussion, pulmonary embolism is confined to the thrombus which breaks loose, not a fat or air embolism.

OCCURRENCE OF PULMONARY EMBOLISM

It is estimated that there are more than 500,000 nonfatal pulmonary emboli annually in the United States. There are an additional 150,000 fatal pulmonary emboli each year. The more massive the emboli, the greater the risk of death. Recurrent emboli are common and have a 25% mortality rate. If diagnosed and treated properly to resolution, chances of a complete recovery are good.

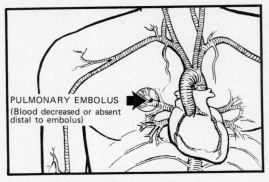

PULMONARY EMBOLUS
(Blood decreased or absent distal to embolus)

Figure 7-1.   Pulmonary embolism.

PATHOPHYSIOLOGY OF PULMONARY EMBOLISM

There are three conditions which tend to precipitate thrombus formation. These three conditions are referred to as Virchow's triad.

1. Damaged endothelium of veins
2. Venous stasis
3. Hypercoagulability of the blood

With these three conditions present, a thrombus has a great chance of developing.

Some mechanism causes the dislodgment of some or all of the thrombus formed. Natural processes of clot dissolution may cause release of fragments of the clot, or external mechanisms such as direct trauma, muscle contraction, or changes in perfusion may contribute to the release of the thrombus.

As the thrombus breaks loose, it flows through the venous circulation, entering the right ventricle and then lodging in small pulmonary arteries (Figure 7-1). Normally, more than 50% of the pulmonary bed must be compromised to alter hemodynamics. Compromise will occur more readily if there is underlying COPD, congestive heart failure (CHF), or other chronic conditions.

Pulmonary hypertension is due to pulmonary arterial obstruction. If the obstruction is partial or develops slowly, the patient may survive to be treated. However, if the obstruction is rapid and total, the patient may suffer sudden death. Chronic pulmonary hypertension does not usually occur with a single embolus. It usually results from multiple emboli of middle size vessels.

ETIOLOGY OF PULMONARY EMBOLISM

Ten percent of pulmonary emboli develop in patients with no predisposing factor. However, some predisposing factors include stasis of venous blood due to immobilization in postoperative patients, varicose veins, obesity, pregnancy, and congestive heart failure.

Less commonly, aging, vasculitis, and trauma to the vessel wall during venipuncture or prolonged intravenous therapy are causes of embolism. Venous wall damage due to soft tissue trauma, fractures, or infiltration by malignant cells may cause thrombi. Hypercoagulability is related to thrombocytosis, increased platelet activity following surgery, trauma, parturition, polycythemia, and hemoconcentration. All of these may be factors, and patients with any of these conditions or diagnoses should be considered at high risk for developing pulmonary emboli.

Rare causes of thrombus formation include thrombus formation in the heart secondary to acute myocardial infarction, atrial fibrillation, subacute bacterial endocarditis, and cardioversion.

CLINICAL PRESENTATION OF PULMONARY EMBOLISM

The signs and symptoms of pulmonary emboli must be divided into the clinical pictures of a massive embolism and a submassive embolism. *Massive embolism* occurs suddenly. The patient may have crushing, substernal chest pain and appear to be in shock. The patient may be hypotensive, dyspneic, cyanotic, apprehensive, or comatose. Respirations are rapid, shallow, and gasping. Arterial pulse is rapid and the volume is diminished. If awake, the patient may express feelings of impending doom. *Submassive embolism* may present only fleeting minimal symptoms. If the submassive embolism has occluded a medium size artery, tachypnea, dyspnea, tachycardia, generalized chest discomfort, and pleuritic-type chest pain may develop within a few hours. Fever, cough, and hemoptysis may occur over several hours (or days). A pleural friction rub and a pleural effusion may develop.

DIAGNOSIS OF PULMONARY EMBOLISM

There are no specific 100% accurate tests to diagnose pulmonary embolism. Routine chest x-ray may be normal or in about 20% of such cases may show some consolidation. EKG may be normal but most often shows sinus tachycardia; it may also show right ventricular strain. Blood chemistries are nonspecific. Arterial blood gases usually reveal a hypoxemia. If the P_{O_2} is above 80 mm Hg on room air, a pulmonary embolism is unlikely.

The most useful tests are nuclear studies and angiography. A lung scan that is normal usually rules out a pulmonary embolism. If a lung scan shows perfusion defects on segments that appear normal on chest x-ray, then pulmonary embolism is likely. A lung scan may be abnormal due simply to COPD. If xenon-133 ventilation scan is done and shows normal ventilation in areas of decreased perfusion, the diagnosis is almost certain.

Pulmonary angiography is the most accurate way to diagnose pulmonary embolism. An angiogram is the standard by which other tests are compared. An angiogram should be obtained before surgical therapy is instituted.

COMPLICATIONS OF PULMONARY EMBOLISM

Complications of pulmonary embolism may be pulmonary infarction due to extension of emboli. Any embolus that is large enough to alter hemodynamics can result in any and every complication. These include stroke, myocardial infarction, cardiac dysrhythmias that are not amenable to our available drugs, liver failure and necrosis secondary to congestion, pneumonia, pulmonary abcesses, ARDS, shock, and death.

TREATMENT OF PULMONARY EMBOLISM

Drug Therapy

Heparin is the immediate drug of choice with an intravenous bolus of 5,000–10,000 units. Within 30 minutes of this bolus, anticoagulation should be documented. Lee-White time of 20–25 minutes or a partial thromboplastin time (P.T.T.) of 55–85 seconds is adequate anticoagulation. Heparin impedes clotting by preventing fibrin formation. It is metabolized by the reticuloendothelial cells and some by the liver, and small amounts are excreted by the kidneys unchanged.

Anticoagulation is continued by a heparin bolus every 4–6 hours *or* a continuous intravenous heparin drip (usually 20,000 units of heparin per 1,000 ml of intravenous fluid). Continuous intravenous heparin is preferred for the high risk patient, the massive embolus, or the high risk bleeder. A continuous infusion maintains a steady therapeutic blood level in contrast to the heparin bolus every 4–6 hours. The bolus causes peak levels for short times and subtherapeutic levels for the remaining time before another bolus is due. Heparin is usually continued for 5–7 days or when oral anticoagulation can become effective.

Oral anticoagulants are often started 3–4 days before stopping the heparin to avoid a period of no anticoagulant therapy. Oral anticoagulants are usually given for 6–8 weeks if the patient is asymptomatic. They *may* be given indefinitely or for the remainder of the patient's life for multiple reasons.

Streptokinase and urokinase are thrombolytic enzymes being used to "dissolve" or lyse the emboli. Streptokinase interrupts the plasminogen activation of converting plasminogen to plasmin in two different steps. Urokinase activates plasminogen in one step by separating it from its peptide bond in two different sites. This would increase pulmonary capillary perfusion and decrease hemodynamic abnormalities. These two thrombolytic enzymes are administered *only* by intravenous infusion. Therapeutic action begins immediately and ceases with the interruption of the intravenous administration. However, residual effects may last for as long as 12 hours, as indicated by blood coagulation studies. Results are controversial.

Low molecular weight dextran at 500 ml daily *may* prevent extensions and/or help lyse present emboli by reducing blood sludging. Results are controversial.

Surgery

This is reserved for those patients who do not respond to anticoagulants, who have "rebound" effects to heparin, or who have recurrent emboli. Procedures may include ligation or clipping of the inferior vena cava, filter placement in the vena cava, and embolectomy. Embolectomy is a serious operation and is usually reserved for the massive emboli or for the decompensating patient that cannot be stabilized.

The vena caval umbrella may filter emboli *and* obviate the necessity of major surgery in select patients.

NURSING INTERVENTION IN PULMONARY EMBOLISM

These measures will help prevent emboli in potential patients. Ambulate patients within physician guidelines. Nonambulating patients may have regular active and passive exercises assisted by the nurse or physical therapist. Elevating legs, *refusing* to gatch the knees, and the use of antiembolic hose will help prevent stasis of venous blood. Deep breathing exercises and adequate fluid intake will help to maintain adequate ventilation, circulation, and expectoration of pulmonary secretions. Fear and anxiety need to be reduced as much as possible. A quiet room, a calm nurse, and family members present may help as much, if not more than, sedation. Some patients will require sedation and every other nursing intervention imaginable to survive a submassive or massive pulmonary embolism. If they survive, patient and family teaching to decrease the risk of another embolus is essential.

Chest Trauma

Chest injuries are almost always seen in multiple trauma. The more systems involved in the trauma, the more critical each injury becomes. Chest injuries are especially serious in elderly people, obese people, and people with cardiac or pulmonary disease. The older the patient, the more likely the presence of underlying health problems; and thus, physiologic reserve or "ability to spring back" is diminished.

Statistically, if there is a chest injury alone, there is a 5–10% mortality rate. If there is a chest injury and another injury, the mortality rate is 30%. There is chest trauma in 6 out of 10 auto accidents.

CLASSIFICATIONS OF CHEST TRAUMA

Chest trauma can be classified into one of three categories: (1) closed chest injury, (2) open chest injury, and (3) visceral injuries. Any chest injury interrupts the normal thoracic pressures and movements. Treatment of *all* chest injuries is to re-establish normal and adequate ventilatory function. The type and location of the trauma determine the presentation, diagnosis, treatment, and complications of chest trauma. Diagnosis and treatment of chest trauma MUST be delayed until it is certain that an *adequate and patent* airway exists. If the airway is not patent and multiple trauma exists, insertion of a large bore needle (size 14) into the cricothyroid membrane will suffice until cervical spine injuries have been ruled out and endotracheal intubation or tracheostomy may be performed. Some hospitals will perform a tracheostomy or cricoidotomy prior to ruling out cervical spine injuries rather than use a large bore needle to assure airway patency.

The most common injuries in chest trauma are fractured ribs and pneumothoraces.

Closed Chest Injuries

These are usually the result of a blunt force which does not penetrate the chest wall. Vehicular accidents, falls, and sometimes violence are the common causes of closed chest injury.

One of the most common closed chest injuries is rib fractures. Symptoms will be pain, dyspnea, ecchymosis, and splinting on movement (if alert).

Fracture of the First Rib. It is not common to have a fracture of the first rib. When a very strong force is applied to the upper thoracic cage, the result is a "star burst" fracture, that is, pieces of bone going in all directions.

Examination for neck injuries, brachial plexis injury, pneumothorax, aortic rupture or tear, and very often thoracic outlet syndrome is a must. Fracture of the first rib is life-threatening and indicates severe underlying thoracic and/or abdominal injuries.

Fracture of the Second Rib. This is commonly termed "the hangman's fracture" and is covered in Chapter 19.

Fractures of Ribs 3–8. These ribs are the most commonly fractured. If the rib fractured is a single rib, pain relief is usually the only treatment necessary. The intact rib on each side of the fractured rib stabilizes the fracture and keeps it in alignment for healing.

Fractures of Ribs 9–12. These fractures arouse suspicion of the possibility of laceration and/or rupture of the spleen and liver.

Specific Treatment and Nursing Interventions: The objective is to relieve the pain of fractured ribs without compromising ventilatory efficiency. Intercostal nerve block is most efficient in relieving pain, without interfering with coughing, sighing, and deep breathing. Bronchial hygiene and physical therapy are often used. Binders should not be used at all because they decrease excursion over a wide area of the chest. This predisposes the patient to hypoxemia and atelectasis.

Flail Chest. If two or more adjacent ribs have segmental fractures (fractures at two or more sites on the same rib), the involved portion of the chest wall may be so unstable that it will move paradoxically or opposite to the rest of the chest wall when the patient breathes. This is known as a flail chest or flail segment (Figure 7-2). The flail chest may be especially severe if it is associated with a transverse fracture of the sternum.

Symptoms: Symptoms of flail chest include rapid, shallow respirations, cyanosis, severe chest wall pain, shock, bony crepita-

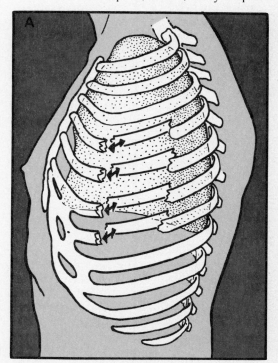

Figure 7-2a. Flail chest segment.

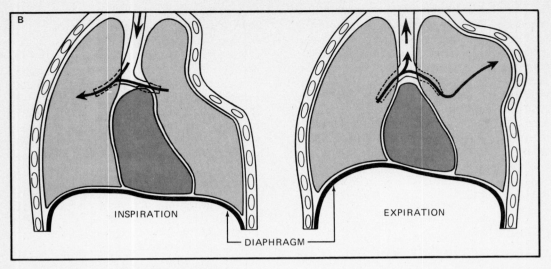

Figure 7-2b. The mechanics of flail chest.

tion at the site of fracture, and paradoxical chest movement. There may be signs of pulmonary contusion. It is quite common for the pulmonary status to progress to ARDS. Mortality is high.

Treatment and Nursing Interventions: Specific treatment is to stabilize the flail segment and to restore more normal breathing. In an emergency, anything can be used to stabilize the chest wall and help immobilize the segment—sandbags, hands, and so on. Hospital care is usually intubation, positive pressure ventilation, and PEEP as indicated.

Fracture of the Sternum. Sternal fracture is suspected when there is paradoxical movement of the anterior chest wall. It may be stabilized with traction or with endotracheal intubation, mechanical ventilation, and PEEP.

Nursing Intervention: A major nursing function is to explain that the endotracheal tube and ventilator are temporary *and* that while the tube is in place, the patient cannot talk. A communication system acceptable to the patient MUST be established. Blinking of the eyes once for yes and twice for no, squeezing the hand in the same pattern, or if the patient is capable and literate, writing may be the method of choice. Questions for the patient must be simple and answerable by yes or no unless the patient can write. The nurse call bell placed in the patient's hand may relieve anxiety when the nurse must leave the patient for a minute.

Lung Contusion. This may occur as the result of blunt chest trauma or penetrating lung trauma. Pulmonary contusion is damage to the lung parenchyma, resulting in localized edema and hemorrhage. Vehicular accidents are the most common cause of lung contusion since the chest hits the steering wheel during an accident and compresses the lung against the thoracic cage, the sternum, and/or the vertebrae. It is assumed that the pressure of striking the steering wheel compresses the thoracic cage, diminishing its size and compressing the lungs due to the increased intrathoracic pressure. As the pressure from hitting the steering wheel decreases, the thoracic cage increases in size, decreasing the intrathoracic pressure and the pressure on the lung parenchyma. This allows expansion of the lung parenchyma (under pressure), rupturing capillaries and resulting in hemorrhage. Figure 7-3 shows the mechanics of pulmonary contusion and the consequences.

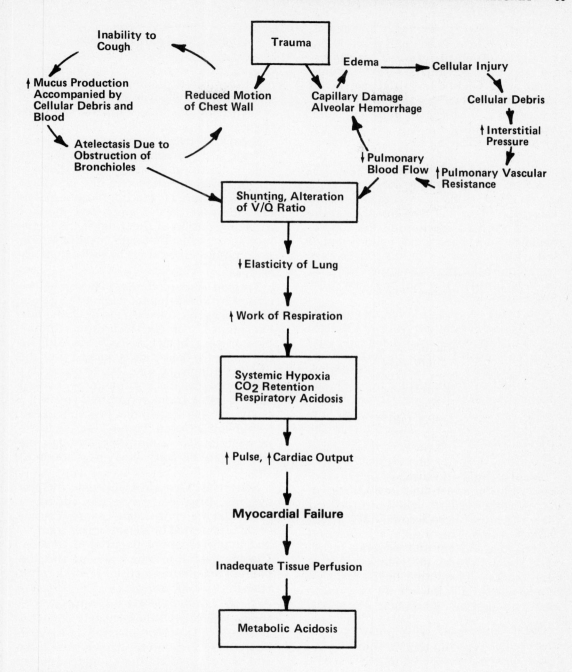

Figure 7-3.   Mechanics of pulmonary contusion.

Diagnosis: The diagnosis of pulmonary contusion due to blunt trauma is difficult since symptoms may not occur for from 4 to 72 hours posttrauma. X-rays may be normal or may reveal a complete "white out" de-pending upon the severity of the trauma and the time elapsed since the trauma was sustained.

Symptoms: Depending upon the severity of the trauma, symptoms almost always include tachypnea, tachycardia, and blood-tinged secretions. The cough reflex is impaired, resulting in retained secretions, and rales can normally be heard throughout all lung fields due to retained secretions. Arterial blood gases reveal a decreased Pa_{CO_2} and P_{O_2}. As hypoventilation progresses, there is an increase in the $A - aDO_2$, indicating severe respiratory failure.

Treatment and Nursing Interventions: The objectives of treating lung contusion are a patent airway, adequate oxygenation, and restoration of normal lung function. If the contusion is mild, monitoring and supplemental oxygen by mask may be sufficient. If deterioration occurs with this conservative treatment, many physicians prefer to treat the lung contusion as ARDS to arrest the progressive deterioration.

Controversy exists over the use of steroids and crystalloid (Ringer's lactate) versus colloid (Dextran, Plasmanate, etc.) fluid replacement. Since moderate-to-severe pulmonary contusions are often accompanied by multisystem injuries, the treatment must be balanced. If the vascular system needs fluid, a respirator with the use of PEEP can control the fluid in the lungs and thus prevent cardiovascular compromise.

Nasotracheal suctioning, aggressive chest physiotherapy, and humidification may help the patient expel secretions and allow the nurse more accurate assessment of the situation. The onset of agitation and anxiety may indicate the presence of hypoxia and may be a first sign of impending deterioration. A fever may be the first sign of infection, and culture of the sputum to identify a specific organism is warranted.

Chest Contusions. These may occur as the result of a penetrating injury as well as a blunt injury. Penetration of the parietal pleura or lung parenchyma by a sharp rib edge or a knife will cause both a contusion and a pneumothorax or hemothorax.

Simple Closed Pneumothorax. This can be a result of blunt or penetrating trauma resulting in subcutaneous air buildup in the pleural cavity, decreasing vital capacity. Diagnosis is by physical exam and chest x-ray.

Symptoms: These include dyspnea and restlessness (classic signs), cardiac pain radiating throughout the chest, diminished or absent breath sounds on the affected side, decreased chest wall movement, signs of increasing respiratory distress, and tracheal shift toward the UNAFFECTED side.

Specific Treatment: If the patient is symptomatic, a chest tube is inserted in the second or third intercostal space at the *midclavicular line* to drain out the air. Chest tubes are sutured in place and connected to an underwater seal. Daily x-rays monitor the re-expansion of the lung. If the pneumothorax is small enough, needle aspiration or thoracentesis may be sufficient treatment.

Tension Pneumothorax. These may be caused by blunt trauma tearing the pleura or by iatrogenic causes. This is a bona fide emergency. Air can accumulate in the pleural space, but it CANNOT ESCAPE! As the patient inhales, air is sucked into the pleura through the tear. As the patient begins to exhale, the torn pleura is "sucked back" against the parenchyma, creating a one-way valve system that prevents the air from being exhaled (Figure 7-4). On inspiration, more air is drawn in through the tear. Severe hemodynamic imbalances occur.

Symptoms: General symptoms include dyspnea, progressive cyanosis, and chest pain. On the *affected* side, symptoms include diminished or absent breath sounds, and hyperressonant percussion sounds. The mediastinum, the trachea, and the point of maximum intensity (PMI) all shift *away from the affected side.*

Specific Treatment: Air under tension in the pleural cavity is immediately removed. A large (14G) needle is inserted midclavicular in the second and third intercostal space and aimed towards the shoulder (Figure 7-5). The chest tube is usually connected to a water seal or suction drainage. The insertion site of the tube is covered with a sterile dressing. Once the immediate crisis is over, x-rays are used to determine if the chest tube is properly positioned and/or if additional tubes are indicated.

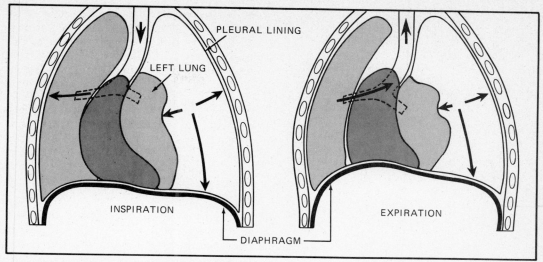

Figure 7-4.   Tension pneumothorax mechanics.

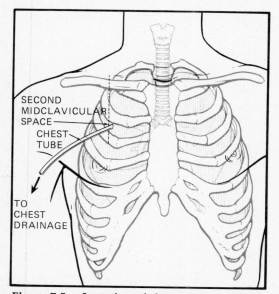

Figure 7-5.   Insertion of chest tube for tension pneumothorax.

Hemothorax. This may develop from blunt or penetrating chest trauma, or iatrogenic causes. The two major effects of a hemothorax are the accumulation of blood in the lungs, collapsing alveoli, and systemic hypovolemia.

Symptoms: The symptoms of a hemothorax depend upon the size of the blood accumulation. Small amounts of blood (400 ml or less) will cause minimal symptoms and minimal chest x-ray changes. Larger amounts of blood usually present signs of shock including tachycardia, tachypnea, hypotension, and nervousness. Breath sounds may be diminished or absent, and there is dullness to percussion.

Treatment and Nursing Interventions: Small hemothoraces may resolve spontaneously because of low pulmonary system pressure and the presence of thromboplastin in the lungs. Large hemothoraces are treated with the insertion of one or more chest tubes in the fifth or sixth intercostal space in the *midaxillary* line (Figure 7-6). The chest tube is sutured in place and covered with a sterile dressing after connection to an underwater seal with suction. Severe or uncontrollable hemothoraces may require a thoracotomy to arrest the bleeding.

It is now controversial to "milk" chest tubes every hour to prevent occlusion due to the presence of fibrin. "Milking" the tubes may increase intrathoracic pressures. Monitoring the patient's ability to expel secretions and suctioning when necessary are important in preventing hypoxia and atelectasis. Bronchial hygiene and aggressive chest physical therapy will help avoid infection. Analgesic medications will make these nursing procedures more tolerable for the patient. Sputum cultures should be

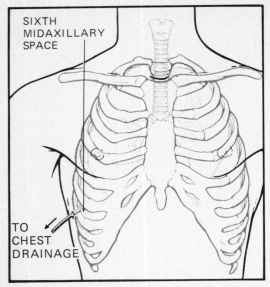

Figure 7-6.   Insertion of chest tube for hemothorax.

performed if fever develops. Psychological support of the patient and reassurances that the tubes are only temporary will help decrease the patient's anxiety.

Open Chest Injury

Open Sucking Chest Injuries. These occur as the result of blunt, penetrating, or deceleration forces. As the chest wall is opened, due to the injury, air rushes in and collapses the exposed lung. The mediastinum is pushed towards the opposite lung, preventing it from functioning normally. Unless rapidly corrected, severe and often fatal hemodynamic compromise occurs.

Open Tension Pneumothorax. This is the presenting problem in "sucking chest wounds" (Figure 7-7). Immediate treatment consists of covering the wound. Vaseline gauze is the covering of choice, but a hand, towel, or anything similar will suffice until appropriate treatment can be obtained.

Symptoms: The symptoms of open tension pneumothorax are obviously the appearance of the chest wall *and* the distinctive sound of air being sucked into the chest. The chest wall appears to "cave-in" or to have been pushed in at the injury site. The patient has dyspnea, tachycardia, hypoxia, and is usually hyperventilating severely. Subcutaneous emphysema is present and spreads very rapidly.

Treatment and Nursing Interventions: Treatment is to stop the inrushing air as described. Once this has been accomplished, chest tubes are inserted to drain the air if the wound is small. If the wound is large, thoracotomy will be required to debride the wound and repair the damage from the injury.

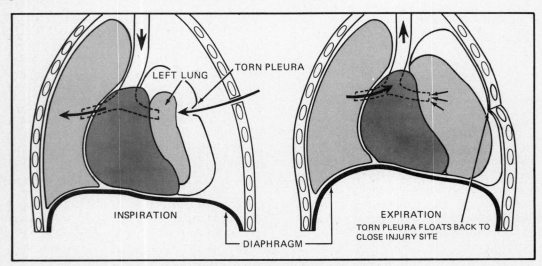

Figure 7-7.   Open tension pneumothorax ("sucking chest wound").

Nursing interventions include close monitoring for signs of increasing respiratory distress, extension of the pneumothorax, and possible cardiac involvement previously undetected.

Suctioning may be required to prevent atelectasis and hypoxia, and to decrease the chance of infection from retained secretions. In addition to the pneumothorax, a hemothorax may develop requiring immediate treatment if the patient is deteriorating and/or going into shock. Nursing care of the chest tubes and psychological support are the same as for patients with closed pneumothoraces.

Visceral Injuries

The most common visceral injury is pulmonary contusion, which was covered under closed chest injury. The next most common visceral injury is pulmonary laceration, which results in pneumothoraces and was covered under closed chest injury. If the force of the injury is sufficient to lacerate the lungs, cardiac injury is quite likely to have occurred.

Cardiac Contusion. This is the most common blunt injury to the heart. It is only rarely fatal. Signs and symptoms are the same as for myocardial ischemia and/or infarction.[1] Specific treatment is to monitor cardiac status with daily electrocardiograms since some ST and T wave changes may not become apparent for up to 48 hours, and to treat dysrhythmias as they occur.

Severe visceral injury may result in delayed cardiac rupture, ventricular septal defect (VSD), and ventricular aneurysm, all of which would receive conventional treatment.

Symptoms: These include angina-like chest pain, tachycardia, and after some time lapse, a pericardial friction rub.

Cardiac Rupture. This is a blunt trauma injury and is the most common cause of death. In sequence of frequency of rupture, it is right ventricle, left ventricle, right atrium, and left atrium. There is no treatment for cardiac rupture.

[1]Shires TG: Care of the Trauma Patient, 2nd ed. New York: McGraw-Hill, p. 270, 1979

Valvular Injury. This is a blunt trauma injury. The aortic valve is the most commonly injured valve. Signs and symptoms are regurgitation and congestive heart failure. Specific treatment could include valve replacement or the normal medical treatment for congestive heart failure.

Cardiac Tamponade. This may result from blunt or penetrating trauma. Blood gets into the pericardial sac, but cannot get out. As more blood enters the sac, more pressure is placed against the heart, decreasing venous return and cardiac output (Figure 7-8).

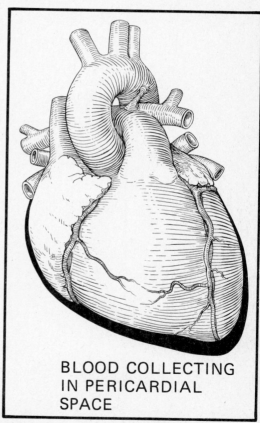

BLOOD COLLECTING IN PERICARDIAL SPACE

Figure 7-8.   Cardiac tamponade.

Signs and Symptoms: Beck defined a triad of symptoms indicating cardiac tamponade. They are hypotension, muffled or distant heart sounds, and distended neck veins. Additional clues are a falling systolic blood pressure, narrow pulse pressure, pulsus paradoxus (more than a 10 degree drop in systolic blood pressure during inspiration and expiration), elevated central venous pressure, and various degrees of shock.

Treatment and Nursing Intervention: The objective of treatment is to confirm the diagnosis *and* relieve the tamponade. This is best accomplished by a pericardiocentesis. Anesthesia is achieved with xylocaine, and then a three-inch spinal or a cardiac needle is introduced at a 35 degree angle in the right paraxiphoid space (Figure 7-9). An electrocardiographic lead is attached to the needle. This will show by cardiac monitoring if the needle tip enters the myocardium (S-T segment elevation). The needle can be withdrawn slightly and the diagnosis confirmed by aspiration of pericardial fluid (pericardiocentesis). This also relieves symptoms *if* it is a slowly developing tamponade. If pericardiocentesis does not relieve the tamponade, thoracotomy for direct repair of the pericardial wound is indicated.

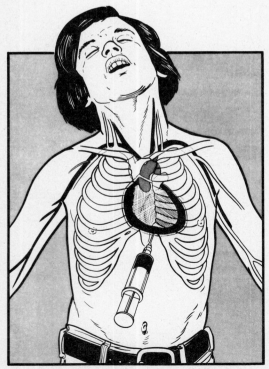

Figure 7-9.   Paraxiphoid approach to pericardiocentesis.

Nursing interventions include monitoring of the respiratory and cardiovascular systems especially closely for early signs of deterioration, assisting with preparations for the pericardiocentesis and the procedure itself, providing emotional support for the patient, and continuing close monitoring after the procedure for recurring signs of tamponade.

Diaphragmatic Rupture and/or Herniation. This is associated with both blunt and penetrating trauma. It is almost always accompanied by multisystem injuries. Ninty percent of the time, the left hemidiaphragm is the one injured. (Perhaps the more solid liver protects the right hemidiaphragm.)

Signs and Symptoms: These include marked or increasing respiratory distress, severe shoulder pain on the *same* side as the tear (due to air entering the thoracic cavity), an inability to insert a nasogastric tube (it cannot pass the kinked esophagus), and increasing signs of cardiopulmonary collapse. The immediate result of a significant tear in the diaphragm is the herniation of the abdominal contents into the thoracic cavity. Bowel sounds heard in the chest are pathognomonic of diaphragmatic rupture and herniation.

Diagnosis: The diagnosis is established if bowel sounds are heard in the chest. X-ray may reveal an elevated, arched shadow of a high left hemidiaphragm, a shift of the heart and mediastinum to the right, shadows appearing above the diaphragm, and abnormal air/fluid levels. Diagnosis is aided by water-soluble contrast studies and fiberoptic endoscopy.

Treatment and Nursing Interventions: Immediate treatment is to establish adequate respiratory function. This is most frequently accomplished by endotracheal intubation and mechanical respiration. Stabilizing a patient in shock prior to surgery may or may not be possible, depending upon the severity of the rupture. Definitive therapy consists of surgical repair of the torn diaphragm and replacement of the abdominal organs in the abdominal cavity. Gastrointestinal obstruction and/or bleeding is treated by conventional methods.

The nursing intervention of the highest priority is to monitor the patient's respiratory status to ensure adequate oxygenation. Cardiovascular monitoring is the next priority since the increased pressure and contents of the thoracic cavity will usually cause marked hemodynamic compromise, and cardiovascular collapse is not uncommon. Attempts to decrease the patient's anxiety by assuring him or her that the endotracheal tube is temporary and by establishing a means of communicating with the patient will provide much needed emotional support.

Esophageal Perforation. Esophageal perforation is due to penetrating injuries or iatrogenic causes. Perforation is suspected when there is posterior injury to the mediastinum or an unexplainable pneumothorax. Early diagnosis and treatment may be life-saving, while a delayed or missed diagnosis may cause permanent disability or death.

The possibility of severe morbidity and mortality is related to the degree of contamination, the site of the perforation, and the delay in diagnosis and initiation of treatment.

Diagnosis: A definitive diagnosis is made by having the patient swallow a water soluble contrast medium under fluoroscopy, which will reveal any esophageal tear or leak. Chest x-ray may reveal a widening mediastinum, rib fractures, pleural effusions, pulmonary contusion, and/or hydropneumothorax among other things.

Symptoms: These include most commonly pain, choking, hoarseness, dysphagia, dyspnea, and upper abdominal pain. Stridor, decreased breath sounds, cyanosis, or shock not consistent with the apparent degree of injury suggests an esophageal tear.

Treatment and Nursing Interventions: Specific treatment includes insertion of a nasogastric tube, endotracheal intubation, and surgical repair of the tear *if* diagnosis is made within 6–12 hours. After that timelapse, edema, necrosis of tissue, and infection will probably prevent primary healing since suturing the tear may well not hold. In these instances, the esophagus may be ligated above the tear and oral secretion drainage achieved with a cervical esophagostomy. The esophagus is also ligated below the tear and stomach drainage is achieved by a gastrostomy. The tear then heals by secondary intention, and at a later date, the esophagus may be reopened and reconstructed if necessary. Massive broad-spectrum antibiotic therapy is maintained until the situation has resolved.

Nursing interventions include close monitoring of the respiratory system since it is frequently damaged and usually infected from the esophageal contents. Secretions must be continuously drained both from the mouth and the endotracheal tube. Infection is monitored by the administration of antibiotics and the nurses' report of the patient's response to them. Nutritionally, it is important to maintain a positive nitrogen balance to promote healing; this may be accomplished by gastrostomy feedings or hyperalimentation. Physical therapy, as soon as tolerated by the patient, will help avoid musculoskeletal problems. Passive range of motion progressing to active and resistive exercise is the usual sequence of physical therapy. Psychological support of the patient and reassurances that the situation will be temporary will help alleviate the patient's fears and anxieties.

Tracheobronchial Injuries. This type of injury may be the result of blunt or penetrating trauma. Shearing forces are the cause of these injuries since the trachea is "fixed" (attached) in the cervical outlet and the thoracic inlet, whereas the rest of the airways are not as fixed in the chest and significant movement is likely. The movement of non-fixed airways will result in a shearing effect on the portion of the airways that is fixed and secured to other tissues.

Diagnosis: Diagnosis of a tracheal or bronchus tear is made by careful bronchoscopy which allows the physician not only to identify the source of the tear, but also to rule out abnormalities in the trachea and bronchus and plan the best surgical approach for repairing the tear.

Symptoms: Symptoms include failure of a lung to re-expand after proper treatment of pneumothorax, increasing subcutaneous emphysema, occasionally hemoptysis, the development of a pneumomediastinum, and a deterioration of the patient's condition that is out of proportion to the known injuries.

Treatment and Nursing Interventions: Treatment consists of intubation, ventilatory support, and surgical repair of the injury.

Nursing interventions include close monitoring of the respiratory and cardiovascular systems. Control of respiratory secretions to prevent hypoxia, atelectasis, and infection is of paramount importance. Alterations in the cardiovascular status may indicate fresh bleeding and impending shock. If not in a coma, the patient must have a communication system with the nurse to alert the nurse of his or her needs and to decrease the patient's fear and anxiety. It is important to stress to the patient that the endotracheal tube is a temporary measure to help him or her breathe and will be removed as soon as possible. Knowledge that the removal of the tube will allow him or her to talk will help to reassure the patient.

Aortic Rupture. This injury is the result of blunt trauma, usually a deceleration injury, and most patients with this injury die immediately; however, some 10–12% survive to reach a hospital because a tamponade occurs around the rupture. This allows some blood to leave the left ventricle and pass beyond the distal end of the rupture.

Diagnosis: Aortic rupture is diagnosed by aortogram. X-ray may reveal a widened mediastinum, which indicates a suspicion of aortic rupture. The aortogram will identify the area of rupture. Figure 7-10 identifies the most common sites of aortic rupture.

Symptoms: Symptomology may include an increased blood pressure and pulse in the upper extremities, a decreased blood pressure and pulse in the lower extremities, and the x-ray picture of a widened mediastinum. Shortness of breath, weakness, chest or back pain, and varied abnormalities involving the lower extremities may be present.

Treatment and Nursing Interventions: Treatment consists of thoracotomy to repair the

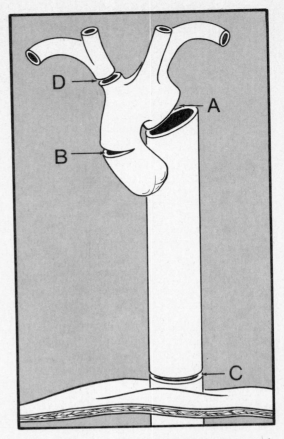

Figure 7-10.   Sites of aortic rupture. (A = arch of aorta, B = area just above aortic valve, C = end of thoracic aorta, D = subclavian vein. A is the most common, D is the least common.)

rupture. If the thoracotomy cannot be performed immediately, the patient is medically treated as a patient with dissecting aortic aneurysm until surgery.

Nursing interventions include monitoring the respiratory, cardiovascular, neurologic, and renal systems since these suffer first due to the decreased blood flow. Sodium nitroprusside is usually administered until the patient can be taken to surgery. Nursing care of the patient on ventilatory support and in need of close monitoring before and after surgery applies to the patient with a ruptured aorta. Emotional support should be given as previously listed in this section on chest injuries.

Pulmonary Bibliography

Anderson JM: Occupational Lung Disease: An Introduction. New York: American Lung Association, 1979

Borg N, Mikas DL, Stark J, Williams SM (eds): Core Curriculum for Critical Care Nursing, 2nd ed. American Association of Critical-Care Nurses. Philadelphia: W. B. Saunders, pp. 2–76, 1981

Bushnell SS: Respiratory Intensive Care Nursing. Boston: Little, Brown and Co., 1973

*Divertie MB, Petty TL: Adult respiratory distress syndrome. In Current Concepts, a Scope publication. Kalamazoo, MI: The Upjohn Co., 1979

Freitag JJ, Miller LW (eds): Manual of Medical Therapeutics, 23rd ed. Boston: Little, Brown and Co., pp. 143–174, 1979

Genton E: Pulmonary embolism. In Chung EK (ed): Quick Reference to Cardiovascular Disease. Philadelphia: J. B. Lippincott, pp. 177–184, 1977

Grant JCB, Basmajian JV: Grant's Method of Anatomy by Regions, 7th ed. Baltimore: Williams and Wilkins, pp. 463–499, 1965

*Guyton AC: Textbook of Medical Physiology, 6th ed. Philadelphia: W. B. Saunders, pp. 289–297, 476–538, 1981

*Huber GL: Arterial blood gas and acid-base physiology. In Current Concepts, a Scope publication. Kalamazoo, MI: The Upjohn Co., 1978

Hudak CM, Lohr TS, Gallo BM (eds): Critical Care Nursing, 3rd ed. Philadelphia: J. B. Lippincott, pp. 175–256, 1982

Jay SH, Stonehill RB (eds): Manual of Pulmonary Procedure. Philadelphia: W. B. Saunders, 1980

Kinney MR, Dear CB, Vorrman DMN (eds): AACN's Clinical Reference for Critical-Care Nursing. New York: McGraw-Hill, pp. 15–32, 363–387, 485–542, 1981

Morris JD: Patterns of thoracic trauma. In Frey C (ed): Initial Management of the Trauma Patient. Philadelphia: Lea and Febiger, pp. 311–327, 1976

Morris JF (ed): Chronic Obstructive Pulmonary Disease. New York: American Lung Association, pp. 60–106, 1977

*Morrison ML: Respiratory Intensive Care Nursing, 2nd ed. Boston: Little, Brown and Co., 1979

Muir BL: Pathophysiology: An Introduction to the Mechanisms of Disease. New York: John Wiley and Sons, 1980

Naclerio EA: Chest trauma. In Clinical Symposia, Vol. 22, No. 3. Summit, NJ: CIBA Pharmaceutical Co., 1970

*A Programmed Approach to Anatomy and Physiology of the Respiratory System. Bowie, MD: Robert J. Brady Co., 1972

Rellar LB, Sahn SA, Schrier RW (eds): Clinical Internal Medicine. Boston: Little, Brown and Co., pp. 58–121, 1979

*Said SI: Metabolic and endocrine functions of the lungs. In Current Concepts, a Scope publication. Kalamazoo, MI: The Upjohn Co., 1979

*Shapiro BA, Harrison RA, Trout CA: Clinical Application of Respiratory Care. Chicago: Year Book Medical Publishers, 1975

Traver GA (ed): Symposium on care in respiratory disease. In The Nursing Clinics of North America, Vol. 9, No. 1. Philadelphia: W. B. Saunders, pp. 97–206, March 1974

West HB: Respiratory Physiology—The Essentials. Baltimore: Williams and Wilkins, 1974

Wilson RF (ed): Principals and techniques of critical care. In Critical Care Manual, Vol. 1, Sec. F. Kalamazoo, MI: The Upjohn Co., pp. 5–13, 1977

Wilson RF, Steiger Z, Hirsch D, Thoms N, Arbulu A: Thoracic injuries. In Walt AJ, Wilson RF (eds): Management of Trauma: Pitfalls and Practice. Philadelphia: Lea and Febiger, pp. 303–321, 1975

Worthington L: What those blood gases can tell you. In RN, Vol. 42, No. 10, pp. 23–27, October 1979

*Zarren HS: The Respiratory System: Disease, Diagnosis, Treatment. Bowie, MD: Robert J. Brady Co., 1977

II

The Cardiovascular System

8

Cardiac Anatomy

Learning Objectives

By the end of this chapter, the nurse will be able to:

1. State the two basic functions of the heart.
2. State the location and boundary marks of the heart.
3. Describe the fibrous skeleton and identify its components.
4. List the four layers of the heart wall.
5. Identify two functions of the pericardium.
6. Define papillary muscle and chordae tendineae.
7. State the relationship between papillary muscle and the chordae tendineae.
8. Define the following parts of the cardiac muscle cell and state the function of each.
   a. Sarcomere
   b. Sarcolemma
   c. Intercalated discs
   d. Sarcoplasma
   e. T-tubule
   f. Sarcoplasmic reticulum
   g. Actin
   h. Myosin
   i. Troponin
   j. Tropomyosin
9. List the four chambers of the heart.
10. Identify three sources of blood entering the right atrium.
11. State the function and describe the structure of the right ventricle.
12. Identify the source of blood entering the left atrium.
13. Explain the function and describe the structure of the left ventricle.
14. List the four valves in the heart.
15. Compare the structure of the arterioventricular valves and the semilunar valves.
16. Trace the conduction system of the heart.
17. Trace the coronary, pulmonary, and systemic circulatory systems.

There are two basic functions of the heart. The first function is to circulate blood throughout the body without interruption. The second function is to adjust the blood flow in response to many factors in the body. The heart is superbly designed to accomplish these functions.

Normal Location and Size of the Heart

The heart lies in the mediastinum, with the lungs on either side and the diaphragm below. If one looks at a frontal (anterior) view, the heart resembles a triangle (Figure 8-1). The base of the heart is parallel to the right edge of the sternum, whereas the lower right point of the triangle represents the apex of the heart. The apex is usually at the left midclavicular line at the fifth intra-

clavicular space. The average adult heart is about 5 inches long and 3½ inches wide. This corresponds to an average man's clenched fist. The heart weighs about 2 grams for each pound of ideal body weight.

Normal Anatomy of the Heart

The heart is supported by a fibrous skeleton (Figure 8-2) composed of dense connective tissue. This fibrous skeleton connects the four valve rings (annuli) of the heart, that is, the tricuspid, mitral, pulmonic, and aortic valves. Attached to the superior (top) surface of this fibrous skeleton are the right and left atria, the pulmonary artery, and the aorta. Attached to the inferior (lower) surface of the fibrous skeleton are the right and left ventricles and the mitral and tricuspid valve cusps.

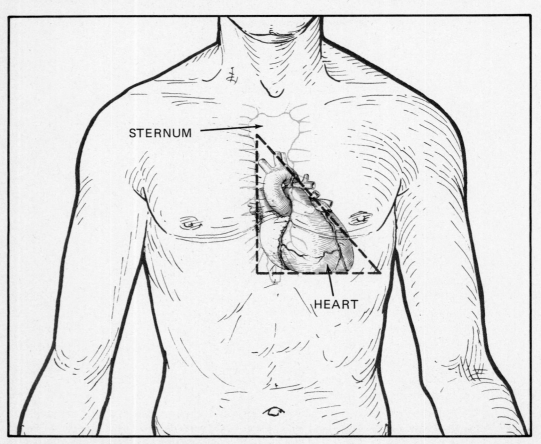

STERNUM

HEART

Figure 8-1.   Frontal view of the heart.

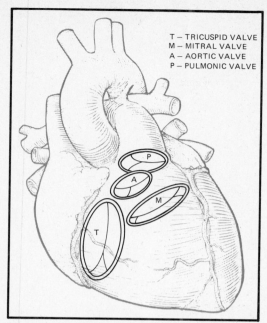

Figure 8-2.   Fibrous skeleton of the heart (frontal view).

T — TRICUSPID VALVE
M — MITRAL VALVE
A — AORTIC VALVE
P — PULMONIC VALVE

The heart can be studied as two parallel pumps: the right pump and the left pump. Each pump receives blood into its atrium. The blood flows from atria through a one-way valve into the ventricles. From each ventricle, blood is ejected into a circulatory system. (There are four circulatory systems in the body.) Although the right and left heart have major differences, the gross anatomy of each is similar. Structural differences will be examined for each individual chamber.

Structure of the Heart Wall

The heart per se is enclosed in a fibrous sac called the pericardium. The pericardium is composed of two layers. The fibrous pericardium is the outer layer that helps support the heart. The inside layer is a smooth fibrous membrane called the parietal (serous) pericardium.

Next to the parietal serous layer of the pericardium is a visceral layer, which is actually the outer heart surface. It is most often termed the epicardium. Between the epicardium and the parietal pericardium are 10–20 milliliters of fluid which prevents

friction during heart contraction and relaxation.

The myocardium is the muscle mass of the heart composed of cardiac muscle, which has characteristics of both smooth and skeletal muscles. The endocardium is the inner surface of the heart wall. It is a membranous covering that lines all the heart chambers and the valves. The endocardium is simple squamous epithelium.

Papillary muscles originate in the ventricular endocardium and attach to chordae tendineae (Figure 8-3). The chordae tendineae attach to the inferior surface of the triscupid and mitral valve cusps to enable the valves to function. The papillary muscles are in parallel alignment to the ventricular wall.

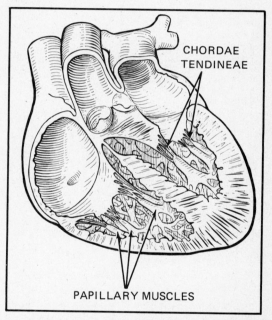

CHORDAE TENDINEAE

PAPILLARY MUSCLES

Figure 8-3.   Papillary muscles and chordae tendineae.

Cardiac Muscle Cells

The sarcomere (Figure 8-4) is the contracting unit of the myocardium. The outer covering of the sarcomere is the sarcolemma, which surrounds the muscle fiber. The sarcolemma covers a muscle fiber which is composed of thick and thin fibers often col-

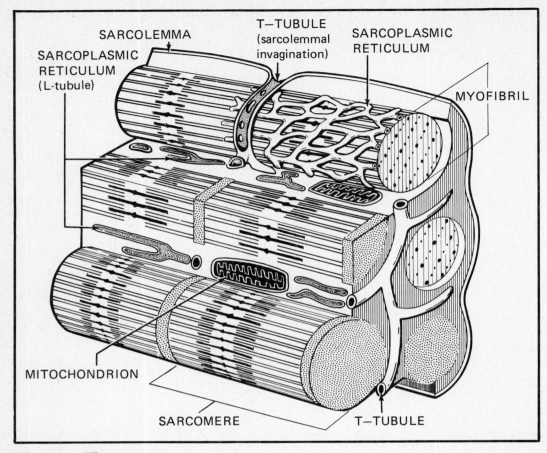

Figure 8-4.   The sarcomere.

lectively called myofibrils. Sarcomeres are separated from each other by a thickening of the sarcolemma at the *ends* of the sarcomere. These thickened ends are called intercalated discs and are actively involved in cardiac contraction. Each sarcomere has a centrally placed nucleus surrounded by sarcoplasma.

The sarcolemma invaginates into the sarcomere at regular intervals, resulting in a vertical penetration through the muscle fibrils coming into contact with both the thick and thin fibrils. These invaginations form the T-tubules. Closely related, but not continuous with the T-tubule system, is the sarcoplasmic reticulum. The sarcoplasmic reticulum (containing calcium ions) is an intracellular network of channels sur-

rounding the myofibrils. These channels comprise the longitudinal (L-tubule) system of the myofibrils.

Myofibrils are thick and thin parts of the muscle fiber. Thick fibrils are myosin filaments. They have regularly placed projections which form calcium gates to the thin myofibrils. The thin myofibrils are actin. The myosin and actin myofibrils are arranged in specific parallel and hexagonal patterns (Figure 8-5). This arrangement of fibers forms a syncytium that results in *all* of the fibers depolarizing when even one fiber is depolarized. This is known as the "all or none" principle. All fibers depolarize *or* no fibers depolarize. Troponin and tropomyosin are regulatory proteins attached to or affecting actin. These thick and thin myofibrils slide back and forth over each other, resulting in contraction and relaxation of the sarcomeres and thus, the heart. The mechanisms of action will be covered in Chapter 9.

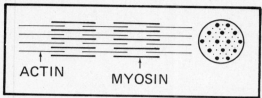

Figure 8-5. **Arrangement of myosin and actin myofibrils.**

Heart Chambers

There are four chambers in the heart (Figure 8-6). The atria are superior to the ventricles and are separated from them by valves. The right atrium and ventricle are separated from the left atrium and ventricle by the atrial and ventricular septum.

RIGHT ATRIUM

The right atrium (R.A.) is a thin-walled chamber exposed to very low blood pressures. Systemic venous blood from the head, neck, and thorax enters the right atrium from the superior vena cava. Sys-

temic venous blood from the remainder of the body enters from the inferior vena cava. Venous blood from the heart itself enters the right atrium through the thesbian veins which drain into the coronary sinus. The coronary sinus is located on the medial atrial wall just above the tricuspid valve.

RIGHT VENTRICLE

The right ventricle (R.V.) is the pump for the right heart. The right ventricle contracts to pump *venous* blood into the pulmonary *artery* and to the lungs. The lungs are a low pressure system normally. The right ventricle is shaped and functions like a bellows to propel blood out during contraction.

LEFT ATRIUM

The left atrium (L.A.), just like the right, is thin-walled. Blood flowing passively from the low lung pressure area does not stress the walls of the left atrium. The left atrium receives *oxygenated* blood from the four pulmonary *veins*.

LEFT VENTRICLE

The left ventricle (L.V.) is the major "pump" for the entire body. As such, it must have thick, strong walls. To overcome the high pressure of the systemic circulation, the left ventricle is shaped like a cylinder. As it contracts (starting from the apex), it also narrows somewhat. This cylindrical shape provides strong physical forces to propel blood into the aorta with sufficient force to overcome the aortic valve pressure and the high systemic pressure.

HEART VALVES

There are two types of valves in the heart: the atrioventricular and the semilunar valves. All valves in the heart are unidirectional, unless they are not competent.

ATRIOVENTRICULAR VALVES

The atrioventricular valves of the heart are the tricuspid and the mitral valves. These valves allow blood to flow from the atria

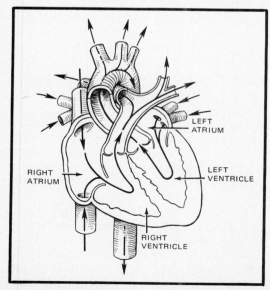

Figure 8-6. **Four chambers of the heart.**

into the ventricles during atrial contraction and ventricular diastole. Mnemonics may help you remember which valve is on which side of the heart. Consider the following: "L" and "M" come together in the alphabet and in the heart. The left heart contains the mitral valve. Likewise, "R" and "T" are close in the alphabet. The right heart contains the tricuspid valve. Both the mitral and the tricuspid valves have two *large opposing* leaflets and small intermediary leaflets at each end.

MITRAL VALVE

The mitral valve's two large leaflets are not quite equal in size (Figure 8-7). The chordae tendineae from adjacent leaflets are inserted upon the same papillary muscles. This physical feature helps to assure complete closure of the valve. When the mitral valve is open, the valve, chordae tendineae, and the papillary muscle look like a funnel.

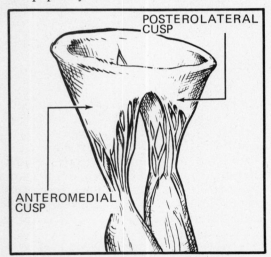

Figure 8-7.   Side view of the mitral valve.

TRICUSPID VALVE

The tricuspid valve differs from the mitral valve in that it has one larger leaflet than the mitral valve. Also, the tricuspid valve has three papillary muscles instead of two. Otherwise, these structures and the functions of these valves are similar.

SEMILUNAR VALVES

The semilunar valves (Figure 8-8) of the heart are the aortic and the pulmonary valves. Each has three symmetrical valve cusps to provide for complete opening without stretching of the valve. The pulmonary valve is located between the right ventricle and the pulmonary artery. The aortic valve is located between the left ventricle and the aorta.

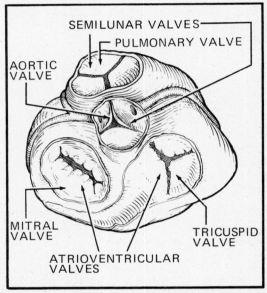

Figure 8-8.   The semilunar valves and the atrioventricular valves (posterior view).

The Normal Conduction System of the Heart

The conduction of an electrical impulse normally follows an orderly, repetitive pattern from the right atrium, through the heart, and into the myocardium where the impulse usually results in ventricular contraction (Figure 8-9).

The sinoatrial (SA) node is at the junction of the superior vena cava and the right atrium. The SA node is a group of specialized heart cells that are self-excitatory. All self-excitatory cells have automaticity; that is, if the cells can excite themselves, they require NO stimulus and may excite them-

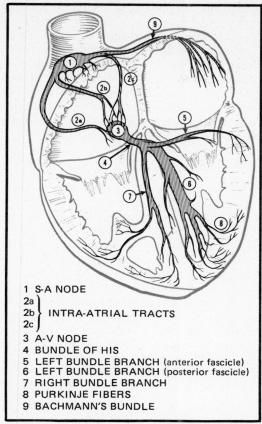

1 S-A NODE
2a
2b ⎬ INTRA-ATRIAL TRACTS
2c
3 A-V NODE
4 BUNDLE OF HIS
5 LEFT BUNDLE BRANCH (anterior fascicle)
6 LEFT BUNDLE BRANCH (posterior fascicle)
7 RIGHT BUNDLE BRANCH
8 PURKINJE FIBERS
9 BACHMANN'S BUNDLE

Figure 8-9.   Conduction system of the heart.

selves at will. This is termed "inherent automaticity." The SA node excites itself faster than any other cardiac cells under normal conditions. For this reason, the SA node becomes the heart's normal pacemaker.

Once the impulse originates in the SA node, it spreads through the atria along three paths called internodal tracts. The impulse continues from the internodal tracts into the atrioventricular junction. The area of the atrioventricular node (AV node) is located at the superior end of the junctional tissue. The AV node is located near the tricuspid valve ring just above the ventricular septum. There is a slight pause in the impulse at the upper portion of the AV node to allow for completion of atrial contraction. The impulse traverses the AV node, the junctional tissue, and then reaches the bundle of His.

The bundle of His carries the impulse to the bundle branches very quickly. The bundle of His divides into right and left bundle branches.

The left bundle branch (LBB) continues along the ventricular septum, dividing into two subdivisions called fascicles. The left anterior fascicle excites the anterior and superior surfaces of the left ventricle. The left posterior fascicle excites the posterior and inferior surfaces of the left ventricle. The right bundle branch (RBB) continues as a single branch to innervate the right ventricle.

Having passed through the bundle of His and the bundle branches, the impulse arrives at the Purkinje fibers, which spread into the ventricular myocardium. The impulse spread usually is followed by ventricular contraction, and thus the cycle repeats.

Disturbances in this conduction system will be reviewed as to the specific resulting dysrhythmias (Chapters 11 and 12).

Circulatory Systems of the Body

Circulatory paths can be remembered by the mnemonic that "a" for artery means "a" for away. ALL arteries carry blood, either arterial or venous (pulmonary) AWAY from the heart. Conversely, all veins carry blood either arterial (pulmonary) or venous TO the heart.

There are four circulatory systems in the body. The heart must pump blood through three of the four systems in the amount needed by the body to maintain optimal function. The four systems are the coronary, the pulmonary, the systemic, and the lymphatic systems. The lymphatic circulation will be covered in Chapter 35.

THE CORONARY CIRCULATION

The coronary circulatory system begins with the inflow of oxygenated blood into the coronary arteries. The opening of these arteries are located near the cusps of the aortic valve. These arteries fill during ventricular diastole, except after bypass surgery. After bypass surgery, these arteries fill during both diastole and systole with the blood present in the aorta.

The right coronary artery (RCA) supplies the posterior and inferior myocardium with oxygenated blood. The left coronary artery starts at the valve cusp as the left *main* coronary artery and bifurcates to form the left anterior descending (LAD) and the circumflex arteries. The LAD artery supplies the anterior and septal myocardium. The circumflex artery supplies the lateral myocardium. These arteries then follow the normal sequence of becoming arterioles, capillaries, venules, and veins as they course through the myocardium. The veins empty into thesbian veins which in turn empty into the coronary sinus. Blood from the coronary sinus joins the venous blood in the right atrium.

THE PULMONARY CIRCULATION

The pulmonary system is unique in that this is the only system (excluding the fetal) in which the pulmonary artery carries unoxygenated blood away from the heart to the lungs, and the four pulmonary veins carry oxygenated blood from the lungs to the left atrium. The right ventricle sends venous blood into the main pulmonary artery, which divides into the right and left pulmonary arteries. These arteries follow the normal blood vessel path, that is, arteries to arterioles to capillaries (where the blood becomes oxygenated) to venules to veins.

THE SYSTEMIC CIRCULATION

The aorta is the only artery that the left ventricle normally ejects blood into and it arches over the pulmonary artery. The aorta gives off many branches as it traverses down the body to bifurcate into the iliac arteries. All of the arteries follow the normal vessel paths. In the capillaries the blood surrenders oxygen and picks up carbon dioxide. The inferior and superior venae cavae are the final veins returning blood to the right atrium. Effects of the vessels on cardiac function will be covered in Chapters 9, 15, and 16.

9

Physiological and Mechanical Events of the Cardiac Cycle

Learning Objectives

By the end of this chapter, the nurse will be able to:

1. Explain the sliding action of myosin and actin.
2. State the function of troponin and tropomyosin.
3. Explain the mode of action of actin and myosin.
4. State two functions of calcium in cardiac contraction.
5. Explain the ion activity occurring in phase 0.
6. Explain the ion activity occurring in phase 1.
7. Explain the ion activity occurring in phase 2.
8. Explain the ion activity occurring in phase 3.
9. Explain the ion activity occurring in phase 4.
10. Define inotropism.
11. Explain the Frank-Starling law.
12. List three factors affecting inotropism.
13. Identify autonomic regulation of peripheral vessels.
14. Explain the baroreceptor control of peripheral vessels.
15. Explain chemoreceptor control of the peripheral vessels.
16. Define arterial pressure.
17. Identify six factors affecting arterial pressure.
18. List the three MAJOR influences on systemic blood pressure.
19. Define cardiac output.
20. Define stroke volume.
21. Define pulse pressure.
22. Explain autonomic control of the heart.
23. Explain atrial pressure curves in relation to cardiac blood flow.
24. Explain ventricular pressure curves in relation to cardiac blood flow.
25. Define eddy currents.

The study of physiology of the cardiac cycle examines the means in which the heart pumps blood and the various mechanisms which control the heart pump. Before looking at the heart as a whole, let us examine the contraction of a single sarcomere.

Contraction of the Sarcomere

The components of a single sarcomere were identified in Chapter 8. The sarcomeres are much like striated muscles, but they have far more mitochondria than striated *or* smooth muscles. The mitochondria provide the energy for the sarcomeres to contract. This energy is released by converting adenosine triphosphate (ATP) into adenosine diphosphate (ADP). This chemical change releases oxygen (aerobic condition) and provides energy. Energy *can* be produced by anaerobic conditions but not as efficiently.

In the sarcomere, thick (myosin) and thin (actin) fibrils are arranged side by side in parallel rows. The myosin fibrils have projections which make contact with actin at specific points. These contact points are referred to as calcium gates (Figure 9-1). During cardiac contraction, the myosin and actin slide together and overlap to as great

an extent as possible (Figure 9-2). (In the normal resting state, there is some overlapping of the myosin and actin fibrils.) Troponin and tropomyosin are protein rods interwoven around the actin fibril, having a regulatory effect upon the actin and its ability to connect with the calcium gates in the presence of calcium ions.

At the start of cellular excitation leading to a contraction, calcium ions (Ca^{++}) attach to troponin molecules around the actin fibril. This enables the projections (calcium gates) of the myosin fibril to attach to the actin. These projections twist around causing a sliding of the fibers over each other. The calcium is removed from the calcium gates by calcium pumps located throughout the sarcoplasmic reticulum. As soon as the calcium is removed, the myosin and actin fibers slide back to their original position. This process repeats, causing contraction and relaxation of the cardiac cell.

It is important to remember that calcium initiates and regulates the sarcomere depolarization and repolarization. Even though calcium ions initiate the sliding movement of the fibrils, calcium *alone* is not able to cause the contraction.

In addition to the presence of calcium, an exchange of ions (creating electrical energy) must occur during phases of depolarization

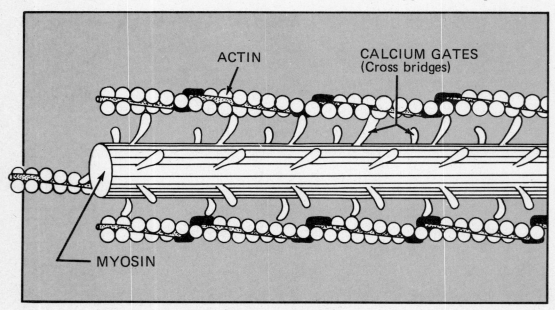

Figure 9-1.   Myosin and actin fibrils with calcium gates.

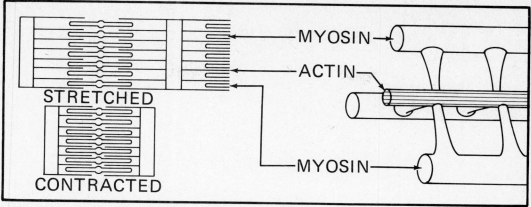

Figure 9-2.   Contraction of the myosin and actin fibrils.

and repolarization. This ionic exchange is mainly between sodium and potassium, which creates an ionic action potential. The exchange of chemical elements occurs across the semi-permeable cell membrane in three ways: filtration, osmosis, and diffusion (active or passive).

Action Potential of the Cardiac Cell

There are four phases of activity during the cardiac cell cycle. The exhange and concentration of ions differ in each phase. Mainly four ions are involved: sodium (Na^+), potassium (K^+), calcium (Ca^{++}), and chloride (Cl^-). Normally, there is more sodium, calcium, and chloride *outside* the cell, and more potassium *inside* the cell. Since all ions have an electrical charge, an electrical gradient is established. (In a state of ionic electrical neutrality, there is a relative impermeability of the cell membrane known as the resting potential.) The presence of an electrical gradient plus a chemical (ion) gradient and membrane selectivity establishes an action potential.

PHASE 0 (ZERO)

Due to the presence of sodium and potassium outside and inside the cell respectively, an electronegative gradient occurs. A depolarizing stimulus is caused by efflux of potassium from the cell, increasing the cell permeablility for sodium. Calcium ions in

the T-tubule and L-tubule systems of the sarcomere are at Ca^{++} gates on the cell membrane and "open" the gates for the influx of sodium. When this gradient reaches about -90 mV (millivolts) inside the cell, there is a rapid increase of the action potential (zero on Figure 9-3). The result of the depolarization stimulus is an increase in the cell permeability for sodium. As the sodium threshold (the point at which sodium moves most freely) is reached (about -55 mV), sodium rushes into the cell and depolarizes it. Actually, more sodium rushes in than the amount required to reach electrical neutrality (zero). The cell becomes electropositive at about $+20$–30 mV, causing a spike on the action potential diagram.

PHASE ONE

This is the spike phase of positive electrical charge. There is a brief period of *rapid repolarization* (tip of spike to #1 on Figure 9-3), which is probably due to a flow of chloride ions into the cell.

PHASE TWO

This is a plateau phase of repolarization. Calcium entering the cell and potassium leaving the cell balance each other, so there is no net electrical change and thus a flat line (plateau) appears. Sodium entry into the cell is almost completely inactivated. A slow movement of calcium into the cell begins (#2 on Figure 9-3). Also, a small

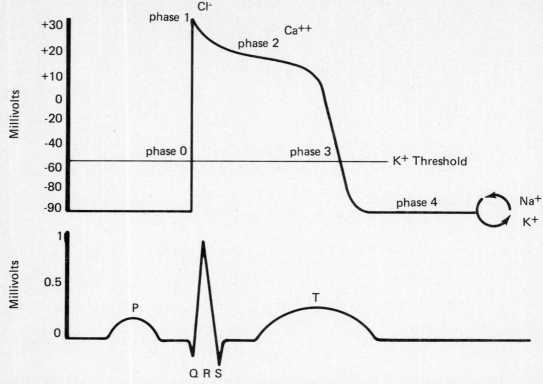

Figure 9-3.   Phases of the cardiac action potential and ion movement correlated with the EKG tracing.

amount of potassium begins leaving the cell at this point.

PHASE THREE

This is a rapid decline phase of repolarization (#3 on Figure 9-3). Potassium *loss* from the cell is greatest in this phase. This potassium loss returns the cell to electronegativity. Sodium and calcium currents are completely inactivated.

PHASE FOUR

This is the resting interval between action potentials (#4 on Figure 9-3). The sodium/potassium pumps (diffusely spread throughout the sarcomere) are the most active here in effecting an exchange of position of these ions across the cell membrane. Potassium continues to leave the cell, and when electronegativity reaches −90 mV, phase zero starts again if a stimulus occurs.

Variables Affecting Contractility

Inotropism is the ability of something to influence the contractility of muscle fibers. If the cardiac inotropic factor is positive, myocardial contractility will increase. If the cardiac inotropic factor is negative, myocardial contractility will decrease.

The *Frank-Starling law* is a basic principle of cardiac muscle function. Essentially, the Frank-Starling law (Figure 9-4) states that the more muscle fibers are stretched during diastole, the stronger the next contraction. This is true WITHIN LIMITS. Fibers can be streched only so far and for so long before they lose their resilience and ability to return to their prestretched length. Once this limit is reached, contractility decreases. Prior to this limit, certain factors (such as increased venous return) will improve cardiac contractility by increasing fiber length. Unfortunately, in clinical practice, the limit for the individual is not known before it is reached.

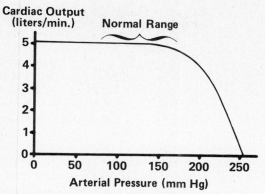

Figure 9-4.   The Frank-Starling law curve.

The greatest control one can exert on inotropy is in the use of drugs. Positive inotropic drugs include digitalis glycosides, calcium, isoproterenol hydrochloride (Isuprel®), and the catecholamine drugs. Negative inotropic drugs include quinidine sulfate (Quinidine®), propranolol hydrochloride (Inderal®), and the barbiturates.

The amount of oxygen and carbon dioxide in the blood affects the contractility of the heart. Elevation of carbon dioxide above 45 mm Hg and hypoxia (less than 50% oxygen saturation) both exert a negative inotropic effect, decreasing contractility of the heart.

Electrolyte disturbances alter cardiac inotropy. The most common are hyponatremia and hyperkalemia, which exert a negative effect, and hypercalcemia, which exerts a positive inotropic effect. A positive inotropic effect may NOT always be a desirable effect since increased contractility means an increased demand for oxygen and usually a faster heart rate, resulting in more cardiac work.

Myocardial infarction leaves scar tissue at the site of the infarction. Scar tissue has a negative inotropic effect because it limits the actual amount of myocardial tissue that can contract.

Changes in cardiac rate and rhythm may first exert a positive effect (an increase in rate means an increase in contractility) followed by a negative effect. If the rate is too fast for too long, the myocardium becomes exhausted and effective contractility decreases.

The autonomic nervous system has inotropic effects upon cardiac contractility. The sympathetic nervous system has a positive inotropic effect. The parasympathetic nervous system has a *negative* inotropic effect through the *vagus* nerve.

Control of Peripheral Blood Vessels

Peripheral blood vessel status may influence cardiac contraction and cardiac function by controlling the amount of blood returned to the heart. There are three proven controls of peripheral blood vessels and one hypothetical control.

1. Autonomic Regulation of Peripheral Vessels

The sympathetic nervous system has an adrenergic effect upon peripheral vessels. The norepinephrine released by the sympathetic system causes a vasoconstriction. This vasoconstriction prevents pooling of blood in the peripheral vessels and augments the return of blood to the heart.

The parasympathetic nervous system has a cholinergic effect upon peripheral vessels. Acetylcholine is released by the parasympathetic nervous system. This causes a vasodilatation of peripheral vessels. With dilatation, more blood can remain in the peripheral vessels, and less blood is returned to the heart.

2. Baroreceptor Control

Baroreceptors are also called pressoreceptors or stretch receptors since these areas respond to a stretching of arterial and venous vessel walls. These receptors are specialized cells located in the aortic arch, carotid sinus, atria, venae cavae, and pulmonary arteries. These receptor sites are responsive to mean arterial pressure greater than 60 mm Hg. When stimulated by an elevated pressure, these receptors send signals to the medulla oblongata in the brain. The medulla then inhibits sympathetic nervous system activity, which allows the vagus nerve of the parasympathetic nervous system to assume control. This results in vasodilatation of peripheral vessels and a decreased heart rate. Under normal circumstances, this will allow the blood pressure to return to normal.

Conversely, if pressure is low, vagal tone is decreased, which allows the sympathetic nervous system to assume control. This results in vasoconstriction of the peripheral vessels and an increased heart rate. Under normal circumstances, this will allow the blood pressure to return to normal.

3. Vasomotor Center of Regulation

There are two areas of vasomotor control in the medulla oblongata: a vasoconstrictor area and a vasodilator area. The vasomotor center responds to baroreceptors and chemoreceptors in the aortic arch and carotid sinus.

If the vasoconstrictor area is stimulated, normally an increased heart rate, stroke volume, and cardiac output will result due to peripheral vasoconstriction. As the peripheral vessels constrict, more blood is forced from these vessels and returned to the heart. This normally restores arterial blood pressure.

If the vasodilator area is stimulated (by inhibition of the vasoconstrictor area), a decrease in stroke volume and cardiac output will normally occur. The vasodilatation allows for more blood to remain in peripheral vessels; and therefore, less blood is returned to the heart. The normal end result will be a decrease in blood pressure.

Chemoreceptors are activated by a decreased oxygen saturation, an increased carbon dioxide level, and/or a decreased pH. Once activated, the chemoreceptors stimulate the vasoconstrictor area. The events that normally occur with such stimulation are then set into action.

LOCAL CONTROL MECHANISMS

Three *hypothetical* mechanisms for control of peripheral vessels *may* exist: myogenic, metabolic, and tissue pressure. More data are needed to verify the existence of these

mechanisms and how they function in both the healthy heart and the diseased heart.

Control of Arterial Pressure

Arterial pressure can be defined as that pressure within the arterial system that serves as a driving force to propel blood through vessel channels. The actual pressure is determined by the left ventricular contraction and the elasticity in the arterial channels themselves. Cardiac output and the total peripheral resistance determine systemic arterial pressure. Systolic pressure increases with age due to a loss of elasticity in the vessel walls. A blood pressure of $\frac{60 \pm 10}{40}$ is considered critical since below this level pressure is insufficient to adequately perfuse the brain and the kidneys. A decreased level results in sensorium changes and acute renal failure.

Many physiologic factors interact to influence blood pressure. These are shown in Figure 9-5. Other factors such as age, emotions, diet, environment, exercise, and weight will affect the blood pressure. The major influences on blood pressure are the cardiac output, the peripheral resistance, and the blood volume.

Cardiac output is the heart rate times the stroke volume. Stroke volume is the end-diastolic volume minus the end-systolic volume (the amount of blood in the ventricle at the end of diastole minus the amount of blood remaining in the ventricle after systole). An increase in either the heart rate or the stroke volume without significant change in other factors will cause an increase in blood pressure (within the limits of the Frank-Starling law). Stroke volume may be increased by sympathetic stimulation, alterations in preload, and/or alterations in afterload. Cardiac output can be measured (directly and indirectly) in both the right heart and the left heart. The outputs *must* be nearly identical in the normal, healthy heart.

Preload is the intramyocardial wall tension at rest, that is, the amount of blood in the ventricle at the end of diastole and the extent that this amount of blood has

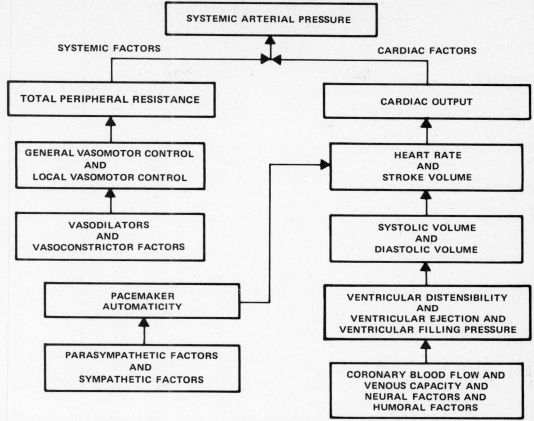

Figure 9-5. The physiological factors influencing blood pressure (Adapted from Rushmer RF: Cardiovascular Dynamics, 4th ed. Philadelphia: W. B. Saunders, p. 177, 1976)

stretched myocardial fibers. The factors which affect the amount of blood in the ventricle and the amount of stretch to the myocardial fibers will alter preload.

Afterload is the resistance to the ejection of blood from the left ventricle. The systemic blood pressure is the major force resisting ejection of blood. Factors which alter this resistance to the ejection of blood may be manipulated to alter afterload.

Peripheral resistance is regulated mainly by three factors:

1. *Autonomic nervous system.* The sympathetic nervous system causes vasoconstriction, and the parasympathetic nervous system causes vasodilatation.

2. *Circulating hormones.* The kidney secretes renin which is converted to an-giotensin II. This is the most potent vasoconstrictor known. This increases blood pressure (see Chapter 25).

3. *Blood volume and viscosity.* Increases in blood volume and/or viscosity will increase blood pressure. Blood volume may be directly related to kidney function.

Control of the Heart

The heart is controlled in part by a balance between the sympathetic and parasympathetic nervous systems, by chemoreceptors, baroreceptors, and miscellaneous factors.

The sympathetic nervous system causes two types of effects due to its neurotransmitter, norepinephrine. One effect is termed alpha-adrenergic, which causes arteriolar vasoconstriction. The second effect is termed beta-adrenergic, which increases the SA node discharges, AV conduction, and contractility. Such effects increase the heart rate and contraction.

The parasympathetic nervous system has one effect on two different tissue masses. The acetylcholine it releases has a cholinergic effect. It slows the rate of discharges from the SA node through its actions on the right vagus nerve. This will cause a bradycardia, and if strong enough, a sinus arrest. Through the left vagus nerve, acetylcholine will slow the conduction time through the AV node tissue, causing various degrees of AV block. This effect also slows the heart rate.

Baroreceptors and chemoreceptors and their effect upon the heart were discussed under control of peripheral blood vessels and will not be repeated here.

Miscellaneous factors that affect cardiac function include hormones that increase pacemaker activity. A modified baroreceptor is the respiratory stretch reflex. Inspiration expands the lungs and chest, thus stimulating stretch receptors which increase the heart rate. During expiration, the stretch stimulation abates and the heart rate slows. (This is demonstrated by the slight variation in heart rate related to inspiration and expiration in normal sinus rhythm.) In the healthy heart, this is normal. A Bainbridge (atrial) reflex occurs when pressure in the atria increases and stimulates the heart to increase its rate. Return of atrial pressure to normal terminates the Bainbridge (atrial) reflex.

Relationship of Blood Flow and Pressure in Cardiac Cycle

The pressure of a fluid in a chamber depends upon the size of the chamber, the amount of fluid, the distensibility of the chamber, and whether the chamber is open or closed.

The atria (both right atrium and left atrium) are open chambers. The venae cavae in the right atrium and the pulmonary veins in the left atrium are always open.

Thus, pressures in these chambers will remain low unless something occludes the openings or prevents them from emptying.

The anatomic structure of the right ventricle contributes to its low pressure. The right ventricle normally empties into a low pressure system—the lungs.

The left ventricle has a high pressure. Its anatomic structure contributes to the high pressure. It empties into a high pressure, closed system—the aorta. Let us trace the flow of blood through the chambers and examine its relationship to the cardiac valves and the chamber pressures. These relationships are shown in Figure 9-6.

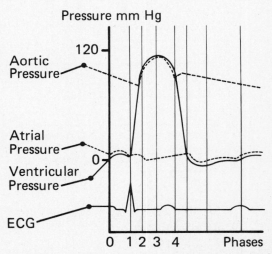

Figure 9-6.   Blood flow and pressure during the cardiac cycle.

ATRIAL PRESSURE CURVE

Throughout diastole, pressure slowly increases in the atria due to the influx of blood. The volume of blood increases in relation to the chamber size. With atrial contraction (first curve on the atrial line in Figure 9-6), there is a sudden increase in pressure because the contraction decreases the size of the atrium. During atrial contraction, pressure is greater in the atrium than the ventricle. This higher pressure causes the AV valves to open. Atrial blood flows through the open AV valves into the ventricles.

As the ventricles begin the systolic phase, blood flow is reversed. As soon as the blood flow reverses, the blood completely closes the partially closed AV valves. The ventricle pressure increase is so sudden that the AV valves bulge into the atria, increasing the intra-atrial pressure (second curve on atrial line in Figure 9-6). Following this second curve, there is a sharp fall in atrial pressure. This pressure drop is caused by two factors:

1. The AV septum is pulled down by the contracting ventricular walls. This increases the size of the atrial chamber.

2. Ejection of 30–40 ml of blood from the chest cage via the aorta causes a pressure drop because the thoracic cavity is a closed system.

Gradually, the atrial pressure rises again during the next period of diastole, and the cycle repeats.

VENTRICULAR PRESSURE CURVE

During diastole, the ventricular pressure is less than the atrial pressure. Just before atrial systole occurs, the AV valves open and blood flows into the ventricles. As soon as the ventricles fill, the blood flow reverses and closes the AV valves. At this point, the ventricles become closed chambers. The ventricle walls contract against the volume of blood in the ventricle. Since the ventricle is a closed chamber, pressure rises rapidly. Aortic pressure during diastole has fallen to about 80 mm Hg. As ventricle pressure builds from near-zero to 80 mm Hg, it is termed the isometric contraction phase (ventricle curve between lines 1 and 2 in Figure 9-6). The left ventricle continues to contract strongly and the pressure rises to 110 mm Hg. Since left ventricular pressure exceeds the aortic pressure of 80 mm Hg, the aortic valve is forced open, and blood is ejected into the aorta. These same mechanisms are occurring concurrently in the right ventricle, only under much lower pressures. This is called the rapid ejection phase (ventricle curve between lines 2 and 3

in Figure 9-6). Pressure begins to drop in the ventricle because blood is being ejected faster than the ventricle is contracting. This is called the reduced-ejection phase (ventricular curve between lines 3 and 4 in Figure 9-6). Ventricular contaction ceases and the ventricle relaxes. Since the ventriclar pressure has dropped rapidly, the blood flow starts to reverse at about 80 mm Hg in the aorta. This backward flow closes the aortic valve. The ventricle again becomes a closed chamber, but since no blood is entering, the pressure does not rise. The fall of pressure in the ventricle continues until it is less than atrial pressure. Then the cycle begins again.

EDDY CURRENTS

Blood does not flow from the atria into the ventricles in a centered column of blood. Rather, as blood enters, it spreads out, hits the ventricle walls, and swirls around. As the ventricles fill, the swirling blood starts to "float out" the valve cusps. This swirling of blood is called an eddy current. By the time the ventricles are almost full, the valve cusps have floated into an almost closed position. Thus, the eddy currents prevent regurgitaion through wide-open valves when contraction starts; and the eddy currents save a lot of energy and wear-and-tear on the valve cusps.

The Electrical Axis of the Cardiac Muscle

The direction of the electrical impulse in the heart is termed axis. In the normal heart, the electrical impulse flows from the SA node to the apex of the heart (negative depolarized cells to positive polarized cells). The normal axis of the heart is from 30° to 60° or 0° to 90°, depending upon the text you are reading.

Axis deviation is a situation in which the impulse travels outside these degrees due to mechanical or physiological causes. Refer to the cardiac section of Appendix I to determine the degree, direction, and extent of deviation.

— 10 ———————————————

Diagnostic Studies and the Normal EKG

Learning Objectives

By the end of this chapter, the nurse will be able to:

1. Identify three enzymes normally studied in cases of myocardial infarction or suspected myocardial infarction.
2. State the hours and days of increase, peak, and decrease for each of the enzymes: SGOT, LDH, and CPK.
3. Define phonocardiography.
4. Define echocardiography.
5. Define cardiac nuclear studies.
6. Define vectorcardiography.
7. Distinguish between invasive and noninvasive studies.
8. List indications for the use of pulmonary arterial catheter monitoring.
9. Identify the normal values of PA diastolic, PA systolic, PA mean, and PCWP.
10. Explain the significance of each of the measurements listed in number 9.
11. Define cardiac catheterization.
12. Define electrophysiologic studies.
13. Define intracardiac phonocardiography.
14. List the uses of a 12-lead EKG.
15. State the value in time of each vertical line on standard EKG paper.
16. State the value in voltage of each horizontal line on standard EKG paper.
17. List the three main deflections in the normal cardiac cycle.
18. Describe the normal shape, size, and significance of a P wave.
19. Describe the normal shape, size, and significance of a QRS complex.
20. Describe the normal shape, size, and significance of a T wave.
21. List five essential steps when interpreting a rhythm strip.

Laboratory Diagnostic Studies

It is routine to have a complete blood count, clotting profile, blood chemistries, and iso-enzyme studies performed on all cardiac or suspected cardiac patients. Lipid profiles are frequently done to ascertain the extent of cholesterol and triglyceride levels. Urinalysis, with or without urine electrolytes, are also usually performed. For the cardiac patient, cardiac profile or cardiac iso-enzyme studies are of paramount importance.

CARDIAC ISOENZYMES

These are the most useful adjuncts known, along with the EKG, to the diagnosis of myocardial infarction. The specific enzymes are serum glutamate-oxaloacetate transaminase (SGOT), lactic dehydrogenase (LDH), and creatinine phosphokinase (CPK). The normal values for these enzymes are found in Table 10-1.

SGOT enzymes are found in tissues of the heart, liver, skeletal muscle, kidney, and pancreas (in descending order of concentrations). LDH is found in all tissues. The largest amounts are found in red and white blood cells, skin, heart muscle, kidney, liver, and brain. CPK is found mainly in skeletal and cardiac muscle and the brain.

An increase above normal range in enzyme activity occurs with damage to cells sufficient to cause the cell membrane to become so permeable that enzymes leak out. Ischemia is sufficient to cause this leaking. Necrosis of the cells is not a require-ment for elevated serum enzyme levels. An index to the extent and severity of cell membrane damage is the amount of increase above normal for each enzyme. Within a specified number of days (Table 10-1), enzyme levels will return to normal. Consequently, enzyme studies give an up-to-date picture. Both enzyme studies and EKGs are performed to obtain maximum information. Enzyme studies augment EKG knowledge and are especially helpful in patients with known previous infarctions.

SGOT has been measured since 1954, and the higher SGOT level, the greater the damage. Since SGOT is associated with many other diseases, the cardiac isoenzymes are relied upon more now.

LDH has been found to have five isoenzymes, labeled LDH_{1-5} respectively. LDH_1 is specific for myocardial tissue. After infarction, LDH_1 becomes elevated in 8–12 hours, peaks in 24–48 hours, and starts to decrease after 5 or more days. Table 10-1 gives values for LDH, not LDH_1, since many hospitals do not yet routinely use the isoenzyme tests.

Creatinine phosphokinase (CPK) is present in three parts of the body and exhibits different properties in each area. This means that CPK has isoenzymes (substances that have the same chemical components but different properties). CPK is found in the heart, the brain, and skeletal muscle. The CPK isoenzyme found only in the heart is termed CPK-MB (myocardial band); that found in the brain, CPK-BB (brain band); and that found in skeletal muscles, CPK-MM (muscle mass). Each isoenzyme can be differentiated in the labora-

Table 10-1.   Cardiac enzyme activity levels following ischemia or infarction.*

Enzyme	Begins to Increase (hours)	Maximum Level Reached (hours)	Return to Normal (days)	Normal Value (units)
SGOT	4–6	24–48	5	10–40
LDH	8–12	48–72	14	165–300
CPK	2–4	24–36	3	0–200

*Data from: Hurst JW: The clinical recognition and medical management of coronary atherosclerotic heart disease. The Heart, 3rd ed. New York: McGraw-Hill, pp. 1044–1049, 1977.

tory. So the CPK-MB is specific for cardiac cell damage.

Noninvasive Diagnostic Studies

PHONOCARDIOGRAPHY

This records heart sound waves produced by muscular valve movement. This procedure graphically records the position and motion of heart walls as well as internal heart structures. Movement of the heart and fluid results in a sound wave. This sound wave is transmitted through the chest wall. It is used to diagnose mitral valve disease, aortic stenosis, and idiopathic hypertrophic subaortic stenosis (IHSS), and to assess left ventricular function.

ECHOCARDIOGRAPHY

This is the procedure of introducing a high intensity sound wave into the body. As this ultrasonic sound wave contacts solid material (heart tissue), it bounces back and is recorded. It is used to evaluate valve function, atrial tumors, chamber size, and pericardial effusions.

NUCLEAR STUDIES

A radioactive isotope is injected intravenously into the bloodstream and is absorbed by the tissues. Special machines trace the radioactive isotope and form pictures of the areas of isotope concentration by use of a computer. This is radioactive scanning and is sometimes called nuclear imaging. It is used to evaluate multiple facets of cardiac function including aneurysms, perfusion, obstructions, contraction (of the left ventricle), ejection fractions, and effusions.

VECTORCARDIOGRAPHY

This is the recording of the direction and magnitude (vector) of the electromotive forces in a loop display on an oscilloscope during one complete heart cycle utilizing EKG leads. This is used to help diagnose bundle branch and fascicular blocks as well as atrial and ventricular hypertrophy and atrial septal defects.

ELECTROCARDIOGRAPHY

This measures electrical activity of the heart and records the activity on special paper. It is used mainly to determine cardiac rhythms, myocardial ischemia, and myocardial infarction.

Invasive Diagnostic Studies

PULMONARY ARTERY CATHETER

This form of monitoring is probably the most frequenty used invasive monitoring system, although central venous pressure (CVP) monitoring is still very popular. The pulmonary artery catheter, of which the Swan-Ganz is one brand, has up to four lumens and a balloon at the end of the catheter to enable the catheter to "float" into a pulmonary artery with the flow of blood. The pulmonary artery catheter allows *continuous* evaluation of the hemodynamic status of the patient. This includes vascular tone, fluid balance, and myocardial contractility. With a pulmonary artery catheter, the pulmonary artery (PA) pressure and pulmonary capillary wedge pressure (PCWP) can be measured.

The PA systolic pressure reflects pressure of the right ventricle and is normally 20–30 mm Hg. The PA diastolic pressure represents left ventricular end-diastolic pressure (LVEDP) since during diastole the mitral valve is open and there is no resisting force. The PA diastolic pressure is normally less than 10 mm Hg. The PA mean equals the average PA systolic and PA diastolic and is related to the relative lengths of systole and diastole. It is normally less than 20 mm Hg.

The PCWP is the pressure within the pulmonary arteriole. The pressure difference from the pulmonary arteriole to the pulmonary vein in the absence of lung disease is minimal. Thus, PCWP is equal to left atrial pressure and left ventricular end-diastolic pressure. The PCWP is normally 4–12 mm

Hg. The mean PCWP should normally approximate the PA diastolic pressure.

The values obtained from the pulmonary artery catheter readings monitor fluid balance and give an indication of the existence of a hypovolemic state, signs of impending cardiogenic shock, or the existence of pulmonary hypertension.

Complications may occur but are *rare* as the result of using a pulmonary artery catheter. These include thromboemboli, balloon rupture causing emboli or infarction, infection, pulmonary infarction if the balloon remains wedged, dysrhythmias during and after insertion of the catheter, and perforation of the right atrium, right ventricle, or pulmonary artery with subsequent hemorrhage.

CARDIAC CATHETERIZATION

This is a common invasive cardiac study performed (usually) by introducing a catheter into the left femoral artery and feeding it into the left ventricle. Other arteries may be used for the procedure. Cardiac catheterization provides visualization and evaluation of ventricular function of both the right and left sides of the heart and of the presence and severity of coronary artery disease. It enables one to determine the degree of ventricular function by measuring pressures in the heart and the cardiac output. Ventriculography (study of the left ventricle) is a common part of cardiac catheterization. Aortography (study of the aorta and aortic valve leaflets) is frequently performed as a part of cardiac catheterization.

Complications of cardiac catheterization include cardiac dysrhythmias, pain (angina), congestive heart failure (CHF) due to the dye, allergic reactions to the contrast media, thrombosis, emboli, and rarely, perforation of the ventricle and/or arteries. Infection at the site of catheter introduction, hypovolemia, and acute renal failure may occur. (Acute renal failure occurs if the catheter diminishes the supply of blood to the renal artery for a sufficient time and to a sufficient degree to decrease renal perfusion, or as a consequence of reaction to the dye which has a very high iodide salt content.)

ELECTROPHYSIOLOGY STUDIES

These studies are normally performed by introducing a pulmonary artery catheter into the right ventricle. These studies are used to identify specific cell groups in the AV node, His bundle, or bundle branches that may be causing blocks. These studies are also used to determine sites of abnormal excitation resulting in paroxysmal atrial tachycardia, recurrent ventricular tachycardias, Wolff-Parkinson-White syndrome, and sometimes atrial flutter or atrial fibrillation. Electrophysiology may be used in studying drug effects.

Complications of electrophysiology studies are most frequently cardiac dysrhythmias.

INTRACARDIAC PHONOCARDIOGRAPHY

This is an investigative technique for studying heart sounds and murmurs in congenital heart disease and some acquired cardiac myopathies. A catheter that has a microphone on the end of it is introduced into the heart and the sounds of the chambers and valves are recorded for study and diagnosis.

The Components of the Normal Electrocardiogram

The electrocardiograph is a machine which records the electrical activity of the heart on special paper resulting in an electrocardiogram (EKG or ECG). The electrical activity measured is the electrical potential between two points on the body. One point is a positive pole and the other point is a negative pole.

The 12-lead EKG is the graphic recording of the electrical output of the heart from 12 different positions. A 12-lead EKG can be diagnostic in drug toxicity, conduction disturbances, electrolyte imbalances, ischemia, infarction, size of the heart chambers, and axis orientation of the heart.

Cardiac monitoring uses rhythm strips to assess heart rate, rhythm, and dysrhythmias. Rhythm strips may be run on any one of the 12 leads used in a 12-lead EKG and several other special leads.

The most common leads used to monitor patients are leads 2 and MCL_1. Lead 2 is a standard lead with the negative pole attached to an electrode placed on the upper chest near the right arm and the positive pole attached to an electrode placed on the lower left side of the chest.

MCL_1 is a modified chest lead representative of V_1 of the 12-lead EKG. In MCL_1, the negative pole is attached to an electrode placed on the upper left chest and the positive pole is attached to an electrode placed to the right of the sternum at the fourth intercostal space.

Lead 2 is especially useful in assessing P waves, and MCL_1 is particularly valuable in assessing dysrhythmias.

EKG PAPER

This is special paper (Figure 10-1) that is treated to respond to the heat produced by the electrocardiograph or monitoring stylus touching it. The EKG paper has a series of horizontal lines exactly one millimeter apart (Figure 10-1). The horizontal lines represent voltage (or amplitude). EKG paper also has vertical lines which represent time. Each vertical line is 0.04 seconds apart. To help in measuring wave forms, every *fifth* line is darker than the other lines, *both* horizontally and vertically. The intersection of these lines produces both small boxes (the lighter lines) and large boxes (the darker, bolder lines). Horizontally,

each small box represents 1 mm (0.1 mV) and each large box represents 5 mm (0.5 mV). (Note that each large box is made up of five small boxes.) Vertically, each small box represents 0.04 seconds and each large box represents 0.20 seconds. Because of the design of EKG paper, one can measure the duration of impulses (wavelengths) and the amplitude (height) of impulses. All waves will be either isoelectric (no net electrical activity = flat), or positively deflected (upright towards the positive pole), or negatively deflected (downward towards the negative pole).

Components of a Cardiac Cycle

Before a rhythm strip can be labeled, a systematic analysis of each portion of the strip *and* the relation of each wave to the electrical activity in the cardiac cycle is made. The interpretations will be made using lead 2 in this text. It is conventional to label the components of the cardiac cycle P, QRS, and T. There is no reason these specific letters were chosen. There are three prominent deflections in the EKG: the P wave, the QRS complex, and the T wave (Figure 10-2).

P WAVE

This represents the generation of an electrical impulse and depolarization of the atria (Figure 10-3). The P wave is extremely important in determining if the impulse started in the SA node or elsewhere in the atrium.

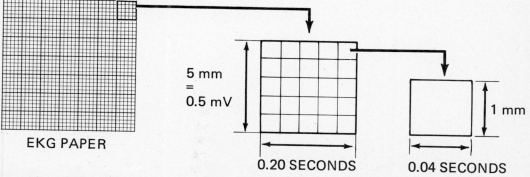

EKG PAPER

5 mm = 0.5 mV

0.20 SECONDS

1 mm

0.04 SECONDS

Figure 10-1.   EKG paper.

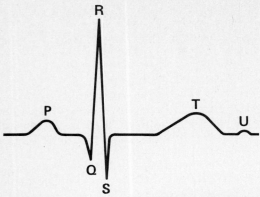

Figure 10-2. The normal PQRST deflections, lead 2.

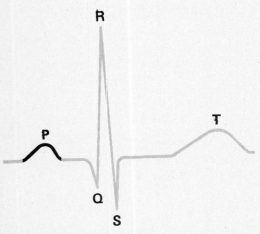

Figure 10-3. The P wave.

QRS COMPLEX

The QRS complex is composed of three separate wave forms which represent ventricular depolarization (Figure 10-4). Multiple variations exist in the shape of the QRS complex. A Q wave is the first *negative* deflection and may or may not be present. The R wave is the first *positive* deflection in the complex. The S wave is the first negative deflection following the R wave.

T WAVE

The T wave is the third major deflection in the EKG (Figure 10-5). It represents repolarization of the ventricles. In lead 2 of a healthy heart, the T wave is positively deflected. In ischemia or infarction, the T wave may be inverted.

There are four other parts of a rhythm strip and an EKG that must be identified.

P-R INTERVAL

The P-R interval (Figure 10-6) represents the time for the electrical impulse to spread from the atrium to the AV node and His bundle. It is measured from the beginning of the P wave to the beginning of the QRS complex. Normally, this interval is 0.12–0.20 seconds.

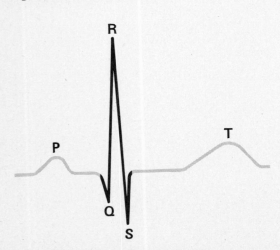

Figure 10-4. The QRS complex.

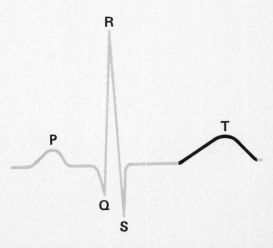

Figure 10-5. The T wave.

S-T SEGMENT

The S-T segment (Figure 10-7) represents the time from complete depolarization of the ventricles to the beginning of repolarization (recovery) of the ventricles. In the healthy heart, the S-T segment is flat or isoelectric. Since no net electrical activity is going on during the recovery phase of the cardiac cycle, the wave is not deflected in either direction. In injury or ischemia, the segment may be elevated or depressed.

P-R SEGMENT

This segment (Figure 10-8) represents the normal delay in the conduction of the electrical impulse in the AV node. It is normally isoelectric and is measured from the *end* of the P wave to the beginning of the R wave. Duration of the P-R segment varies.

Q-T INTERVAL

This interval (Figure 10-9) represents the total period of time required for depolarization and repolarization (recovery) of the ventricles. It is measured from the beginning of the QRS complex to the end of the T wave. It is normally less than 0.40 seconds, but is dependent upon heart rate, sex, age, and other factors.

Occasionally another wave is seen after the T wave and before the next P wave. This is called a U wave (Figure 10-10). Some au-

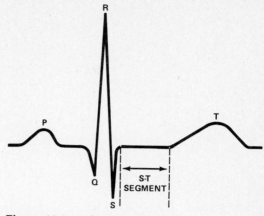

Figure 10-7.   The S-T segment.

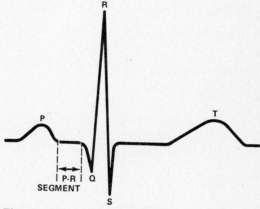

Figure 10-8.   The P-R segment.

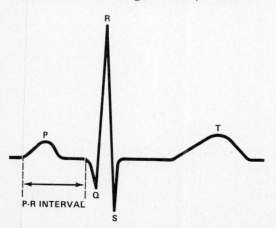

Figure 10-6.   The P-R interval.

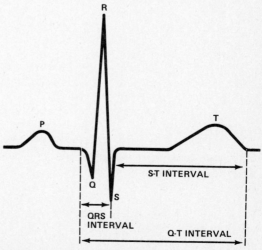

Figure 10-9.   The QRS, S-T, and Q-T intervals.

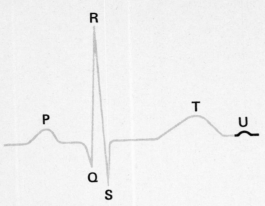

Figure 10-10.   The U wave.

thorities believe it represents repolarization of the Purkinje fibers. It may or may not be seen.

Interpretation of a Rhythm Strip

There are five basic steps to be followed in analyzing a rhythm strip (or an EKG) to aid in the interpretation and identification of a rhythm. Each step should be followed in sequence. Eventually this will become a habit and will enable one to identify a strip correctly, accurately, and quickly.

STEP ONE

Determine the rate at which the atria and the ventricles are depolarizing. This may not be the same. To count the rate of the atria, count the number of P waves present in the 6-second rhythm strip and mutiply by 10. (Each mark at the top edge of the EKG paper represents 3 seconds and each inch of EKG paper equals 1 second.) This gives the atrial rate per minute for irregular rhythms.

Count the number of QRS complexes in a 6-second strip and multiple by 10. This gives the ventricular rate per minute for irregular rhythms.

For regular rhythms, determine the rate by counting the number of small boxes between each P wave and divide into 1,500 or count the number of large boxes between each P wave and divide into 300. Do the same thing to determine the ventricular rate by counting QRS complexes.

STEP TWO

Determine if the rhythm is regular or irregular. The most accurate method of determining this is to measure the interval from one R wave to the next R wave. (Set one point of the cardiac calipers on the tip of the first R wave and the other point on the tip of the next R wave.) Then move the cardiac calipers from R to R. If the measurement is the same (or varies less than 0.04 seconds between beats), the rhythm is regular. If the intervals vary more than 0.12 seconds, the rhythm is irregular. Often one can tell by simply looking at the strip that it is irregular. However, IF it looks regular, it is best to measure the R to R intervals to be certain.

STEP THREE

Analyze the P waves. A P wave should precede every QRS complex. All the P waves should be identical in shape. The normal P wave is fairly sharply curved, less than 3 mm in height, and less than 0.1 seconds in width in lead 2. If the P wave is abnormally shaped or varies in shape from wave to wave, the stimulus may have arisen from somewhere in the atrium other than in the SA node. Almost all impulses that originate in the SA node will meet the "normal" shape and size previously stated if heart function is normal. A biphasic P (a single P wave moves above and below the baseline) may indicate left atrial enlargement; a peaked P may indicate right atrial enlargement, and both of these P waves originate in the SA node. If there is no P wave or if the P wave does not precede the QRS complex, the impulse did not originate in the SA node.

STEP FOUR

Measure the P-R interval. This is measured from the beginning of the P wave to the beginning of the QRS complex. It should measure between 0.10 and 0.20 seconds. Intervals outside of this range indicate a conduction disturbance between the atria and the ventricles.

STEP FIVE

Measure the width of the QRS complex. This is measured from the beginning of the Q (if present, otherwise the R) to the end of the S wave. The normal duration is 0.06 to 0.10 seconds. If the QRS is greater than 0.10 seconds, it indicates an intraventricular conduction abnormality.

Figure 10-11 is a 6-second, lead 2 rhythm strip. Let us analyze this rhythm strip by applying the five steps just mentioned.

Step One: The atrial rate is 80 (eight P waves in 6 seconds). The ventricular rate is 80 (eight R waves in 6 seconds). The heart rate is 80.

Step Two: There is less than a 0.12 second variation from R wave to R wave so the rhythm is regular.

Step Three: The P waves are all the same shape, size (in height), and duration. Each P wave appears immediately before a QRS complex. These factors indicate the impulse starts in the SA node.

Step Four: The P-R interval is 0.12 seconds. This is within the normal duration range indicating normal conduction of the impulse from the SA node to the AV node.

Step Five: Each QRS complex is less than 0.10 seconds in duration, which is normal.

Interpretation of the Strip: Normal sinus rhythm (NSR)

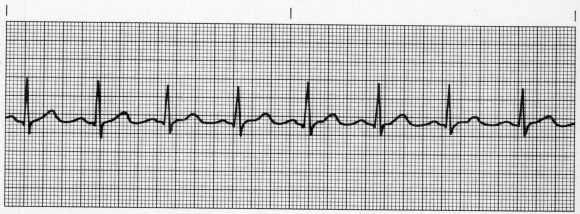

Figure 10-11.   Lead 2 normal sinus rhythm.

— 11

Sinus and Atrial Dysrhythmias

Learning Objectives

By the end of this chapter, the nurse will be able to:

1. List the identifying characteristics of:
   a. Sinus arrhythmia
   b. Sinus bradycardia
   c. Sinus tachycardia
   d. Sinus pause/arrest and block
   e. Paroxysmal atrial tachycardia (PAT)
   f. Atrial tachycardia
   g. Premature atrial contraction (PAC)
   h. Wandering atrial pacemaker
   i. Atrial flutter
   j. Atrial fibrillation
2. Identify the risk of each of the aforementioned dysrhythmias.
3. Identify the appropriate drug and/or method of treating each of the aforementioned dysrhythmias.
4. List the nursing interventions for each of the aforementioned dysrhythmias.

All dysrhythmias occur due to a disturbance in the formation of the cardiac impulse *or* due to a disturbance in the conduction of the impulse. The classification of the dysrhythmias is shown in Table 11-1.

Every dysrhythmia has specific identifying characteristics associated with it. The first four dysrhythmias discussed in this chapter originate in the SA node. The next six dysrhythmias originate in the atrium—but not in the SA node. (Note: All rhythm strips are 6 seconds, lead 2.)

Sinus Arrhythmia

ETIOLOGY

Variations of impulse formation in the SA node are caused by the vagus nerve. This results in an irregular rhythm with alternating fast and slow rates (see Figure 11-1).

IDENTIFYING CHARACTERISTICS

The rate varies, usually between 60 and 100. The rate increases with inspiration and de-

Table 11-1. Classification of dysrhythmias.*

Dysrhythmias Due to Disorders in Impulse Formation	Dysrhythmias Due to Conduction Disturbances
Sinoatrial (SA) Node Dysrhythmias	**Sinoatrial Block**
Sinus Tachycardia	
Sinus Bradycardia	**Atrioventricular (AV) Blocks**
Sinus Arrhythmia	First-Degree AV Block
Wandering Pacemaker	Second-Degree AV Block
Sinoatrial Arrest	Third-Degree (Complete) AV Block
Atrial Dysrhythmias	**Intraventricular Blocks**
Premature Atrial Contractions	Left Bundle Branch Blocks
Paroxysmal Atrial Tachycardia	Right Bundle Branch Blocks
Atrial Flutter	Bilateral Bundle Branch Blocks
Atrial Fibrillation	Ventricular Standstill
Atrial Standstill	
AV Nodal Area (Junctional) Dysrhythmias	
Premature Junctional Contractions	
Passive Junctional Rhythm	
Paroxysmal Junctional Tachycardia	
Nonparoxysmal Junctional Tachycardia	
Ventricular Dysrhythmias	
Premature Ventricular Contractions	
Ventricular Tachycardia	
Ventricular Fibrillation	

*Adapted from: Meltzer LE et al.: Intensive Coronary Care: A Manual for Nurses, 3rd ed. Bowie, MD: Charles Press, p. 133, 1977.

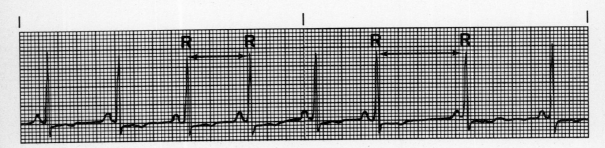

Figure 11-1.   Sinus arrhythmia.

creases with expiration due primarily to vagal influences. Both atrial and ventricular rhythms are regularly irregular. The P waves are normal. The P-R interval is within normal limits. The QRS complex is normal. Conduction is normal. The difference between normal sinus rhythm and sinus arrhythmia is the variation of the R to R intervals. In sinus arrhythmia, the variation is at least 0.12 seconds between the shortest and the longest R to R intervals. The variation in normal sinus rhythm is less than 0.12 seconds.

RISK

No risk exists for the patient because this dysrhythmia is a normal variant and causes no hemodynamic compromise.

TREATMENT

No treatment is needed.

NURSING INTERVENTION

Document the dysrhythmia with a rhythm strip. This interpretation can be substantiated if the patient holds his or her breath and the rate stabilizes. A 12-lead EKG will provide a definite diagnosis.

Sinus Bradycardia

ETIOLOGY

Parasympathetic (vagal) control over the SA node due to ischemia, pain, drugs, sleep, or athletic conditioning decreases the formation of electrical impulses (see Figure 11-2).

IDENTIFYING CHARACTERISTICS

The rate is less than 60 but usually more than 40. Both atrial and ventricular rhythms are usually regular. P waves are normal. The P-R interval is within the upper limits or is slightly prolonged. The QRS complex in normal. Conduction is normal.

RISK

This dysrhythmia may lead to syncopal attacks, CHF, angina, premature beats, ventricular tachycardia, congestive heart failure, and cardiac arrest. This is a serious warning dysrhythmia if the rate is low (about 40).

TREATMENT

No treatment may be necessary if the rate is close to 60 or if the patient is asymptomatic. If the rate is low and/or the patient is symptomatic, atropine intravenously is the drug of choice to increase the heart rate. If unsuccessful, isoproterenol hydrochloride (Isuprel®) by intravenous drip may be tried. A pacemaker may be required.

NURSING INTERVENTIONS

Document the dysrhythmia with a rhythm strip. Monitor and document effectiveness of drug therapy. Do not administer drugs such as digitalis, morphine sulfate, or propranolol hydrochloride (Inderal®) which may further slow the heart rate. Be especially alert for PVCs. If PVCs occur, obtain a rhythm strip and notify the physician.

Sinus Tachycardia

ETIOLOGY

Cardiac decompensation (heart failure) is the most serious cause of sinus tachycardia. It may also be caused by any factor which stimulates the sympathetic nervous system, such as anxiety, exertion (physical), and fever (see Figure 11-3).

IDENTIFYING CHARACTERISTICS

The rate is usually 100–160. Both atrial and ventricular rhythms are regular. The P wave

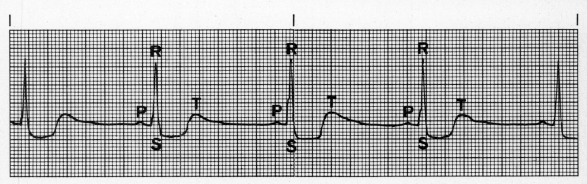

Figure 11-2.   Sinus bradycardia.

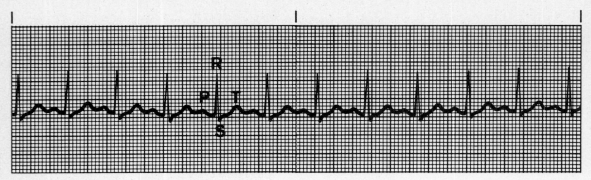

Figure 11-3.   Sinus tachycardia.

is normal but may be difficult to identify because of the rapid rate. (Note: Look for the P wave superimposed on the T wave with fast rates.) The P-R interval is usually at the lower limits of normal. The QRS is normal. Conduction is normal.

RISK

If the etiolgy is not cardiogenic, sinus tachycardia may precipitate cardiac decompensation in patients with borderline cardiac function. If the cause is cardiogenic, left ventricular failure may occur rapidly (cardiac decompensation).

TREATMENT

Effective treatment depends upon treatment of the underlying cause. Digitalis may be indicated.

NURSING INTERVENTION

Document dysrhythmia with a rhythm strip. Monitor the patient for signs of left ventricular failure (restlessness, orthopnea, cough, shortness of breath, and such). Nursing attempts to calm the patient and to decrease the patient's stress are helpful.

Sinus Pause/Arrest, SA Block

ETIOLOGY

Ischemic injury to the SA node is the most common and important cause of SA block.

A technical, but not clinical, difference exists between sinus pause/arrest and SA block. In the pause/arrest, the SA node does not form an electrical impulse. In SA block, the node initiates an impulse, but the impulse is prevented from leaving the node and thus it cannot be visualized. Regardless of this difference, the end result is that no impulse stimulates the atria or the ventricles. The terms pause and block are often used interchangeably. Vagal effect, digitalis toxicity, quinidine sulfate (Quinidine®), and isoproterenol hydrochloride (Isuprel®) may be causes of SA block (see Figure 11-4).

IDENTIFYING CHARACTERISTICS

The rate is usually slower than normal. Rhythm (both atrial and ventricular) is generally regular except for the arrest/block complex. P waves are absent in arrest and block for a specific time period. Otherwise, P waves are normal. The P-R interval is absent in the arrest/block complex. The QRS complex may be normal or abnormal in arrest, depending on the escape site. It is absent in block. Conduction depends on the escape site in arrest and is absent in sinus block for that specific interval.

RISK

The greatest risk is that both sinus pause/arrest and sinus block may proceed to cardiac arrest if the arrest or block is frequent. If the arrest or block is infrequent and self-limiting, it is not dangerous.

TREATMENT

If the arrest or block is rare, it does not require treatment. If the arrest is frequent, treatment is essential. If drugs are the underlying cause, they should be evaluated and stopped. Atropine, isoproterenol, or epinephrine may be effective in increasing the heart rate. If these are not effective and the patient is symptomatic, a pacemaker may be inserted.

NURSING INTERVENTION

Document the dysrhythmia with a rhythm strip. If drugs are the possible underlying cause, withhold the drug until reordered. Monitor the patient closely to determine if the frequency of arrest or block is increasing. If so, document with rhythm strips and notify the physician; a pacemaker may be indicated.

Paroxysmal Atrial Tachycardia (PAT)

ETIOLOGY

An irritable focus in the atrium becomes excited due to sympathetic stimulation and initiates impulses faster than the SA node. This irritable focus then takes over as pacemaker (see Figure 11-5).

IDENTIFYING CHARACTERISTICS

Three key characteristics identify PAT.

1. It starts suddenly.
2. It ends abruptly.
3. The ventricles respond to every impulse created by the focus (1:1 conduction).

The rate is usually 150–250—*both* atrial and ventricular. The rhythm is perfectly

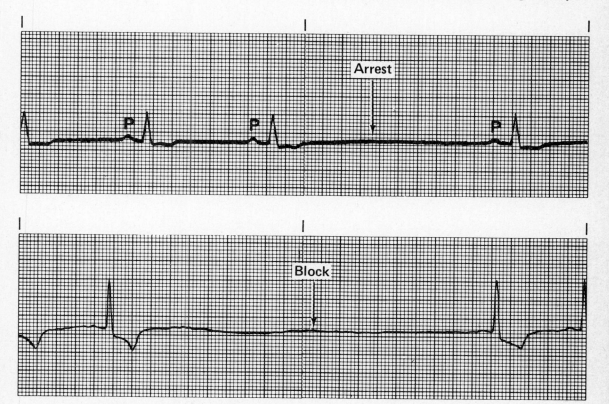

Figure 11-4. Sinoatrial arrest or block.

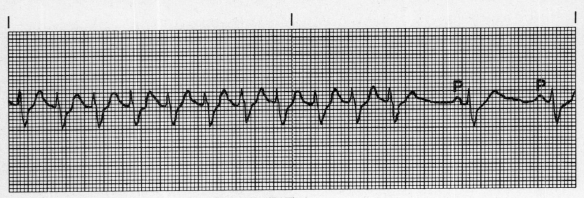

Figure 11-5.   Paroxysmal atrial tachycardia (PAT).

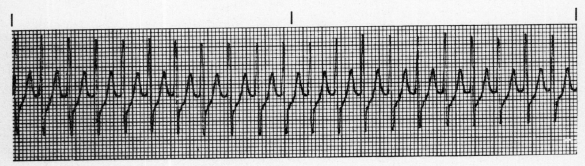

Figure 11-6.   Atrial tachycardia.

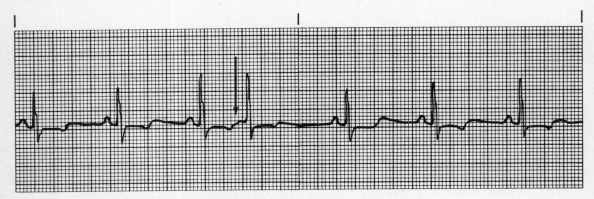

Figure 11-7.   Premature atrial contraction (PAC).

regular. P waves are always present but may be very difficult to identify. The P wave will not have the normal, smooth, rounded shape of a sinus P wave since this impulse originates in the atrium. The P-R interval is within normal limits and is usually greater than one expects for the rate. The QRS complex is normal. Conduction originates in an abnormal focus (the atrium—not the SA node) but then continues through normal pathways.

RISK

PAT frequently stops spontaneously. If it does not, the rapid rate may lead to myocardial ischemia and, eventually, cardiac decompensation. If PAT occurs post-M.I., it may rapidly lead to increased myocardial ischemia and injury, left ventricular failure, and cardiac decompensation.

TREATMENT

Vagal stimulation and other vagal maneuvers such as coughing may terminate the dysrhythmia. Having the patient perform a Valsalva maneuver stimulates the vagus nerve. If this fails to terminate the rhythm, carotid massage by the doctor (or nurse if allowed) often terminates PAT. If this fails *and* the patient is asymptomatic, drug therapy may be tried. Propranolol hydrochloride (Inderal®) intravenously, digoxin, or verapamil hydrochloride (Isoptin®) intravenously may terminate PAT. If the patient is symptomatic (complains of angina, becomes diaphoretic, short of breath, and hypotensive), cardioversion may be used immediately. Cardioversion almost always terminates PAT. Quinidine sulfate (Quinidine®) may be used prophylactically if PAT occurs frequently.

NURSING INTERVENTION

Document the dysrhythmia with a rhythm strip. Assess and monitor the patient for signs of ischemia and decompensation. Medicate as ordered by the physician. Be prepared for cardioversion but do not lower the head of the bed until necessary since these patients are usually dyspneic.

Atrial Tachycardia

The impulse of atrial tachycardia originates in the atrium. The *rate* of atrial tachycardia is constant. The difference between PAT and atrial tachycardia is *only* that PAT starts and stops suddenly. Atrial tachycardia is a *constant* rhythm, not irregular. All other parameters of PAT apply to atrial tachycardia (see Figure 11-6).

Premature Atrial Contraction (PAC)

Note: Premature atrial contractions are also called atrial premature beats—APBs.

ETIOLOGY

On occasion, an irritable focus in the atrium fires off before the next expected complex initiating depolarization. The irritable focus does not become the heart's pacemaker except for this single beat (see Figure 11-7).

IDENTIFYING CHARACTERISTICS

The underlying rate is usually normal. The rhythm has an occasional irregularity due to the earliness of the beat and a brief pause after the premature beat. The P wave is abnormally shaped for only the premature beat. The P-R interval is usually prolonged but may be normal or shortened. The QRS complex is normal. PACs may be blocked or may have an aberrant conduction. Conduction below the atria (junctional and ventricular) is normal.

RISK

If PACs occur infrequently, there is no risk. If they occur six or more times per minute, they indicate that atrial flutter, atrial fibrillation, or other atrial dysrhythmias may occur.

TREATMENT

PACs of less than six per minute do not need treatment. With more than six PACs per minute, the physician may elect to control them with quinidine sulfate, propranolol hydrochloride (Inderal®), disopyramide phosphate (Norpace®), or other antidysrhythmic drugs.

NURSING INTERVENTION

Document the dysrhythmia with a rhythm strip. Monitor the patient for increasing frequency of PACs. Increasing PACs may cause anxiety, some hemodynamic compromise, hypotension, and dyspnea. Document an increase with rhythm strips and notify the physician of the increase.

Wandering Atrial Pacemaker

ETIOLOGY

Various foci within the atrium or from the AV node supercede the SA node as the pacemaker for a variable number of beats (see Figure 11-8).

IDENTIFYING CHARACTERISTICS

Rate is usually normal but may be slow. Rhythm is frequently regular. P waves are abnormal and change in size, shape, and deflection. The P-R interval may vary or may be constant. The QRS complex is normal. Conduction is abnormal in the atrium and sometimes in the AV node. From the AV node on, conduction is normal.

RISK

Generally there is no risk. However, in some instances, an atrial flutter or atrial fibrillation may occur.

TREATMENT

Usually no treatment is necessary; but sometimes digitalis may be given (although digitalis toxicity can be the cause of the dysrhythmia). If the AV node is the site of frequent impulse formation, atropine may be needed to increase a slow sinus rate.

NURSING INTERVENTION

Document the dysrhythmia with a rhythm strip. Monitor for an unacceptably low ventricular rate (below 50 beats per minute) and treat as necessary.

Atrial Flutter

ETIOLOGY

A very irritable atrial focus supercedes the SA node. This is a fairly common dysrhythmia in atherosclerotic heart disease (ASHD) and some congenital heart diseases (see Figure 11-9).

IDENTIFYING CHARACTERISTICS

The atrial rate is rapid, usually 250–350 beats per minute. Atrial rhythm is regular,

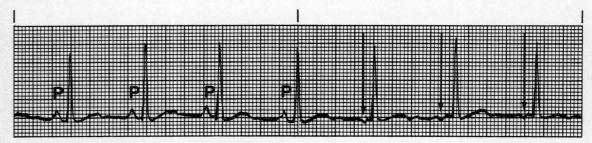

Figure 11-8.   Wandering atrial pacemaker.

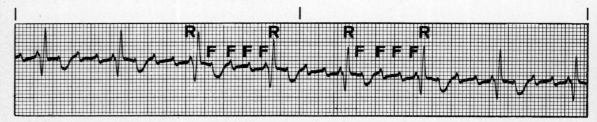

Figure 11-9.   Atrial flutter.

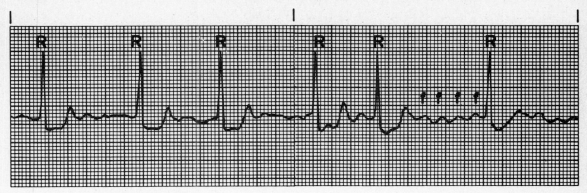

Figure 11-10. Atrial fibrillation.

and ventricular rhythm varies with the number of impulses transmitted through the AV node. The P wave is replaced by a flutter wave (F waves). Flutter waves have no isoelectric interval between the waves. The P-R interval is absent. The QRS is normal. Conduction is abnormal in the atria, and the AV node normally blocks many of the F waves.

RISK

Congestive heart failure may occur *within minutes*, especially if the AV node conducts almost all the F waves. There is the possibility of severe hemodynamic compromise. If the ventricular response is rapid, there is insufficient filling time for the ventricle. This decreases cardiac output. Rapid response of the ventricle increases myocardial oxygen demand which cannot be met due to the decreased cardiac output. If severe, the hemodynamic compromise may lead to cardiogenic shock.

TREATMENT

Digitalis may be used in treating this dysrhythmia if the ventricular response is slow. If the ventricular response is rapid, cardioversion with low voltage is the preferred treatment. Atrial flutter is converted to atrial fibrillation and then normal sinus rhythm (NSR). Persistent atrial flutter is a poor prognostic sign.

NURSING INTERVENTION

Document the dysrhythmia with a rhythm strip. Monitor the patient closely for signs of hemodynamic compromise. The physician *should* be notified when this dysrhythmia develops.

Atrial Fibrillation

ETIOLOGY

Many highly irritable foci develop in the atrium to the extent that atrial contraction is an impossibility. It may be caused by rheumatic heart disease, coronary disease, hypertension, thyrotoxicosis, and congenital heart disease (see Figure 11-10).

IDENTIFYING CHARACTERISTICS

The atrial rate is not measurable but is probably greater than 350. The atrial rate is so high that the AV node cannot accept all the stimuli it receives. Consequently, the atrial and the ventricular rates are markedly different. The atrial and ventricular rhythms are grossly irregular. P waves are nonexistent and are replaced by fibrillatory waves. There is no true P-R interval. The QRS complex may be normal or abnormal. Ventricular response may be slow, normal, or very rapid. Conduction is abnormal in both the atria and the AV node. The number of impulses that the AV node transmits determines the degree of AV block.

RISK

There may be a rapid development of CHF. Atrial thrombi may form, leading to embolization. Marked hemodynamic disturbance is common if the rhythm is of recent onset. Angina and increased myocardial ischemia may occur.

TREATMENT

If the dysrhythmia is not causing hemodynamic compromise, digitalis is the drug of choice, along with quinidine sulfate (Quinidine®), in treating this dysrhythmia. If hemodynamic compromise develops, cardioversion is essential to reduce and control the ventricular response—providing the dysrhythmia has not been present for 72 or more hours. The risk of atrial thrombus development after the first 72 hours contraindicates the use of cardioversion to terminate the dysrhythmia since it may produce embolization.

If there is hemodynamic compromise within the first 72 hours, cardioversion is essential to reduce and control a rapid ventricular response. This is considered an acute form of atrial fibrillation.

A chronic form of atrial fibrillation is considered to exist if there is NO hemodynamic compromise, if the dysrhythmia has been present for more than 72 hours, and if the patient is asymptomatic *and* has a ventricular response greater than 50 complexes per minute but less than 100 complexes per minute. In these instances, treatment may not be needed.

NURSING INTERVENTION

Document the dysrhythmia with a rhythm strip. Notify the physician if atrial fibrillation develops suddenly. Monitor the patient carefully for hemodynamic compromise and embolization. Contact the physician *if* rapid ventricular response develops or if an unacceptably low ventricular response develops (less than 50 beats per minute).

12

Junctional and Ventricular Dysrhythmias

Learning Objectives

By the end of this chapter, the nurse will be able to:

1. List the identifying characteristics of:
   a. Junctional rhythm (idiojunctional)
   b. Premature junctional contraction (PJC)
   c. Paroxysmal junctional tachycardia
   d. Conduction defects
      (1) First degree block
      (2) Second degree block (Mobitz I and Mobitz II)
      (3) Third degree block (Complete heart block)
      (4) AV dissociation
      (5) Bundle branch blocks
   e. Idioventricular rhythm
   f. Accelerated idioventricular rhythm
   g. Premature ventricular contraction (PVC)
   h. Ventricular tachycardia
   i. Ventricular fibrillation
   j. Escape beats
2. Identify the risk of each of the aforementioned dysrhythmias.
3. Identify the appropriate drug and/or method of treatment of each of the aforementioned dysrhythmias.
4. List the nursing intervention for each of the aforementioned dysrhythmias.
5. State the *major* difference between complete heart block and atrioventricular dissociation.

It was once thought that the AV node itself could initiate impulses. Such rhythms were termed nodal rhythms. Research has shown that the AV node *itself* does not initiate an electrical impulse but that an electrical impulse *is* initiated in the junctional tissue around the AV node. This has resulted in changing the term nodal rhythm to the more accurate term of junctional rhythm. All rhythm strips in this chapter are 6 seconds, lead 2.

Junctional Rhythm

ETIOLOGY

This dysrhythmia is often due to an acute myocardial infarction, an SA block, digitalis toxicity, or treatment with quinidine and procainamide (Figure 12-1).

IDENTIFYING CHARACTERISTICS

The rate is usually 40–60 beats per minute. The rhythm is usually regular. P waves are abnormal in shape and size and may precede or follow the QRS complex or be buried in it. If seen, the P wave is usually inverted (negatively deflected). This inversion is caused by the electrical impulse originating in junctional tissue and moving *both* down into the ventricles (a normal path) and back up into the atrium (retrograde movement, which is an abnormal path). The P-R interval, if present, is less than 0.10 seconds and often is immeasurable. The QRS complex is normal, unless a P wave is buried in it. Conduction to the atria is abnormal due to its retrograde depolarization of the atria.

RISK

The junctional impulse formation is slow. This allows other foci to enter and initiate depolarization. This may lead to a series of dangerous and lethal dysrhythmias including ventricular tachycardia, ventricular fibrillation, or cardiac arrest. Hemodynamic balance may be compromised by a slow ventricular rate leading to poor cardiac output and perhaps ventricular failure.

TREATMENT

A pacemaker will override the slow rate. If drug toxicity is the underlying cause, the drug should be stopped immediately.

NURSING INTERVENTION

Document the dysrhythmia with a rhythm strip. Monitor the patient closely. (PVCs are a common occurrence and do not respond well to lidocaine in this dysrhythmia but may be eliminated by a pacemaker.) Monitor for signs of hemodynamic compromise. Notify the physician *immediately* if compromise occurs.

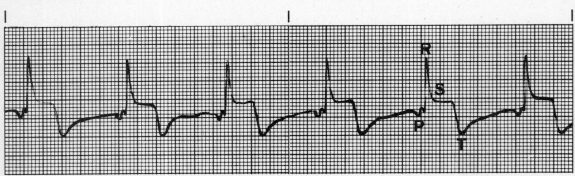

Figure 12-1.   Junctional rhythm.

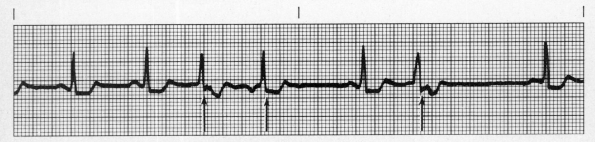

Figure 12-2.   Premature junctional contraction (PJC).

Premature Junctional Contraction (PJC)

ETIOLOGY

An irritable focus in the junctional tissue initiates an impulse early. The impulse depolarizes the ventricles normally and the atria in a retrograde fashion. Coronary artery disease, acute myocardial infarction, and digitalis toxicity are frequent causes. Any factor that increases junctional ischemia may produce a PJC (Figure 12-2).

IDENTIFYING CHARACTERISTICS

The underlying rate may be normal or slow. The rhythm is regular *except* for the premature (early) beat. P waves are abnormal, inverted, and may precede, follow, or be buried in the QRS complex of the PJC. The P-R interval varies with the position of the pacemaker and is frequently immeasurable. The QRS complex is normal unless the P wave is buried in it or aberration occurs. Conduction is normal through the ventricles and retrograde through the atria.

RISK

PJCs may lead to a supraventricular tachycardia if frequent. If rare, PJCs do not pose a threat for the patient.

TREATMENT

If PJCs are infrequent or the patient is asymptomatic, no treatment is necessary. If frequent, PJCs may be controlled by digitalis or quinidine.

NURSING INTERVENTION

Document the dysrhythmia with a rhythm strip (to justify junctional origin rather than ventricular origin). Monitor the patient for increasing frequency of PJCs and notify the physician if the frequency does increase.

Paroxysmal Junctional Tachycardia (PJT)

ETIOLOGY

A highly irritable junctional focus becomes the pacemaker for the heart. The most common causes are metabolic imbalances and increased catecholamine secretion. Acute myocardial infarction, ischemia of the AV node, and digitalis toxicity may also precipitate paroxysmal junctional tachycardia (Figure 12-3).

IDENTIFYING CHARACTERISTICS

The rate is usually 140–220 beats per minute. The rhythm is usually regular. P waves are abnormal, inverted, and may precede, follow, or be buried in the QRS complex. The P-R interval, if present, is shortened or immeasurable. The QRS complex is normal unless the P wave is buried in it or it is aberrantly conducted. Conduction of the QRS may be normal. Atrial conduction is retrograde. PJT may be difficult to distinguish from PAT. They are often called SVT (supraventricular tachycardia).

This is a serious warning of lethal ventricular dysrhythmias. It *begins suddenly* and if it ends, it *ends suddenly*. It may progress to ventricular tachycardia, ventricular

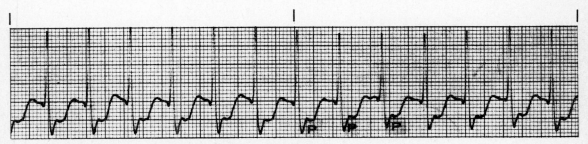

Figure 12-3. Paroxysmal junctional tachycardia (PJT).

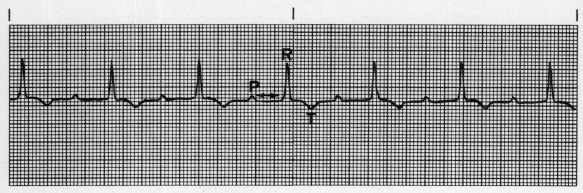

Figure 12-4.   First degree AV heart block.

fibrillation, and cardiac arrest. Even short runs of PJT cause serious hemodynamic compromise leading rapidly to left ventricular failure and circulatory collapse.

TREATMENT

Vagal maneuvers may be tried. If the patient is tolerating the dysrhythmia, digitalis and/or quinidine may be tried. More commonly, intravenous pressor drugs are employed. If hemodyamic compromise occurs, synchronized cardioversion is indicated.

NURSING INTERVENTION

Document the dysrhythmia with a rhythm strip. Assess the patient for hemodynamic compromise. If compromise occurs, notify the physician and medicate as ordered. Monitor the patient for progression to a lethal dysrhythmia and treat accordingly.

First Degree Block

ETIOLOGY

First degree AV junctional block may be caused by arteriosclerotic heart disease (ASHD), acute myocardial infarction, AV node ischemia, and drugs (digitalis, quinidine, and procainamide). It may also be congenital. The AV node delays the pro-gression of the impulse from the SA node for an abnormal length of time (Figure 12-4).

IDENTIFYING CHARACTERISTICS

The rate is normal. The rhythm is regular. P waves are normal. The P-R interval is prolonged beyond 0.20 seconds. The QRS complex is normal. Conduction is normal except for the prolonged delay at the AV node.

RISK

First degree block is not a serious dysrhythmia itself. It may warn of an impending second or third degree block.

TREATMENT

If the P-R interval is less than 0.25 seconds and if it does not increase, no treatment may be required. If the P-R interval is 0.26 seconds or more, atropine is indicated to accelerate the conduction. If the first degree block is progressive, a prophylactic pacemaker may be warranted.

NURSING INTERVENTIONS

Document the dysrhythmia with a rhythm strip. Monitor the patient closely for a sudden progression to second or third degree heart block. If progression develops, document with a rhythm strip and notify the physician immediately.

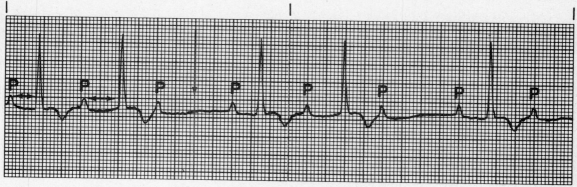

Figure 12-5.   Second degree AV block—Mobitz Type I (Wenckebach).

Second Degree Block—Mobitz Type I and Mobitz Type II

Both Mobitz I (Wenckebach) and Mobitz II are AV junctional blocks. The AV node delays the progression of the SA node impulse for a longer-than-normal time. The characteristics, treatment, and prognosis in these two forms of second degree AV block differ. The Mobitz I (Wenckebach) form of second degree block will be considered first.

MOBITZ I

Etiology

Conduction arises normally from the SA node and progresses to the AV node. With each succeeding impulse, it becomes more difficult for the AV node to conduct the impulse. Eventually, one impulse is not conducted and a QRS complex does not occur. The progression then begins again. Ischemia or injury to the AV node is the cause of this progression (Figure 12-5).

Identifying Characteristics

Atrial rate may be normal. The ventricular rate is slower than the atrial rate. Atrial rhythm is regular and ventricular rhythm, irregular. P waves are normal. The P-R interval becomes *progressively* prolonged, with a decreasing R to R interval, until a P wave is not conducted and a QRS complex does not occur. The QRS complex is normal (with an occasional complex dropped).

Conduction is normal in the atria and delayed or blocked in the AV node.

Risk

Wenckebach is often a temporary block following an acute myocardial infarction. It may, however, progress to a complete (third degree) block. For this reason, Wenckebach is considered a *potentially* dangerous dysrhythmia.

Treatment

Frequently, no treatment is indicated. If the ventricular rate is slow, atropine may increase AV conduction. Isoproterenol is the second drug of choice to increase the SA node rate and thus the overall rate. On occasion, a pacemaker may be inserted.

Nursing Interventions

Document the dysrhythmia with a rhythm strip. Monitor the patient closely, especially the width of the QRS complex. A widening of the complex often precedes complete heart block. If widening of the QRS occurs, document with a rhythm strip and notify the physician.

Now let us look at second degree AV block, Mobitz II.

MOBITZ II

Etiology

An impulse originates in the SA node and progresses normally to the AV node. Below the AV node in the common bundle or bundle branches, impulses are blocked on a *regular* basis with every second, third, or fourth impulse not being conducted. In this block, a QRS complex is regularly missing. This is due to injury of the AV node, the AV junctional tissue, or the His-Purkinje system (Figure 12-6).

Identifying Characteristics

Atrial rate may be normal. Ventricular rate is 2:1, 3:1, or 4:1. The ventricular rate depends on the frequency of the block. (In 4:1 block, there are four atrial beats to every one QRS complex.) The atrial rhythm is regular. Ventricular rhythm is regular or irregular, but slow. P waves are normal. *The P-R interval is constant.* The QRS complex may be normal or widened. Conduction in the atria is normal and may be abnormal in the ventricles. The indicator for Mobitz II is its sudden occurrence, not the regularity or irregularity.

Risk

Type II block is unpredictable and may *suddenly* advance to complete heart block or ventricular standstill, especially common after inferior infarction. This is a dangerous warning dysrhythmia.

Treatment

If the ventricular response is slow, atropine or isoproterenol may be tried. Because it is so unpredictable, a temporary pacemaker is often the treatment of choice. A permanent pacemaker is frequently necessary.

Nursing Interventions

Document the dysrhythmia with a rhythm strip. Determine the width of the QRS complex. The wider the width, the more dangerous the dysrhythmia. Monitor the patient closely for a widening of the QRS complex. The width of the QRS complex indicates the location in the conduction system of the block. The wider the complex, the lower the block is in the bundle branch system. Document the widening, if it occurs, with a rhythm strip; notify the physician immediately; and prepare for the insertion of a transvenous pacemaker. Assess the patient frequently for hemodynamic compromise if the ventricular response is slow (3:1 and 4:1 block).

Third Degree Block—Complete Heart Block

ETIOLOGY

Ischemia or injury to the AV node, junctional tissue, or His-Purkinje tissue is the cause of complete heart block. The ischemia may be secondary to ASHD, acute myocardial infarction, drugs use (digitalis toxicity, quinidine, or procainamide), systemic disease, or electrolyte imbalances (especially in renal patients) (Figure 12-7).

IDENTIFYING CHARACTERISTICS

Atrial rates are faster than ventricular rates. P waves are not conducted. The ventricular

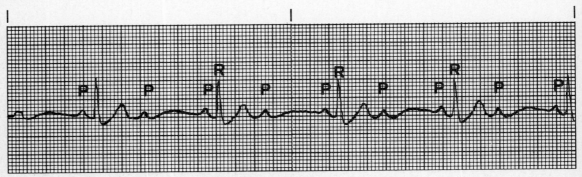

Figure 12-6.   Second degree AV block—Mobitz Type II.

rate is 30–40 (unless there is a junctional escape mechanism). The rhythm is *regular* for both the atria and the ventricles even though they are depolarizing completely independently of each other. P waves are normal and *not* associated with a QRS complex. The P-R interval is not constant. QRS complexes are close to normal if they arise near the AV node. The QRS complex may be wide and bizarre if the impulse arises from the ventricles. There is no AV conduction: The atrial pacemaker controls the atria and the ventricular pacemaker controls the ventricles.

RISK

Because of the slow ventricular rate, ectopic foci often release an impulse (PVC) that may lead to ventricular fibrillation. Complete heart block is a very dangerous, ominous rhythm indicating an impending ventricular fibrillation or asystole.

TREATMENT

Immediate pacemaker insertion is the treatment of choice. Usually complete heart block is temporary after a myocardial infarction, and pacing ability should be available for several days after the return of a normal sinus rhythm.

NURSING INTERVENTION

Document the dysrhythmia with a rhythm strip and notify the physician immediately.

Monitor the patient for ventricular failure, Stokes-Adams attacks, and convulsions. Hemodynamic status is compromised by the slow ventricular rate, and circulatory collapse is not uncommon.

Atrioventricular Dissociation— AV Dissociation

Atrioventricular dissociation is a *symptom* or description of a disorder rather than a dysrhythmia per se.

ETIOLOGY

The many causes of atrioventricular dissociation include anesthesia, drugs (digitalis, quinidine, atropine, procainamide, and salicylates), infections, rheumatic fever, acute inferior infarction, and ischemic heart disease (Figure 12-8).

IDENTIFYING CHARACTERISTICS

The relationship in AV dissociation is from P to P, which is regular, and from R to R which is regular. The P-R interval is nonexistent. (Some texts refer to a P-R distance.) Ventricular rate is greater than atrial. The P wave, usually normal in form, may vary slightly in measurements. The P may fall immediately before, during, or after a QRS complex during the absolute refractory period of the ventricles (the period in which they *cannot* depolarize). The QRS complex may be normal or abnormal. Conduction is abnormal, with no relationship between

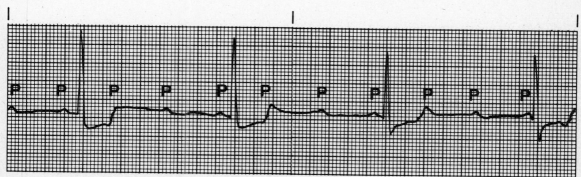

Figure 12-7.   Third degree (complete) AV block.

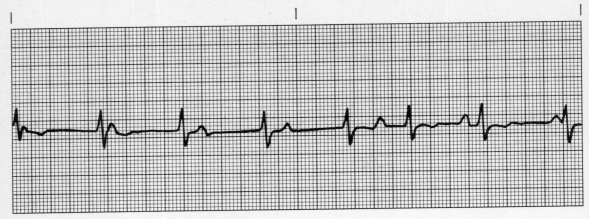

Figure 12-8. Atrioventricular dissociation.

atria and ventricles. The differentiation between complete heart block and AV dissociation is that the ventricular rate in complete heart block is normally 30–40 and is much faster in AV dissociation.

RISK

AV dissociation may develop a slow ventricular response and may require treatment as a third degree heart block.

TREATMENT

Close monitoring for progression of heart block is necessary. A pacemaker may not be indicated if the ventricular rate is adequate.

NURSING INTERVENTION

Monitor the patient closely for signs of cardiac decompensation and progression of the dysrhythmia. Document the dysrhythmia with a rhythm strip and notify the physician if the ventricular rate drops below 50 beats per minute. Be prepared for the insertion of a transvenous pacemaker. Attempt to calm the patient and avoid additional stress.

Bundle Branch Blocks

Bundle branch blocks are also termed intraventricular or subjunctional blocks. There may be a right bundle branch block (RBBB) or a left bundle branch block (LBBB). Since the left bundle branches into fascicles, these fascicles may also become blocked. These are termed hemiblocks. There may be a left anterior hemiblock (LAH) of the anterior fascicle of the left bundle branch or there may be a left posterior hemiblock (LPH) of the posterior fascicle of the left bundle branch. Trifascicular blocks involve both left bundle fascicles and the right bundle branch. Bifascicular blocks usually involve the right bundle branch and one fascicle of the left bundle branch, or both fascicles of the left branch.

Bundle branch blocks CANNOT be diagnosed by a rhythm strip, *only* suspected. A 12-lead EKG is essential.

ETIOLOGY

Three different factors may cause a bundle branch block. First, an acute myocardial infarction may cause ischemia in the intraventricular conduction system. Second, chronic degeneration with fibrous scarring may permanently block the bundle branches. Third, right bundle branch blocks may be congenital (Figure 12-9).

IDENTIFYING CHARACTERISTICS

Bundle branch blocks cannot be diagnosed by a rhythm strip. Rate is usually normal, although it may vary if the bundle branch block varies. Rhythm is regular. P waves

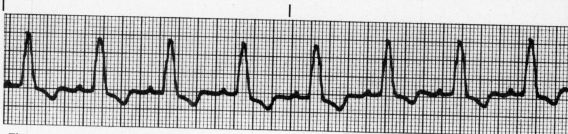

Figure 12-9. Bundle branch blocks.

may be normal. The P-R interval is normal. The QRS complex is *ALWAYS* wide (greater than 0.12) and may be notched, depending upon the lead viewed. Ventricular conduction is abnormal.

RISK

The development of bundle branch blocks indicates marked ischemia of the intraventricular conduction system, and bundle branch blocks are potentially more dangerous than AV blocks since these blocks are subjunctional. The involvement of more than one fascicle often progresses to complete heart block. In these instances, the prognosis is poor.

TREATMENT

There is no effective drug therapy. A temporary pacemaker may be inserted to prevent ventricular standstill if the block is secondary to acute myocardial infarction. In chronic block, the use of a pacemaker is controversial.

NURSING INTERVENTION

If a wider QRS develops suddenly, document this with a rhythm strip. Notify the physician. Obtain a 12-lead EKG. Monitor the patient's condition *closely*. Serious, lethal dysrhythmias are not uncommon.

Idioventricular Rhythm

ETIOLOGY

There is no functioning pacemaker above the ventricles. A focus somewhere in the ventricle initiates an impulse. All diseases and injuries that cause loss of function from the SA node down are etiologic factors (Figure 12-10).

IDENTIFYING CHARACTERISTICS

The ventricles initiate a rate at their inherent ability, usually 20–40 beats per minute. The rhythm is regular but may slow as a "dying heart syndrome" progresses. There

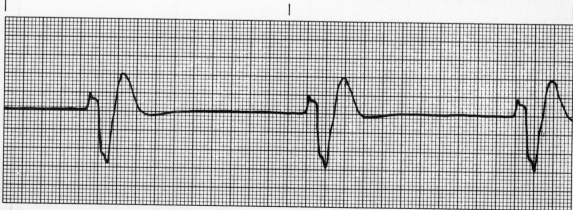

Figure 12-10. Idioventricular rhythm.

is no P wave. There is no P-R interval. The QRS complex is wide and bizarre measuring 0.12 or more. Conduction is abnormal.

RISK

The imminent danger is ventricular standstill. It is possible that the electrical event is not leading to an effective contraction, which means that electrical mechanical dissociation has developed.

TREATMENT

A pacemaker is the only reliable and totally effective form of treatment. In a crisis until a pacemaker can be inserted, isoproterenol hydrochloride (Isuprel®) may accelerate the heart rate. Epinephrine is less reliable in this dysrhythmia but is used if isoproterenol hydrochloride (Isuprel®) is not effective.

NURSING INTERVENTION

Document the dysrhythmia with a rhythm strip. Notify the physician immediately. Assess and treat the patient continuously for cardiac arrest and/or circulatory collapse. Prepare for a pacemaker insertion.

Accelerated Idioventricular Rhythm

ETIOLOGY

The etiology is the same as for the idioventricular rhythm (Figure 12-11).

IDENTIFYING CHARACTERISTICS

These are the same as those of an idioventricular rhythm with the exception that the rate is usually 60–100 beats per minute.

RISK

The immediate risk is that the accelerated focus may cease and the dysrhythmia may convert to an idioventricular rate or cardiac standstill.

TREATMENT

This is the same as for idioventricular rhythm. A pacemaker may not be indicated if the patient is not compromised.

NURSING INTERVENTION

This is the same as for idioventricular rhythm.

Premature Ventricular Contraction (PVC, PVB, VPC)

ETIOLOGY

An irritable focus in the ventricle initiates a contraction before the normally expected beat. The irritability may be due to acute myocardial infarction (most common), ASHD, CHF, drug toxicity, hypoxia, electrolytes, acidosis, or bradycardia (Figure 12-12).

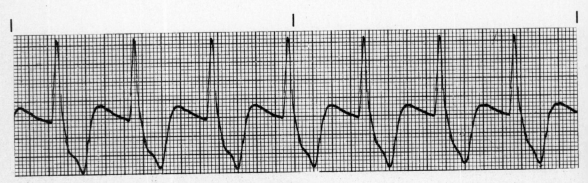

Figure 12-11.   Accelerated idioventricular rhythm.

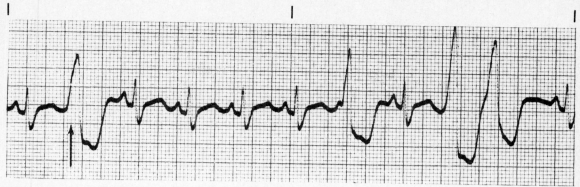

Figure 12-12.   Premature ventricular contraction (PVC, PVB, or VPC).

IDENTIFYING CHARACTERISTICS

The rate is variable. Rhythm is irregular due to the premature beat. P waves are not present in the PVC unless retrograde conduction occurs or unless they are buried in the QRS complex. The P-R interval is immeasurable in the PVC complex. The QRS complex is wide and bizarre. It usually has a compensatory pause which is equal to two R-R distances following the PVC. Ventricular conduction is abnormal.

RISK

The danger of a PVC is the possibility of increasing myocardial irritability leading to an increasing frequency of PVCs. With an increased occurrence of PVCs, ventricular tachycardia and/or ventricular fibrillation may occur. There is a special danger of a fatal dysrhythmia when (a) PVCs occur from more than one focus (multifocal PVCs), (b) PVCs occur more often than six per minute, (c) bigeminy is present (every other beat is a PVC), (d) short runs of PVCs occur frequently (two to four sequential PVCs every few beats; in actuality, three consecutive PVCs constitute a salvo of ventricular tachycardia), and (e) the PVC occurs on the T wave of the preceding complex (described as the R on T phenomenon). If the PVC occurs on the T wave, it may precipitate ventricular fibrillation.

TREATMENT

Lidocaine bolus followed by a lidocaine drip is the treatment of choice. (Note: If a lidocaine bolus has been given and 10–15 minutes have elapsed, another bolus must be administered before hanging the drip to establish and maintain therapeutic blood levels of the drug.) If hypokalemia is present, potassium may terminate the PVCs. If lidocaine is an unsuccessful treatment, procainamide may be tried. Oxygen therapy may eliminate or prevent hypoxia.

NURSING INTERVENTION

Document the dysrhythmia with a rhythm strip. Determine the origin of the PVC. A 12-lead EKG may be helpful. Monitor the patient closely for increasing frequency of PVCs or the development of multifocal PVCs and document. Bolus with lidocaine, document the effect, and prepare a lidocaine drip if indicated. Notify the physician. Observe the patient and monitor closely for ventricular tachycardia and ventricular fibrillation.

Ventricular Tachycardia

ETIOLOGY

Advanced irritability of the ventricles allows a ventricular focus to become the heart's pacemaker. The myocardial irritabil-

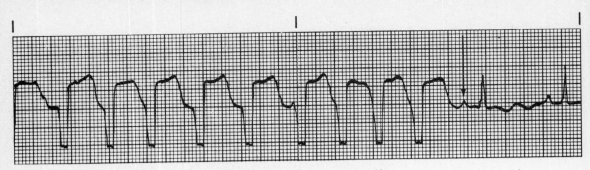

Figure 12-13.   Ventricular tachycardia terminating spontaneously.

ity may be due to ASHD, CHF, acute myo-cardial infarction, electrolyte imbalance, hypoxia, acidosis, or occasionally drugs (Figure 12-13).

IDENTIFYING CHARACTERISTICS

The rate is greater than 100, often 120–220 beats. The rhythm is regular or only slightly irregular. P waves are not discernible and may be referred to as Dressler beats. No measurable P-R interval exists. The QRS complex is wide and bizarre, resembling essentially a salvo (or burst) of premature ventricular contractions. There is no nor-mal conduction. A ventricular focus initi-ates ventricular depolarization.

RISK

If ventricular tachycardia is not terminated, ventricular fibrillation usually develops. Hemodynamic status is so markedly com-promised that cardiogenic shock or sudden death occur. *Ventricular tachycardia is an abso-lute emergency.*

TREATMENT

Although the American Heart Association changed its position on precordial thumps, in a monitored, witnessed development of ventricular tachycardia, a precordial thump is warranted. It may temporarily terminate the ventricular tachycardia.

Immediate intravenous lidocaine bolus is given. If this does not convert the dys-rhythmia, then defibrillation may terminate this dysrhythmia. Treatment to correct a potassium imbalance is essential. Recur-rent ventricular tachycardia *may* be avoided with a lidocaine drip. (Note: If it has been 15 minutes since a bolus was given, a repeat bolus must be given before starting the drip due to the short half-life of lidocaine.) Bre-tylium tosylate (Bretylol®), procainamide hydrochloride (Pronestyl®), and phenytoin sodium (Dilantin®) may all be used if lido-caine is ineffective. In some centers, bre-tylium tosylate is the first line drug of choice over lidocaine.

NURSING INTERVENTIONS

Document this dysrhythmia with a rhythm strip *AND* leave the chart recorder running continuously until the dysrhythmia is ter-minated. If the patient is unconscious, im-mediate defibrillation and institution of car-diac arrest procedures are essential. If the patient is conscious, administer a lidocaine bolus (usually 100 mg or 1 mg/kg of body weight) and prepare a lidocaine drip. If the patient is conscious, prepare for defibrilla-tion and notify the physician. If uncon-sciousness develops, defibrillate stat.

Ventricular Fibrillation

ETIOLOGY

Due to extensive ventricular irritability, ventricular fibers fail to depolarize in se-quence; instead they depolarize individu-ally at random instead of following the all-or-none law of depolarization. This com-monly occurs shortly after an acute myocar-dial infarction. It may, however, occur as a

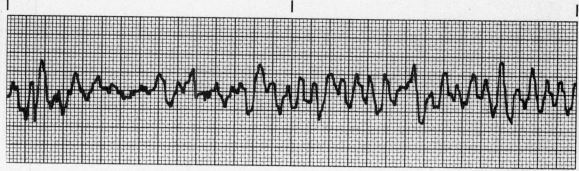

Figure 12-14.   Ventricular fibrillation.

result of ASHD, CHF, digitalis or other drug toxicity, electrolyte imbalance, and such (Figure 12-14).

IDENTIFYING CHARACTERISTICS

There is no identifiable rate. The rhythm is irregular and immeasurable. P waves are replaced by undulating waves as the baseline. The P-R interval is nonexistent or immeasurable. The QRS complex is an undulating, asymmetrical line. There is no conduction.

RISK

The development of cardiac standstill may occur *within* seconds. Circulatory collapse occurs within approximately 2 minutes and is followed by death.

TREATMENT

Immediate defibrillation is the only possibility of establishing a viable cardiac rhythm. Initiate CPR immediately.

NURSING INTERVENTION

Document the dysrhythmia with a rhythm strip and keep the monitor recorder running throughout the dysrhythmia. Initiate cardiac arrest procedures and defibrillate the patient *immediately*. CPR is instituted until the defibrillator is ready and is continued in between attempts at defibrillation. The cardiac arrest protocol is followed until a rhythm is established or a physician pronounces the patient dead.

Escape Beats

A dominant rhythm, essentially regular but with intermittent interruptions, may contain escape beats. This results in an occasional prolonged R-R interval. Several areas may produce escape beats.

Atrial escape beats have an abnormal P wave, a normal P-R interval and a normal QRS complex. Junctional escape beats have an abnormal P wave, a short P-R interval, and usually a normal QRS complex. Ventricular escape beats have an abnormal QRS complex without a preceding P wave.

Escape beats usually occur with an associated prolonged R-R interval (but not long enough to be compensatory).

Escape beats are of minor significance and usually require no treatment. It is important not to suppress an escape beat; this might allow a ventricular foci of a more serious nature to develop.

13

Atherosclerosis, Angina Pectoris, and Myocardial Infarction

Learning Objectives

By the end of this chapter, the nurse will be able to:

1. Differentiate between arteriosclerosis and atherosclerosis.
2. Explain the differences in the four grades of atherosclerosis.
3. List four risk factors for coronary artery disease that cannot be altered.
4. List three risk factors for coronary artery disease that may be altered with appropriate medical treatment.
5. List four risk factors for coronary artery disease that *can* be altered by the individual.
6. Define angina pectoris.
7. Identify the primary presenting symptom of angina pectoris.
8. Differentiate between the pathophysiology of angina pectoris and that of a myocardial infarction.
9. List the usual presenting signs of a myocardial infarction.
10. Identify the three primary goals in the treatment of an acute myocardial infarction.

A series of physiologic changes within the body and heart starts with arteriosclerosis and advances (without intervention) to coronary artery disease (CAD). The first symptoms of coronary artery disease are usually those of angina pectoris, but may be myocardial infarction or sudden death. Without intervention, angina frequently results in a myocardial infarction (M.I.).

Arteriosclerosis/Atherosclerosis

Arteriosclerosis is the name applied to a group of three chronic disease states. One of these three states is termed atherosclerosis. Frequently, the terms arteriosclerosis and atherosclerosis are used interchangeably to mean that fatty acid placques have adhered to the intimal layer of the arteries.

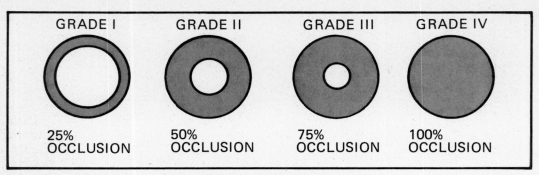

Figure 13-1.   The four grades of coronary artery occlusion.

Although atherosclerosis occurs throughout the body, our study in this chapter is of the effect of atherosclerosis upon the heart and the coronary arteries.

CLASSIFICATION OF ATHEROSCLEROSIS

In the coronary arteries, there are four grades of atherosclerosis as classified by cardiac catheterization (Figure 13-1). Normally (i.e., ideally), atherosclerosis is not present.

1. *Grade one* atherosclerosis is minimal; that is, less than 25% of the lumen of the coronary artery is occluded.

2. *Grade two* atherosclerosis is present when 50% of the lumen of the coronary artery is occluded.

3. *Grade three* is severe atherosclerosis with 75% of the lumen of the coronary artery occluded.

4. *Grade four* is complete occlusion of the coronary artery resulting in myocardial infarction.

Obstruction by atherosclerotic placques may (and does) occur in any or all of the coronary arteries. It is thought that grade three atherosclerosis must be present before *significant* symptoms develop. Specific factors tend to be related to the development of atherosclerosis.

ETIOLOGY

Four Unalterable Risk Factors

1. *Hereditary predisposition* to the development of atherosclerosis seems to be a factor in developing atherosclerosis.

2. *Age* appears to influence the development of atherosclerosis by the fact that it is more prevalent in older persons than in younger persons.

3. *Sex* seems to be a factor in the development of atherosclerosis since more men than women develop atherosclerosis (at least prior to menopause).

4. *Race* influences atherosclerosis. It is more common in Caucasians than in any other race.

Three Medically Alterable Risk Factors

1. *Hypertension* has been shown to be related to the development of atherosclerosis. Close medical treatment of hypertension may retard the development of atherosclerosis.

2. *Diabetics* develop atherosclerosis five times more often than nondiabetics. Close medical treatment and control of diabetes may retard the atherosclerotic process.

3. *Hyperlipidemia*, when accompanied by high serum cholesterol levels, *may* have a bearing on the development and/or progression of atherosclerosis. Medical treatment of hyperlipidemia

may help retard the atherosclerotic process.

Four Alterable Risk Factors

These factors can be altered *by the individual* to decrease the possibility or progression of atherosclerosis.

1. *Obesity* can be reduced if the individual is motivated.

2. *Cigarette smokers* have an increased incidence of atherosclerosis over non-smokers.

3. *Emotional tension and stress*, such as experienced by Type A personalities are influential in increasing one's chances of developing atherosclerosis. The greater the tension and stress, the greater the incidence of atherosclerosis. Research continues to look at the cause/effect relationship since these factors are associated with increased atherosclerosis.

4. *Sedentary life-styles* predispose one to developing atherosclerosis.

If an individual is sufficiently motivated, these last four risk factors can be modified.

RESULTS OF ATHEROSCLEROSIS

One cannot change some risk factors; one can alter other risk factors with medical treatment; and one can eliminate some risk factors if so motivated. The progression of atherosclerosis is from the development of angina, to ischemia, to myocardial infarction, to congestive heart failure or sudden death. In spite of the prognosis with alterable risk factors, coronary atherosclerosis is still responsible for one-third of *all* deaths in the United States.

Angina Pectoris

If atherosclerosis has developed to between grade two and grade three, the individual will probably develop signs of angina. Angina is chest pain due to cardiac ischemia and is usually related to atherosclerosis.

PATHOPHYSIOLOGY

Any factor that results in diminished blood flow and, therefore, decreased oxygen to the heart muscle may produce angina and its symptoms.

ETIOLOGY

Arteriosclerotic heart disease (ASHD) is probably the leading cause of angina. Hypertension, tachydysrhythmias, and some bradydysrhythmias, CHF, and shock are also prominent causes of angina. Thyrotoxicosis, aortic and mitral valvular disease, and anemia less commonly cause angina.

PRECIPITATION OF ANGINAL ATTACKS

The four Es are the most important factors to consider in predicting one's chances for an anginal attack. The four Es are exercise, eating, emotions, and environmental exposure (to extremes of hot and cold temperatures). Persons with severe ASHD may have anginal attacks when they smoke (since smoking increases heart demands for oxygen and simultaneously lowers the available oxygen).

Nocturnal angina occurs with marked ASHD anytime the person lies down. When a person lies down, there is a decrease in metabolic activity and in cardiac output and thus coronary perfusion. The decreased perfusion limits the oxygen available to the myocardium, and angina results.

PRESENTING SYMPTOMS OF ANGINA

Pain is the primary symptom. It may be described as burning, squeezing in a tight band, or extreme heaviness or pressure on the lower sternum. It may radiate to the neck, jaws, shoulders, arms, and stomach.

Characteristically, the pain begins after eating or physical activity and subsides with rest. The pain usually lasts 1–4 minutes but it may require as long as 10 minutes to subside completely. The pain occurs when the supply of oxygen does not meet the oxygen demands of the myocardium.

TREATMENT OF ANGINA

Sublingual nitroglycerin (NTG) usually relieves the angina within 1½ minutes. Nitroglycerin taken *before* an activity may prevent an attack. Alteration of one's life-style to eliminate the alterable risk factors may help decrease the severity and frequency of attacks. If the angina attacks increase in frequency or intensity (crescendo angina), stress testing and/or cardiac catheterization to determine the extent of the disease is indicated. The patient may be a candidate for transluminal angioplasty or coronary bypass surgery, which will stop the angina and decrease the risk of myocardial infarction. The patient is advised to exercise within his or her pain limits and obtain adequate rest.

If atherosclerosis is present, the patient *has* coronary artery disease (CAD). Angina is a symptom of CAD.

VARIANTS OF ANGINA

There are two variants of angina. Nocturnal angina occurs with the patient at rest, often waking him or her. Prinzmetal angina is a form of angina due to coronary artery spasm and *not* ASHD, although ASHD may be present. Prinzmetal angina is also not related to exercise, but appears to be related to emotional stress.

Acute coronary insufficiency is a synonym for angina. Other frequently applied terms include unstable angina, impending myocardial infarction, and preinfarction angina. In these states, anginal attacks are more frequent, more severe, and longer-lasting than in "simple" angina pectoris. These are all symptoms of coronary artery disease (CAD) and may terminate in an acute myocardial infarction or sudden death.

Myocardial Infarction (M.I., A.M.I.)

An M.I. is the actual necrosis or death of myocardial tissue because of no blood supply (and thus, no oxygen) to a specific area of the heart.

ETIOLOGY

In 90% of all M.I.s, ASHD is present. The remaining 10% of M.I.s are due to coronary artery spasm (Prinzmetal angina) in which the artery spasms sufficiently to prevent blood from reaching the myocardium. Any occlusion of the coronary arteries will also cause an M.I.

PRESENTING SYMPTOMS OF AN M.I.

Chest pain with nausea (and maybe vomiting), diaphoresis, and weakness are the most common symptoms of an M.I. The infarct pain differs from anginal pain. With an M.I., the chest pain is constant, severe, and *not* relieved with nitroglycerin. The location of the pain is similar to anginal pain. It is, however, *not* relieved with rest or lying down. In fact, it often occurs at rest without a clear precipitating event.

As the pain, nausea, weakness, and diaphoresis continue, patients become dyspneic and often develop severe apprehension which may be accompanied by a sense of impending doom.

A 12-lead EKG or a rhythm strip may show dysrhythmias and marked QRST changes dependent upon the site of infarction. The typical changes in an EKG are found in Appendix I and many other cardiology texts.

Occlusion of the right coronary artery results in an inferior infarction and may include posterior portions of the heart. Occlusion of the left main artery is known as the "widow maker" since it normally results in sudden death. Occlusion of the circumflex artery results in a lateral infarction. Occlusion of the left anterior descending artery results in an anterior infarction, which may include some inferior parts of the heart.

TREATMENT AND COMPLICATIONS OF AN M.I.

The goals of treating an infarction are to increase coronary blood flow and decrease oxygen demand to prevent death or extension of injury to the myocardium, and to control or correct dysrhythmias that occur.

Pain relief is a prime objective and is usually accomplished with I.V. morphine sulfate (drug of choice), I.V. hydromorphone hydrochloride (Dilaudid®), or I.V. meperidine hydrochloride (Demerol®). (I.M. injections are avoided since they raise the SGOT and LDH enzyme blood levels.)

Continuous cardiac monitoring is used to provide for the early identification and intervention of dysrhythmias. If the patient survives the initial infarction and subsequently dies, death is usually due to a shock syndrome. Dysrhythmias of all types including conduction disturbances occur.

Oxygen therapy is usually started to ensure that sufficient oxygen content is available for myocardial needs.

An intravenous (life-line) is started and kept patent for use in emergency situations.

Diet, usually low sodium, is given as tolerated. A majority of hospital CCUs prohibit caffeine-containing drinks and food. Caffeine is a stimulant and may add stress to an already injured heart.

Hemodynamic monitoring must be continuous for early intervention in congestive failure, ventricular failure, circulatory collapse, pulmonary edema, and cardiogenic shock.

Bedrest and emotional support of the patient are necessary for healing the injured myocardium. It may be *most* difficult to promote such rest, especially in Type A personality patients. Tranquilizers and sedatives may be useful.

Venous pooling may result in thromboembolism. Passive and active range of motion exercises and support hose help prevent this pooling. Emboli may also occur due to a phlebitis from an infiltrated intravenous line.

Less common but equally lethal complications of an M.I. include pericarditis, papillary muscle rupture, ventricular aneurysm, and ventricular rupture. Sudden death commonly occurs with the last three of these complications.

RECOVERY FROM AN M.I.

Recovery begins as soon as myocardial injury and necrosis stops. Scar tissue develops (Figure 13-2) at the necrotic area. This process takes 6–8 weeks to complete.

Emotional support of the patient and family is a key factor in recovery. Patients often feel that their active and productive lives are over. It is not uncommon to see the patient and family members going through the stages of grief following an M.I. Chapter 47 on psychosocial ramifications deals with this in more detail.

Education of the patient and family in ways of changing their life-styles to eliminate alterable risk factors is an essential role of the nurse and helps the patient and family work through the emotional grieving process.

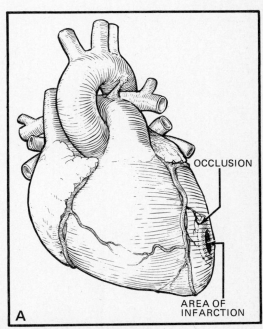

Figure 13-2a. Myocardial infarction.

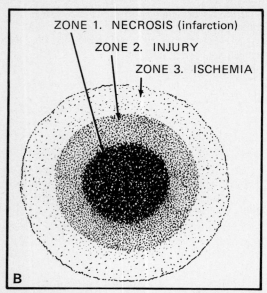

Figure 13-2b. The development of scar tissue following myocardial infarction.

— 14

Acute/Chronic Heart Failure, Pulmonary Edema, Pleural Effusion, and Pericarditis

---

Learning Objectives

By the end of this chapter, the nurse will be able to:

1. Differentiate between acute and chronic heart failure.
2. Explain the pathophysiology and progression of heart failure.
3. List three methods of treating heart failure.
4. Define pulmonary edema.
5. List the presenting symptoms of pulmonary edema.
6. Explain the pathophysiology of pulmonary edema.
7. List three treatment modalities for pulmonary edema.
8. Define pleural effusion.
9. Identify the presenting symptoms of a pleural effusion.
10. Explain the treatment for pleural effusion.
11. Define pericarditis.
12. List the presenting symptoms of pericarditis.
13. Identify three complications of pericarditis.
14. Explain the treatment of pericarditis.

All of the disease entities in this chapter may develop rapidly except chronic heart failure. Chronic heart failure may rapidly convert to acute heart failure. Early recognition and rapid intervention are the key factors to a successful outcome.

Acute/Chronic Congestive Heart Failure (CHF)

Acute heart failure is a severe inability of the heart to pump blood through the systemic circulation in an amount sufficient to meet the body's needs.

Chronic heart failure is the gradual development of this failure of the heart to pump sufficient blood to meet body demands. Chronic heart failure can become acute without an obvious cause.

Heart failure may be classified as right or left heart failure in addition to acute or chronic.

PATHOPHYSIOLOGY OF HEART FAILURE

Left ventricular pump failure usually occurs before right ventricular pump failure. The left ventricular myocardium weakens to the extent that it cannot eject blood in the normal amount. This reduces the cardiac output.

If the left ventricle cannot pump out all of the blood it receives from the atrium, a buildup of blood and pressure occurs in the left atrium. As the pressure increases in the left atrium, it becomes more difficult for blood to enter the atrium from the pulmonary veins. As the blood in the pulmonary veins becomes unable to flow into the left atrium, blood backs up in the lung vessels. When pressure in the lungs exceeds 10–25 mm Hg, fluid from the pulmonary capillaries leaks into the interstitial spaces. (This results in the development of pulmonary edema.)

Since the lung vasculature is distensible, it can accept a moderate amount of blood back up. But without intervention, the pressure in the lungs increases to the point that the right ventricle cannot eject its blood into the lungs for oxygenation. As the backflow pressure increases, the right ventricle fails. Then blood from the right atrium cannot drain completely and consequently cannot accommodate all the blood entering it from the vena cavae. Since venous blood flow to the heart is impeded, venous pooling and eventual organ congestion with venous blood occurs.

ETIOLOGY

Left heart failure is most often caused by acute myocardial infarction. Arteriosclerot-

ic heart disease, dysrhythmias, and increased circulating blood volume are the next most frequent causes of left pump failure. Less commonly, myocarditis and valvular diseases precipitate heart failure.

Right heart failure is most commonly caused by left heart failure and then by all the factors that cause left heart failure. Right failure may also be caused by pulmonary emboli, essential pulmonary hypertension, and COPD.

PRESENTING SYMPTOMS

The left heart failure patient usually demonstrates restlessness followed by anxiety, dyspnea, paroxysmal nocturnal dyspnea (PND), orthopnea, diaphoresis, a gallop rhythm, and elevated pulmonary artery (PA) diastolic and pulmonary capillary wedge presssure (PCWP) values. As the left pump failure advances, additional pulmonary signs develop. These include basilar rales, bronchial wheezing, hyperventilation, cyanosis, hypoxia, and coughing with a frothy sputum. A sinus tachycardia and pulsus alternans (the palpation of alternating strong and weak pulse beats) are common.

Right heart failure symptoms include pitting dependent edema, hepatosplenomegaly, jugular venous distension (JVD), elevated right atrial pressure (CVP), oliguria, and bounding pulsus. Dysrhythmias may occur in both left and right heart failure.

TREATMENT AND NURSING INTERVENTIONS

The goal of treating left heart failure is to improve ventricular function and to prevent the progression towards right heart failure. Three methods of treatment exist.

1. Improve contractility of the ventricle. This is attempted by drug therapy (with positive inotropic agents), most commonly with digitalis or ouabain. Within the limits of Starling's law, this method of treatment is very effective.

2. Decrease afterload. Afterload is the pressure resistance of the blood in the

aorta which the left ventricle must overcome to eject blood. Decreasing this pressure will decrease afterload. Through the dilatory effects of nitrates and sodium nitroprusside (Nipride®), the lumen size of the ateries can be increased. Intra-aortic balloon pumps are also used for this in some centers.

3. Decrease preload. If one can lower the volume of blood entering the right atrium, the stress on the left ventricle is reduced. Diuretic therapy (furosemide and the thiazides), intravenous nitroglycerin, fluid and sodium restrictions, and rotating tourniquets will all alter preload.

Close monitoring of the patient and the patient's response to these treatments are very important in early detection of a deteriorating state requiring more aggressive therapy.

COMPLICATIONS OF HEART FAILURE

The major complications of heart failure are the progression of failure and the development of lethal dysrhythmias, resulting in cardiac and pulmonary deterioration ending in death. Therapies to treat heart failure may cause drug toxicity (including oxygen toxicity) and fluid and electrolyte imbalances.

Pulmonary Edema

Pulmonary edema occurs when pressure in the pulmonary vasculature exceeds 30 mm Hg. This results in extravasation of fluid from pulmonary capillaries into interstitial tissue and intra-alveolar spaces.

ETIOLOGY

Acute pulmonary edema is usually the result of rapid left ventricular failure. Pulmonary edema also develops when sudden decompensation occurs in the chronic heart failure patient, as a result of increased permeability of the alveolar cell membrane, and from other diseases.

CLINICAL PRESENTATION

Dyspnea, PND, and orthopnea are common signs. As pulmonary edema increases, bibasilar rales may be heard. Bronchial wheezing, which is due to constriction (spasm) of the bronchioles secondary to increased congestion in the bronchioles, occurs. Hyperventilation and agitation are common. Cyanosis may or may not be present.

X-RAY CHANGES

Changes due to pulmonary edema occur on x-rays in stages equal to the progression and/or severity of the pulmonary edema. The first change is an enlargement of the pulmonary veins. As interstitial edema occurs, the vessels become poorly outlined and foggy. This is frequently referred to as hilar haze. As intra-alveolar edema develops, the x-ray shows a density in the inner middle zone. This gives the appearance of a "bat wing" or "butterfly" at the hilum. Interlobar fluid is often seen in this stage.

TREATMENT AND NURSING INTERVENTIONS

The goal of therapy is to resolve the pulmonary edema by improving cardiac function which will improve renal function while supporting respiratory needs.

Renal function improvement is attempted by diuretic therapy. Furosemide and ethacrynic acid are potent, fast-acting diuretics.

Morphine sulfate intravenously is used to correct pulmonary vasoconstriction caused by alveolar hypoxia and to increase venous capacitance. It also eliminates anxiety and agitation.

Cardiac function may be improved with rapid digitalization, using digitalis or deslanoside (Cedilanid-D®). The goal is to decrease preload, decrease afterload, and increase contractility.

Correction of hypoxia is essential. An IPPB treatment with alcohol (a de-sudsing agent) is controversial but may be tried. Oxygen therapy by mask at 100% concentration may correct the hypoxia. Intubation with CPAP or PEEP may be necessary for some patients.

Rotating tourniquets will often be used in patients already digitalized and on diuretics. Use of rotating tourniquets will decrease the volume of circulating blood volume and "buy time" for the other treatment modalities to resolve the pulmonary edema.

Nursing interventions include monitoring of all body systems to ensure adequate ventilation, adequate cardiac function and treatment of developing dysrhythmias, electrolyte and acid/base balance with the use of diuretics, and adequate tissue perfusion to the extremities if rotating tourniquets are used.

Emotional support of the patient with pulmonary edema is made difficult by the patient's fear of suffocation; but it is of paramount importance to decrease this fear along with concurrent treatment modalities being used.

Pleural Effusion

A pleural effusion is the presence of fluid in the pleural space. It must be determined if the fluid is a transudate or an exudate. A transudate is highly fluid and has a low content of cells, protein, and other cellular elements. The specific gravity will be less than 1.015. An exudate has a high content of cells, protein, and other cellular debris. Its specific gravity will be greater than 1.015.

ETIOLOGY

Exudates are caused by bacteria, viruses, tuberculosis, pulmonary infarction, and many other conditions. Transudates are the result of congestive heart failure, cirrhosis, and the nephrotic syndrome.

CLINICAL PRESENTATION

Chest x-ray will normally show transudate fluid on the right side or exudate fluid bilaterally. The patient will have orthopnea, PND, dyspnea, tachycardia, perhaps a cardiomegaly, a gallop rhythm, murmurs, rales, and peripheral edema.

TREATMENT

The objective of therapy is to treat the underlying condition causing the exudate or transudate. The treatment of pleural effusion is similar to the treatment for congestive heart failure with one addition. If the effusion is large, it normally is drained. If the effusion is small, it will probably resolve with the appropriate treatment for heart failure.

Pericarditis

Pericarditis is *any* alteration in the pericardium.

ETIOLOGY

Pericarditis may be present or may develop in essentially *any* disease process. It may be infectious (most common) due to a virus or bacteria. It may be metabolic such as seen in uremia or it may be drug-related due to such drugs as hydralazine and procainamide. Pericarditis may be idiopathic. It may be secondary to systemic disease or it may occur in trauma cases and may follow acute myocardial infarction.

CLINICAL PRESENTATION

Symptoms vary with the etiology of the pericarditis. Most commonly, pain is present. The pain may mimic an acute M.I., angina, or pleurisy. It usually increases with deep respiration and when lying supine. Sitting up and leaning forward usually diminishes the pain. Fever is usual. Pericardial friction rub may be present for only a few days (post-M.I.) or prolonged for many days (uremia). The pericardial friction rub is a scratchy, superficial sound with three components best heard at the lower left sternum. Classical EKG changes are S-T segment elevation in all leads except aVR and V_1. S-T segment depression occurs in these leads (aVR and V_1).

TREATMENT

Pain relief is essential to promote normal and adequate ventilation. Anti-inflammatory drugs such as indomethacin may be tried. Steroid therapy may be used. Treatment of the underlying cause is imperative. Antipyretic agents will control the fever. Pericardiocentesis may be performed if the possibility of developing a tamponade is present. (Refer to Chapter 7 for the explanation of the pericardiocentesis procedure.) Treatment may consist of pericardiectomy if the pericarditis is severe or recurrent. Anticoagulants are contraindicated.

COMPLICATIONS

Complications of pericarditis include dysrhythmias, tamponade, and constriction. Each complication must be treated promptly. Hemodynamic monitoring with a pulmonary artery catheter is useful in early detection of tamponade. Auscultation of heart sounds is essential on a regular and frequent schedule.

NURSING INTERVENTIONS

These include continuous EKG monitoring for signs of dysrhythmias that may indicate the early development of cardiac tamponade. Monitoring with a pulmonary artery catheter is preferred over only EKG monitoring in some centers. The standard nursing interventions involved with PA monitoring are employed in these instances. The nurse should be prepared to set up and assist with an emergency pericardiocentesis if it becomes warranted. Especially close auscultation of cardiac sounds is imperative for early intervention.

Medications to relieve pain and fever are administered as ordered.

Arterial blood gases should be monitored at regular intervals to determine ventilatory status and to allow early intervention if hypoxia develops.

Emotional support of the patient and explanations of the close monitoring will help to alleviate some of the patient's anxiety.

— 15 —

Cardiogenic Shock, Intra-Aortic Balloon Pump, and Hypertensive Crisis

---

Learning Objectives

By the end of this chapter, the nurse will be able to:

1. Define cardiogenic shock.
2. List several causes of cardiogenic shock.
3. Discuss the progressive pathophysiologic cycle of cardiogenic shock.
4. List four compensatory mechanisms of cardiogenic shock.
5. List five or more "early" and five or more "late" signs of cardiogenic shock.
6. Describe the purpose of six or more specific steps in treating cardiogenic shock.
7. List at least four complications of cardiogenic shock.
8. List the uses of the IABP and explain the insertion and placement of the IABP.
9. Describe the function of the IABP in correlation to the cardiac cycle.
10. List two major complications of IABP.
11. Define hypertensive crisis.
12. List five etiologies of hypertension.
13. Identify at least three presenting symptoms of a hypertensive crisis.
14. Differentiate between hypertensive encephalopathy and malignant hypertension.

Cardiogenic Shock

Cardiogenic shock exists when the heart is unable to pump sufficient oxygenated blood to all parts of the body.

ETIOLOGY

Any condition that leads to a decreased cardiac output can cause cardiogenic shock. Left myocardial infarction is the most common cause. Other causes include dysrhythmias, decompensated congestive heart failure, coronary or pulmonary embolus, rupture of any heart structure (chordae tendineae, papillary muscle, septum, valves), dissecting aortic aneurysm, and tension pneumothorax.

PATHOPHYSIOLOGY

Cardiogenic shock secondary to myocardial infarction follows the same pathophysiologic cycle as acute heart failure (Chapter 14). To review: Decreased strength of the left ventricular myocardium results in incomplete systolic emptying of the left ventricle (which increases left ventricular end-diastolic pressure or LVEDP). Less blood from the left atrium can enter the left ventricle which increases the pressure in the left atrium. The increased left atrial pressure inhibits blood inflow from the four pulmonary veins. The pulmonary veins become engorged. This engorgement leads to pulmonary edema resulting in pulmonary insufficiency. The increased pulmonary pressure prevents the right ventricle from emptying completely. Pressure builds in the right ventricle preventing complete emptying of the right atrium. As pressure increases in the right atrium it impedes entry of venous blood from the venae cavae. Concurrently, the decreased cardiac output activates several compensatory mechanisms.

COMPENSATORY MECHANISMS

1. Stimulation of the sympathetic nervous system by the baroreceptors releases norepinephrine and epinephrine from the adrenal medulla. Epinephrine is responsible for an increased heart rate and both epinephrine and norepinephrine increase vasoconstriction of vessels throughout the body EXCEPT the cerebral and coronary vessels.

2. Decreased cardiac output of oxygenated blood to the brain results in hypercardia, which stimulates respiratory centers in the medulla oblongata to compensate for the pulmonary dysfunction. Cerebral ischemia results in sympathetic stimulation of the vasomotor center producing a further generalized vasoconstriction.

3. Decreased renal perfusion activates the renin-angiotensin system (Chapter 25) to increase blood pressure and to promote retention of sodium by the kidneys. The increased sodium increases serum osmolality, which stimulates the pituitary gland to release ADH, and water is reabsorbed.

4. Marked vasoconstriction of blood vessels in the splanchnic region, subcutaneous tissue, and pulmonary veins helps to maintain cardiac filling pressure.

These compensatory mechanisms cannot function indefinitely. If intervention to support the weakening myocardium is not prompt and aggressive, the shock becomes irreversible and the patient dies. Even with prompt and aggressive treatment, more than 80% of the patients who develop cardiogenic shock will die.

FAILURE OF COMPENSATORY MECHANISMS

The vasoconstriction of the splanchnic area is presumed to result in the release of a myocardial toxic factor (MTF) which is probably an enzyme. The MTF has a negative inotropic effect depressing myocardial contractility by interfering with the calcium role in depolarization. Other toxic factors, such as endotoxins from dead bacteria in the constricted intestines, result in depression of cardiac function and vasodilatation.

Severe and/or sustained cerebral ischemia eventually affects the vasomotor center by depressing its sympathetic action. In the late stages of shock, there will be no vasomotor center activity. The end result is a pooling of blood in the periphery as vasoconstriction fails and vasodilatation begins.

Arterial blood pressure falling below a critical point $\left(\frac{60 \pm 10}{40}\right)$ reduces myocardial contractility, which results in a decreased perfusion of the coronary arteries. This decreased perfusion causes further weakening of the myocardium. This becomes a vicious cycle.

Progression of shock may be caused, in part, by sludged blood. Tissue metabolism continues in spite of a slow blood flow. This metabolism releases large amounts of acid (lactic and carbonic) which promotes microthrombi and blood agglutination. The thrombi may actually occlude capillaries and result in increased agglutination of RBCs, WBCs, and platelets, which will impede the circulation.

A generalized cell deterioration occurs as the shock state becomes severe. The liver is especially affected since its normally high metabolic activity cannot be supported by the decreased perfusion with poorly oxygenated blood. Due to its vascular construction, the liver is also in contact with all the abnormal chemicals and toxins present in the blood. This contact with toxins causes a marked decrease in energy for the active transport of sodium and potassium. The result is sodium and chloride accumulating inside the cell and potassium accumulating outside the cell. Mitochondrial activity is severely depressed. Lysosomes split, releasing hydrolases which cause a further deterioration of intracellular structures.

Severe shock causes a tissue necrosis. The necrosis occurs first in the tissues most poorly perfused. Necrosis develops as a result of the tissues' *anaerobic* metabolism instead of their normal aerobic metabolism.

Acidosis occurs as a result of both pulmonary dysfunction and pump failure that decreases tissue perfusion. Insufficient tissue perfusion results in cells obtaining energy from anaerobic glycolysis. This form of energy production releases large quantities of lactic acid. Lactic acidosis depresses the myocardium even further and this becomes another vicious cycle.

Vascular failure occurs in severe shock, resulting in venous dilatation and pooling of blood. This pooling of blood further diminishes cardiac output by decreasing preload and becomes a cycle.

As compensatory mechanisms fail, the shock state rapidly becomes irreversible.

PRESENTING SYMPTOMS

Signs and symptoms can be divided into early signs and late signs. However, the patient who develops cardiogenic shock may deteriorate very rapidly and die before the sequence of signs and symptoms are observed. *Early signs* include tachycardia, gallop rhythm, dyspnea, orthopnea, PND, rales, restlessness, and fatigue. *Late signs* include extreme restlessness, oliguria, anuria, nausea, vomiting, anorexia, hypotension, Cheyne-Stokes respirations, cough with production of frothy mucus, pulmonary edema, distended jugular veins, hepatojugular reflux, and pulsus alternans. Left ventricular hypertrophy and hepatomegaly are sometimes seen.

TREATMENT OF CARDIOGENIC SHOCK

Treatment methods of cardiogenic shock differ from area to area. Some generalizations can be made.

1. *Patient position* is a controversial issue. In comatose, unintubated patients, the necessary position is supine. In the conscious patient, a low Fowler's position may be preferred. In this position, return cerebral venous flow is facilitated, preventing stagnant anoxia of brain tissue. The brain is higher than in a Trendelenberg position, increasing cerebral venous return. A low Fowler's position aids in ventilation since abdominal contents are not pressing against the diaphragm, which results in greater pulmonary expansion. Gravity of the low Fowler's position helps drain blood from the four pulmonary veins into the left atrium. Finally, venous return from the lower trunk and legs is impeded, mimicking to some extent the effect of rotating tourniquets.

2. *Pain relief* to decrease anginal pain will also help allay apprehension and anxiety. With relief of pain, the patient will breathe slowly and deeply. This helps decrease pulmonary edema (especially using morphine sulfate) and dyspnea.

3. *Respiratory insufficiency* is treated by administering oxygen. Some physicians order oxygen by mask. Others prefer oxygen delivered under pressure, either frequent IPPB treatments or intubation and a ventilator. Use of pressure may aid alveolar expansion and exchange of gases by forcing accumulated fluid from alveoli back into the pulmonary capillaries.

4. *Renal output* must be maintained in an attempt to avoid pulmonary edema and extra strain on the heart due to fluid overload and to maintain electrolyte balance. Intravenous furosemide (Lasix®) is the drug of choice, in most cases, to help maintain intake and output balance. Output should be measured and recorded every 30 minutes.

5. *Administration of drugs* is vital in cardiogenic shock. Digitalis is often the first drug given. It slows and strengthens the myocardial contraction. Vasopressors may be used. Dopamine hydrochloride (Intropin®) has positive inotropic and chronotropic effects *without* constricting the renal arteries in low doses. Isoproterenol (Isuprel®) has a positive effect and dilates the coronary arteries. However, isoproterenol hydrochloride increases myocardial oxygen needs by increasing heart rate. Norepinephrine (Levophed®) has a positive inotropic effect and causes a peripheral vasoconstriction. This vasoconstriction increases circulatory volume (afterload) and may be avoided for that reason. Vasodilators may also be used. Sodium nitroprusside (Nipride®) alone or with dopamine will reduce arterial pressure. Dobutamine hydrochloride (Dobutrex®) may be used in place of sodium nitroprusside and dopamine hydrochloride (Intropin®). Intravenous nitroglycerin is gaining acceptance to reduce afterload, which will decrease the strain on the myocardium. It is essential that the patient be monitored very closely while vasoactive drugs are being administered. (Newer cardiac drugs are covered in Chapter 16.) A pulmonary artery catheter is most adequate and preferred. However, sometimes an arterial line is the only available monitoring source.

6. *Metabolic needs* must be decreased to a minimum. Physical and/or emotional needs of the patient should be reduced to a minimum, and the nurse should assume responsibility for *all* the physical needs. The metabolic needs of a patient increases seven times for every one degree centigrade increase in temperature. The patient frequently complains of being cold. But he or she should NOT be covered unless actual shivering occurs. Raising the patient's temperature will cause a peripheral dilatation and decrease circulating blood volume.

7. *Acid-base disturbances* occur early in shock and often are complex. Treatment of acid-base states is covered in Chapter 3.

8. *Steroid* use is controversial in treatment of cardiogenic shock. If used, usually one gram of a corticosteroid is administered by intravenous bolus.

COMPLICATIONS OF CARDIOGENIC SHOCK

The most common complication of cardiogenic shock is death (in more than 80% of all cases). The development of shock lung—ARDS—is covered in Chapter 5. Renal failure may occur and is discussed in Chapter 27. Liver dysfunction is discussed in Chapter 46. Disseminated intravascular coagulation (D.I.C.), Chapter 42, is not an infrequent cause of death. Cerebral infarction (due to ischemia) may occur. Extension of an acute M.I. may occur and result in death. Cardiac dysrhythmias are common and require prompt intervention to prevent a progression to death.

Intra-Aortic Balloon Pump (IABP)

Use of the aortic counterpulsation balloon, or the intra-aortic balloon pump (IABP), is available in some hospitals. The IABP reduces the strain against the left ventricle and increases blood flow into the coronary arteries, which makes it useful in treating refractory cardiac failure and cardiogenic shock.

INSERTION OF THE IABP

The IABP is inserted in the femoral artery after local anesthesia is achieved. It is advanced up the artery until it is in the descending thoracic aorta (Figure 15-1). The IABP is synchronized with the patient's own heart rate.

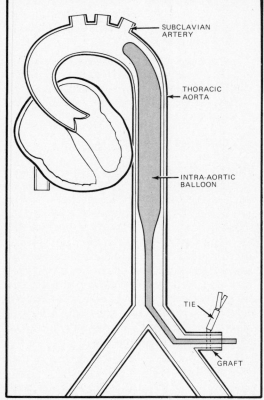

Figure 15-1.   The IABP in the thoracic aorta.

PRINCIPLES OF THE IABP

The IABP decreases strain on the left ventricle by lowering the pressure in the aorta (afterload). With a lower pressure, the ventricle does not have to contract as forcibly to expel its blood into the aorta.

During ventricular diastole, the balloon inflates (Figure 15-2). With inflation, the blood distal to the balloon is forced back towards the aortic valve. Thus, the coronary arteries are supplied with additional oxygenated blood to meet myocardial needs.

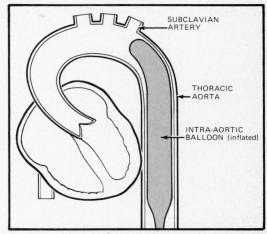

Figure 15-2.   IABP inflated during ventricular diastole.

Prior to ventricular systole (Figure 15-3), the balloon deflates decreasing the pressure in the aorta. This makes it easier for the left ventricle to contract and expel its normal amount of blood.

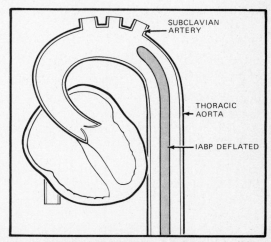

Figure 15-3.   IABP deflated prior to ventricular systole.

COMPLICATIONS OF IABP

There are two major complications associated with the use of the IABP.

1. Circulation to the leg inferior to the insertion site is compromised to varying degrees. Monitoring and documenting the pulses, temperature, and appearance of the leg below the insertion site is extremely important. A comparison to the unused extremity should be made.

2. Weaning the patient off the IABP is usually accomplished by changing the ratio of IABP function to the cardiac function. The ratio with insertion is normally 1:1. To effect weaning, the ratio first becomes 2:1, then 4:1, and then 8:1, as the patient tolerates it. Weaning may also be achieved by decreasing balloon volume depending upon the model of the IABP machine in use. There are times when the left myocardium is so severely damaged that it cannot function adequately without the support of the IABP. At some point, use of the IABP must be terminated, regardless.

As a minor complication, the balloon may rupture. For this reason, carbon dioxide gas is used to inflate the IABP.

Contraindications of IABP include the presence of aortic or ventricular aneurysms, ventricular septal defects, and such.

Hypertensive Crisis

Hypertension is not a disease by itself, but is a symptom of a disease. "Normal" blood pressure range is $\frac{110-130}{60-80}$. Hypertension is considered present if systolic pressure is 140 mm Hg or higher (in the adult) and/or if the diastolic pressure is greater than 90 mm Hg. Hypertensive crisis is the sudden, sustained increase in systemic arterial pressure as indicated by a diastolic increase above 120 mm Hg.

ETIOLOGY

There are five major classifications of hypertension by etiology.

1. *Unknown origin* accounts for 90% of all hypertension identified. This is termed *essential hypertension*.

2. *Adrenal origin* results from a tumor (pheochromocytoma) secreting epinephrine and norepinephrine, Cushing's disease, or a brain tumor.

3. *Renal origin* is due either to an interruption of blood supply or to a disease state of the kidney itself (e.g., pyelonephritis).

4. *Cardiovascular origin* is a result of either degenerative changes (atherosclerosis) or congenital origin (coarctation of the aorta).

5. *Lack of compliance* with medical therapy in "known" hypertensives or inadequate treatment in "known" hypertensives, or certain drugs may cause hypertension.

PRESENTING SYMPTOMS

The most common symptom is severe headache accompanied by nausea, vomiting, restlessness, and mental confusion, which may rapidly advance to coma and/or convulsions. Signs of a developing or progressing cerebrovascular accident (CVA), an M.I., or a pulsating mass indicative of an aneurysm may be present. The blood pressure suddenly increases in hypertensive encephalopathy and in malignant hypertension. The diastolic pressure is greater than 120 mm Hg. Retinopathy and renal dysfunction are common.

PATHOPHYSIOLOGY

Pathophysiology should be examined from two perspectives: (a) hypertensive encephalopathy, and (b) malignant hypertension.

1. *Hypertensive encephalopathy* results from prolonged, high blood pressure. The extreme pressure results in an inability of the autoregulatory system of the brain to regulate cerebral blood pressure. This results in an increased cerebral perfusion causing increased cerebral capillary pressure. The increased capillary pressure causes cerebral edema. Untreat-

ed, this may terminate in cerebral hemorrhage.

2. *Malignant hypertension* is thought to have its origin in renal dysfunction even though it frequently occurs in the presence of other primary disease states. For some unknown reason the renin-angiotensin cascade is turned on and some factor prevents the turn-off of this cascade. The renin-angiotensin cascade is covered in Chapter 25.

TREATMENT

Treatment must encompass three areas.

1. Administration of antihypertensive medications depends upon the extent and nature of the crisis. In a severe crisis, intravenous sodium nitroprusside (Nipride®) in a continuous drip usually lowers the blood pressure. The patient receiving intravenous sodium nitroprusside *must* be continuously monitored by EKG and pressure monitoring to detect hypotension and allow appropriate interventions.

Diazoxide (Hyperstat®) by *rapid* intravenous push and hydralaxine hydrochloride (Apresoline®) intravenously are also used in severe crisis. Patients receiving diazoxide must be monitored for transient hyperglycemia, sodium retention, and nausea and vomiting. Patients receiving hydralazine hydrochloride must be EKG monitored for tachycardia. They may also be uncomfortable due to flushing and/or headache, which are common side effects of this drug.

Hypertensive crisis that is not immediately life-threatening may be treated with reserpine, methyldopa, prazosin hydrochloride (Minipress®), and clonidine hydrochloride (Catapres®).

2. Administration of diuretics to increase urinary output is a common practice. The loop diuretics (furosemide and ethacrynic acid) are widely used because of their rapid action and relatively few side effects.

3. Elimination of the aggravating factors, such as obesity, stress, cigarettes, and such is important along with treating the underlying disease.

COMPLICATIONS

Untreated hypertensive crisis will ultimately result in death due to CHF, CVA, intracerebral hemorrhage, kidney failure, or dissecting aneurysms.

— 16

Pacemakers, Cardiac Surgery, and Cardiac Drugs

Learning Objectives

By the end of this chapter, the nurse will be able to:

1. Define pacemaker.
2. Describe the difference between temporary and permanent pacemakers.
3. List three or more indications for use of a pacemaker.
4. Identify four modes of pacing.
5. List three complications of pacing.
6. Identify essential teaching needs of the patient and family when permanent pacing is instituted.
7. Identify three pathologies that benefit from open chest or open heart surgery.
8. List and explain six postoperative nursing interventions.
9. List four ways drugs influence autonomic nervous system function.
10. Identify three drugs that alter the relative refractory phase of the cardiac cycle.
11. Describe the action of vasoactive drugs.
12. Describe the action of catecholamines.
13. Describe the action of vasodilators and name three.

Pacemakers

There are many pathologic states that may be most efficiently treated by the use of an artificial pacemaker.

DEFINITION

A pacemaker is a system consisting of a lead and a pulse generator. The generator is capable of producing repeated, short (3–5 milliseconds), and rhythmic bursts of electric current for a prolonged period of time. The bursts of electric current are of sufficient magnitude to initiate depolarization of the heart.

MODES OF PACING

There are two modes of pacing. Temporary pacing is one mode used mainly to manage emergencies such as acute heart block and cardiac arrests. The lead is inserted into the right atrium or ventricle. The pulse generator is external. Insertion routes include the transvenous (brachial via cut-down), subclavian, femoral, or jugular (via percutaneous entry), post-surgery (endocardial), and transthoracic (needle through chest into heart muscle). The power supply for temporary pacing is external batteries (the pulse generator). For a specific insertion procedure, the nurse is referred to his or her institution policy.

Permanent pacing with a fully implantable system is a second mode. The pulse generator contains the circuit for the specific pacing mode selected and cells that provide energy to the circuit. The components are encased in a nonconductive plastic material that does not react with body fluids.

INDICATIONS FOR PACING

The major indication for pacing is the development of third degree heart block. The heart rate is slow and fixed. Ineffective cardiac rhythms develop leading to cardiac standstill.

Chronic heart block of varied degrees may be treated by pacing if the patient has syncopal episodes, congestive heart failure, convulsions, or evidence of cerebral dysfunction.

Intermittent complete heart block (third degree) is often treated with a pacemaker. Usually, there is evidence of block in one or two of the three bundle branches (fascicles). Thus, these patients rely solely on the third fascicle, which may become dysfunctional at any time.

Complete heart block that develops in conjunction with an acute myocardial infarction *may* be an indication for pacing. If the infarction is anterior, the involved artery is usually the left anterior descending. This results in ischemia or necrosis of part of the ventricular septum with damage to the intraventricular conduction system below the His bundle. These patients frequently die in spite of a pacemaker due to the extent of myocardial damage. If the infarction is posterior or inferior, the artery involved is usually the right coronary (90%

of the time), and the circumflex (10% of the time). The area of damage is the AV node area. Mobitz I and II may be indications for pacing. Mobitz I may progress into a Mobitz II (2:1) or higher block. Mobitz II, due to the block occurring below the AV node, often progresses into third degree heart block. A block that develops postinfarction is usually transient and responds to atropine or a brief period of time with a temporary pacemaker.

Heart block may occur after a cardiac surgical procedure. It occurs most often with repair of a ventricular septal defect.

Pacemakers may be used in rhythm disturbances. Sick sinus syndrome indicates dysfunction of the SA node. This may occur as sinus bradycardia, sinus arrest, and/or brady-tachy syndromes. Pacemakers may also be used to inhibit ventricular dysrhythmias and to terminate tachycardias.

Pacemakers may be used as a diagnostic aid to evaluate SA node function and AV node function. They may be used to eliminate multiple ectopic foci by overriding the rate of the foci or they may be used to abolish re-entry phenomena by delivering a premature stimulus which breaks the re-entry pattern.

TYPES OF PACING

There are several types of pacing.

1. Asynchronous—This type is used in both temporary and permanent pacing. The pulse generator is set at a predetermined rate. It delivers an impulse at a regular rate *regardless* of the heart's intrinsic rhythm.

2. Ventricular inhibited—This type is also used in both temporary and permanent pacing. It is the most common type for permanent pacing and is often called "demand" pacing. The pacemaker contains a circuit which senses the electrical change generated by ventricular contraction. If there is no ventricular contraction for 800 milliseconds (depending on the setting), the pacemaker fires (i.e., initiates an impulse).

3. Ventricular triggered—This type is noncompetitive and may be termed R wave triggered standby, or ventricular synchronous. In this type, a natural QRS triggers the pacemaker to fire in synchrony with the heart's inherent rhythm. If the heart rate drops below the rate of the pacemaker, the pacemaker depolarizes the ventricles at a fixed rate.

4. P wave synchronous pacing—In this type, a circuit "senses" atrial depolarization and, after an appropriate delay, delivers a ventricular pacing impulse. If atrial depolarization does not occur, the ventricular pacemaker will fire at a fixed rate. If the atrial rate increases, the ventricular pacer will block ventricular response. The degree of block (2:1, 4:1, etc.) will be controlled by the ventricular electrode.

5. Asynchronous atrial pacer—In this type, the AV conduction is intact and the atrial electrode stimulates the atria at a fixed rate.

6. P wave inhibited pacing—This type is a demand pacing. When atrial depolarization occurs, the pacemaker does not fire. If atrial depolarization fails to occur, the pacemaker will fire.

There are many other types of pacemakers used. These are simply the most commonly used. There are also two types of leads which may be used, unipolar and bipolar. A unipolar lead has a positive pole (charge). The bipolar lead contains both the positive and negative poles within the lead itself.

COMPLICATIONS

Catheter dislodgment, prolonged battery failure, and infection are important and not infrequent problems of pacemakers. Failure of the pacemaker to sense and/or capture (stimulate) is common. In failure to sense, the pacing artifact is seen on a rhythm strip to occur *irregularly* throughout the cardiac cycle. In failure to capture, the pacing artifact is seen but not followed by depolarization. Many pacemakers may be externally reprogrammed, decreasing the number of repeat or repositioning procedures needed.

Less commonly, ventricular perforation, diaphragmatic stimulation, and lead disconnection may occur. Figure 16-1 shows pacing artifacts.

NURSING INTERVENTIONS

Patient and family teaching is essential to prevent infection by appropriate care of implant site. It is also essential to teach the patient and family about situations of daily living which might affect pacemaker function adversely such as microwave ovens

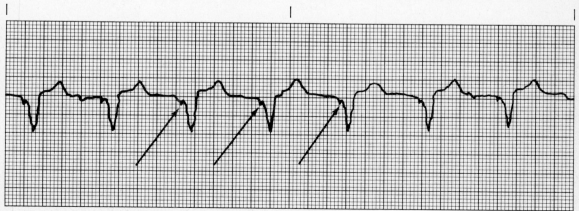

Figure 16-1. Pacing artifacts.

(older models), magnetic fields, and electrical hazards. Irritation over the generator implant site should be avoided by women NOT carrying shoulder strap purses on the implant side and men avoiding suspenders and such.

If traveling by airplane, the patient with a pacemaker should not walk through the detection alarm path. Showing the pacemaker card will allow passage through another walkway.

Adult Cardiac Surgery

This surgical specialty may be subdivided into open chest surgery and open heart surgery. Open chest surgery includes myocardial revascularization, aortic surgery, and excision of ventricular aneurysm. Open heart surgery includes repair of septal defects, valvular surgery, and correction of congenital abnormalities.

ETIOLOGY

Coronary artery disease (CAD) results in partial or total occlusion of one or more of the major coronary arteries and often the diagonal and marginal arteries. Transluminal angioplasty or coronary artery bypass surgery is performed for these diseases.

Acute myocardial infarction is the major cause of ventricular aneurysm. Treatment consists of reinforcing the aneurysmal section with a patch or surgically removing the aneurysm.

Rheumatic fever is the primary disease entity that results in valvular malfunction through partial fusion of leaflets or dilatation of the valve. Calcification of the valves may occur. Syphilis is the cause of some valvular dysfunction but is far less common an etiology today than 20 years ago. Subacute bacterial endocarditis (SBE) is also a common cause of valve disease due to bacterial vegetation on the valve leaflets. Treatment may consist of valve commissurotomies or valve replacements.

Septal defects are most commonly a congenital malformation. However, trauma and/or disease may cause a septal defect.

Rarely, a myocardial infarction may cause a septal defect. These are most often treated by a surgical patch.

CLINICAL PRESENTATION

The presenting signs and symptoms vary according to the disease or congenital anomaly.

POSTOPERATIVE NURSING INTERVENTIONS AND COMPLICATIONS

Complications may occur in almost every body system. Complications may be due to the disease or defect, the surgical procedure, and/or to utilization of the heart/lung pump.

1. Pulmonary interventions include maintaining a patent airway, ensuring adequate ventilation, and preventing occlusion of chest tubes if present. These nursing interventions will help prevent hypoxemia, hypoxia, pulmonary edema, pneumothorax, infections, and acid-base imbalances. Endotracheal tubes are commonly used for up to 24 hours postoperatively and removed only when the stable patient is alert enough to breathe adequately without assistance.

2. Cardiac interventions include continuous monitoring for dysrhythmias and signs of cardiac failure. Monitoring usually includes frequent checks and recording of the B/P (by cuff), PAP, PCWP (by pulmonary artery catheter), and arterial pressure (via arterial line). Intravenous fluids and administration of drugs are closely monitored. Arterial blood gases are usually monitored via the arterial line. Other monitoring modes include central venous presure, left atrial pressure, and cardiac outputs.

3. Renal function is monitored by urinary output measured hourly in the fresh postoperative patient. Oliguria may represent acute renal failure which will be accompanied by electrolyte, acid-base, and fluid imbalances.

4. Neurologic function is assessed by the patient's reorientation to person, place, and thing. Checking pupil responses may help identify early signs of increased intracranial pressure secondary to cerebral edema. CVAs may occur intraoperatively and postoperatively. Inability to move the extremities on one side and altered mental status are clues that a CVA has occurred, *providing* sufficient time has elapsed for the patient to be rid of the effects of general anesthesia.

5. Vascular functions such as clotting mechanisms may be altered resulting in clotting dyscrasias, hemorrhage, and thrombus formation. Monitoring nasogastric drainage, urine, and feces for occult blood will help detect clotting dyscrasias and aid in blood component therapy. Confirmation of dysfunction will be found in laboratory test results.

6. Infections are extremely dangerous and the postoperative patient is at high risk because of the multiple ports for entry of bacteria (I.V. lines, Swan-Ganz and arterial catheters, endotracheal tubes, urinary catheters, and incision sites). Cultures of all sites of possible infection are made if a febrile state develops. Specific antibiotic therapy is started as soon as the infecting organism is identified.

7. Emotional stress for the patient and family is extremely high and must be acknowledged. Nursing interventions that encourage the patient and family to express their feelings will help the patient recuperate. These interventions should begin *before* the surgery if at all possible. Psychosocial aspects of critical illness are covered in Chapter 47.

Vascular Surgery

Endarterectomy, aneurysm repair, and vascular bypass are the three types of surgery which are commonly seen in critical care areas.

ETIOLOGY

Arteriosclerotic disease is the underlying etiology for endarterectomies. Aneurysms may occur secondary to a congenital anomaly or as a result of prolonged, sustained hypertension. Vascular bypass may be needed secondary to embolism, thrombi, aneurysms, or traumatic injury.

PATHOPHYSIOLOGY

The pathophysiology is the same as for coronary artery disease, but it occurs most often in the carotid arteries and then in the aortoiliac bifurcations.

PRESENTING SIGNS AND SYMPTOMS

Presenting signs and symptoms depend upon which arteries are most affected. For example, partial carotid artery occlusion causes transient ischemic attack (TIA). The most common arteries affected are the aortoiliac, renal, popliteal, and femoral.

POSTOPERATIVE NURSING INTERVENTIONS AND COMPLICATIONS

Postoperative nursing interventions and complications are the same as any postoperative care *plus*:

1. Patency of the artery or graft must be maintained. This is accomplished by positioning the patient so that the graft site is as straight as possible for a minimum of 24–48 hours. Knees are not bent. Some physicians keep the patient's blood pressure *slightly* high for several days to keep the suture line taut.

2. Bleeding at the graft site may be controlled with appropriate drugs depending upon the reason for the bleeding.

3. If a graft clots and impedes circulation to an extremity, the extremity may become gangrenous resulting in amputation. Monitoring appearance, color, temperature, and pulses distal to the graft site and comparing these findings to the other extremity will allow for early intervention.

4. Acute renal failure may occur (and fairly often following resection of an abdominal aortic aneurysm). This is caused by the necessity of cross clamping the aorta to repair or remove the aneurysm which interferes with the circulation to the kidneys. Recording hourly urine output and serum creatinine levels will facilitate early intervention.

Carotid endarterectomy patients should *NOT* receive IPPB therapy for a minimum of 48 hours following surgery to avoid high pressure in the pulmonary vascular tree, which could easily tear the carotid suture line.

Cardiac Drugs

Included in this section are the most commonly used drugs and the newest approved drugs as of the publication of this textbook. Since new cardiac drugs are constantly being aproved for use by the FDA, not all drugs can be included.

A few of the more commonly used drugs will be discussed. For more detail, the reader is referred to basic pharmacology and cardiology texts.

Some drugs are specifically antidysrhythmic agents and will affect excitability, contractility (inotropism), and conductivity. Other drugs act on the autonomic nervous system in one of four ways:

1. They stimulate the parasympathetic nervous system, which releases the catecholamine acetylcholine. This is called a cholinergic effect.

2. They block the parasympathetic nervous system prohibiting the release of acetylcholine and are termed anticholinergic drugs.

3. They stimulate the sympathetic nervous system which releases the catecholamine norepinephrine. This is called an adrenergic effect.

4. They block the sympathetic nervous system prohibiting the release of norepinephrine and are called antiadrenergic drugs.

A major group of antidysrhythmic drugs are those which decrease cardiac excitability. This group includes lidocaine (Xylocaine®), propranolol hydrochloride (Inderal®), phenytoin sodium (Dilantin®), disopyramide phospate (Norpace®), and bretylium tosylate (Bretylol®).

Some antidysrhythmic drugs prolong the relative refractory period which slows the rate of conduction. Lidocaine, procainamide, propranolol, and quinidine are the most commonly used drugs in this group.

Inotropes are a group of drugs which influence the strength of cardiac contraction. Digitalis glycosides and catecholamines are the most common positive inotropic agents. The digitalis glycosides include digoxin (Lanoxin®), lanatoside C (Cedilanid®), ouabain, and digitoxin (Crystodigin®).

Vasoactive drugs are drugs which act on the smooth muscle layer of blood vessels. This group includes drugs that primarily affect preload and afterload. The drugs are vasodilators or vasoconstrictors.

Vasopressors (vasoconstrictors) include epinephrine (Adrenalin®), norepinephrine (Levophed®), metaraminol bitartrate (Aramine®), isoproterenol hydrochloride (Isuprel®), dopamine hydrochloride (Intropin®), and dobutamine hydrochloride (Dobutrex®). These drugs mimic the sympathetic nervous system and may be referred to (as a group) as catecholamines. By mimicking the sympathetic nervous system, they provide a positive inotropic effect. However, they also increase myocardial oxygen needs and this *may* not be a desired effect for the patient.

Vasodilators cause dilatation of veins, arterioles, and coronary arteries. The dilatational effects may be blocked in atherosclerotic vessels since the sclerotic placques cannot dilate. Vasodilators decrease preload, increase blood supply to healthy coronary arteries and the extremities, decrease afterload, and decrease blood pressure. The most common vasodilators are nitroglycerin, isosorbide dinitrate (Isordil®), and sodium nitroprusside (Nipride®).

DRUG THERAPY

Dosages vary according to the hospital.

Atropine increases AV conduction due to vagal blockade and increases SA node firing. It does not have a marked hemodynamic effect. It is used mainly in bradydysrhythmias and CHF. Side effects include nausea, vomiting, diarrhea, central nervous system (CNS) changes, and all types of dysrhythmias if digitalis toxicity occurs. A late sign of digitalis toxicity is the patient seeing greenish-yellow objects.

Phenytoin sodium (Dilantin®) increases the speed of conduction through the atria and AV node tissue. It is mainly used in treating digitalis-toxic dysrhythmias. Side effects include hypotension, bradydysrhythmias, CNS disorientation, and local thrombophlebitis. (Note: It must be given *slowly* when an I.V. route is used (50 mg/minute). I.V. drip is *not* recommended because of easy precipitation of the drug in a solution.) Diphenylhydantoin has been the generic name for dilantin. Phenytoin sodium is now the generic name used.

Lidocaine (Xylocaine®) decreases excitation, conduction (slightly), and contractility. It is used with PVCs, ventricular tachycardia, and ventricular defibrillation. Side effects include hypotension, heart block, CNS disorientation, and convulsions.

Isoproterenol hydrochloride (Isuprel®) increases excitation, conduction, and contractility. It is used mainly in heart block and sinus or junctional bradycardia. Side effects include angina, and atrial and ventricular ectopy.

Procainamide hydrochloride (Pronestyl®) decreases excitation, conduction, and contractility. It is used with PVCs and ventricular tachycardia. It increases the effect of antihypertensive drugs and other anticholinergic drugs. Side effects include nausea, vomiting, drug rash, hypotension, AV block, bundle branch block, and lupus-type reaction.

Propranolol hydrochloride (Inderal®) decreases excitation, conduction, and contractility (markedly). Its main use is to decrease oxygen demand of the myocardium by decreasing contractility and by terminating digitalis-induced ventricular tachydysrhythmias. It is also used to control supraventricular tachydysrhythmias and ventricular ectopy when other drugs have failed. Side effects include hypotension, shock, bradycardia, heart block, CHF, and a worsening of underlying asthma and allergic rhinitis. CAUTION: *DO NOT STOP THE DRUG SUDDENLY.* It may cause a rebound effect in patients with unstable angina. *DO NOT USE THIS DRUG FOR PATIENTS WITH ASTHMA.* Propranolol is a BRONCHOCONSTRICTOR.

Quinidine decreases excitation, automaticity, conduction, and contractility. In small doses, it is vagolytic and may enhance AV conduction. It is primarily used in atrial tachydysrhythmias. It may be used with atrial and ventricular premature beats. (Note: I.V. and I.M. administration are *NOT* recommended.) Side effects include nausea, vomiting, diarrhea, hypotension, SA and AV blocks, and CNS disturbances. An *ABSOLUTE CONTRAINDICATION* for the use of quinidine is second or third degree heart block.

New Cardiovascular Drugs

Amiodarone is used to supress supraventricular tachydysrhythmias. It slows the sinus node discharge rate and lengthens the AV nodal conduction time. It antagonizes the chronotropic and inotropic effects of glucagon. Amiodarone also increases coronary blood flow and thus decreases cardiac work and myocardial oxygen consumption needs.

Side effects are few and include nausea, vomiting, and constipation. A slate-gray or bluish discoloration of the skin may occur and may take months to disappear after the drug is discontinued. Rarely, thyroid dysfunction may occur.

Nifedipine (Procardia®) is a calcium channel blocker producing an antianginal effect. Nifedipine inhibits the influx of calcium ions into cardiac and smooth muscle without altering the serum calcium level. It relaxes and prevents coronary artery spasms and reduces afterload. This decreases the work of the heart and decreases the myocardial oxygen consumption needs.

Hypotension is the most serious side effect and the patient must be closely monitored until stabilized. Other side effects may include shortness of breath, nasal congestion, abdominal cramps, diarrhea, constipation, and central nervous system dysfunction including ataxia. Dermatitis, pruritis, and urticaria may also occur.

Verapamil hydrochloride (Isoptin®, Calan®) is a calcium inhibitor or antagonist. It inhibits the influx of calcium ions into specific cardiac cells, slowing conduction through the atrioventricular node. It dilates arteries and diminishes myocardial contractility. It is used to reduce supraventricular tachydysrhythmias and to decrease a rapid ventricular response in atrial flutter and atrial fibrillation.

Side effects are few since the drug is well tolerated. If side effects occur, they may include nausea, headache, dizziness, hypotension, abdominal discomfort, bradycardia, or severe tachycardia. CAUTIONS: Do not use in patients with severe hypotension, cardiogenic shock, congestive heart failure, or second or third degree heart block. If an *INTRAVENOUS* beta-blocking drug has been administered, verapamil hydrochloride must not be given for several hours. Disopyramide phosphate (Norpace®) should not be given for 48 hours prior to the use of verapamil hydrochloride nor for 24 hours after verapamil hydrochloride has been discontinued.

Diltiazem hydrochloride (Cardizem®) is the third calcium channel blocker. It is less potent than verapamil hydrochloride and nifedipine and has fewer side effects. It functions in the same manner as verapamil and nifedipine by its role as a calcium antagonist.

Timolol (Blocadren®) is a beta blocker inhibiting the nervous system response to adrenalin and stimulating hormones. It decreases the strength and rate of cardiac contractions. It is used for the same indications of propranolol hydrochloride (Inderal®) with the same precautions and side effects.

Atenolol (Tenormin®) is a beta-adrenergic blocking agent. It is similar in efficiency to propranolol hydrochloride (Inderal®), Timolol (Blocadren®), and Metoprolol (Lopressor®). It is an oral antihypertensive medication frequently used in conjunction with diuretic therapy.

Side effects include postural hypotension, bradycardia, nausea, diarrhea, dizziness, dyspnea, and depression. CAUTION: Atenolol is contraindicated in bradycardias, second and third degree heart block, heart failure, and cardiogenic shock. Dosages must be reduced in patients with renal disease. Termination of drug therapy must be tapered to prevent increased angina and thyroid storm.

Captopril (Capoten®) is a new antihypertensive medication that suppresses the renin-angiotensin-aldosterone mechanism.

Side effects include the development of serum hyperkalemia. Potassium supplements or potassium conserving diuretics should be given *only* after a hypokalemic state has been documented. Proteinuria, neutropenia, tachycardia, palpitations, chest pain, and decreased taste sensation have occurred. CAUTION: If possible, all other antihypertensive medications should be discontinued for one week prior to initiating captopril therapy.

Amiloride hydrochloride (Midamor®) is a potassium sparing diuretic (antikaliuretic). It is similar to triamterene (Dyrenium®) and spironolactone (Aldactone®). It is used with thiazide diuretics and other potassium wasting diuretics. It prevents hypokalemia in digitalized or dysrhythmic patients and helps to correct hypokalemia in other patients on certain diuretics.

Side effects include nausea, vomiting, diarrhea, constipation, weakness, dyspnea, fatigue, and muscle cramps. CAUTION: It is contraindicated in patients with renal disease and should be used very cautiously in diabetic patients. Patients should be monitored for hyperkalemia.

Cardiac Bibliography

Berne RM, Levy MN: Cardiovascular Physiology, 3rd ed.   St. Louis, MO: C. V. Mosby, pp. 1–114, 1977

Bordicks KJ: Patterns of Shock: Implications for Nursing Care, 2nd ed. New York: Macmillan Publishing, pp. 207–234, 1980

Borg N, Mikas DL, Stark J, Williams SM (eds): Core Curriculum for Critical Care Nursing, 2nd ed. American Association of Critical-Care Nurses. Philadelphia: W. B. Saunders, pp. 77–171, 1981

Braunwald E (ed): Heart Disease: A Textbook of Cardiovascular Medicine, Vol. 1. Philadelphia: W. B. Saunders, pp. 70–951, 1980

Chung EK (ed): Quick Reference to Cardiovascular Diseases. Philadelphia: J. B. Lippincott, pp. 17–50, 107–118, 282–318, 338–353, 1977

Foster WT: Principles of Acute Coronary Care. New York: Appleton-Century-Crofts, 1976

*Guyton AC: Textbook of Medical Physiology, 6th ed. Philadelphia: W. B. Saunders, pp. 150–205, 1981

Hurst JW, Logue RB: The clinical recognition and medical management of coronary atherosclerotic heart disease. In Hurst JW, Logue RB, Schlant RC, Wenger NK (eds): The Heart, 3rd ed. New York: McGraw-Hill, pp. 1038–1041, 1974

*Jackle M, Marney H: Cardiovascular Problems: A Critical Care Nursing Focus. Bowie, MD: Robert J. Brady Co., 1980

Meltzer LE, Pinneo R, Kitchell JR: Intensive Coronary Care: A Manual for Nurses, 3rd ed. Bowie, MD: Charles Press, 1977

*A Programmed Approach to Anatomy and Physiology: The Cardiovascular System, 2nd ed. Bowie, MD: Robert J. Brady Co., 1970

*Rushmer RF: Cardiovascular Dynamics, 4th ed. Philadelphia: W. B. Saunders, 1976

*Swan KG: The Cardiovascular System: Disease, Diagnosis, Treatment. Bowie, MD: Robert J. Brady Co., 1973

Verel D, Smith GH: Basic Cardiology. Lancaster, England: MTP Press Limited International Medical Publishers, 1979

Walraven G: Basic Arrhythmias. Bowie, MD: Robert J. Brady Co., 1980

Wilson RF (ed): Principals and techniques of critical care. In Critical Care Manual, Vol. 1, Sec. A through Sec. E. Kalamazoo, MI: The Upjohn Co., 1977

III

The Neurological System

— 17 —

Anatomy of the Nervous System

> ## Learning Objectives
>
> By the end of this chapter, the nurse will be able to:
>
> 1. Identify the components of the central, peripheral, and autonomic nervous systems.
> 2. Explain the construction of the cranium including the diploic space.
> 3. List the meningeal membranes, from outside to inside, that cover the brain and spinal cord.
> 4. Identify the four processes formed by the inner layer of the dura mater.
> 5. List the six major divisions of the brain and the functions of each.
> 6. Describe the formation, circulation, and absorption of the cerebrospinal fluid.
> 7. List the normal characteristics of CSF.
> 8. Identify the arteries of the circle of Willis and the portions of the brain supplied by each artery.
> 9. List two types of cells in the brain.
> 10. Describe the structure and function of each cell type listed in 9.
> 11. Identify the four types of fibers comprising the spinal nerves.
> 12. List the cranial nerves and identify the function of each.
> 13. Differentiate between the sympathetic and parasympathetic nervous system in relation to ganglions and functions.

It is customary to divide the nervous system into three segments to facilitate learning and comprehension of the system and its dysfunctions. The three segments are the central nervous system (composed of the brain and spinal cord), the peripheral nervous system (composed of the cranial, spinal, and peripheral nerves), and the autonomic nervous system (composed of the sympathetic and parasympathetic systems).

The Central Nervous System

The skull is the bony structure of the head. The cranium refers to the bones of the head excluding the facial bones and the mandible. The cranium is covered by the scalp.

THE SCALP

The letters in the word scalp form a mnemonic for remembering the cranial coverings (Figure 17-1). "SCA" actually forms a single layer of *s*kin, *c*utaneous, and *a*dipose tissue. This layer contains blood vessels, but these cannot contract. Consequently, when the scalp is lacerated, it bleeds more than an identical cut elsewhere on the body. The "L" is the dense, fibrous ligament-like layer called the *galea aponeurotica*. This layer helps to absorb the forces of external trauma. The "P" represents the pericranium, which contains less bone-forming elements than the periosteum.

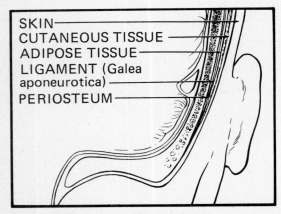

Figure 17-1. Layers of the scalp.

THE CRANIUM

The scalp covers the cranium, which is a part of the skull. The cranium is hollow and very rigid. It provides strong protection to the head without being heavy. To achieve this, there is an outer and an inner layer of regular bone structure. The middle layer is called the diploë (or diploic space), which is spongy and lightweight.

Cranial Bones

The cranium consists of two single and four pairs of bones fused together (Figure 17-2). They are the frontal (single), occipital (single), and pairs of parietal, temporal, sphenoid, and ethmoid bones. The fusion of these bones form three landmarks. The coronal suture is the fusion of the frontal and parietal bones. The sagittal suture is the fusion of the two parietal bones. The lamboidal suture is the fusion of the parietal bones and the occipital bone.

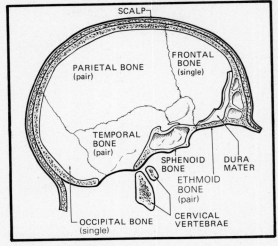

Figure 17-2. The cranium.

The Fossae

The internal surface of the cranium has three distinct ridges on it that serve to divide the brain area into anterior, middle, and posterior segments called fossae (plural; singular is fossa).

THE MENINGES

The three membranes covering the entire brain surface, the spinal cord, and the spinal canal below the cord are the meninges (Figure 17-3). A mneumonic (PAD) may help distinguish the meningeal coverings: the *p*ia mater, *a*rachnoid, and *d*ura mater. The meningeal layers absorp shocks from sudden movements or trauma. The meninges literally "PAD" the brain. In between each layer of the meninges is a space containing certain structures.

Starting from the brain per se, the first meningeal layer is the pia mater. The pia mater is contiguous with the brain surface and its convolutions.

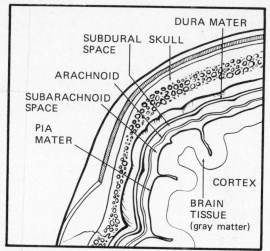

Figure 17-3. The meninges.

The "A" of "PAD" represents the arachnoid layer of the meninges. It looks much like a lacy spiderweb with projections onto the pia mater, forming a space. This space, the subarachnoid space, contains many cerebral arteries and veins which are bathed by cerebrospinal fluid (CSF). The arachnoid membrane also has projections called arachnoid villi which absorb CSF. The subarachnoid space enlarges at the base of the brain to form the subarachnoid cisterns.

The most exterior layer of the meninges is the dura mater. The dura mater is actually two layers of tough fibrous membrane. The outermost layer forms the periosteum of the cranial cavity. The inner layer folds to form four processes: the *falx cerebri*, the *tent-*

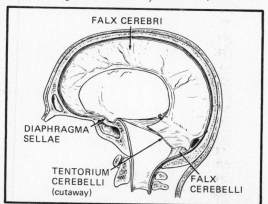

Figure 17-4. Sagittal section showing processes formed by the inner layer of the dura mater.

orium cerebelli, the *falx cerebelli*, and the *diaphragma sellae* (Figure 17-4). The space formed by the two layers of the dura mater contains meningeal arteries and venous sinuses.

THE BRAIN

The brain is nervous tissue that fills up the cranial vault. It weighs about three pounds in the adult male. Although it is an integrated unit, for study purposes, it may be divided into six major parts (Figure 17-5). These parts are the cerebrum (telencephalon), diencephalon, midbrain (mesencephalon), pons, cerebellum, and medulla oblongata.

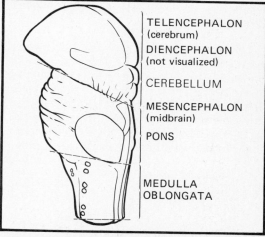

Figure 17-5. Gross anatomical sections of the brain.

The Cerebrum

The cerebrum is contained in the anterior and middle fossae of the cranium. It is divided into two halves by a longitudinal fissure. The fissure is formed by the sagittal folds of the dura mater. The fissure is called the falx cerebri. The two cerebral hemispheres are joined by the corpus callosum (Figure 17-6).

In addition to this function, the corpus callosum also provides a path for fibers to cross from one hemisphere to the other. Each hemisphere has a lateral ventricle. These two hemispheres are sometimes referred to as the telencephalon.

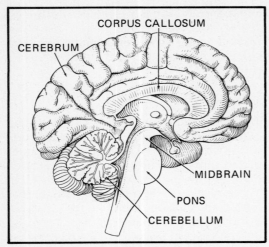

Figure 17-6. Midsagittal section showing the corpus callosum.

The cerebral surface is covered with convolutions which give rise to gyri (raised portions) and sulci (depressions in the surface). The cerebral surface is about six cells deep and is called the cerebral cortex. It normally appears gray and thus these six layers (Figure 17-7) are called gray matter. The cerebral cortex receives sensory infor-mation from the body.

Looking at a lateral view of the cerebral hemispheres, we see two fissures dividing the hemisphere (Figure 17-8). The lateral fissure (also called the fissure of Sylvius) divides the frontal lobe and the temporal lobe (named for the overlying bones). This area contains the primary auditory center. The central sulcus, also known as the fissure of Rolando, divides the frontal lobe from the parietal lobe. Immediately in front of the central sulcus is the precentral gyrus, which is the primary motor area. Immediately posterior to the central sulcus is the postcentral gyrus, which is the primary sensory cortical area.

NOTE: In looking at pictures of the brain surface which do *not* show the cerebellum, imagine the brain as a boxing glove. The thumb of the boxing glove always points towards the frontal area of the brain.

The basal ganglia, or basal nuclei, are also part of the telencephalon. The basal ganglia include the caudate nucleus, puta-men, globus pallidus, claustrum, subthala-mic nucleus, and the substantia nigra (Fig-ure 17-9). Specific functions of the brain segments are listed in Table 17-1.

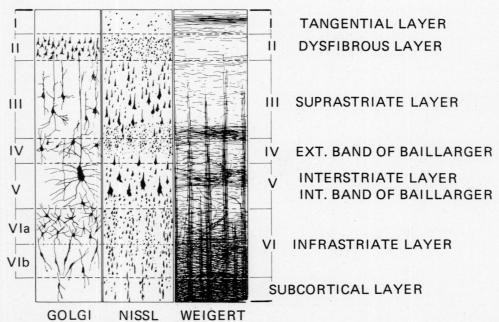

Figure 17-7. The six layers of the cerebral cortex.

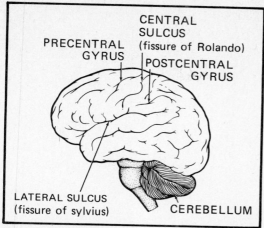

Figure 17-8. Fissures, sulci, and gyri dividing the cerebral hemisphere.

The Diencephalon

The diencephalon is the most superior portion of the brain stem and is covered by the cerebrum (Figure 17-10). It is a paired structure with a thin fluid space between the two sides. The diencephalon is composed of the thalamus, hypothalamus, and the limbic system. The thalamus is the largest structure in the diencephalon and it integrates all body sensations except smell. It is also the major relay area for all neuronal impulses. The hypothalamus connects with the limbic system, thalamus, mesencephalon, and the hypophysis (pituitary gland).

The Mesencephalon

This is the midbrain. It is located between the diencephalon and the pons. It contains the major motor nerves for eye movement, carries impulses down from the cerebrum, and controls the wakefulness of the brain through the reticular activating system.

The Pons

This is situated between the midbrain and the medulla oblongata. The pons forms a bridge (thus its name from the latin word for bridge) between the cerebellar hemispheres and contains the neurons for sensory input and motor output for the face.

The Medulla Oblongata

This is located between the pons and the spinal cord. It is the structure that marks the change between the spinal cord and the brain per se. Collectively, the mesencephalon, pons, and the medulla oblongata are termed the *brain stem*.

The Cerebellum

This is situated in the posterior fossa of the

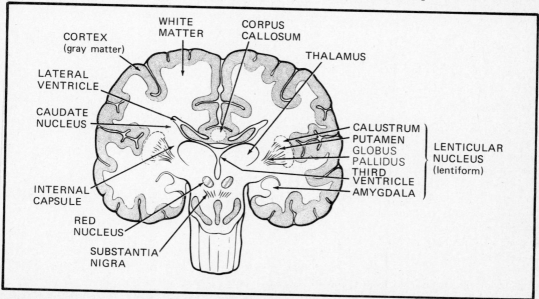

Figure 17-9. Coronal section of the brain showing internal parts of basal ganglia of the telencephalon.

Table 17-1. Function of specific brain structures.

Structure	Function
Cerebrum (divided into cerebral hemispheres)	Governs all sensory and motor thought, and learning; analyzes, associates, integrates, and stores information.
Cerebral cortex (4 lobes) 1. Frontal lobe	Motor function; motor speech area; controls morals, values, emotions, and judgment.
2. Parietal lobe	Integrates general sensation; governs discrimination; interprets pain, touch, temperature, and pressure.
3. Temporal lobe	Auditory center, sensory speech center.
4. Occipital lobe	Visual area.
Basal ganglia	Central motor movement.
Thalamus (diencephalon)	Screens and relays sensory impulses to cortex. Lowest level of crude conscious awareness.
Hypothalamus (diencephalon)	Regulates autonomic nervous system, stress response, sleep, appetite, body temperature, water balance, and emotions.
Midbrain (mesencephalon)	Motor coordination, conjugate eye movements.
Pons	Contains projection tracts between spinal cord, medulla, and brain.
Medulla oblongata	Contains all afferent and efferent tracts, and most pyramidal tracts, and cardiac, respiratory, vasomotor, and vomiting centers.
Cerebellum	Connected by cerebellar peduncles to other parts of CNS; coordinates muscle movement, posture, equilibrium, and muscle tone.
Limbic system	Regulation of some visceral activities; some function in emotional personality.

cranial cavity. It is separated from the cerebrum by dura mater folds forming the tentorium cerebelli. The cerebral hemispheres are above the tentorium cerebelli and are thus supratentorial structures. The two cerebellar hemispheres are connected to each other by a structure called the vermis. They are connected to the brain stem by cerebellar peduncles. There are three cerebellar peduncles (Figure 17-11). The superior cerebellar peduncles send impulses from the cerebellum to the thalamus. The middle cerebellar peduncles receive cerebral cortex information from nuclei in the pons. The inferior cerebellar peduncles receive impulses that reveal body and extremity positions.

There are two structures within structures that must be recognized. Within the medulla oblongata some motor and sensory fibers (tracts) will cross to the opposite hemisphere. This crossing is termed *decussation*. This is responsible for specific symptoms of dysfunction to occur ipsilaterally

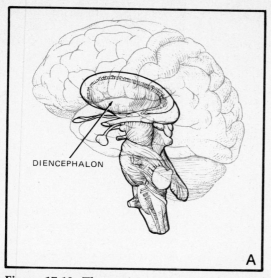

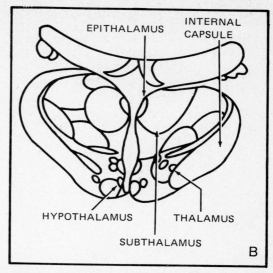

Figure 17-10. The position of the diencephalon (A) and the internal components of the diencephalon (B).

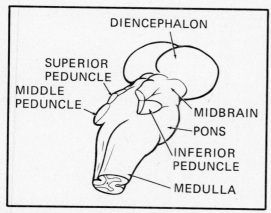

Figure 17-11. Cerebellar peduncles.

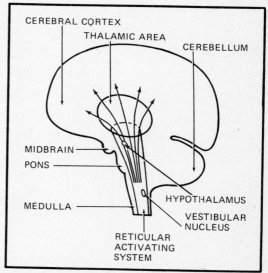

Figure 17-12. Reticular activating system.

Circulation and Formation of Cerebrospinal Fluid

(same side as the lesion or injury) or contralaterally (opposite side of lesion or injury). Note that the terms *homolateral* and *ipsilateral* are synonymous.

The second structure is the reticular activating system (RAS). The RAS (Figure 17-12) is a complex system that occupies a large portion of the mesencephalon (midbrain). RAS fibers connect with the thalamus, the cerebral cortex, the cerebellum, and the spinal cord.

There are four ventricles (cavities) involved in the cerebrospinal fluid (CSF) system (Figure 17-13). CSF is synthesized by the choroid plexus. This is an area of modified epithelial cells covering tufts of capillaries found in all ventricles but predominating in the anterior segment of the lateral ventricles. CSF is a clear, colorless liquid having a

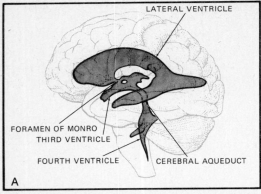

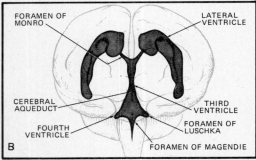

Figure 17-13. Lateral view of the ventricular system of the brain (A) and anterior view of the ventricular system of the brain (B).

few cells, some protein, glucose, and a large amount of sodium chloride. There is a lateral ventricle in each hemisphere of the cerebrum.

The foramen of Monro allows the CSF to leave the lateral ventricles and flow into the third ventricle. From the third ventricle, CSF flows through the aqueduct of Sylvius into the fourth ventricle. Foramina of Luschka and Magendie direct the CSF from the fourth ventricle into the cisterns and subarachnoid space.

After circulating (in the subarachnoid space) over the entire brain and spinal cord, the CSF is reabsorbed by the arachnoid villi in dural sinuses and by pacchionian bodies found in the superior sagittal sinus.

The CSF "cushions" the brain and spinal cord to protect them from colliding with the cranium and vertebrae in response to moving forces. The CSF also reduces the gravitational weight of the brain. To a limited extent, the CSF adjusts to changes in the intracranial vault's pressure and volume. If the pressure or volume increases in the vault, more CSF will be absorbed and/or pushed into the spinal canal in an attempt to maintain normal pressure. Normally, 125–150 ml of CSF are in the ventricles and the subarachnoid space. An average of 500 ml of CSF is produced in 24 hours. The CSF also participates in the exchange of nutrients and waste material between the blood and the CNS cells.

Cerebral Blood Supply

The brain is supplied with oxygenated blood from two arterial systems: the internal carotid arteries and the vertebral arteries. As a reserve to these two systems, the circle of Willis helps provide adequate circulation through its anastomoses. The circle of Willis anastomoses are between the two vertebral arteries and the two carotid arteries (Figure 17-14).

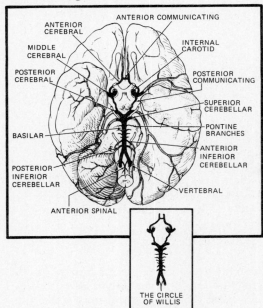

Figure 17-14. The circle of Willis.

EXTERNAL CEREBRAL BLOOD SUPPLY

The external carotid arteries bifurcate and form the occipital, temporal, and maxillary arteries. The occipital arteries supply the posterior fossa. The temporal arteries supply the temporal region. The maxillary arteries form the middle meningeal arteries which supply the anterior, middle, and posterior portions of the meninges and the fossae.

INTERNAL CEREBRAL BLOOD SUPPLY

The internal carotid arteries bifurcate to form the anterior cerebral arteries, the anterior communicating arteries, the middle cerebral arteries, the posterior communicating arteries, and the anterior choroidal arteries. The anterior communicating artery connects the left and right anterior cerebral arteries. The posterior communicating artery connects the internal carotid arteries to the basilar artery. These communicating arteries do not supply any part of the brain directly, but some are collateral channels helping to form the circle in the circle of Willis.

The vertebral arteries enter the posterior fossa and join to form the basilar artery. The basilar artery bifurcates to form the superior cerebellar arteries and the posterior cerebral arteries. The superior cerebellar arteries supply the pons and the cerebellum. Posterior cerebral arteries supply the posterior one-third of the cerebrum.

Some of these arteries anastomose with each other to form the circle of Willis. They are the anterior cerebral artery, the anterior communicating artery, the posterior communicating arteries, and the posterior cerebral arteries. All of these arteries are involved in supplying blood to the anterior two-thirds of the cerebrum.

Only about 50% of all people have a "classic" circle of Willis. The most common difference is that the posterior communicating artery is not present and the posterior cerebral artery comes directly from the internal carotid artery.

Veins run parallel with many of the arteries. The middle meningeal arteries are special in that the veins that accompany these arteries are positioned between the arteries and the bones of the cranium. This helps protect the middle meningeal artery, which is frequently torn in skull fractures of the temporal bones.

As there is an internal and external arterial blood supply, there is a corresponding internal and external venous return system. Many of the veins are important in aneurysms and as surgical landmarks. The veins which drain the dura mater and diploë of the skull (external) empty into venous sinuses which are located between the layers of the dura mater. Internal cerebral veins also empty into venous sinuses.

Venous sinuses are lined with epithelium; they have no valves and no muscle in the walls. The sinuses connect with emissary veins which in turn connect with external cranial veins that empty into the *internal jugular veins*. The superior sagittal sinus receives venous blood from the superior cerebral veins. The inferior sagittal sinus receives venous blood from the medial cerebral hemisphere veins. The straight sinus receives venous blood from the internal cerebral veins. There are many other sinuses that receive venous blood from other areas of the brain.

Components of Nervous Tissue

There are two main types of cells in the brain: neurons (Figure 17-15) and neuroglia (glial cells). The neuron is the functioning unit of the nervous system and its function is to transmit impulses. There are more than 10 billion neurons in the CNS and three-fourths of them are in the cerebral cortex.

Neurons are categorized in two ways: by the direction of impulse flow and/or by the number of processes emanating from the neuron cell body.

Neurons that transmit impulses *to* the spinal cord or brain are afferent sensory neurons. Those transmitting impulses *away* from the brain or spinal cord are called efferent motor neurons. Interneurons transmit impulses from sensory neurons to motor neurons. The mnemonic "SAME" helps maintain correct direction and type of neuron. The "SA" of SAME stands for sensory afferent and the "ME" stands for motor efferent.

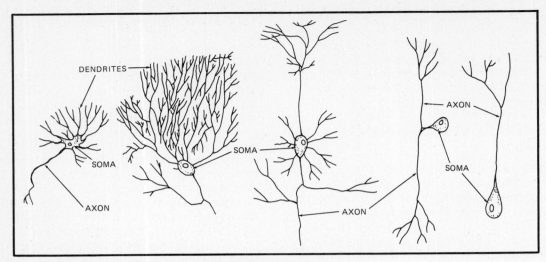

Figure 17-15. Various shapes of neurons and neuroglia.

Neurons will be one of three types according to the number of processes that exist. Unipolar neurons have one process coming from the cell body. After a short distance, this one process will split to form one axon and one dendrite. Bipolar neurons have one axon and one dendrite coming from the cell body. Multipolar neurons have one axon and multiple dendrites.

Regardless of the category of neurons, they all have certain unique structures common only to neurons (Figure 17-16), that is, axons, dendrites, neurofibrils, nissl bodies, myelin, neurilemma, and nodes of Ranvier.

The cell body of a neuron is called a *soma* or *perikaryon*. It contains a nucleus and many cytoplasmic organelles. The axon

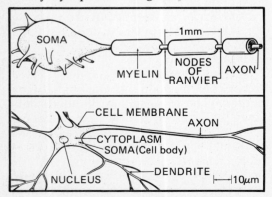

Figure 17-16. Schematic diagram of the structures of the neuron.

originates from a thickened area of the soma called an axon hillock. The axon transmits impulses away from the soma. There is one axon per neuron. Dendrites are short processes that transmit impulses to the soma. Multipolar neurons have many dendrites. The branching of dendritic processes is termed *arborization* since the processes look like tree branches. Neurofibrils are thin, threadlike fibers forming a network in the cytoplasm. Nissl bodies specialize in protein synthesis with RNA to maintain and regenerate the neuronal processes.

Myelin is a protein-lipid compound that covers some axons. In the CNS, myelin is produced by oligodendrocytes. In the peripheral nervous system, myelin is produced by Schwann cells. Myelin covers axons of nerve cells in between the nodes of Ranvier. The nodes of Ranvier are *bare* spots at regular intervals that speed the conduction of impulses.

The neurilemma is an outer coating of the neurons outside of the CNS. The neurilemma encompasses all structures, even myelin. It is the neurilemma that provides for peripheral nerve regeneration. Since the neurilemma is *not* found on neurons of the brain and spinal cord, these neurons *cannot* regenerate.

Neurons require an extensive support system to maintain optimal function. The neuroglia are responsible for this support system (Figure 17-17). Neuroglia are composed of glial cells and they outnumber the neurons by ten to one. Four types of specific cells comprise the glial support system.

1. Astrocytes are star-shaped cells that form the actual tissue support system. Astrocytes, which may be protoplasmic or fibrous tissue, constitute part of the blood-brain barrier by sending foot processes to the blood vessels.

2. Microglia are tiny cells that lie quiescent until nervous tissue is damaged. Because of their origin, microglia are part of the reticuloendothelial cell system. They wander in and out of the CNS in response to need. When damage occurs, the microglia become mobile and travel to the damaged tissue. They enlarge and phagocytize the debris.

3. Oligodendroglia help support the nervous tissue, but their primary function is the original formation of myelin in the CNS during fetal, neonatal, and early years. Once the myelin has been formed, the oligodendroglia *cannot* form it again.

4. Ependyma are special glial cells that are found lining the ventricles of the brain and the central canal in the spinal cord.

The spinal cord is the second part of the central nervous system. It is examined in Chapter 19.

The Peripheral Nervous System

The peripheral nerves, the spinal nerves, and the cranial nerves form the peripheral nervous system. There are 31 pairs of spinal nerves and 12 pairs of cranial nerves.

The 31 pairs of spinal nerves are numbered in relation to the vertebral level at which they emerge from the spinal cord instead of being named. Spinal nerves do not attach directly to the spinal cord. Instead, the spinal nerves attach to a short anterior (ventral, motor) root and a short posterior (dorsal, sensory) root (Figure 17-18). The posterior root has a bulge which consists of neuron cell bodies. This bulge is called a *spinal ganglia*. There are eight cervical, twelve thoracic, five lumbar, five sacral, and one coccygeal spinal pair of ganglia.

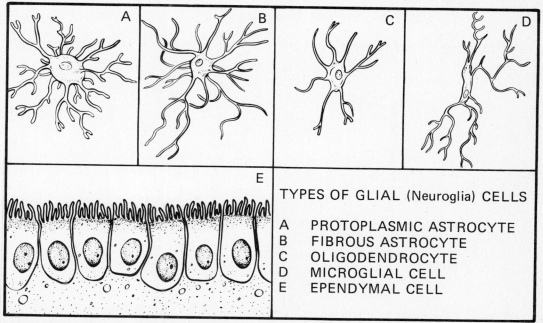

TYPES OF GLIAL (Neuroglia) CELLS

A   PROTOPLASMIC ASTROCYTE
B   FIBROUS ASTROCYTE
C   OLIGODENDROCYTE
D   MICROGLIAL CELL
E   EPENDYMAL CELL

Figure 17-17. Types of glial (neuroglia) cells.

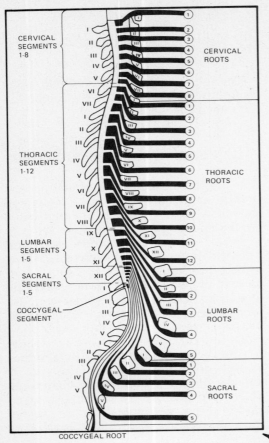

CERVICAL
SEGMENTS
1-8

CERVICAL
ROOTS

THORACIC
SEGMENTS
1-12

THORACIC
ROOTS

LUMBAR
SEGMENTS
1-5

SACRAL
SEGMENTS
1-5

COCCYGEAL
SEGMENT

LUMBAR
ROOTS

SACRAL
ROOTS

COCCYGEAL ROOT

Peripheral nerves often encompass more than one spinal nerve root. The sciatic nerve is a good example. It includes all the spinal nerve roots in the sacrum.

SPINAL NERVE FIBERS

There are four types of nerve fibers comprising the spinal nerves.

1. Motor fibers originate in the ventral (anterior) horn of the spinal cord with efferent fibers relaying motor impulses from the CNS to peripheral skeletal muscles.

2. Sensory fibers originate in the dorsal (posterior) horn of the spinal cord with afferent fibers relaying sensory impulses from organs and muscles to the CNS.

3. Meningeal fibers transmit sensory and vasomotor innervation to the spinal meninges.

4. Autonomic fibers will be considered separately.

DERMATOMES

Each spinal nerve dorsal root innervates a specific portion of skin. The skin regions are called dermatomes (Figure 17-19).

▼**Figure 17-18. Spinal nerve roots and their attachment to the spinal cord.**

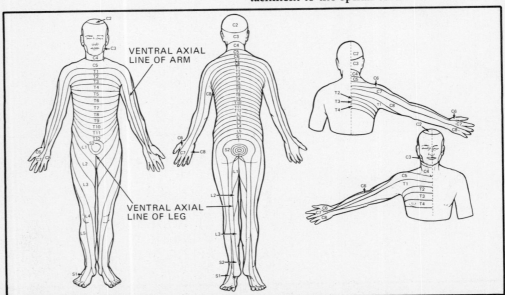

VENTRAL AXIAL
LINE OF ARM

VENTRAL AXIAL
LINE OF LEG

Figure 17-19. Dermatomes.

These are clinically important in identifying areas of spinal cord injury.

PLEXUSES

The spinal nerves interweave in three areas that are termed plexuses—the cervical, brachial, and lumbosacral plexuses (Figure 17-20). The cervical plexus involves spinal nerves C-1 to C-4. It sends motor impulses to neck muscles and the diaphragm. It receives sensory impulses from the neck and head. The brachial plexus is composed of spinal nerves C-4 to C-8 and T-1. It innervates the arms. The lumbosacral plexus is formed by spinal nerves L-1 to L-5 and S-1 to S-3. This plexus innervates the legs.

CRANIAL NERVES

Twelve pairs of cranial nerves complete the peripheral nervous system. Three pairs of cranial nerves are totally sensory, five pairs are totally motor, and four pairs are combined sensorimotor. Origin of the nerves is seen in Figure 17-21. By convention the cranial nerves are numbered by roman numerals as well as named.

The cranial nerves are summarized in Table 17-2. The standard mnemonic may help keep them in order: *On Old Olympus Tippy Top A Finn And German Vaulted Some Hops.*

The Autonomic Nervous System

The sympathetic nervous system and the parasympathetic nervous system together form the autonomic nervous system. Technically, the autonomic nervous system is part of the peripheral nervous system. However, it seems easier to understand the autonomic nervous system if it is looked at as a separate system.

The sympathetic nervous system releases norepinephrine, which stimulates and prepares our bodies for "fight or flight." Norepinephrine is categorized as an adrenergic chemical (hormone). Fibers originating in the thoracic and lumbar areas form the peripheral sympathetic nervous system division.

The parasympathetic nervous system releases acetylcholine, which is categorized as a cholinergic chemical (hormone). In reality, the parasympathetic system is an antagonist to the sympathetic system and mediates or slows body responses when the "fight, fright, or flight" situation no longer exists. Fibers originating in the cranial and sacral areas form the peripheral parasympathetic nervous system division.

NERVE STRUCTURES OF THE AUTONOMIC NERVOUS SYSTEM

The sympathetic nervous system has a chain of ganglia situated on both sides of the vertebrae (Figure 17-22). Nerve fibers between the spinal cord and the ganglia are termed preganglionic fibers (or axons). The nerve fibers between the ganglia and visceral end organ are called postganglionic fibers (or axons). The norepinephrine that

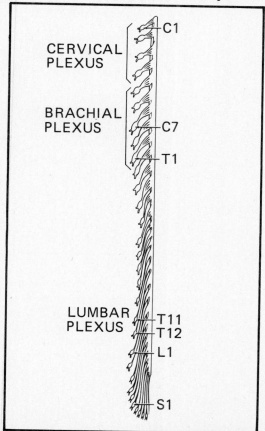

Figure 17-20. The three spinal nerve plexuses.

CERVICAL PLEXUS — C1

BRACHIAL PLEXUS — C7 — T1

LUMBAR PLEXUS — T11 — T12 — L1 — S1

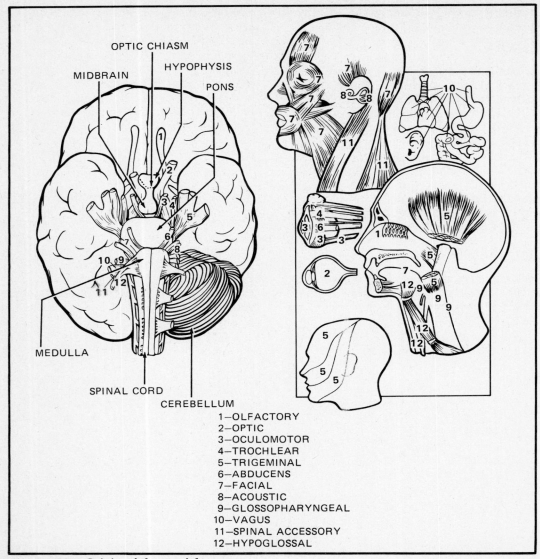

OPTIC CHIASM
HYPOPHYSIS
MIDBRAIN
PONS

MEDULLA

SPINAL CORD

CEREBELLUM

1—OLFACTORY
2—OPTIC
3—OCULOMOTOR
4—TROCHLEAR
5—TRIGEMINAL
6—ABDUCENS
7—FACIAL
8—ACOUSTIC
9—GLOSSOPHARYNGEAL
10—VAGUS
11—SPINAL ACCESSORY
12—HYPOGLOSSAL

Figure 17-21. Origin of the cranial nerves.

is released to maintain body function is not easily nor rapidly neutralized, so the effect is sustained for a period of time. The sympathetic system may be referred to as the thoracolumbar system since *major ganglia* arise in the thoracic and lumbar regions.

The parasympathetic nervous system does not have a chain of ganglia next to the vertebral column. The preganglionic fibers (or axons) originate in the brain and sacrum (Figure 17-23). These axons are long to allow them to reach specific organs. Ganglia

are found adjacent to or within specific organs. So postganglionic fibers (or axons) are short. The chemical released by the parasympathetic system, acetylcholine, is rapidly neutralized by cholinesterase. Because of this, the parasympathetic effect is brief and must be renewed fairly regularly to counter the sympathetic stimulation. This system may be referred to as the craniosacral system since the preganglionic fibers arise from certain cranial nerves and in the sacral spinal cord.

Table 17–2. Summarization of cranial nerves.

Number	Name	Major Functions
I	Olfactory	Sense of smell
II	Optic	Central and peripheral vision
III	Oculomotor	Eye movement, elevation of upper eyelid Pupil constriction
IV	Trochlear	Downward and inward eye movement
V	Trigeminal	Touch, pain, temperature Jaw and eye muscle proprioception Mastication
VI	Abducens	Abduction of the eye
VII	Facial	Close eyelid, muscles of facial expression Secretion by glands of mouth and eyes Taste (anterior two-thirds of tongue)
VIII	Acoustic: Vestibular branch Cochlear branch	Equilibrium Hearing
IX	Glossopharyngeal	Movement of pharyngeal muscles Secretion by parotid glands Pharyngeal and posterior tongue sensation
X	Vagus	Pharyngeal and laryngeal movement Visceral activities Pharyngeal and laryngeal sensation, taste
XI	Spinal Accessory	Pharyngeal, sternocleidomastoid, and trapezius movement
XII	Hypoglossal	Tongue movement

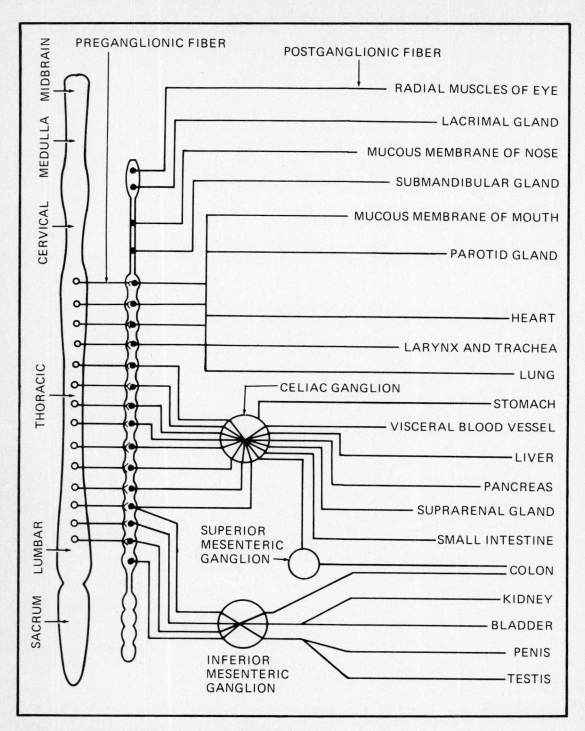

Figure 17-22. Sympathetic nervous system ganglia.

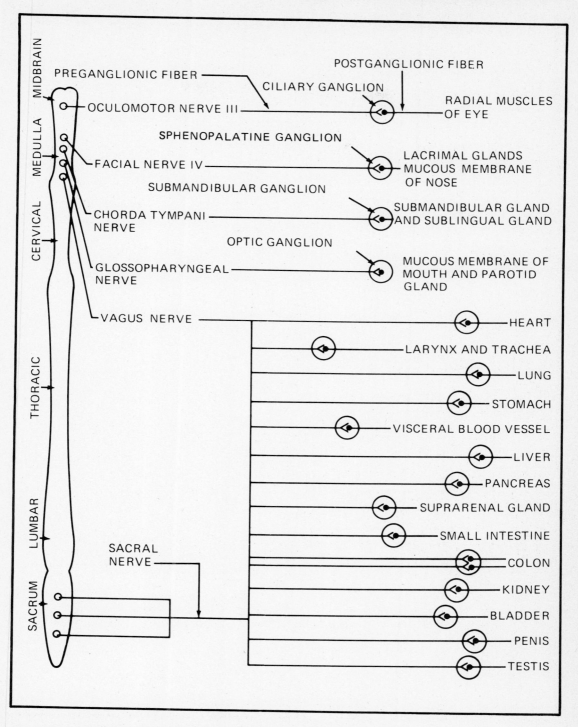

Figure 17-23. Parasympathetic nervous system ganglionic fibers.

18

Physiology of the Nervous System

Learning Objectives

By the end of this chapter, the nurse will be able to:

1. Define the following:
   a. Depolarization
   b. Repolarization
   c. Action potential
2. Explain summation and facilitation.
3. Explain saltatory conduction.
4. Identify and explain the function of:
   a. Synaptic knob
   b. Synaptic vesicles
   c. Synaptic cleft
   d. Subsynaptic membrane
   e. Neuromuscular end-plate or junction
5. List five neurotransmitters.
6. Describe the release and termination of action of acetylcholine.
7. Compare the termination of action of acetylcholine and the monoamine transmitters.
8. Define reflex.
9. Trace the path of the impulse in a monosynaptic reflex arc and polysynaptic reflex arc.
10. List the oxygen, nutritional, and vitamin needs for brain metabolism.
11. Identify circulatory needs of the brain.
12. Explain the blood-brain barrier.

Integrity of the nervous system in its entirety is essential for optimal neural function. Certain components must be present in specified amounts. These components initiate impulses and assist in transmission of impulses. It is the integrity of the nervous system that integrates and mediates these impulses.

Neural Cell Depolarization and Repolarization

Depolarization and repolarization of the nerve cell follow the same principles as depolarization and repolarization of the cardiac cell.

DEPOLARIZATION

The neuron in a resting state (resting membrane potential or RMP) is positively charged outside the cell membrane and negatively charged on the inner surface of the cell membrane. When the cell is stimulated, sodium rapidly enters the cell and potassium leaves the cell. This produces a positive ionic charge at the entry site and decreases the resting membrane potential. This positive ionic charge is transmitted along the length of the neuron and is termed *a wave of depolarization*.

REPOLARIZATION

As soon as potassium reenters the cell and sodium leaves the cell, the resting state of the cell is re-established. This is called *repolarization*. A specific mechanism exists to force the sodium ions that entered the cells' cytoplasm back into the extracellular fluid. The mechanism is termed the *sodium pump*. Without the sodium pump, ion homeostasis could not be preserved. At the same time, a potassium pump exists to maintain potassium ion homeostasis by forcing potassium ions back into the cell.

An *action potential* exists when an ionic charge on one side of the membrane is different from an ionic charge on the other. Depolarization occurs when a stimulus is strong enough (threshold) to alter the cell membrane permeability to sodium, allowing a change in the ionic charge. (Sodium ions enter and potassium ions leave the cell interior.) Once an action potential exists and a stimulus of threshold level magnitude occurs, the neuron totally depolarizes. The neuron depolarizes following the all-or-none principle. It depolarizes in its entirety or else it does not depolarize at all. As with the cardiac cell, the neuron has a complete refractory period during which it is repolarizing and cannot be stimulated. Also like the cardiac cell, the neuron has a relative refractory period. During this period, the neuron can be stimulated (or excited), but only when the stimulus is at a threshold level.

Two terms are important in relation to action potentials. *Summation* refers to repetitive, accumulated discharges that eventually reach threshold level (much like building blocks one on top of the other until the top is reached). *Facilitation* is an increase in every subsequent neuron stimulus even though the stimulus remains below threshold levels. No action potential occurs in facilitation. Action potential does occur in summation.

The rapid velocity of conduction of the impulse is due in part to the neuron structure (Figure 18-1) and the size of the nerve fiber. Myelin is a protective, lipid insulation of the neuron that is nonconductive. This prevents an easy flow of ions into the nerve fiber. The myelin sheath is segmented. At specified intervals the myelin sheath is *totally* absent. These noninsulated points are called nodes of Ranvier. Ions flow easily around the nerve fiber at the nodes of Ranvier. The action potential on myelinated nerve fibers jumps from one node of Ranvier to the next node of Ranvier. This is called *saltatory conduction* and is far faster than conduction in an unmyelinated fiber. In unmyelinated fibers, the impulse must travel the entire length of the neuron.

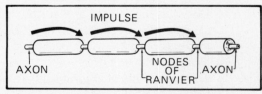

Figure 18-1. Nodes of Ranvier providing saltatory conduction.

Chemical Synapses

A synapse is a point of junction, but not of contact, between one neuron and another neuron, a muscle cell, or a gland cell. Synapses differ in shape and size, but function similarly in transmitting impulses.

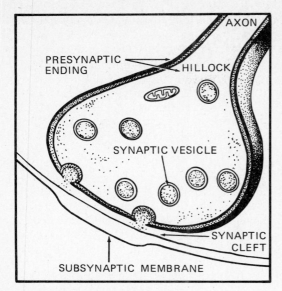

Figure 18-2. A chemical synapse.

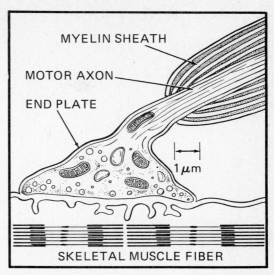

Figure 18-3. The neuromuscular junction or neuromuscular end plate.

The neuron's axon enlarges at its end forming a "synaptic knob." This knob may be called a terminal button or a presynaptic terminal (Figure 18-2). The synaptic knob contains vesicles which are filled with specific neurotransmitter chemicals. When the axonal knob is stimulated, these chemicals are released from the vesicles. The presynaptic terminal is separated from the postsynaptic side by a minute space termed the *synaptic cleft*. The postsynaptic membrane is slightly thicker at the synaptic cleft than elsewhere and is termed the *subsynaptic membrane*. The extra thickness is thought to be due to an increased number of receptor sites for the neurotransmitter.

When the axons of a motor neuron synapse with skeletal muscle, the presynaptic terminal (synaptic knob) is called a *neuromuscular junction* or a *neuromuscular endplate* (Figure 18-3). At this specific synapse, the presynaptic terminal looks like a plate. The neuromuscular junction is the only synapse specifically named.

Neurotransmitters

1. *Acetylcholine* is the neurotransmitter chemical found in the vesicles of neuro-muscular junctions and in the parasympathetic system. As the action potential in the axon reaches the neuromuscular junction, the neuromuscular junction is stimulated to release the chemical in its vesicles. The chemical diffuses across the synaptic cleft coming in contact with receptors on the postsynaptic membrane. Acetylcholine acts on the postsynaptic membrane briefly before it is neutralized by the enzyme acetylcholinesterase (ACH). The milliseconds that acetylcholine is in contact with the postsynaptic membrane are enough to propagate conduction of an impulse. Acetylcholinesterase is found in abundance in skeletal muscles and blood, so it very rapidly breaks down acetylcholine into acetic acid and choline. This rapid degradation of acetylcholine assures that only one action potential occurs at a time at the receptor sites on the postsynaptic membrane. The end products (acetic acid and choline) are resynthesized in the synaptic vesicles for use again.

The end result of the release of acetylcholine at many peripheral synapses is muscular contraction. The amount of acetylcholine released is determined in part by calcium ion diffusion into the presynaptic terminal. Calcium ions are necessary for depolarization at other peripheral synapses, so it is assumed that calcium plays a similar role at *all* chemical synapses.

Acetylcholine is a cholinergic neurotransmitter. It is felt that more cholinergic synapses exist in the central nervous system, but they have not been positively identified.

2. *Epinephrine, norepinephrine,* and *dopamine* are classified as catecholamines. These catecholamines and *serotonin* are further classified as monoamines. Epinephrine and norepinephrine are found in adrenergic fibers of the sympathetic nervous system. They exert a generalized "fight, flight, or fright" response in the body.

3. *Dopamine* is a precursor to adrenalin and norepinephrine. Dopamine acts as an inhibitory chemical transmitter and is one of the most important chemicals involved in basal ganglionic functions. (Acetylcholine is the other important transmitter in basal ganglionic functions.) Dopamine is decreased in the brains of patients with parkinsonism. It may play a role in eating, drinking, and sexual behavior.

4. *Serotonin* is also a monoamine chemical. It is an inhibitory transmitter and is linked to slow wave sleep patterns.

The aforementioned monoamines (epinephrine, norepinephrine, dopamine, and serotonin) all function much like acetylcholine in synthesis, storage, and release of chemicals when the axons are stimulated. The termination of action of monoamines is *markedly different* than that of acetylcholine. Instead of breaking down into inactive chemicals, the monoamines' function is terminated by being reabsorbed into the presynaptic terminals. The uptake of monoamines rapidly terminates the chemical action and concurrently prevents depletion of the transmitter.

5. *GABA (gamma-aminobutyric acid)* is a neutral amino acid that has an inhibitory effect on synaptic function.

Reflexes

A reflex is a stereotypical reaction of the central nervous system to specific sensory stimuli. There are two types of reflexes: the monosynaptic reflex and the polysynaptic reflex.

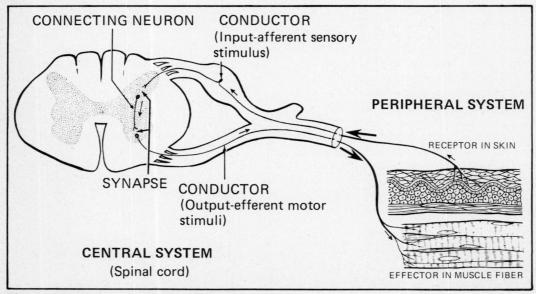

Figure 18-4. The monosynaptic reflex arcs.

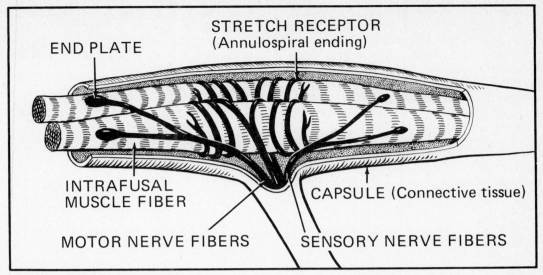

Figure 18-5. The muscle spindle.

MONOSYNAPTIC REFLEX ARCS

This constitutes the simplest reflex in the body and is depicted in Figure 18-4. Inside every group of muscles is a structure called a muscle spindle. The muscle spindle is made of small fibers that are bound together by afferent sensory fibers (Figure 18-5). As a muscle spindle is stretched, an action potential develops and a sensory impulse travels to the dorsal root ganglion. From the ganglion the impulse enters the spinal cord. In the gray matter (unmyelinated) of the spinal cord, the impulse synapses with interneurons in the anterior portion of the cord. These interneurons have efferent (motor) fibers that leave the spinal cord through the anterior (ventral) root. The efferent fibers carry an impulse back to the original muscle. The muscle contracts upon receiving this impulse.

The monosynaptic reflex arc is more important in research than in practice. However, the muscle stretch reflex (knee jerk) is the most commonly tested reflex.

POLYSYNAPTIC REFLEX ARCS

The withdrawal reflex is a common example of the polysynaptic reflex (Figure 18-6). Afferent nerve fibers in the peripheral mus-

cles are excited, producing an impulse. This impulse enters the spinal cord via a dorsal root ganglion. This excited neuron will synapse with appropriate interneurons within the gray matter of the spinal cord.

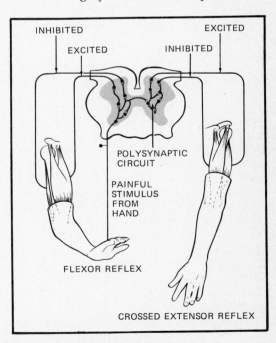

Figure 18-6. Polysynaptic reflex arcs.

The interneurons in the anterior (ventral) horn emerge from the spinal cord through efferent (motor) fibers. These fibers transmit the motor impulse to the original muscle that produced the sensory impulse. The muscle then contracts. There are literally hundreds of interneurons with which the impulse could and does snyapse, and thus the name polysynaptic reflex arc.

When impulses effect a muscular contraction, other impulses must negate the function of opposing muscle groups. For the knee to bend, extensor muscles are inhibited and concurrently flexor muscles are excited. This is termed *the law of reciprocal innervation*.

Metabolism in the Brain

Both white matter (myelinated) and gray matter (unmyelinated) have the same metabolic needs.

OXYGEN NEEDS

The brains's need for oxygen does not decrease in a resting state. Even though it weighs only about three pounds (2% of the body weight), brain tissue requires about 20% of the body oxygen supply. The brain needs a constant supply of oxygen, but it is unable to store oxygen for future use. Energy is necessary for metabolic functions of the brain and this energy is obtained from the oxidation of glucose. All oxidative reactions require oxygen. Hypoxia may occur without irreversible anoxic injury to brain cells. If the anoxic state lasts four or more minutes at normal body temperature, cerebral neurons are destroyed. Once destroyed, cerebral neurons cannot regenerate. The most sensitive area of the brain to hypoxia is the cerebral hemispheres, particularly the hippocampus, which is most likely to be damaged by small amounts of decreased oxygen. Since the cerebral *cortex* is only six layers (cells) deep (see Figure 17-7), the entire cerebral cortex, especially layer four, is very sensitive to decreases in oxygen. Damage here results in the so-called *laminar cortical necrosis*.

The brain stem is the most resistant area to hypoxic damage. If hypoxia occurs in this area beyond the four or five minute limit, irreversible coma or a persistent vegetative state usually develops.

NUTRITIONAL NEEDS

The extensive, continuous activity of the brain results in very high metabolic energy needs. Glucose, a carbohydrate, is the main source of energy (ATP) for cellular activity. Glucose and oxygen are essential for reestablishing electrochemical gradients for impulse transmission, for the synthesis of neurotransmitters, and for maintaining cellular integrity. If the cerebral glucose level is less than 70 mg/100 ml, confusion results. With a glucose level of less than 20 mg/100 ml, coma develops followed by death (without treatment). Whereas hypoglycemia causes confusion, coma, and death, hyperglycemia does not appear to have a direct influence on nervous system functions.

Certain vitamins are essential in adequate amounts to ensure normal central nervous system functions.

Vitamin B_1 (thiamine) is important in the Krebs cycle of energy production. Insufficient B_1, common in alcoholics, causes the Wernicke-Korsakoff's syndrome, which in late stages causes cerebellar degeneration.

Vitamin B_{12} function is not understood. However, insufficient B_{12} results in a gradual degeneration of the brain, optic nerves, spinal cord (especially posterior and lateral columns), and the dorsal root entry zone of the peripheral nerves. Degeneration often starts with the spinal cord. Pernicious anemia is the dominant systemic disease with vitamin B_{12} deficiency. A deficiency is also present in alcoholism and other malnutritional states.

Pyridoxine is a coenzyme and participates in many enzymatic reactions in the central nervous system. Pyridoxine deficiencies produce polyneuropathies, seborrheic dermatitis, glossitis, and conjunctivitis.

Nicotinic acid is needed for synthesis of coenzymes. Insufficient nicotinic acid results in altered mentation leading to coma, extrapyramidal rigidity, and tremors of the extremities. This form of encephalopathy seems to be becoming nonexistent in the United States. There may be a relationship between inadequate nicotinic acid and pellagra.

CIRCULATORY NEEDS

The brain needs a more continuous supply of oxygenated blood, even during sleep, than any other organ since the brain's needs are never decreased. The cerebral blood flow (CBF) is determined in part by the cerebral perfusion pressure. This pressure is the difference between mean arterial (systemic) pressure and intracranial pressure. The size of the cerebrovascular system, activity, disease, fever, injury, and other factors determine the actual amount of blood needed at any given time.

Hypercapnia and hypoxia will cause an arteriolar dilatation of the cerebral arteries increasing the amount of blood flowing into the brain regardless of the *actual* amount needed. This may cause an increased intracranial pressure that the healthy brain could accommodate but that an injured or diseased brain may not be able to accommodate.

Increases in intracranial pressure will result in a decrease in blood perfusion to the brain due to compression of the arteries, veins, and brain mass as a whole.

The brain has its own autoregulatory mechanism which functions mainly by increasing (constricting arteries) resistance to blood flow or by decreasing (dilatation of arteries) resistance to blood flow, thus altering the diameter of the vessels. This system works well until the intracranial pressure increases beyond a certain unknown point. Then the system fails.

Blood-Brain Barrier

A barrier is known to exist between the blood and brain which controls the diffusion of substances from the blood into the extracellular fluid or the cerebrospinal fluid of the brain. The location and structure of this carrier is thought to be related to the "tight junctions" of cerebral endothelial cells. The permeability of cerebral capillaries and the choroid plexus controls the movement of specific substances.

Water, oxygen, glucose, and carbon dioxide move quickly through the blood-brain barrier. Other substances either move slowly or not at all across the barrier. This control determines the level of metabolism, ionic composition, and the homeostasis of cerebral tissue.

In addition to a blood-brain barrier, there is a blood-cerebrospinal fluid barrier. This barrier functions like the blood-brain barrier in controlling the composition of the cerebrospinal fluid. This is a vitally important function because substances in the cerebrospinal fluid are rapidly absorbed into the interstitial brain fluid.

— 19

The Vertebrae and the Spinal Cord: Function and Dysfunction

Learning Objectives

By the end of this chapter, the nurse will be able to:

1. Identify the divisions of the vertebral column.
2. List the anatomical components of a typical vertebra.
3. Describe intervertebral discs.
4. Identify the location of the spinal cord.
5. Explain the gross anatomy of the spinal cord.
6. Differentiate between gray and white matter.
7. List at least four important ascending tracts and their functions.
8. List at least four important descending tracts and their functions.
9. Describe at least four classifications of spinal cord injuries.
10. List three pathologies other than trauma which will alter spinal cord function.
11. Compare central cord syndrome, anterior cord syndrome, and Brown-Sequard syndrome.
12. Define spinal shock.
13. List precipitating causes of spinal shock.
14. Identify nursing interventions to prevent and/or treat complications of spinal cord injuries relating to: respiratory, cardiovascular, renal, G.I., musculoskeletal, and metabolic systems.
15. Explain autonomic dysreflexia—its causes, symptoms, and nursing interventions.

Vertebral Column

The spinal cord is protected by and housed by the vertebrae. There are a total of 33 vertebrae.

DIVISIONS OF THE VERTEBRAL COLUMN

There are eight cervical vertebrae. Some texts state that there are seven cervical vertebrae. These texts apparently count the atlas and axis as one since they articulate directly with each other. There are twelve thoracic vertebrae, five lumbar, five sacral, and three to five fused as the coccygeal segment.

THE TYPICAL VERTEBRA

The body of a typical vertebra (Figure 19-1) is the solid portion which lies anteriorly. Opposite the vertebral body is the spinous process (the bony segment felt down the back). Projecting laterally from each side of the vertebra is the transverse processes. The lamina is the curved portion of bone joining the transverse processes to the spinous process. The lamina is the most frequently fractured portion of the vertebra. The vertebrae may sustain any fracture of any type in ways that other bones in the body can. Between the vertebral body and the spinous process is the spinal foramen—the cavity through which the spinal cord passes.

THE CERVICAL VERTEBRAE

The cervical vertebrae are the smallest. Figure 19-2 shows the atlas vertebra (C-1) which articulates with the occipital bone and the axis vertebrae (C-2). The axis has an odontoid process (the only one) which permits C-1 to articulate directly and to provide rotation of the head. Trauma to the odontoid process is sometimes called the "hangman's" fracture when this process is broken

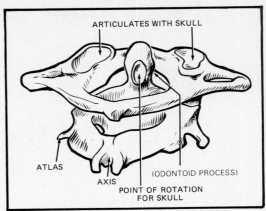

Figure 19-2. Articulation of C-1 and C-2 vertebrae.

and the head is no longer stabilized by C-1's articulation. If C-2 is fractured, the required force is so great that the vertebra bursts like a star. This causes multiple bone fragments which may penetrate the spinal cord nerves and vascular structures, too.

THE THORACIC VERTEBRAE

The twelve thoracic vertebrae (Figure 19-3) have points of attachment for the ribs to help support the chest musculature.

THE LUMBAR VERTEBRAE

The five lumbar vertebrae (Figure 19-4) are the largest and they support the back muscles. These vertebral discs are the most frequently herniated.

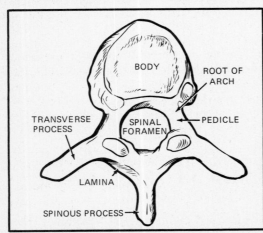

Figure 19-1. A typical vertebra.

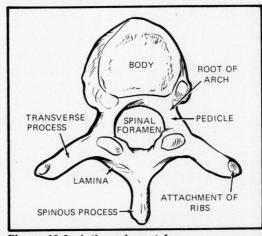

Figure 19-3. A thoracic vertebra.

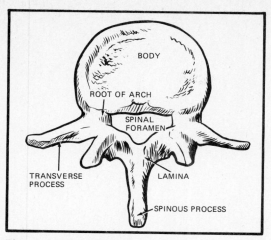

Figure 19-4. A lumbar vertebra.

THE SACRAL VERTEBRAE

The five sacral vertebrae (Figure 19-5) are fused forming the sacrum—a frequent point of low back pain.

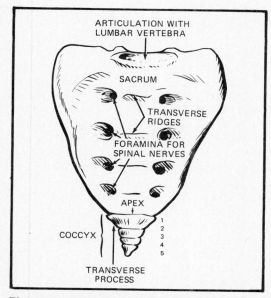

Figure 19-5. The sacral vertebrae and the coccyx.

THE COCCYX VERTEBRAE

Depending upon the individual, three to five vertebrae are fused to form the coccyx (as seen in Figure 19-5).

INTERVERTEBRAL DISCS

In between each of the lumbar, thoracic, and cervical vertebrae, excluding the atlas and axis, is an intervertebral disc. The disc is a fibrocartilaginous material designed to absorb the shocks or pressure between one vertebra and another. The center portion of the disc is a gelatinous layer called the nucleus pulposus. Unexpected movement and/or force may "rupture" the disc forcing the nucleus pulposus out of position—the so-called "slipped disc." When out of position, the disc may impinge upon the spinal canal, the spinal cord, or the emerging spinal nerves.

Unfortunately, it is very common for the spinal cord to be damaged by extreme hyperextension or hyperflexion forces (Figure 19-6). Damage may occur with or without fracture of the vertebrae.

The Spinal Cord

The spinal cord is the second major component of the central nervous system (the brain is the other). The spinal cord is vital for life and is protected by vertebrae.

LOCATION OF THE SPINAL CORD

The spinal cord (Figure 19-7) is continuous with the medulla oblongata in the brain stem. It is located in the spinal canal of the vertebrae. The vertebrae extend from the foramen magnum to the coccyx. Within the vertebrae, the spinal cord extends from the foramen magnum to the first lumbar vertebra. The caudal end of the spinal cord is called the conus medullaris. The filium terminale is a group of fibers extending from the conus medullaris at the L-1 vertebral level to the first coccygeal vertebra.

STRUCTURE OF THE SPINAL CORD

The spinal cord is oval and is surrounded by the meninges that also encase the brain. Between the first lumbar and second sacral vertebrae, the arachnoid membrane enlarges somewhat to form the space known

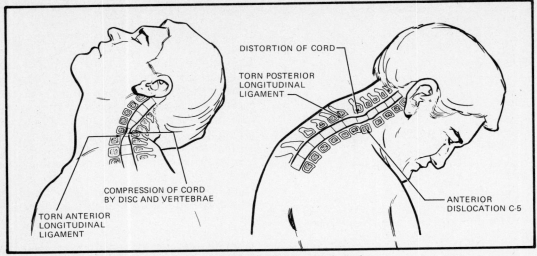

Figure 19-6. Hyperextension and hyperflexion of the spinal cord.

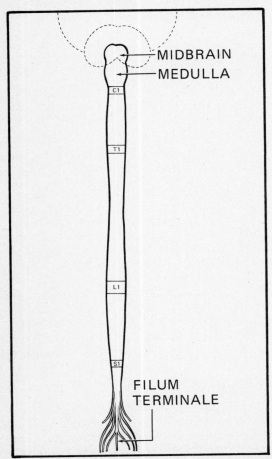

Figure 19-7. The spinal cord.

as the lumbar cistern used for lumbar punctures. The spinal cord has a minute cavity in its center—the central canal. This canal is an extension of the fourth ventricle and contains CSF.

The spinal cord is composed of both white (myelinated) and gray (unmyelinated) tissue. The gray matter appears (with a little imagination) to be shaped like an H which is surrounded by white matter (Figure 19-8). The amount of gray matter varies with its location in the vertebral column. A mnemonic may help distinguish white/gray matter and myelinated/unmyelinated fibers. The fourth letter of gray is "y" as is the fourth letter of unmyelinated. So gray matter is unmyelinated fibers.

Gray matter is composed of nerve cells and unmyelinated fibers arranged in three columns (Figure 19-9). The anterior gray columns are also known as the anterior horns. They contain cell bodies of efferent (motor) fibers. The middle gray columns are known as the lateral columns which contain preganglionic fibers of the autonomic nervous system. The lateral columns are largest in the upper cervical, thoracic, and midsacral regions. The posterior columns, also known as the posterior horns, contain cell bodies of afferent (sensory) fibers.

The white matter (myelinated) is arranged in three columns each called

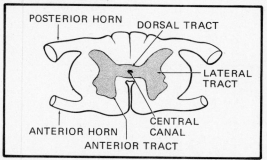

Figure 19-8. Gray and white matter of the spinal cord (cross section).

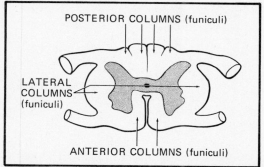

Figure 19-9. Columns (tracts) of gray matter in the spinal cord (cross section).

funiculus (singular)—the anterior, lateral, and posterior funiculi (Figure 19-10). Within these columns or funiculi are ascending (sensory) and descending (motor) tracts termed fasciculi.

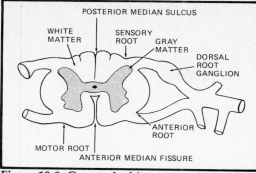

Figure 19-10. The funiculi of white matter in the spinal cord.

The significant ascending tracts (Figure 19-11) are the fasciculus gracilis, fasciculus cuneatus, lateral spinothalamic tract, anterior spinothalamic tract, dorsal and ventral spinocerebellar tracts, and the spinotectal tract. These tracts carry sensory impulses and are identified in Figure 19-11.

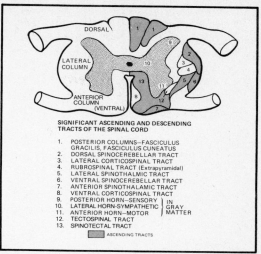

SIGNIFICANT ASCENDING AND DESCENDING TRACTS OF THE SPINAL CORD

1. POSTERIOR COLUMNS—FASCICULUS GRACILIS, FASCICULUS CUNEATUS
2. DORSAL SPINOCEREBELLAR TRACT
3. LATERAL CORTICOSPINAL TRACT
4. RUBROSPINAL TRACT (Extrapyramidal)
5. LATERAL SPINOTHALAMIC TRACT
6. VENTRAL SPINOCEREBELLAR TRACT
7. ANTERIOR SPINOTHALAMIC TRACT
8. VENTRAL CORTICOSPINAL TRACT
9. POSTERIOR HORN—SENSORY   } IN
10. LATERAL HORN-SYMPATHETIC } GRAY
11. ANTERIOR HORN—MOTOR   } MATTER
12. TECTOSPINAL TRACT
13. SPINOTECTAL TRACT
    ASCENDING TRACTS

Figure 19-11. Significant ascending and descending tracts of the spinal cord. The left half of the picture is a mirror image of the right half.

The significant descending tracts (Figure 19-11) are the rubrospinal tract, ventral and lateral corticospinal tracts, and the tectospinal tract. These carry motor impulses and are identified in Figure 19-11.

Spinal Cord Injuries

Spinal cord injuries are more and more common and are a result mainly of auto accidents, diving accidents, and athletic accidents. Spinal injuries may be classified by many criteria.

CLASSIFICATION OF SPINAL CORD INJURIES

1. The level of injury may be cervical, thoracic, or lumbar injury. The cervical injury is the most common.
2. Degree of spinal cord involvement may be either complete or incomplete. Complete cord involvement by lesion (or transection) results in total loss of sensory and motor function below the level of the lesion. This loss is a result of irreversible damage to the spinal cord. If the cervical cord is involved, quadriplegia is the common result. If the thoracic or lumbar cord is involved, paraplegia is the common result.

Incomplete cord lesion involvement (or partial transection) leaves some tracts intact. The degree of sensory/motor loss is variable dependent upon the level of lesion. Three syndromes are commonly the result of incomplete lesions.

a.   *The central cord syndrome* is characterized by microscopic hemorrhage and edema to the central cord (Figure 19–12). When the damage is in the cervical central cord, it is termed central cord syndrome. There is motor weakness in both the upper and lower extremities, but the weakness is much greater in the upper extremities than in the lower ones.

Sensory dysfunction varies according to the site of injury or lesion. Bladder dysfunction is common. This syndrome is frequently due to hyperextension of an osteoarthritic spine. The extent of recovery depends upon the resolution of edema and the intactness of the spinal cord tracts.

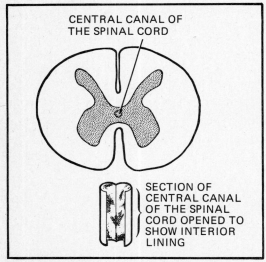

CENTRAL CANAL OF THE SPINAL CORD

SECTION OF CENTRAL CANAL OF THE SPINAL CORD OPENED TO SHOW INTERIOR LINING

Figure 19-12. The central cord syndrome.

b.   *Anterior cord syndrome* is characterized by injury resulting in an acute compression of the anterior portion of the spinal cord, often a flexion injury (Figure 19-13). Compression is usually caused by a disc or bony fragment. It may also be caused by an actual destruction of the anterior cord by an anterior spinal artery occlusion caused by a thrombus. Symptoms include immediate anterior paralysis which is complete from the injury or compression down. Hypesthesia (decreased sensation) and hypalgesia (decreased pain sensation) occur below the level of injury. Since the posterior cord tracts are not injured, there are sensations of touch, position, vibration, and motion. If the syndrome is caused by the compression of the anterior cord from bony fragments, surgical decompression is indicated.

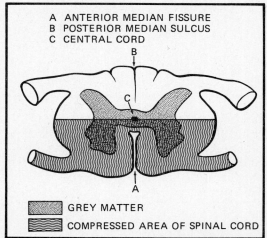

A ANTERIOR MEDIAN FISSURE
B POSTERIOR MEDIAN SULCUS
C CENTRAL CORD

GREY MATTER
COMPRESSED AREA OF SPINAL CORD

Figure 19-13. The anterior cord syndrome.

c.   *Brown-Sequard syndrome* is due to transection or lesion of one-half of the spinal cord (Figure 19-14). There is a loss of motor function (paralysis) and position and vibratory sense, as well as vasomotor paralysis on the same side (ipsilateral) and below the hemisection. On the opposite (contralateral) side of the hemisection, there is loss of pain and temperature sensation below the level of the lesion or hemisection.

3.   Spinal cord injuries may be categorized as stable (vertebral column is aligned) or unstable (vertebral column is not aligned).

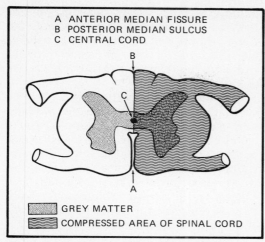

A ANTERIOR MEDIAN FISSURE
B POSTERIOR MEDIAN SULCUS
C CENTRAL CORD

◾ GREY MATTER
〰 COMPRESSED AREA OF SPINAL CORD

Figure 19-14. Brown-Sequard syndrome.

4. Injuries may be classified according to the injury to the vertebral column. Such types include dislocation, subluxation, compression fracture, and "hangman's" fracture (C-2).

5. Injuries may be classified in relation to the specific level of injury. These injuries are summarized in Table 19-1.

6. The final classification of spinal cord injuries is in relation to the mechanism involved. This is either hyperextension or hyperflexion. Rarely, rotational injuries may occur.

Spinal cord injuries are frequently associated with head or other systems trauma.

Disease states may relate specifically to the spinal cord, for example, tumor, arteriovenous malformations, and infections. In these instances, treating the underlying condition may result in improvement in spinal cord function.

SPINAL SHOCK

Spinal shock is a state that exists when irreversible damage has occurred to the spinal

Table 19-1. Classification of injury according to specific vertebral level.

Injury Level	Intact Function	Lost Function
Below L-2	Mixed motor/sensory dependent on intact nerve fibers	Mixed motor/sensory, possible loss of use of bladder, bowels, and sexual functioning
T-1 to L-1 or L-2	Arm function	Leg functions, bladder, bowels, and sexual functioning
C-7, C-8	Triceps muscle, Head rotation, Respiration	No intrinsic muscles of hand, no other function retained
C-6, C-7	Biceps muscle, Head rotation, Respiration	No triceps, no other function retained
C-5, C-6	Gross arm movement, Head rotation, Diaphragmatic respiration	No other function retained
C-4, C-5	Head rotation, Diaphragmatic respiration	No other function intact
C-3, C-4	Head rotation	No other functions intact (many die)
C-1, C-2	None	Most die

cord resulting in areflexia and flaccid paralysis below the level of injury.

Spinal shock may affect any and all body systems and is more severe in cervical vertebral injuries than other vertebral injuries. Spinal shock lasts about 7–10 days. One knows that spinal shock is resolving when flaccid paralysis becomes a spastic paralysis and reflexes return.

COMPLICATIONS OF SPINAL CORD INJURY

Immediate post-injury problems are (a) maintaining a patent airway, (b) maintaining adequate ventilation, (c) maintaining an adequate circulating blood volume, and (d) prevention of an extension of cord damage.

Respiratory System: Cervical injury or fracture above C-4 presents special problems in that total respiratory function is lost. Artificial ventilation will be required to keep the patient alive; however, most of these patients will die. Injury or fracture of C-4 or the lower cervical vertebrae will result in diaphragmatic breathing if the phrenic nerve is functioning. Hypoventilation almost always occurs with diaphragmatic respirations because there is a decrease in vital capacity and tidal volume.

Since cervical fractures or severe injuries cause a paralysis of abdominal musculature and frequently intercostal musculature, the patient is unable to cough effectively enough to remove secretions; this leads to atelectasis and pneumonia. Artificial airways provide direct access for pathogens, so bronchial hygiene and chest physiotherapy become extremely important. If multiple trauma is involved, a neurogenic pulmonary edema may result from the sudden changes in thoracic pressures at the time of the injury. The occurrence of pulmonary edema (as opposed to neurogenic pulmonary edema) is probably due to fluid overload.

Cardiovascular System: Any cord transection above the level of T-5 abolishes the influence of the sympathetic nervous system. Consequently, immediate problems are bradycardia and hypotension. If the bradycardia is only slight, close cardiac monitoring may reveal a stable cardiac condition. Junctional escape beats may be observed and a junctional rhythm may become established. If the bradycardia is marked, appropriate medications to increase the heart rate and avoid hypoxia will be necessary.

With the abolition of the influence of the sympathetic nervous system, vasodilatation occurs, decreasing venous return of blood to the heart. This decreases cardiac output and hypotension results. Intravenous fluids may resolve the problem or vassopressor drugs may be required.

Renal System: Urinary retention is a common development in acute spinal injuries and spinal shock. The bladder is hyperirritable. There is a loss of inhibition of reflex from the brain. Consequently, the patient will void small amounts of urine frequently. In spite of this, the bladder becomes distended since this is actually urinary retention with overflow. Urinary retention increases the chance of infection. In addition, urinary calculi are likely to develop in a distended bladder retaining urine. Catheterization is indicated.

Gastrointestinal System: If the cord transection has occurred above T-5, the loss of sympathetic innervation may lead to the development of an ileus or gastric distention. A nasogastric tube to intermittent suction may relieve the gastric distention, and standard treatment will be used for an ileus. A common occurrence in the past has been the development of biochemical stress ulcers due to excessive release of hydrochloric acid in the stomach. Cimetidine (Tagamet®) is frequently used to prevent the occurrence of these ulcers during the initial extreme body stress. It is quite effective. Because of the absence of clinical signs, intra-abdominal bleeding may occur and be difficult to diagnose. There will be no pain, tenderness, guarding, or such. Continued hypotension in spite of vigorous treatment is suspicious. Expanding girth of the abdomen may be ascertainable, but not always. If the rectum is not emptied on a *regular* basis, the patient may develop a fecal impaction.

Musculoskeletal System: The integrity of the patient's skin is of primary importance. The deterioration of denervated skin can occur very quickly leading to major, life-threatening infection. The use of Roto-Beds (Figure 19-15) and their variations help to prevent the breakdown of the skin. A certain degree of muscle atrophy will occur during the flaccid paralysis state, while contractures tend to occur during the spastic paralysis stage.

Poikilothermism is the adjustment of the body temperature towards the room temperature. This occurs in these injuries because the interruption of the sympathetic nervous system prevents its temperature controlling fibers to send impulses that will reach the hypothalamus.

Metabolic Needs: Correcting an existing acid-base disturbance and maintaining acid-base balance will promote the function of other body systems. Recall that nasogastric suctioning may lead to alkalosis, and decreased perfusion may lead to acidosis. Electrolytes must be monitored until a normal diet is resumed and suctioning has been discontinued. A positive nitrogen bal-ance and a high protein diet will help prevent skin breakdown and infections, and will help decrease the rate of muscle atrophy.

Psychologic Needs: These are covered in Chapter 47.

Nursing Interventions: The primary nursing intervention is ensuring a patent airway at ALL times to provide for adequate ventilation. Most patients with cervical fractures will have an endotracheal tube or a tracheostomy. Frequent, gentle suctioning of the nasopharynx, oropharynx, and endotracheal tube or tracheostomy is imperative to help prevent hypoxia secondary to retained secretions. HOWEVER, suctioning must not exceed 10–15 seconds, and the patient should be hyperventilated before and after the procedure to prevent a cardiac arrest which may occur *if* hypoxia develops and the patient has a bradycardia or junctional rhythm. Chest physiotherapy protocols should be followed according to neurologic and cardiovascular parameters. The

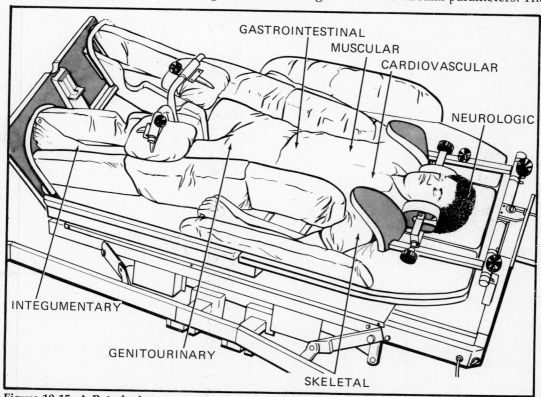

GASTROINTESTINAL
MUSCULAR
CARDIOVASCULAR
NEUROLOGIC
INTEGUMENTARY
GENITOURINARY
SKELETAL

Figure 19-15. A Roto-bed.

patient's vital capacity, tidal volume, and ABGs should be carefully and frequently monitored until the patient is stable and ventilatory support is no longer needed.

Cardiovascular monitoring of dysrhythmias and hypotension is essential. The dysrhythmias which occur may require standard treatment or only continued close monitoring. Hypotension is often controlled with fluids intravenously, which requires that the nurse monitor the patient for the development of pulmonary edema.

The prevention of extension of cord injury is the next major nursing responsibility. If traction is employed, the rope knots should be taped, weights hanging freely, and traction lines kept straight or as positioned by the physician.

Renal status is usually monitored hourly in the first few days following injury. The amount of intravenous fluids necessary to prevent hypotension is usually sufficient to prevent renal complications of oliguria or anuria unless there is multiple trauma involving the kidneys. The common renal problem after vertebral and cord injury above the sacral level is urinary retention. A Foley catheter is often used in the early stages of the injury. If a Foley is not inserted, intermittent catheterization is needed to ensure that an excessive urinary volume is not retained in the bladder, leading to further problems.

Gastrointestinal interventions include initial drainage of the stomach contents, and then the nasogastric tube is usually connected to intermittent suction since gastric distention occurs and acid secretions are increased in the first few days. Contents suctioned should be routinely tested for blood since biochemical stress ulcers may occur.

Musculoskeletal needs of the patient include proper body alignment, support of bony prominences to prevent skin breakdown, and frequent turning (unless on a Roto-Bed) to promote circulation and induce comfort. During the flaccid paralysis stage, extremities should be maintained in a functional position. During the spastic stage of the paralysis, medications and some physical therapy may help control the spasms.

Metabolic needs of the patient are initially met with intravenous fluids. As soon as the patient is stabilized, tube feedings are often started. Depending upon the site of the injury and the residual deficits, the patient may be able to start oral feedings relatively soon after the injury. Rarely is hyperalimentation used unless there are protracted multiple trauma injuries.

Autonomic Dysreflexia

This is also called autonomic hyperreflexia. The condition is a *life-threatening* situation requiring immediate resolution.

The most common precipitating etiologies are a distended bladder or rectum. Contraction of the bladder or rectum, stimulation of the skin, or stimulation of the pain receptors may also cause autonomic hyperreflexia.

Symptoms include hypertension, blurred vision, throbbing headache, marked diaphoresis *above* the level of the lesion, bradycardia, piloerection (body hair erect) due to pilomotor spasm, nasal congestion, and nausea.

Pathophysiology of this condition involves the stimulation of sensory receptors below the level of cord lesion. The intact autonomic system reacts with a reflex arteriolar spasm which increases blood pressure. Baroreceptors in cerebral vessels, the carotid sinus, and the aorta sense the hypertension and stimulate the parasympathetic system. The heart rate is decreased, but the visceral and peripheral vessels do not dilate because efferent impulses cannot pass through the cord lesion.

Nursing interventions in this very serious emergency are notification of the physician and assessment to determine the cause. Abdominal palpation for a distended bladder is done *very gently* to avoid increasing the stimulus. Catheter irrigation performed very slowly and gently may open a plugged catheter. A digital rectal exam should be done only after application of a Nupercainal type ointment to decrease rectal stimulation and to prevent an increase of symptoms.

— 20

Acute Head Injuries and Craniotomies

Learning Objectives

By the end of this chapter, the nurse will be able to:

1. Identify at least six initial major areas of concern in acute head injuries.
2. List and define five levels of consciousness.
3. Explain the process of checking motor function.
4. Identify three classifications of head injuries.
5. Explain the differences in linear, depressed, and basal skull fractures.
6. List and define two types of epidural hematomas.
7. List and characterize two types of subdural hematomas.
8. Identify the significance of "battle sign" and "racoon eyes."
9. Explain the visual field loss that occurs with homonymous hemianopsia.
10. List and explain six nursing interventions in postcraniotomy care.

Acute Head Injuries

Acute head injuries are almost always the result of violence or automobile accidents. A history is often very difficult to obtain, but it can be vital in establishing potential damage done by acceleration/deceleration forces. Acceleration injuries may be called coup (pronounced coo) and deceleration forces, contracoup.

EXAMINATION OF THE PATIENT

Although the physician examines the patient, it is a nursing responsibility to perform a modified examination of the patient as a part of continual neurologic evaluation.

Airway: Always establish a patent airway. Use only an oral airway, NOT an endotracheal tube, until the cross table lateral x-rays confirm NO neck fracture. If the oral airway does not provide a patent airway, an emergency tracheostomy or cricoidotomy is preferable to manipulating the neck for insertion of an endotracheal tube if the x-rays have not been made.

Cardiac and Respiratory Function: Continually monitor these systems to ensure early intervention in cases of dysfunction. Inadequate function of either system may result in extension of neurologic impairment.

Shock: Monitor for signs of impending shock. Be prepared to intervene by establishing an intravenous line while awaiting specific physician instructions. If shock occurs, it is NOT due to intracranial bleeding if the cranium is intact. There is insufficient room in the cranium to contain the volume of blood necessary to cause hypovolemic shock.

Abdomen: Palpate for involuntary guarding and increasing girth which may indicate an intra-abdominal hemorrhage leading to shock.

Long Bones: These need to be checked for fractures. Such fractures may lead to fat emboli, shock, and other complications.

Now, and only now, is one ready for the *neurological exam*.

Scalp: Check for tears and/or swelling which may indicate a subgaleal hematoma.

Face: Palpate eye orbits, nose, teeth, maxilla, and mandible for facial fractures. Some facial fractures may provide for leakage of cerebrospinal fluid, and this would be an entry port for infection.

Ears: Blood in the external canal usually indicates a basal skull fracture.

Carotid Arteries: Palpate each carotid artery by itself to check for cerebral hemorrhage. If the carotids cannot be palpated, check for palpation of the superficial temporal arteries which are a branch of the external carotids.

Mentation: There are five possible states or levels of consciousness (LOC). The definition and/or progression may differ in various institutions.

1. Alert—The patient is oriented to person, place, and time.
2. Lethargic—The patient prefers to sleep and when aroused, the degree of alertness or confusion is variable.
3. Obtunded—The patient can be aroused with minimal stimulation, but will drift off to sleep quickly.
4. Stuporous—The patient is aroused only by constant, deep, and usually painful stimuli. The patient may respond by some attempt to withdraw, moan, or exhibit decerebrate or decorticate positioning.
5. Coma—The patient cannot be aroused.

The Glasgow Coma Scale (Table 20-1) is gaining acceptance for use as a general standard for identifying levels of consciousness (mentation) and for prognosis of the outcome of the injury.

Cranial Nerves: Some of the 12 cranial nerves can be checked during routine patient care and during neurologic checks:

II. *Optic nerve*. (This will be covered in detail at the end of the chapter.) The most common result of injury to the optic tract is homonymous hemianopsia. When looking at the optic disc, it usually has a sharp, clear outline. If pulsations in the veins of the optic disc are visible, there is usually *NO* increased intracranial pressure. Papilledema is present when the head of the optic nerve appears raised or increased (bulging) instead of flat.

Table 20-1. Glasgow Coma Scale.

Eye Opening (E)	Best Motor Response (M)	Verbal Response (V)

spontaneous = 4
to speech = 3
to pain = 2
no response = 1
	obeys = 6
	localizes = 5
	withdraws = 4
	abnormal
	  flexion = 3
	  extension = 2
	no response = 1
		oriented = 5
		confused
		  conversation = 4
		inappropriate
		  words = 3
		incomprehensible
		  sounds = 2
		no response = 1

Note: The lowest score received has the worst prognosis.

III. *Oculomotor nerve*. This controls four of the six eye muscles (except the lateral rectus and superior oblique). The parasympathetic nerves cause pupil constriction. The sympathetic nerves cause pupil dilatation.

IV. *Trochlear nerve*. This controls the superior oblique muscle. It turns the eye down and out.

V. *Trigeminal nerve*. Cornea sensation provides the sensory side of arc for corneal reflex. The seventh nerve (facial) provides the motor side of arc.

VI. *Abducens nerve*. This controls the lateral rectus muscle. It turns the eye out. This is the longest unprotected nerve in the brain. (Some physicians think the trochlear nerve is the longest.)

VII. *Facial nerve*. It exits the skull through the bone in the mastoid area. It controls the muscles of facial expression and plays a part in the production of tears.

X. *Vagus nerve*. This controls palate deviation. If the nerve is damaged, the uvula deviates away from the side of the paralysis. In vagal nerve paralysis, there is ipsilateral paralysis of the palate, pharynx, and larynx muscles. The soft palate at rest is usually lower on the affected side and if the patient says "ah," it elevates on the intact side.

XI. *(Spinal) Accessory nerve*. It turns the head by use of sternocleidomastoid muscles. It has some function with the upper trapezius muscles.

XII. *Hypoglossal nerve*. This controls tongue movement. If this is damaged, the patient cannot move the tongue from side to side, and tongue protrusion results in deviation toward the side of nerve damage.

Motor Function: Check to see if the patient moves all extremities voluntarily *AND* equally. Note a one-sided weakness. If muscle weakness is suspected, have patient close eyes and extend arms directly in front. If there is a muscle weakness, there will be a drifting downward of the weakened extremity. Usually, there is no spasticity immediately after an injury. Flaccidity is usually present for about 10 days.

Sensation: In trauma, patients usually respond only to pain. The response to sensation may include decorticate or decerebrate positioning in the unconscious patient.

CLASSIFICATION OF INJURY

1. Closed Head Injuries

The scalp is intact. The injury can be concussion, contusion, and/or skull fracture.

Concussion. There is an elimination of consciousness due to blunt trauma to the head by an accelerative or decelerative force. Some authorities place artificial time limits on unconsciousness to differentiate concussion from contusion or coma. Clinically, duration of unconsciousness may alter terminology of the injury, but the primary consideration is that of neurological deficits. Concussions usually clear spontaneously after varying time intervals with the patient having no residual neurological deficit other than total amnesia for the time interval of unconsciousness. The patient with a mild to moderate concussion will have recovered consciousness within about 12 hours (as the accepted standard). It may be 2 or 3 days before the patient can recall correctly all the factors leading to the concussion.

Contusion. As with concussion, there is an immediate elimination of consciousness due to accelerative or decelerative blunt trauma forces to the head. These forces propel the brain against the rigid cranium (the coup force). With initial impact, the brain is then rotated or thrown back in the opposite direction (the contracoup force). This is shown in Figure 20-1. This invariably results in cerebral bruising and edema. If the forces are strong enough, lacerations and scattered intracerebral hemorrhages may occur. These usually occur along the axis line of the coup and countracoup forces. In severe contusion, subarachnoid hemorrhage may occur, resulting in coma. Mild contusions will clear as the bruising and

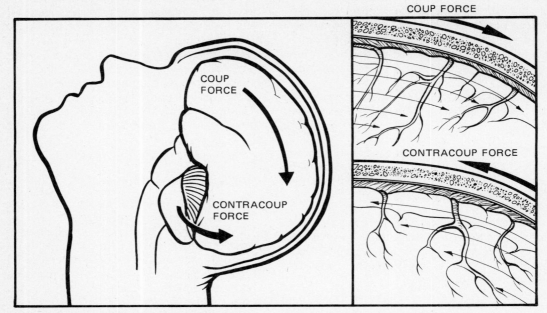

Figure 20-1. Coup and contracoup forces.

edema resolve, leaving no neurological deficit. Severe contusions that do not resolve, as indicated by the patient remaining comatose, indicate that the original bruising and/or lacerations caused a necrosis of brain tissue (possibly secondary to prolonged cerebral hypoxia at the injury sites).

Skull fractures. Skull fractures are usually classified as linear, depressed, or basilar. A *linear* skull fracture that does not tear the dura mater will heal without treatment. If the linear fracture occurs over the temporal lobe and tears the dura (Figure 20-2), there is a chance that the middle meningeal artery will also be torn. This constitutes a medical emergency since the bleeding is arterial and is commonly known as an acute epidural hematoma. The fracture may tear the dura mater over a venous sinus resulting in a slow bleeding causing a chronic (non-acute) epidural hematoma.

A *depressed* skull fracture that is NOT depressed more than the thickness of the skull is usually just monitored. However, a depressed skull fracture greater than the thickness of the skull (usually more than 5 to 7 millimeters) requires surgery to relieve the compression. If the dura is torn, bone fragments may have entered brain tissue,

requiring removal, and the chance of infection is greatly increased.

With a *basilar* skull fracture there is a high risk of: injury to cranial nerves, infection, and residual neurological deficits due to coup and contracoup forces (Figure 20-3). Basilar fractures may occur in the anterior or posterior fossa. Cerebrospinal fluid draining from the nose (rhinorrhea) or the ear canal (otorrhea) are signs of basilar fracture. The "battle sign" is an area of ecchy-

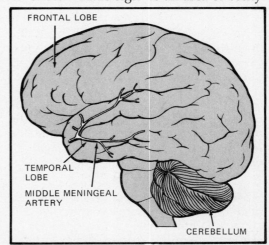

Figure 20-2. Linear skull fracture over the middle meningeal artery.

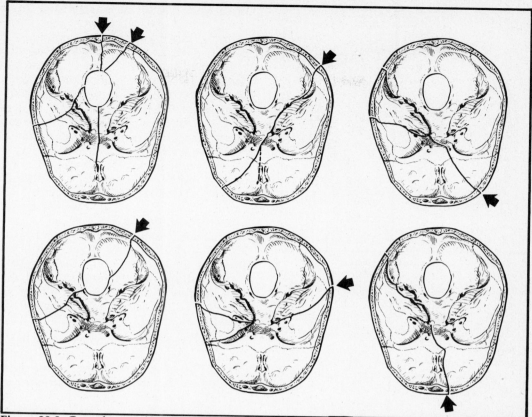

Figure 20-3. Coup forces of basilar skull fractures. Contracoup forces go in the opposite direction along similar paths.

mosis over the mastoid projection and indicates either a temporal or basilar fracture in the posterior fossa. "Raccoon eyes" are a sign of bleeding into the paranasal sinuses with ecchymosis developing around the eyes. This indicates a basilar fracture in the anterior fossa. Other symptoms of basilar fracture include tinnitus, facial paralysis, hearing difficulty, nystagmus, and conjugate deviation gaze. Patients with rhinorrhea will complain of a salty taste as the cerebrospinal fluid drains into the pharynx. Otorrhea can be tested with Tes-tape for glucose. If glucose is present, the drainage is cerebrospinal fluid. Severe neurological deficits are common with basilar fractures.

2. Compound Injuries

This includes a laceration of the scalp with a head injury or skull fracture. If there is a laceration with a head injury (depressed fracture), surgery is usually performed immediately because of the threat of infection.

3. Intracranial Mass Lesions

Acute Epidural Hematoma. This occurs at the time of the injury (Figure 20-4) and is usually associated with a temporal or parietal skull fracture with laceration of the middle meningeal artery (and often vein). There is usually a loss of consciousness which may be followed by a brief period (up to 4–6 hours) of lucidity, then coma. During the lucid period, nausea and vomiting often occur. Other signs may include ipsilateral oculomotor paralysis, contralateral hemiparesis/hemiplegia, and positive Babinski reflexes.

In one type of epidural hematoma, the linear fracture occurs across the sagittal

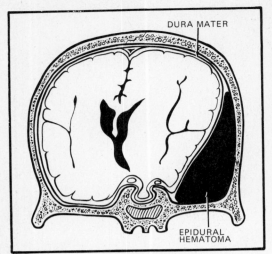

Figure 20-4. An epidural hematoma.

sinus or the transverse sinus. In this instance, *venous* blood oozes into the area *above* the dura mater, producing a chronic epidural hematoma. Symptoms may be delayed for several days.

Subdural Hematomas. There are two types of subdural hematomas: an acute and a chronic form. In the acute subdural hematoma (Figure 20-5), symptoms may occur from the first 2 or 3 days up to 2 weeks. The hematoma consists of some gel and some xanthochromic liquid. Symptoms include headaches, slowness in thinking, confu-

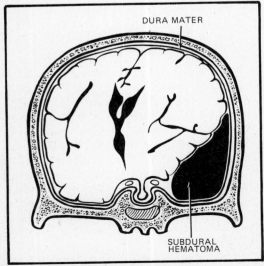

Figure 20-5. A subdural hematoma.

sion, and sometimes agitation. These symptoms progressively worsen.

In the chronic subdural hematoma, a period of weeks may follow the injury before symptoms occur. These symptoms include giddiness, exaggeration of certain personality traits, confusion, occasionally headaches, and rarely a seizure. The cerebrospinal fluid may be clear, bloody, or xanthochromic. Intracranial pressure may be normal, elevated, or decreased. If symptoms do not occur for several weeks, a membrane forms around the subdural hematoma walling it off from the rest of the brain. (In some cases, this walled-off section will calcify.)

Subdural hematoma may occur spontaneously without any form of injury in patients on anticoagulant therapy or in those with clotting dysfunction. CAT scan will provide a diagnosis. Surgery is the treatment of choice in both forms of subdural hematomas.

Intracerebral Hemorrhage. (ICH; Figure 20-6). Many intracerebral hemorrhages occur as hypertensive strokes. Other causes include skull fracture, penetrating trauma (bullets), contracoup decelerative forces, and systemic disease such as leukemias and aplastic anemias. If the hemorrhage occurs in the internal capsule of the brain, paralysis results. If the hemorrhage occurs in the dominant hemisphere, dysfunction is variable, dependent upon the location of hemorrhage. Signs and symptoms include nausea, vomiting, dizziness, headache, signs of increasing intracranial pressure, and a contralateral hemiplegia. A delayed intracerebral hemorrhage may occur hours to days after a closed head injury.

Subarachnoid Hemorrhage (SAH). This may occur after trauma due to hypertension with atherosclerosis or due to a congenital aneurysm or arteriovenous malformation. Symptoms usually include headache, dizziness, tinnitus, facial pain (pressure on the fifth cranial nerve), ptosis, a unilaterally dilated pupil, nuchal rigidity, and hemiparesis or hemiplegia.

Areas and function affected by a subarachnoid hemorrhage on the dominant hemisphere are shown in Figure 20-7.

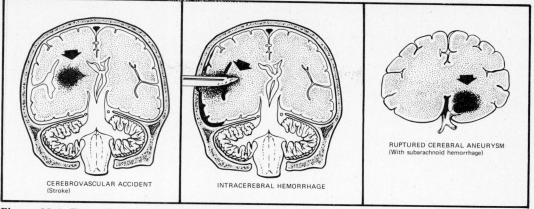

CEREBROVASCULAR ACCIDENT
(Stroke)

INTRACEREBRAL HEMORRHAGE

RUPTURED CEREBRAL ANEURYSM
(With subarachnoid hemorrhage)

Figure 20-6. Examples of intracerebral hemorrhages.

COMPLICATIONS OF CLOSED HEAD INJURIES

Complications include cerebral edema, contusion (with residual neurologic deficits), and persistent vegetative coma (if contusion is severe). Respiratory hypoxia progressing to failure occurs if the cerebral edema is in the medullary area or generalized enough to compress the brain. Increasing intracranial pressure depends upon the amount of edema and/or bleeding. Stress ulcers are not uncommon in moderate to severe closed head injuries. Seizures occur in about 5% of the cases. If edema, bleeding, or the initial injury result in necrosis of brain tissue, infection often occurs as part of the process.

COMPLICATIONS OF INTRACRANIAL HEMORRHAGE (ICH)

Respiratory hypoxia, secondary to the intracranial hemorrhage, causes hypoxemia and hypercapnia. This results in an increased cerebral blood flow increasing intracranial pressure. The increased pressure results in neurologic dysfunctions. Subarachnoid hemorrhage may occur because

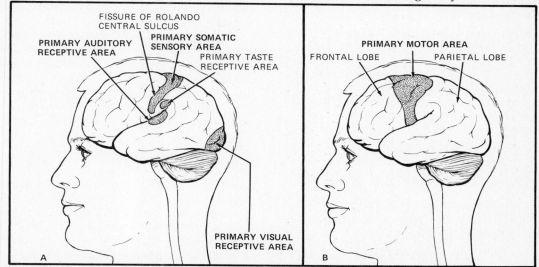

FISSURE OF ROLANDO
CENTRAL SULCUS

PRIMARY AUDITORY
RECEPTIVE AREA

PRIMARY SOMATIC
SENSORY AREA

PRIMARY TASTE
RECEPTIVE AREA

PRIMARY VISUAL
RECEPTIVE AREA

PRIMARY MOTOR AREA

FRONTAL LOBE

PARIETAL LOBE

A

B

Figure 20-7. Areas and function affected by subarachnoid hemorrhage. (A) shows somatic sensory areas. (B) shows primary motor area (strip). Because of rapidly increased intracranial pressures of the subarachnoid hemorrhage, the entire brain can be affected.

of the increased pressure or trauma and a hydrocephalus may result. If the hypothalamus and/or pituitary gland are affected, diabetes insipidus will most likely occur. Biochemical stress ulcers are common and are frequently associated with electrolyte disturbances. Dependent upon the site and degree of injury, seizures may develop. Infections, both cerebrospinal and respiratory, are continuous threats.

COMPLICATIONS OF INTRAVENTRICULAR HEMORRHAGE

These patients usually die. A frequent complication is acute hydrocephalus with increased intracranial pressure. A long-term complication is a communicating hydrocephalus. A drain may be placed. If the P_{O_2} falls below 65 mm Hg, hypoxic brain damage may occur. A rising P_{CO_2} will dilate cerebral vessels, increasing blood flow and pressure. For these reasons, the P_{CO_2} is maintained between 25 and 30 mm Hg.

NURSING INTERVENTIONS

The primary nursing intervention after assurance of a patent airway and the prevention of hypoxia is the frequent neurological assessment. Signs of increasing intracranial pressure may be treated with magnesium sulfate, osmotics, diuretics, or hyperventilation. Intracranial pressure monitoring may be instituted. In some centers, barbiturate coma therapy may be utilized.

Monitoring vital signs and maintaining fluid balance and accurate intake and output records will help in establishing treatment aimed at stabilizing the patient.

Standard procedures to prevent infections are employed.

Diagnostic Tests and Findings

Computerized axial tomography (CAT scan or CT) is the number one diagnostic test in head injuries. It will reveal if:

1. Air has entered the brain from fractures of the eye, mastoid, or sinuses.
2. Blood is present in brain tissue or in the ventricular system.
3. Blood is on the surface of the brain or in the basal cisterns.
4. Ventricles are of normal size and in normal position.
5. The pineal gland has calcified and is in normal position.

Lumbar puncture is contraindicated by increased intracranial pressure and is rarely done in the diagnosis of head injuries.

ABGs in intracranial hematoma reveal respiratory alkalosis (due to hyperventilation). Metabolic acidosis may occur if the patient is in shock, is hypoxic, or has a high level of physical activity (combativeness will produce lactic acidosis as does decerebrate posturing).

In closed head injuries, skull x-ray, brain scan, and angiogram studies may be essentially normal. CAT scan may show cerebral edema and areas of petechial hemorrhage in severe contusions. Hydrocephalus may be present. The echoencephalogram has a high percentage of false results.

In intracranial hematomas, a CAT scan will show increased density that indicates the presence, location, and extent of the hematoma. Skull films may show fractures or increased intracranial pressure, a calcified pineal gland, or a choroid plexus shifted from midline. Cerebral angiography may reveal an avascular mantle with displacement or stretching of vessels. Cervical spine x-rays may show injury. Brain scan may show increased uptake of isotope in the area of hematoma or tumor. Echoencephalogram may reveal a shift of midline structures and is reserved for use in diagnosing the cause of coma in patients where other tests have failed to reveal the cause.

Visual Pathway Defects

Visual field defects may occur due to cranial trauma, various other pathologies, and/or craniotomies. Figure 20-8 demonstrates the most common visual field defects. The key to interpreting visual defects seen in Figure 20-8 is that the left eye is on the *left* and the right eye is on the *right* in the figure. The image is not reversed as with heart drawings.

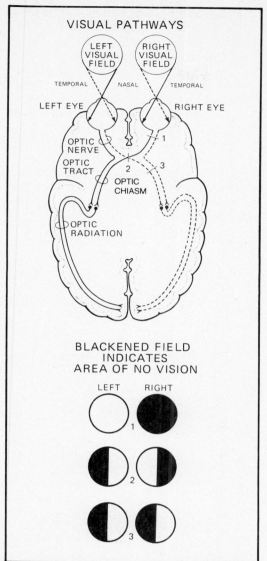

VISUAL PATHWAYS

LEFT VISUAL FIELD   RIGHT VISUAL FIELD

TEMPORAL   NASAL   TEMPORAL

LEFT EYE   RIGHT EYE

OPTIC NERVE   1

OPTIC TRACT   2   3

OPTIC CHIASM

OPTIC RADIATION

BLACKENED FIELD INDICATES AREA OF NO VISION

LEFT   RIGHT

1

2

3

Figure 20-8. Visual field defects. (Adapted from Bates B: A Guide to Physical Examination. Philadelphia: J. B. Lippincott, p. 49, 1974. Reprinted with permission of J. B. Lippincott.)

Visual images from the peripheral field (temporal) hit on the nasal side of each retina. Fibers from the nasal side of each retina carry the visual impulses along the optic nerve towards the optic tract. Just prior to the optic tract, these fibers cross (at the optic chiasm). They then continue on the inside of the optic tract through the optic radiation to the end of the optic tract.

Visual images from the central (nasal) field of vision hit on the outer, temporal side of each retina. Fibers from the outer side of each retina carry the impulses to the optic nerve and follow the optic nerve tract on the outside, through the optic radiation to the end of the tract.

Lesions between the eye and the point where nerve fibers cross cause a blind eye. Lesions of the eye itself will also cause unilateral blindness.

A lesion at the point where the optic nerve fibers cross (the optic chiasm) will result in bitemporal blindness. Images from the periphery of *both* eyes are blocked resulting in bitemporal blindness.

A lesion of the fibers of the right optic tract blocks visual images on the same side of each eye. This is a left homonymous (same side) hemianopsia (one-half the visual field).

In the same way, a lesion of fibers of the left optic tract blocks visual images on the same side of each eye. In this case, a right homonymous (same side) hemianopsia (one-half the visual field) exists. These are the two most common visual defects found associated with optic tract injuries.

A lesion may occur in the optic radiation. If the lesion is completely across the optic radiation, a homonymous hemianopsia develops. However, if the lesion affects only the outer fibers, a homonymous quadrantic defect occurs.

Craniotomies

Craniotomies are performed for many reasons. Postoperative care includes routine postoperative care *plus*:

1. Neurolgoic monitoring compares pre- and postoperative functions, right side to left side function, and hour-to-hour functions.

2. Pain control must be achieved with codeine and not morphine sulfate, which might mask neurologic changes.

3. Intracranial pressure must be maintained within normal range. This is achieved by judiciously using glucocorticoids, by elevating the head of the bed 15–30 degrees, and by keeping P_{CO_2} between 25 and 35 mm Hg.

4. Patent drainage tubes, which may be used for 24–48 hours, help control intracranial pressure and help monitor type and amount of drainage.

5. A clear drainage through dressings may be CSF and should be reported to the physician immediately.

6. Stress ulcers (also known as Cushing's ulcers) are a common occurrence. They may be treated and/or prevented with use of cimetidine (Tagamet®) and antacids.

7. Cardiovascular status is monitored since certain head injuries cause a bradycardia. Bradycardia may be a precursor to other dysrhythmias and cardiac failure. Intravenous fluid needs are calculated daily to prevent fluid overload and to maintain electrolyte balance.

Diabetes insipidus occurs with some head injuries and with other cerebral pathologies. It is covered in section V on the endocrine system.

21

Intracranial Pressure, Aneurysm, Coma, and Brain Herniation

Learning Objectives

By the end of this chapter, the nurse will be able to:

1. Explain the Munro-Kellie hypothesis.
2. Describe two compensatory mechanisms for increasing ICP.
3. Define intracranial compliance.
4. Identify the formula for determining cerebral perfusion pressure.
5. List at least five indications for ICP monitoring.
6. Explain three ICP monitoring techniques, identifying advantages and disadvantages of each.
7. Identify A, B, and C waves of ICP monitoring and list the acceptable characteristics of "A" waves.
8. List four important nursing interventions in ICP monitoring.
9. Define "intracranial aneurysm."
10. List ten symptoms of an intracranial aneurysm.
11. List at least five nursing interventions for the patient with an intracranial aneurysmal bleed.
12. Explain two pathological conditions leading to coma.
13. Identify three disease categories leading to coma.
14. List two routes of herniation and the stages of each.
15. Identify changes in each of the pertinent parameters for each stage of central and uncal herniation.

Within a very narrow range, the contents of the cranial vault can adjust to altering intracranial pressure (ICP). When the limits of the range and time are exceeded, the intracranial pressure rises precipitously.

Components of the Cranial Vault

There are three components which almost completely fill the cranial vault. Brain tissue comprises about 88% of the volume of the cranium. Cerebrospinal fluid comprises about 9–10% of the total volume. Intravascular fluid comprises from 2–11% of the volume of the cranial vault.

Munro-Kellie Hypothesis

This hypothesis is the basis for intracranial pressure monitoring. The hypothesis states that in the adult the cranial vault is nondistensible (it is bone) and the components of the vault are essentially noncompressible. Based on these tenets, a relationship between the vault and its contents can be construed.

An increase in one component of the vault contents necessitates a reciprocal decrease in either or both of the other components. If the reciprocal decrease does not occur, there is a rise in intracranial pressure. This pressure increase is termed *intracranial hypertension*. Normal intracranial pressure is 50–200 cm of water or 4–15 mm Hg. Most practitioners treat a sustained ICP above 25 mm Hg.

Compensatory Mechanisms for Increasing ICP

Initial increases in the volume of the cranium are compensated for by two mechanisms.

1. A decrease in intravascular fluid (blood) occurs by compression of the low pressure venous system. Intravascular volume is the most alterable component of the three in the cranium (brain tissue, CSF, and blood). There is a specific limit to the extent of compressibility. When this limit is exceeded, ICP rises.
2. The CSF is the second compensatory mechanism for increasing ICP. As the ICP rises, CSF is displaced from the cranial vault into the spinal canal. When maxium displacement of CSF has occurred, there is probably an increase in CSF absorption which aids compensatory mechanisms.

These mechanisms function to keep the ICP constant. They function well when the ICP increases slowly. Even then, the mechanisms will lose their compensatory function at a certain point (variable with the individual). If the ICP rises rapidly, the compensatory mechanisms are unable to function.

Intracranial Compliance

The relationship of change in pressure to change in volume is termed *compliance*. When intracranial compliance is low, a small increase in volume causes a large rise in pressure. The ICP provides information about intracranial compliance. Cerebral perfusion pressure (CPP) is equally as important as compliance, or more so. The cerebral perfusion pressure (CPP) can be calculated from the ICP. Cerebral perfusion pressure is the difference between mean arterial pressure (MAP)[1] and the mean ICP.

$$CPP = MAP - ICP$$

Cerebral perfusion pressure (CPP) is the pressure in the cerebral vascular system. This pressure approximates cerebral blood flow (CBF). Decreases in the cerebral perfusion pressure (CPP) reduce cerebral blood flow (CBF). The cerebral blood flow (CBF) affects delivery of both oxygen and glucose to the brain tissue. The normal brain has an extremely good autoregulatory system that maintains normal blood flow with the cerebral perfusion pressure as low as 50 mm Hg. In the injured brain, activity of the autoregulatory system is not known. Thus, many authorities consider a cerebral perfusion pressure of 60 mm Hg to be the least acceptable pressure. If the patient is neurologically unstable, cerebral perfusion pressure is extremely important when the mean arterial pressure (MAP or SAP) is low or when the ICP is high. If the MAP is low or the ICP is high, the brain is NOT being adequately perfused with oxygenated blood.

---

[1] Mean arterial pressure (MAP) is the same as mean systemic arterial pressure (SAP).

Indicators for ICP Monitoring

The outcome of many neurological conditions can be mediated by early recognition and intervention of increasing ICP. Six areas are identified:

1. *Head injuries.* A Glasgow Coma Scale of eight or less indicates significant neurological impairment. The parameters and scoring for the Glasgow Coma Score are shown in Chapter 20, Table 20-1. With ICP monitoring, *early* signs of intracranial problems can be identified and treatment initiated BEFORE clinical signs and symptoms develop.

2. *Treatment of an increasing ICP* can be evaluated for effectiveness. This includes fluid balance, mannitol (Osmitrol®) and dexamethasone (Decadron®) therapy, and hyperventilation.

3. *Postoperative cerebral edema.* Certain brain tumors grow slowly allowing the cranial contents to compensate for the increasing mass volume. After the tumor is removed, cerebral edema may be severe and life-threatening. ICP monitoring will allow early intervention.

4. *Reye-Johnson syndrome.* The mortality of the Reye-Johnson syndrome may be due to cerebral hypoglycemia and ischemia. This could be the result of poor cerebral perfusion and increasing ICP. By monitoring the ICP, therapies can be used to maintain a good cerebral perfusion pressure.

5. *Infections* per se are not always associated with increasing ICP. If coma (and/or brain stem involvement) is present, cerebral edema is a potential problem.

6. *Preoperative and postoperative monitoring* is common in intracerebral hemorrhage. The evacuation of a tumor, treatment of an underlying lesion, and evacuation of the hemorrhagic hematoma may result in cerebral edema and increasing ICP.

Measurement Sites of ICP

The ICP can be measured in many areas: the lumbar sac, cisterna magna, fontanels in newborns, cerebral ventricles, cranial subdural space, and cranial epidural space. The ICP values will depend upon (a) the site selected for monitoring, and (b) the patient's position. The ICP is usually measured supratentorially by an intraventricular cannula or by a subdural catheter or bolt or epidural sensor.

Monitoring Systems

The monitoring system has three parts: a sensor, a transducer, and a recording instrument. It is like an arterial pressure monitoring system *EXCEPT* the ICP monitoring system is *CLOSED* with no continuous flush system and no interflow.

The Sensor. This is a fluid-filled catheter, a cannula, or a bolt which communicates between the epidural, the subdural, or the intraventricular space and the transducer (Figure 21-1).

The Transducer. This converts the pressure signal to an electrical signal that can be recorded.

The Recorder. This is usually a bedside monitor with or without a digital readout and with a waveform display.

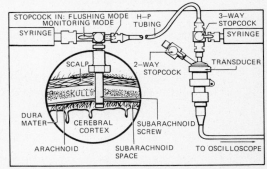

Figure 21-1. An intracranial pressure monitoring system.

Monitoring Techniques

Three common techniques being used are epidural, subarachnoid, and intraventricular monitoring.

1. *Epidural.* The sensor is placed between

the skull and dura with the pressure-sensitive membrane towards the dura (Figure 21-2). The advantage of this device is in leaving the dura intact. Technically, this may protect the patient from intracerebral infection. Disadvantages are summarized in Table 21-1.

2. *Subarachnoid screw.* This may be the most commonly used method of ICP monitoring (Figure 21-3). A hollow screw is inserted into the subarachnoid space and is connected by fluid-filled tubing to the transducer. Advantages of the screw include direct measurement of the CSF and being able to drain or sample the CSF. Disadvantages are summarized in Table 21-1.

3. *Intraventricular monitoring.* This is the most difficult form of monitoring because it involves the insertion of a cannula into one of the lateral ventricles

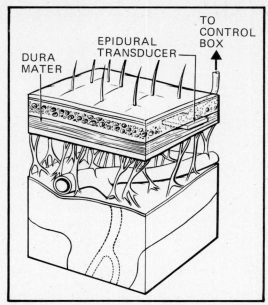

Figure 21-2. Epidural sensor for ICP monitoring.

Table 21-1. Some disadvantages of ICP monitoring.

ALL ICP monitoring has an inherently high risk of infection, some routes more than others.

Intraventricular

May cause increased damage during insertion especially with cerebral trauma, edema, and/or increased ICP.

Increased chance of damage also due to misshapen, tortuous, small, or displaced ventricles.

Statistical increase of infection with this form of monitoring.

Epidural

Wound, bone, and epidural infection may occur and progress to an intracerebral infection and/or a generalized sepsis.

May be plugged by brain tissue.

Waveforms dampened and may give faulty tracing.

Insertion must be in operating room.

Transducer and unit still *very* expensive.

Subarachnoid

Plugging often occurs giving false tracing.

May be flushed AWAY from patient.

Recalibration of transducer with every plugging. This increases chance of infection and chance of false readings.

(Figure 21-4). Insertion is usually performed in the nondominant cerebral hemisphere since brain tissue must be penetrated. The cannula is usually connected to a stopcock or pressure tubing (fluid-filled) to a transducer.

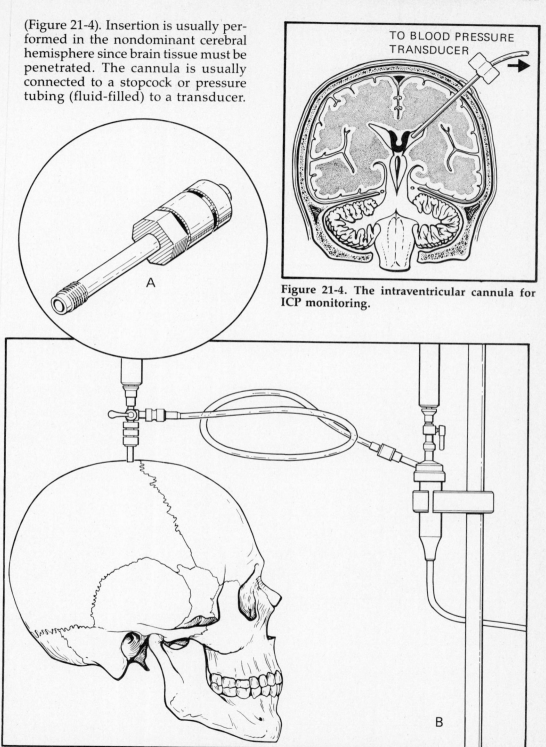

Figure 21-4. The intraventricular cannula for ICP monitoring.

TO BLOOD PRESSURE TRANSDUCER

A

B

Figure 21-3. The subarachnoid screw for ICP monitoring (A) and the subarachnoid screw and monitoring transducer in place (B).

The transducer is positioned at a level of the foramen of Monro. The major advantages of the intraventricular cannula are the ability to measure the CSF directly and to drain or sample the CSF as desired. Disadvantages are summarized in Table 21-1.

ICP Waveforms

There are three waveforms (A, B, and C) seen in ICP monitoring (Figure 21-5). The shape of the waves is affected by both cardiac pulsations and the respiratory cycle.

"A" waves or plateau waves occur when there is a sudden, sustained rise in ICP. "A"

waves may be present for 5–20 minutes. "A" waves are not normally present if the ICP is less than 50 mm Hg.

"B" waves are evident when the ICP rises to approximately 50 mm Hg. These waves are variable in shape and size and usually last for one-half to 3 minutes. They can occur with changes in the cardiac status.

"C" waves have been identified in ICP monitoring. Their significance has not been established.

With intraventricular monitoring, sharp peaked waveforms occur. Systolic and diastolic portions of the wave cycle are "dampened." A dampened waveform is ac-

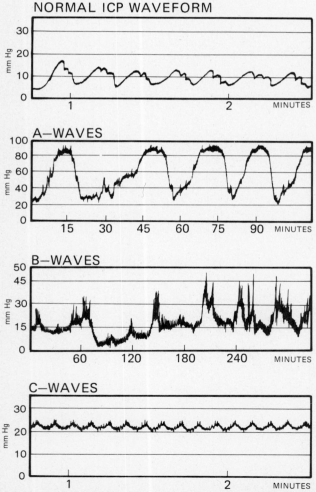

1. NORMAL WAVEFORM HAS STEEP UPWARD SYSTOLIC SLOPE, FOLLOWED BY DOWNWARD DIASTOLIC SLOPE WITH DICROTIC NOTCH. ORDINARILY, THIS WAVEFORM OCCURS CONTINUOUSLY AND INDICATES AN ICP MEASUREMENT BETWEEN 4 AND 15 mm Hg.

2. THE A—WAVES (SOMETIMES CALLED PLATEAU WAVES) TYPICALLY REACH ELEVATIONS OF 50 TO 100 mm Hg AND THEN DROP SHARPLY. IF THEY'RE RECURRING OR ARE SUSTAINED FOR SEVERAL MINUTES, A—WAVES INDICATE A RAPID, DANGEROUS RISE IN ICP AND A DECREASED ABILITY TO COMPENSATE. CONSIDER SUCH WAVES OMNIOUS. SUSTAINED A—WAVES MAY INDICATE IRREVERSIBLE BRAIN DAMAGE.

3. THE B—WAVES ARE SHARP AND RHYTHMIC, WITH A SAWTOOTH PATTERN. THEY OCCUR EVERY 1½ TO 2 MINUTES AND MAY REACH ELEVATIONS OF 50 mm Hg. BUT HIGH ELEVATIONS AREN'T SUSTAINED. THEY SEEM TO OCCUR MORE FREQUENTLY WITH DECREASING COMPENSATION. SOMETIMES THEY PRECEDE A—WAVES. WATCH THEM CLOSELY.

4. C—WAVES ARE RAPID AND RHYTHMIC, LESS SHARP IN APPEARANCE THAN B—WAVES, AND MAY FLUCTUATE WITH RESPIRATIONS OR CHANGING SYSTEMIC BLOOD PRESSURE. C—WAVES AREN'T CLINICALLY SIGNIFICANT.

Figure 21-5. Intracranial pressure waveforms. (Adapted from *Coping with Neurologic Disorders.* Nursing Photobook series. Springhouse, PA: Intermed Communications, Inc., p. 87, 1981.)

ceptable in ICP monitoring because the ICP *mean* is the measurement of significance. CAUTION: Do NOT confuse this with the waveforms of pulmonary artery monitoring where dampened waveforms are NOT acceptable!

Flat line tracings are *unacceptable*. The flat line may be high or low. It indicates occlusion of the monitoring tip. As long as a tracing is scalloped in phase with arterial pulsation, the readings are acceptable.

IMPLICATIONS AND INTERVENTIONS

ICP monitoring is useful in early interventions (stages 1 and 2) to control the ICP.

1. Cellular hypoxia is most likely to occur during the "A" waves (plateau waves). "A" waves indicate sustained pressure peaks up to 100 mm Hg (roughly 1,360 cm H_2O). These waves frequently coincide with headache, decreasing level of consciousness (LOC), and a generalized neurological deterioration. If the patient is on a respirator, hyperventilation will maintain the Pa_{CO_2} between 25 and 35. This will cause a vasoconstriction which may help control ICP.

2. With increasing ICP, the LOC decreases and the reticular activating system (RAS) or "alerting system" fails. Medications such as mannitol, steroids, and diuretics may help decrease the ICP.

3. Motor responses such as hemiparesis or decorticate or decerebrate positioning occur as a result of cortical and midbrain compression of motor tracts. In some centers, barbiturate coma therapy may be tried. Some centers will only continue treatments in the aforementioned 1 and 2.

4. Changes in vital signs and the respiratory pattern are late changes indicating brain stem compression (the pons and medulla oblongata). Interventions will include those listed in aforementioned 1, 2, and 3. Prognosis is poor.

NURSING INTERVENTIONS

Most nursing procedures have an effect on the ICP. Turning the patient may increase the ICP. If the patient can cooperate, having him or her exhale while turning prevents a Valsalva maneuver (Valsalva maneuvers increase ICP). If two nursing actions both increase ICP, space the nursing care to allow the ICP to diminish after the first action before starting the second action.

Suctioning is imperative if the patient cannot clear his or her secretions. Suctioning increases ICP and decreases oxygen availability during the procedure. Limiting suctioning to a maximum of 10 seconds, hyperventilating the patient before and after the procedure, and preventing thick, tenacious secretions limit the increase in the ICP with this procedure.

Dehydration and electrolyte imbalances may occur rapidly in conditions precipitating increased ICP. Careful monitoring of the electrolytes and serum osmolality will allow early interventions to regulate ICP responses.

Infections are a major threat in intraventricular and subdural monitoring. *If* irrigation is performed by the physician, an antibiotic solution may be used. Fever increases cerebral metabolism and may compromise the ICP. Hypothermia blankets may be used to help control febrile states. The most important step in preventing infection is maintaining a "closed" system.

Glucocorticoids may be used to decrease cerebral edema. Maintaining an elevated head (15–30 degrees) is thought to help cerebral edema by promoting venous return from the cranium.

It has become obvious through ICP monitoring that the physical signs of decreasing level of consciousness (LOC), Cushing's triad,[2] and pupillary changes occur late in the course of an increasing ICP. Reliance on only these physical parameters may result in irreversible brain damage and/or death.

---

[2] Cushing's triad is hypertension, bradycardia, and bradypnea.

Intracranial Aneurysms

DEFINITION

An aneurysm is considered to be a congenital developmental defect in the muscle layer of arteries, normally occurring at points of bifurcation. (Recall that there are three layers in the arterial wall: the inner endothelial layer—the intima, a middle smooth muscle layer—the media, and an outer layer of connective tissue—the adventitia.)

PATHOPHYSIOLOGY

The congenital weakness of the arterial wall results in a gradual "ballooning out" of that segment of the artery over a period of years. When an increase in vascular pressure rises to a sufficient (unknown) pressure, the weakened ballooning segment of the artery bursts.

LOCATION, INCIDENCE, AND ETIOLOGY

Most cerebral aneurysms develop in the anterior arteries of the circle of Willis. Aneurysms are the fourth leading cause of cerebrovascular problems. Aneurysms are rare in children and teenagers and most common in the middle age group. Slightly more females than males have aneurysms. Some 10–20% of patients with aneurysms have more than one (may be found on same or opposite side).

Etiological factors may include hypertension (in a majority of cases). *Vigorous* physical activity immediately prior to an aneurysmal bleed is common. Congenital anomalies account for some aneurysms and others occur for unknown reasons.

CLINICAL PRESENTATION

Aneurysms are commonly asymptomatic until a bleed occurs. The exception is a very large aneurysm which may cause symptoms related to pressure against surrounding tissues. *Severe* headache (unlike any other headaches) occurs as the aneurysm starts to bleed. Unconsciousness may occur and be transient or sustained secondary to ischemia and/or necrosis of brain tissue. Nausea and vomiting are common. Transient neurological deficits include numbness, aphasias, and paresis.

Nuchal rigidity, photophobia, diplopia, Kernig's sign (inability to fully extend leg when thigh is flexed to the abdomen), Brudzinski's sign (involuntary adduction and flexion of legs when neck is flexed), and headache are common because of meningeal irritation. All these signs except diplopia are sometimes grouped together under the term meningismus.

DIAGNOSIS

A lumbar puncture is usually performed. Elevated CSF pressure, elevated protein levels, elevated red blood cells, and grossly bloody spinal fluid indicate hemorrhage in the subarachnoid space.

CAT scanning will reveal areas of intracerebral bleed. NOTE: In the adult, an intracerebral bleed is *NEVER* the cause of a hypovolemic shock state if the cranium is intact. The intact cranium does not have sufficient space to accommodate the quantity of blood required to cause a hypovolemic shock state.

Carotid *and* vertebral angiography may reveal the presence of other small aneurysms. Angiography may determine the patient's suitability for preventative measures such as hypotensive drugs or intracranial-extracranial bypass anastomosis, clipping/ligating, reinforcing artery and such.

Classification of Clinical State Post Aneurysmal Rupture

Aneurysms may be placed in one of five categories (grades). These grades are summarized in Table 21-2.

If patients can be stabilized in grade I or II, they may be candidates for surgical intervention.

PROGNOSIS

The prognosis depends upon the site and severity of the bleed. Persistent coma be-

Table 21-2. Grades of aneurysms.

Symptom	Grade I	Grade II	Grade III	Grade IV	Grade V
LOC	alert	decreased	confused	unresponsive	moribund
Headache	slight	mild to severe	—	—	—
Nuchal rigidity	slight	X	X	X	—
Vasospasm	—	—	—	may be present	may be present
Decerebrate Posturing	—	—	—	—	X

Note: X = present; dash = absent

yond 2 days is a poor sign. Rebleeds may occur as the original clot that formed around the bleed is absorbed (or lysed). This usually occurs between the seventh and eleventh days post original bleed and carries a poor prognosis. Increasing and/or persistent vasospasm results in increasing cerebral ischemia. Marked cerebral edema and/or the development of hydrocephalus indicate a poor prognosis.

NURSING INTERVENTIONS

Stabilization of the patient is the primary objective of treatment. Once the patient is stabilized and the condition approaches grade I or II, surgical intervention is usually successful.

1. Complete bed rest with a quiet, dark environment promotes stabilization.
2. Although controversial, the head of the bed may be elevated in an attempt to promote cerebral venous return by gravity. It is usually elevated 15–30 degrees.
3. Dehydrating the patient is avoided, but fluid intake is limited to decrease the possibility of rebleed from hypervolemia or increase intracranial pressure. If vasospasm occurs and is not controlled by other means, short periods of hypervolemia may be tried.
4. If alert, the patient should avoid Valsalva manuevers and any other action

that produces straining, that is, forced cough to clear secretions and such. These actions will increase intracranial pressure and may start a rebleed.

5. Sedating drugs may be used to decrease stress, anxiety, or restlessness of the patient and may have the additional side effect of lowering the blood pressure in a hypertensive patient. Antihypertensive drugs may be used to prevent increases in pressure rather than to bring hypertension down to normal levels.
6. Antifibrinolytic drugs, usually Epsilon-aminocaproic acid (Amicar®), may be given by mouth, if the patient is alert, or intravenously. This drug may delay lysis of the aneurysmal clot. If used intravenously, it is recommended that a continuous infusion be used to assure a continuous therapeutic blood level (130 mg/ml).
7. Antispasmodic drugs (e.g., reserpine) and/or anticonvulsants (e.g., phenytoin) may be used if conditions indicate the need.

SURGICAL INTERVENTION AND NURSING IMPLICATIONS

If an aneurysm is diagnosed prior to a bleed, surgery may be performed to prevent a bleed depending upon the size and location of the aneurysm. If an aneurysmal bleed has occurred and the patient has stabilized in grade I or II, surgery may be performed.

Surgery may consist of one of several procedures:

1. Clipping the aneurysm is probably the oldest and the most frequent surgical treatment (Figure 21-6). If the aneurysm is extremely large, clipping may not be possible.
2. Reinforcing the aneurysm by wrapping some of the new mesh materials around it and the artery may prevent further enlargement or rupture (Figure 21-6). Caution must be taken not to decrease the arterial lumen, especially if atherosclerotic disease is present.
3. Trapping the aneurysm by ligating proximal and distal to the aneurysm may be the procedure of choice if the aneurysm is large (Figure 21-6).
4. Embolization of the aneurysmal clot may be performed once the patient is stabilized, especially if the aneurysmal clot is impinging upon important structures (Figure 21-6).

If the aneurysm cannot be reached and/or surgical risk of one of the above procedures is extremely high, the common carotid artery may be clamped. Prior to this procedure, angiography must demonstrate that vascular perfusion of the involved hemisphere is adequate from the opposite side.

The major nursing responsibilities are assessment of the neurological status for signs of increasing intracranial pressure, observing for signs of impending seizures, and performing the routine postoperative and postcraniotomy care.

Coma and Brain Herniation

Two general types of pathological processes lead to coma. These are (a) conditions which widely and directly depress function of the cerebral hemispheres, and (b) conditions which depress or destroy brain stem activating mechanisms.

Three categories of disease are important in the aforementioned pathological processes leading to coma.

1. A supratentorial mass lesion will encroach on deep diencephalic structures compressing or destroying the ascending reticular activating system.
2. A subtentorial mass or destructive lesion may directly damage the brain stem central core.
3. Metabolic disorders may result in generalized interruption of brain function.

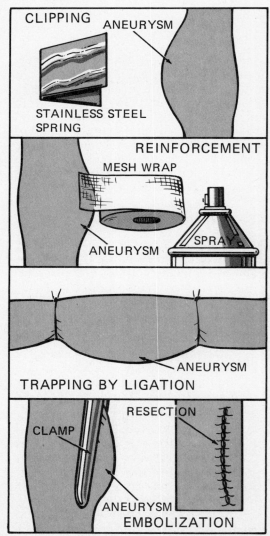

Figure 21-6. Surgical treatment of aneurysms.

Coma does not occur as a result of focal injury or ischemia in a specific lobe. Coma occurs *only* when both cerebral hemispheres or brain stem divisions are dysfunctional. The major catastrophe of coma is death due to brain herniation.

ROUTES OF HERNIATION

There are two main paths of herniation. Brain tissue can herniate through the tentorial notch and/or through the foramen magnum. Herniation through the tentorial notch will be central herniation or uncal herniation. The symptoms differ markedly with each.

Central herniation occurs when the cerebral hemisphere is compressed against the incisura (the opening in the tentorium cerebelli). This compresses the midbrain.

Uncal herniation occurs when the uncus (medial part of the temporal lobe) impacts upon the tentorial notch. This compresses the upper brain stem, especially the cerebral peduncles. This also traps the ipsilateral third cranial nerve.

ETIOLOGY

Herniation is the result of increased intracranial pressure beyond compensatory levels. Papilledema (edema of the optic disc) is a positive sign of increased intracranial pressure. However, in acute intracranial hypertension, papilledema may not occur immediately. In acute cases, elevated ICP may result in herniation *before* sufficient time has elapsed to allow for the development of papilledema.

PATHOPHYSIOLOGY OF CENTRAL HERNIATION

The tentorium cerebelli divides the supratentorial structures from the infratentorial structures. The tentorium cerebelli actually separates the cerebral hemispheres from the cerebellum. The tentorium cerebelli has an opening, the incisura or tentorial notch. The midbrain passes through this opening. Increasing ICP forces the cerebral hemispheres and the basal nuclei through the tentorial notch. This displacement compresses the diencephalon, midbrain, and pons. Divisions of the basilar artery are also displaced causing ischemia and brain stem deterioration.

The displacement also blocks the aqueduct of Sylvius effectively preventing the downward displacement of CSF (a compensatory mechasism of increasing ICP). This further increases ICP. Central herniation usually progresses in a head-to-tail direction. Thus, an alteration in the LOC is often a subtle first sign of impending herniation.

PATHOPHYSIOLOGY OF UNCAL HERNIATION

The uncus is the median portion of the temporal lobe that hangs on the edge of the incisura (that opening known as the tentorial notch). An expanding temporal lobe lesion and/or increasing middle fossa pressure may force the uncus over the edge of the incisura. The movement of the uncus compresses the mesencephalon (midbrain) against the opposite edge of the incisura. Uncal herniation often presses the oculomotor nerve and posterior cerebral artery against the incisura. The earliest consistent sign in uncal herniation is a unilaterally dilating pupil—*not* a change in the LOC.

STAGES OF HERNIATION

There are four distinct stages as central herniation progresses. They are early diencephalic stage, late diencephalic stage, midbrain—upper pons stage, and lower pons—upper medulla stage.

There are three stages in uncal herniation. The first stage is the uncal syndrome—early III nerve. The second stage is the uncal syndrome—late III nerve. The third stage is the same lower pons—upper medulla stage as in central herniation.

MONITORING PARAMETERS IN HERNIATION

Specific parameters can be monitored to indicate impending or active herniation.

In central herniation, the parameters are level of consciousness (LOC), pupillary function (size *and* reaction to light), respiratory pattern, oculocephalic responses (Doll's eyes) and oculovestibular responses (Ice Water Caloric Test), motor response, and ciliospinal reflex.

In uncal herniation, LOC is *not* a primary parameter. Pupillary response and third nerve palsy are early important signs. Then LOC (both content and degree of alertness) or delerium or lethargy suggest impending herniation. Respiratory, oculocephalic, and oculovestibular responses do not come into play until LOC has declined.

PARAMETER NORMS AND TESTING METHODS

1. *LOC*: LOC was discussed in Chapter 20 and will not be repeated here.
2. *Pupils*: Pupillary reaction is controlled by both sympathetic and parasympathetic tracts. These tracts are not easily affected by metabolic states. Therefore, the pupil light reflex is the single most important indicator in differentiating metabolic or structural (neurologic) coma.

   The pupil light reflex (Figure 21-7) is best tested in a darkened room (although not always possible). In a normal state, a pupil will constrict when a light beam is directed into it. Nor-

mally, there is also a consensual response; that is, the eye *NOT* having a light beam directed into it will constrict with the eye being tested.

3. *Ciliospinal reflex*: This is tested by pinching the skin on the back edge of the neck (Figure 21-8). Normally, this action causes ipsilateral pupil dilation.

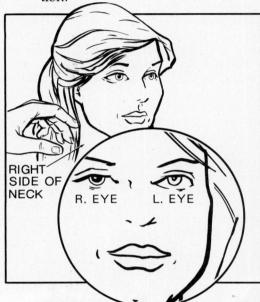

Figure 21-8. Pupil response in the ciliospinal reflex (depicted in inset).

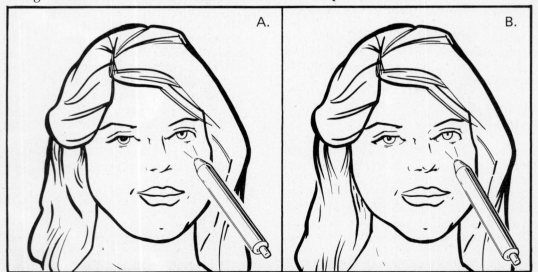

Figure 21-7. The pupillary light reflex (A) and the consensual light reflex (B).

4. *Eye movements*: The key eye movements observed in the comatose patient are the spontaneous motion of each eye, the resting position of each eye, and responses of the eyes to the oculocephalic and oculovestibular tests.

The resting position of the eyes may be conjugate, disconjugate, or skewed. Conjugate position is any resting position with both eyes in the same position. Disconjugate position is a resting position with the eyes in different positions. Right eye midline midposition and left eye midline, fixed to the right side is an example of disconjugate eyes. Skewed eyes are any *vertical* disconjugate positioning. Skewing indicates a brain stem lesion.

The oculocephalic response (Figure 21-9) if often called *Doll's eyes*. Doll's eyes can be tested only in the unconscious patient and is normally recorded as present or absent. To test the oculocephalic response, hold the patient's eyelids open and quickly—but gently—turn the head to one side.

The normal response is for the eyes to conjugately deviate in the contraversive direction of the head turning. Repeat by flexing and extending the head. Again, the normal response is conjugate (parallel) contraversive movement of the eyes in the direction of head movement. This is referred to as Doll's eyes present. Abnormal responses are referred to as Doll's eyes absent. If the eyes move in the same direction of head position (i.e., flex head, eyes go down, or turn head to right, and eyes go right or no further than midline), the test is abnormal. Doll's eyes are absent. Cranial nerves III, IV, and VI are not intact. Cranial nerves III, IV, and VI are responsible for ocular movements. Turning the head to both the right and the left will test each *pair* of these nerves. Doll's eyes must *NEVER* be tested unless cervical spinal cord or vertebral injuries have been ruled out.

The oculovestibular reflex is the Ice Water Caloric Test and is more powerful in eliciting eye movements. An in-

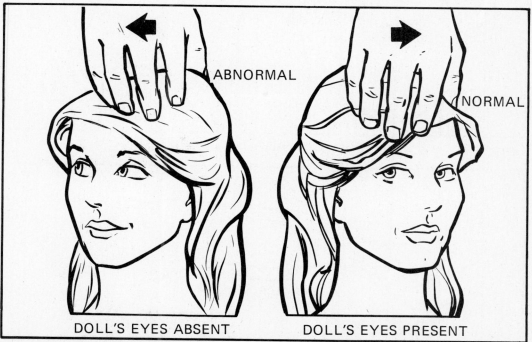

ABNORMAL

NORMAL

DOLL'S EYES ABSENT   DOLL'S EYES PRESENT

Figure 21-9. The oculocephalic response (Doll's eyes phenomenon).

tact tympanic membrane is essential. The head of the bed is elevated about 30 degrees. The physician slowly injects ice water until nystagmus or eye deviation occurs (or until 200 cc of ice water has been used). In the unconscious patient, the eyes move slowly towards the irrigated ear and remain there 2–3 minutes (Figure 21-10). This indicates a supratentorial lesion or a metabolic condition. An extremely abnormal movement (skewing, jerky rotation) usually indicates a cerebellar or brain stem lesion.

5. *Motor responses*: Motor responses are not dependent on LOC. They may and usually do correlate with LOC. These are important sources of infor-

mation concerning the geographical spread of neurological dysfunction.

A cerebral hemisphere frontal lobe dysfunction is characterized by paraplegia in flexion, tonic grasping, and exaggerated snout reflexes.

Decorticate posture (Figure 21-11) is characterized by flexion of the arm, wrist, and fingers. Adduction of arms, extension and internal rotation with plantar flexion of the lower extremities complete the motor responses. Decorticate posturing is synonymous with abnormal flexion response.

Decerebrate posture is characterized by opisthotonos (arching of the back so that the head and heels remain on the surface and the re-

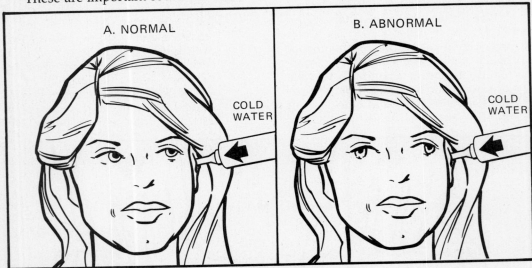

Figure 21-10. Pupil response in the oculovestibular reflex.

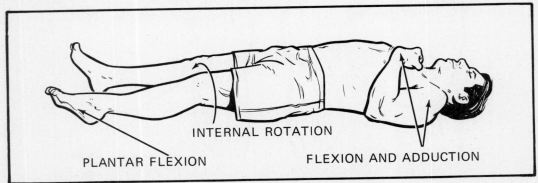

Figure 21-11. Decorticate posture (abnormal flexion response).

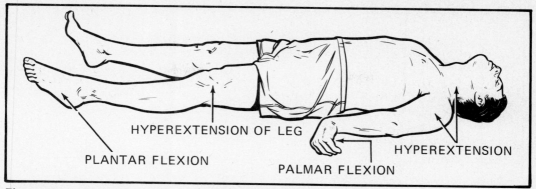

HYPEREXTENSION OF LEG

PLANTAR FLEXION

PALMAR FLEXION

HYPEREXTENSION

Figure 21-12. Decerebrate posture (abnormal extension response).

mainder of the back is raised), arms slightly extended, adducted and hyperpronated (Figure 21–12). The legs are stiffly extended and the feet are flexed in a plantar position. Abnormal extension response is synonymous with decerebrate posture.

6. *Respiratory patterns*: These patterns were discussed in the pulmonary section and will not be discussed again here.

Table 21-3 identifies the stages and parameter responses in central herniation. Table 21-4 identifies the stages and parameter responses in uncal herniation.

Herniation through the Foramen Magnum

If the ICP rises precipitously, the pressure may be of sufficient force to compress the cerebellum and medulla oblongata through the foramen magnum. A lumbar puncture performed in the presence of high ICP may result in brain stem herniation through the foramen magnum as the counterpressure in the spinal canal is lost. Herniation through the foramen magnum results in death secondary to cardiopulmonary arrest. This form of herniation is not clinically separable from central and uncal herniation.

Table 21-3. Stages and parameters of central herniation.

	Central— Early Diencephalic	Central— Late Diencephalic	Midbrain— Upper Pons	Lower Pons— Upper Medulla
Respirations				
Pupillary Response				
Consensual Light Response				
Ciliospinal Reflex				
Oculovestibular Response				
Doll's Eye Response				
Babinski Response				
Body Position Response	REST STIMULUS			

Table 21-4. Stages and parameters of uncal herniation.

	Uncal— Early III Nerve	Uncal Midbrain— Late III Nerve	Lower Pons— Upper Medulla
Respirations			
Pupillary Response			
Consensual Light Response			
Ciliospinal Reflex			
Oculovestibular Response			
Doll's Eye Response			
Babinski Response			
Body Position Response	REST / STIMULUS		

— 22

Seizures, Status Epilepticus, Cerebrovascular Accidents

Learning Objectives

By the end of this chapter, the nurse will be able to:

1. Define seizure.
2. List the characteristics of the following seizures:
   a. Tonic-clonic
   b. Absences
   c. Bilateral myoclonus
   d. Simple motor
   e. Complex psychomotor
   f. Focal motor seizure (Jacksonian)
3. Explain the difference between simple and complex seizures.
4. Explain the difference between partial motor and partial sensory seizures.
5. List four of five major areas of nursing interventions for patients having seizures.
6. Identify the most common drugs used to treat status epilepticus.
7. List three variant types of status epilepticus.
8. Explain the first three steps in the treatment of status epilepticus.
9. Define the following:
   a. CVA
   b. Astereognosis
   c. Autotopagnosia
   d. Anosognosia
   e. Constructional apraxia
   f. Dressing apraxia
   g. Expressive aphasia
   h. Receptive aphasia
10. List five nursing interventions for the patient experiencing a CVA.

Seizures

Seizures are a manifestation of excessive neuronal discharge in the brain. They may be associated with infection, trauma, tumor, cerebrovascular disease, genetic, congenital, or metabolic dysfunction. A convulsion is musculoskeletal contractions accompanying a seizure.

DEFINITION

A seizure is a symptom of paroxysmal electrical discharges in the brain resulting in autonomic, sensory, and/or motor dysfunction. If seizures are recurrent and transient, the condition is classified as epilepsy.

Classification of seizure disorders are summarized in Table 22-1.

TYPES OF SEIZURES

Grand mal seizures may also be termed convulsive or tonic-clonic seizures. These are characterized by a loss of consciousness. *Myoclonic seizures* are characterized by violent contraction of muscle groups, usually without a loss of consciousness. *Petit mal seizures* are common only in the 4–12-year-old range. They are called *absences* rather than seizures since loss of consciousness is for a period of seconds with no generalized motor activity. *Focal (partial) seizures* have a lesion in an identifiable area of the brain. Focal seizures are of two types: *simple seizures* (no loss of consciousness) and *complex seizures* (with loss of consciousness). *Focal motor seizures* are also called *Jacksonian seizures*. *Focal sensory seizures* may involve somatosensory, visual, auditory, olfactory, or vertiginous components. *Psychomotor seizures* are also termed *temporal lobe seizures* and *limbic seizures*. They are characterized by an exaggerated emotional component and a bizarre behavioral component.

PATHOPHYSIOLOGY OF SEIZURES

It is unknown if seizures occur due to an increased neuronal excitability or a decreased neuronal inhibitory force. Focal neurons appear to be unusually sensitive to acetylcholine and possibly a deficit in specific neurotransmitters. Altered cell permeability and/or alteration in electrolytes may have a role in seizure activity. It is logical to assume an electrical threshold for seizures exists in all persons. Factors thought to lower electrical threshold of neurons include fever, fatigue, altered electrolyte and water balance, stress, emotional distress, and/or pregnancy.

Regardless of these factors, hyperexcited neurons become hyperactive. As these localized neuronal discharges become intense, the hyperirritability spreads synaptically to adjacent neurons. In many instances the entire brain is involved. When only one hemisphere is involved, consciousness is preserved. When both cerebral hemispheres are involved, there is usually a loss of consciousness. An exception is a bilateral simple partial seizure.

Table 22-1. Classification of seizures.

A. Generalized Children and Infants	1) Tonic-Clonic	2) Absence	3) Bilateral Myoclonus
	4) Infantile Spasm	5) Atonic Seizures	6) Tonic Seizures
B. Partial Seizures	1) Simple: motor, sensory, affective		
	2) Complex: temporal lobe or psychomotor seizures		
C. Partial (Focal) Seizures with Secondary Generalization			

Also, in a complex partial seizure, consciousness may be altered but not lost since the seizure is in the limbic system (even though it is bilateral).

CLINICAL PRESENTATIONS

Tonic-Clonic (Grand Mal Seizures)

A peculiar sensation or feeling known as an aura (prodroma) may occur at the beginning of a seizure. An aura also accompanies complex partial seizures. For those who do experience an aura, it is almost always the same sensation or feeling. As consciousness is lost, the patient falls (if he or she is upright). The body becomes rigid. Air is forced from the lungs and may result in a high-pitched, loud cry. The jaws become locked and the tongue is often caught between clenched teeth. Pupils dilate and are nonreactive. Apnea results in cyanosis. Bladder incontinence is common. This is the tonic phase of the grand mal seizure and lasts 10–20 seconds.

The clonic phase of the grand mal seizure is a period of violent, rhythmic, symmetric, alternating contraction and relaxation involving the entire body. Increased salivation, mixed with blood if the tongue has been bitten, results in "frothing" at the mouth. The patient has a tachycardia, is profusely diaphoretic, and remains apneic. The tonic and clonic phases last 1–5 minutes.

In the postictal phase, the seizure subsides, the patient resumes breathing, cyanosis clears, and the pupils react. The patient should be bagged with a high volume of oxygen during this stage to help compensate for the period of apnea. The patient is fatigued, has a headache, is sleepy and confused, and may have amnesia of the entire seizure excepting the aura. A residual neurological deficit may continue for several hours (Todd's paralysis).

Absences (Petit Mal Seizures)

These are generalized seizures and consist of frequent episodes of loss of consciousness termed *absences*. The absences last from 2 to 10 seconds and are characterized by the cessation of motor activity, stopping speech in mid-sentence, and/or staring into space. During the seizure, the child (it is rarely seen after age 12) may twitch his or her lips or the lips may droop. The eyes may roll upward. There is no change in muscle tone. The patient may stagger or stumble, but rarely falls. Petit mal is benign neurologically. It may interfere with classroom learning.

Bilateral Myoclonus (Myoclonic Seizures)

These seizures are characterized by sudden, violent contractions of muscle groups. They may be generalized or focal, symmetrical (both sides) or asymmetrical (one side). Loss of consciousness is unusual in certain types of myoclonic seizure activity. The seizures may be a single jerking movement, intermittent periods of active seizure, or present in varying degree all of the waking time. The seizures are absent during sleep, being precipitated by stimulation and intensified with intentional movement.

Atonic Seizures (Akinetic Seizures)

These may occur by themselves or in cases of petit mal epilepsy. There is a sudden, brief loss of muscle tone with or without a loss of consciousness. The child falls often and may be labeled clumsy or awkward. Akinetic seizures may cloud the picture of petit mal epilepsy. These seizures often result from serious neurological disease which cannot be treated.

Simple Partial (Focal) Motor Seizures

These seizures are also known as Jacksonian seizures. The focal point is in the motor strip area—the prerolandic gyrus. The typical seizure starts with a twitching of the fingers or toes or around the lips on one side of the body. The muscle movement becomes more severe and spreads (marches) by involving more muscle groups until one side of the body is totally involved. Consciousness is maintained unless the Jacksonian seizure becomes generalized and spreads to the remainder of the body.

Simple Partial (Focal) Sensory Seizures

These seizures may be described by the patient as a numbness, tingling, or "pins and needles" sensation. If the causative lesion is in the postrolandic gyrus (the sensory strip between the frontal and parietal lobes), the seizure may progress like the Jacksonian seizure. Visual sensations usually indicate an occipital lobe lesion. Auditory sensations are most commonly a buzzing or ringing of the ears. Auditory sensations are often accompanied by olfactory symptoms and dizziness. This indicates a temporal lobe lesion.

Complex Partial Psychomotor Seizures

An aura often precedes a seizure. The aura includes complex visceral and/or perceptual hallucinations. The patient appears to be in an awake but nonresponsive state. Simple or elaborate behavior patterns may be carried out during the seizure. The behavior patterns are automatisms, that is, the patient performs the behavioral pattern like a robot. The average seizure lasts about 5 minutes. Attempts to interrupt the behavior pattern often precipitate violence. The seizure may end abruptly with the patient having complete amnesia or the patient may have a period of headache, confusion, or sleepiness.

ETIOLOGY OF EPILEPSY

Multiple etiologies of epilepsy are known. The most common is the abrupt cessation of antileptic drugs or other chronic sedative medications. Other causes include trauma, tumor, injuries (both perinatal and postnatal), CNS infections, and cerebral vascular disease including A-V malformations. Metabolic and toxic disorders may cause seizures. The role of genetics and heredity is controversial at this time. In a large number of cases, the cause is unknown. These cases are termed *idiopathic epilepsy*.

DIAGNOSIS OF EPILEPSY

The patient's history of seizure activity (duration, frequency, intensity, and progression) is one of the most useful tools in establishing a diagnosis. Physical examination, laboratory studies, radiologic studies, and electroencephalograms may reveal factors supporting a diagnosis of epilepsy or the studies may all be within normal limits.

NURSING INTERVENTIONS AND COMPLICATIONS

There are five major areas of nursing interventions for the patient having seizures.

1. Protect the patient from injury. Remove objects from the immediate environment that might cause injury. Stay with the patient during the seizure. Bedrails should be padded. The patient should not be restrained but efforts to keep the patient's head from injury are appropriate (e.g., if a seizure occurs with the patient out of bed, a pillow may be placed under the head or a nurse may cradle, NOT restrain, the patient's head to protect it). NOTHING should ever be used to pry open the mouth or be forced into the mouth during a seizure. Damage to the mouth and tongue occurs at the start of a seizure and only more damage will occur by forcing objects into the mouth.

2. Observing (and recording) seizure patterns may help identify the seizure focus. Data include precipitating factors, presence and type of aura, duration of unconsciousness, the pattern and progression of seizure activity, body parts involved (generalized or one-sided), incontinence, and postictal activity.

3. Assessment of the respiratory system is extremely important. The danger of a grand mal seizure is that the patient is apneic during the seizure. The respiratory status may be further compromised by aspiration. Oxygen should be at the bedside.

4. Administration of medication on a regularly timed basis and the evaluation

of the effects of the medication on controlling seizures as well as the psychological effects on the patient are important actions and assessments. Teaching the patient the beneficial effects of following the prescribed medication regimen and identifying patient objections will allow teaching that may result in better patient compliance in the future.

5. Promoting physical and mental health may sharply curtail the number of seizures. Regular routines for eating, sleeping, and physical activity should be established. Activity tends to decrease seizure activity. Alcohol, *stress*, and fatigue tend to precipitate seizure activity. Modifying these factors will alter the seizure pattern.

TREATMENT OF EPILEPSY

If seizures are the result of tumor, infection, or metabolic dysfunction, correcting the underlying cause is the goal of therapy. In a majority of cases, an underlying cause may not be identifiable or amenable to curative therapy. These cases are treated with anticonvulsive drugs. It is common to use combinations of drugs to achieve control of seizure activity. The most common drugs include phenytoin sodium (Dilantin®), phenobarbital, primidone (Mysoline®), ethosuximide (Zarontin®), clonazepam (Clonopin®), and carbamazepine (Tegretol®). A recently introduced drug is valproic acid (Depakene®). For the therapeutic serum level of these drugs, their affinity for specific types of seizures, and their side effects, the reader is referred to any standard pharmacology text.

If drug therapy is ineffective *and* if seizures are intractable *and* if the seizures prohibit a normal semblance of life, surgery may be performed. After identifying the specific epileptic focus and the patient's dominant hemisphere, a cerebral lobectomy or hemispherectomy may be done. Seizures may continue for a period after the surgery.

Status Epilepticus

DEFINITION

The state of status epilepticus is present when seizures follow each other so closely that a state of consciousness in not recovered in between seizures. Usually status epilepticus refers to grand mal seizures, but any form of seizures may evolve into status.

ETIOLOGY OF STATUS EPILEPTICUS

Inadequate dosage of antileptic medication in a known epileptic is a common precipitating factor. Other factors include sudden withdrawal of antileptic drugs and other sedative drugs, intercurrent infection (commonly in the CNS), cerebral vascular disease, and cerebral hypoxia, anoxia, and edema. Progressive neurological diseases such as brain tumor and subdural hematoma may cause the status epilepticus. A common triad of causes consists of alcohol abuse, drug abuse, and sleep deprivation. Head trauma or pregnancy (preeclamptic state) may precipitate a status epilepticus state. Metabolic disorders as a cause include hypoglycemia, uremia, and electrolyte imbalances.

INCIDENCE AND PROGNOSIS

Approximatley 6% of the known epileptics will develop status epilepticus. Almost 50% of the cases of status epilepticus occur in known epileptics. From 10 to 30% of the cases of status epilepticus will die. Death is commonly due to respiratory and metabolic acidosis, hypoxemia, hypoglycemia, hyperthermia, electrolyte disturbances, and/or renal failure.

PATHOPHYSIOLOGY OF STATUS EPILEPTICUS

This is the same as the pathophysiology of epilepsy; however, in status the seizures are almost continuous. The rapidly repeating grand mal seizures lead to hypoxemia (patients are apneic during grand mal seizures) and cerebral anoxia. The increased metabolic activity of the brain causes a hypoglycemia and hyperthermic state. Hypoxemia, hypoglycemia, and hyperthermia may themselves precipitate seizure activity resulting in a vicious cycle.

CLINICAL PRESENTATION OF STATUS EPILEPTICUS

There are three variants in the clinical picture of status epilepticus.

1. Grand mal status is a life-threatening emergency. Seizures are the tonic-clonic type without a period of consciousness in between seizures.
2. Petit mal status may exhibit as many as 200–300 "absences" per day.
3. Partial or focal status is termed *epilepsia continua*. Focal seizures occur continuously *or* regularly. Consciousness is usually maintained unless generalization occurs.

Electrical status occurs in every type of status and is not a distinct type. It is always associated with some clinical abnormality. An electroencephalogram shows continuous epileptic activity. There is also a complex partial status.

TREATMENT OF STATUS EPILEPTICUS

The goal of therapy is to restore physiologic homeostasis and to stop the seizures. The first step in treatment is to ensure a patent airway. The second step in the treatment of status is to draw blood (for glucose, electrolytes, BUN, ABGs, and CPK) and establish an intravenous line. (This is often achieved as a one-step process with jelcos or angiocaths.) If there is the slightest possibility of hypoglycemia, 50% glucose is given intravenously. The third step in treatment of status is administering medications to stop seizure activity.

Diazepam (Valium®) intravenously is often the drug of choice in spite of its poten-

tial for suppressing respirations. It very quickly enters the brain and quickly leaves the brain. But these very properties often make diazepam a poor drug for status. After intravenous injection, diazepam will be completely out of brain tissue in 30 minutes.

Phenytoin is given intravenously. It must be injected *slowly* (50 mg/minute) and cardiac monitoring is essential for early intervention in dysrhythmias. Bradycardia and hypotension are especially common in patients over 40. Phenytoin requires 15–20 minutes to peak in brain tissue *and* it remains in brain tissue over a long period.

If seizures persist after 30 minutes, there is a high probability that acute CNS disease caused the seizures. Phenobarbital may be tried. A slow intravenous injection is recommended. Respiratory depression and hypotension may develop. Phenobarbital and diazepam should not be administered concurrently. If diazepam is used to stop seizures, phenytoin is given simultaneously to block recurrence of the seizures.

Lidocaine as a 20% solution in normal saline may be tried. Some medical centers will use general anesthesia (barbiturate coma) to a depth of electroencephalogram silence when other drugs have failed. Pancuronium bromide (Pavulon®) may be used instead of general anesthesia if the patient is on a respirator.

Paraldehyde may be used intramuscularly or rectally. Intravenous administration is hazardous. It must be diluted and given very slowly.

NURSING INTERVENTIONS

Maintaining a patent airway is extremely important. An intravenous line should be maintained. Cardiac drugs should be available as cardiac monitoring may reveal dysrhythmias. Hyperthermia is treated frequently with a hypothermia blanket. Fluid and electrolyte balance is monitored. Neurologic status is monitored continuously.

Cerebrovascular Accident (CVA)

DEFINITION

A cerebrovascular accident (CVA) is a sudden focal neurologic deficit due to cerebrovascular disease. A CVA is the most common cause of cerebral dysfunction in this country.

ETIOLOGY

The end result of any interruption of oxygen to brain tissue for more than a few minutes is the death of those neurons not being oxygenated. The decrease in oxygen may be partial or complete. It is caused by thrombi, emboli, tumor, hemorrhage, hypertension, and compression or spasm of cerebral ateries.

CLINICAL PRESENTATION

The common symptom in CVAs regardless of the etiology is the sudden onset of symptoms. Specific symptomology depends upon location of the injury and the hemispheric dominance of the patient. Homonymous hemianopsia, hemiparesis, and/or hemiplegia are common symptoms.

If the right cerebral hemisphere is involved, there are spatial-perceptual deficits resulting in apraxia. Apraxia may be constructional or dressing. Constructional apraxia is the inability to complete the left half of figures one is drawing or arranging words in an incorrect manner, superimposing words and such. Usually a constructional apraxia will include an inability to complete the drawing of a picture (e.g., clock). Dressing apraxia is the inability to dress oneself properly. Both constructional apraxia and dressing apraxia are common in right cerebral CVAs. Neglect of the paralyzed side, impulsive quick behavior, and poor judgment of abilities and limitations occur with right cerebral CVAs.

Left cerebral hemispheric CVAs have astereognosis and autotopagnosia. Astereognosis is an inability to identify a common object placed in the hand with one's eyes closed. Autotopagnosia is an inability to

determine the *position* of parts of the body in relation to the rest of the body.

In addition, these CVAs tend to cause a finger agnosia (unable to identify a finger being touched) and a right-left disorientation. Behavior is slow, cautious, and disorganized. Aphasia, both expressive and receptive, is common. Expressive aphasia is the inability to express oneself verbally and understandably. Receptive aphasia is the loss of the ability to understand spoken or written word.

Regardless of which hemisphere is involved in a CVA, the patients tend to have a reduced memory span, are emotionally labile, and have spasticity of the affected extremities. Some patients will have an anosognosia, which is the denial of a neurological deficit such as hemiplegia. Anosognosia is different than a psychological denial stage. Deviation of the head and eyes is towards the cerebral hemisphere involved in the CVA of pontine lesions. Frontal lobe lesions produce the opposite signs.

DIAGNOSIS OF CVA

This diagnosis is usually made on the basis of history and clinical symptoms. The history frequently reveals transient ischemic attacks (TIA), reversible ischemic neurological deficits (RIND), and possibly "small" strokes in the past. CAT scan will reveal decreased density in ischemic and infarcted areas. It will reveal increased density in hemorrhage areas. Angiography may show spasms, arteriovenous malformations, and aneurysms.

TREATMENT

In most centers, treatment is supportive. Aminocaproic acid (Amicar®) is thought to help prevent extension of damage in CVAs by preventing extension of a CVA due to bleeding. It helps prevent early lysis of a clot that has formed around a bleeding site. Research is continuing and looks promising for extracranial and intracranial bypass anastomoses in reversible ischemic neurological deficits (RIND). Carotid endarterectomy and bypass patients are seen in critical care areas more than the uncomplicated CVA patient.

NURSING INTERVENTIONS

To some extent nursing interventions (and patient complications) depend upon the site of a CVA, the patient's age, general health, and the extent of neurologic deficit.

Communication with the patient is acheived in any way possible—through writing, pictures, gestures, and so on. Different aphasias make this task difficult.

Monitoring and assessing neurologic status will identify extensions of deficit which may be treatable.

Supportive "comfort" measures are important and include training, positioning, skin care, fluid and nutritional intake, emotional support, and early implementation of rehabilitation.

— 23

Myasthenia Gravis, Meningitis, and Guillain-Barré

Learning Objectives

By the end of this chapter, the nurse will be able to:

1. Define the term myasthenia gravis.
2. Explain the pathophysiology of myasthenia gravis.
3. List three common presenting symptoms.
4. Explain the use of edrophonium chloride.
5. Differentiate between myasthenic crisis and cholinergic crisis.
6. Identify two classes of drugs that must be avoided in myasthenia gravis patients.
7. List three etiologies of meningitis.
8. Explain Kernig's and Brudzinski's signs.
9. List four common presenting symptoms of meningitis.
10. Identify five complications of meningitis.
11. Identify three nursing interventions in meningitis.
12. Define the term Guillain-Barré syndrome.
13. Explain the pathophysiology of Guillain-Barré syndrome.
14. State the objectives of treatment of Guillain-Barré syndrome.
15. Identify six or more nursing interventions in treating patients with Guillain-Barré syndrome.

Myasthenia Gravis and Crisis

DEFINITION

Myasthenia gravis is considered to be an autoimmune disease produced by a defect in neuromuscular transmission resulting in weakness with exercise and improving strength with rest.

PATHOPHYSIOLOGY

Three theories have been proposed as the pathophysiology of myasthenia gravis. Acetylcholine is released at nerve terminals and combines at the postsynaptic muscle membrane producing an electrochemical reaction. The electrochemical reaction results in muscle contraction. In myasthenia gravis, there are either too few postsynaptic receptor sites for the amount of acetylcholine released to bind with to provide for a full muscular contraction, or not enough acetylcholine is released to cause full muscle contraction, or acetylcholinesterase degrades the acetylcholine before sufficient amounts can cause a full muscle contraction.

ETIOLOGY

The most prevalent hypothesis is that myasthenia gravis is an autoimmune process damaging the postsynaptic membrane. A statistically significant number of cases are associated with thymoma and thymic hyperplasia. This is substantiated by finding serum antibodies produced by sensitized lymphocytes or thymocytes that block the action of acetylcholine and the production of immune bodies by the thymus that are capable of reproducing the disease in experimental animal models.

OCCURRENCE

Myasthenia gravis occurs in from one in ten thousand to one in fifty thousand people. It may occur at any age, but it rarely occurs in those under age 10 or over 70. Peak occurrence is in the 20–30 age range. Under the age of 40, the ratio of occurrence in women to men is 3:1; after 40, it is 1:1.

CLINICAL SIGNS, SYMPTOMS, AND COURSE

Pathognomonic signs of myasthenia gravis include uneven drooping of the eyelids, a smile that resembles a snarl, a drooping lower jaw that must be supported by the hand, and a partially immobile mouth with the corners turned downward. However, few patients are first seen with these signs. In more than 90% of the cases, eyebrow and extraocular muscles are involved, accompanied by weakness in eye closure. Ptosis and diplopia are common. The next most commonly affected muscles exhibiting symptoms are those of facial expression, mastication, swallowing, and speaking (dysarthria). Hoarseness occurs after only a few minutes of talking. Neck flexor and extensor muscles, the shoulder girdle, and hip flexors are less frequently involved. There usually is no sensory disturbance.

The course of myasthenia gravis is variable. Remission may occur for no discernible reason in less than half the cases and usually does not last longer than 1–2 months. The disease then becomes progressive. Frequently, the disease is slow but progressive from the onset. The greatest danger of death is during the first year, and again during years 4 through 7 in progressive cases. Stabilization of the disease occurs after this time and severe recurrence is rare. Infection of any kind, but especially respiratory, trauma of any kind, and emotional stress make the disease worse.

ASSOCIATED CONDITIONS

Approximately 15% of cases have a tumor of the thymus. There is an increasing incidence of tumors in older males. Thyroiditis, thyrotoxicosis, lupus erythematosus, and rheumatoid arthritis occur more often than statistically expected. A pregnancy may make the disease worse, better, or may have no effect. Close to 15% of babies born to myasthenic mothers exhibit symptoms of the disease. The symptoms are usually transient and resolve within 1–12 weeks.

DIAGNOSIS

A history of an increasing muscular fatigability which improves with rest is a common characteristic of myasthenia gravis. Various laboratory tests can be used to aid in a diagnosis. However, anticholinesterase tests are considered conclusive.

Edrophonium chloride (Tensilon®) is injected intravenously after the patient's muscle strength has been assessed. Ten milligrams of Tensilon, given in 2–5 mg doses, is the limit used to test for myasthenia gravis. The duration of action for Tensilon is about 5 minutes.

Tensilon is an anticholinesterase agent. When injected, it increases the level of acetylcholine at the myoneural junction by blocking cholinesterase (which breaks down acetylcholine). A clinical increase in muscle strength is positive for myasthenia gravis. No improvement or a deterioration in muscle strength is negative for myasthenia gravis.

If Tensilon is not conclusive, neostigmine bromide 0.5 mg intravenously or 1.5 mg intramuscularly may be used. Atropine sulfate (0.6 mg) should be given *prior* to intravenous neostigmine and *may* be needed with intramuscular injection of neostigmine to counter nausea, vomiting, increased salivation, and sweating. Intravenous neostigmine may cause ventricular fibrillation or cardiac arrest. After intramuscular injection, maximum effect will be apparent within 30 minutes, but effects may last 2–3 hours.

Curare is seldom used because of its paralytic action, but it is a definitive test, if properly done.

TREATMENT

The major objective of therapy is to improve neuromuscular transmission and to prevent complications. Early thymectomy is becoming popular.

Neuromuscular transmission is improved by administration of anticholinesterase drugs. Pyridostigmine bromide (Mestinon®) is a popular choice. If Mestinon is not adequate to establish control of neuromuscular transmission, neostigmine (Prostigmin®) is used. Prednisone has become an adjunctive drug of choice. It is extremely important to medicate the patient on schedule and to document carefully the patient's muscular response. The major difference in Mestinon and neostigmine is their duration of action. Mestinon has a 4-hour effect; neostigmine, 2 hours. Steroids may decrease the amount of anticholinesterase drug required to control myasthenic symptoms. The use of steroids results in suppression of immune responses and the resultant problem of infection and biochemical stress.

Thymectomy produces an improvement in or remission of symptoms in many patients. An improvement may be gradual over several years (up to 10). Frequently, steroid and anticholinesterase drugs are needed in smaller dosages post thymectomy. New treatments include thoracic duct drainage and plasmapheresis.

APHERESIS

This is the general process of separating blood components in order to remove specific portions of the blood. Lymphoresis removes lymphocytes and so forth. Plasmaphoresis removes specific components in the plasma. In myasthenic patients, the plan is to remove auto-antibodies which are believed to cause the disease. Apheresis is a new treatment modality and its effectiveness is still uncertain and all components removed in the plasma (for instance, drugs) are unknown.

NURSING INTERVENTIONS

A major nursing intervention is to maintain adequate ventilation in spite of a weak cough, an inability to clear secretions, and an increased likelihood of aspiration. Vital capacity is checked every 2–4 hours. Ventilators often are set up and kept available.

Prevention of aspiration, infection from any source, and emotional support of the patient are very important. If the patient is on a respirator, a communication system MUST be established. If the patient has had a thymectomy, the monitoring and nursing treatment as of any patient with a thoracotomy must be followed.

Specific drugs that impair neuromuscular transmission must be avoided. The aminoglycoside antibiotics and true mycin drugs are contraindicated. Such drugs include Aureomycin®, Kanamycin®, Polymyxin®, Neomycin®, Streptomycin®, and Gentamicin®.

Ether, quinidine, procainamide, morphine sulfate, and sedatives will aggravate muscle weakness.

Nursing education of the importance of taking prescribed medications *on schedule* is extremely important since an early or late dose may immediately affect muscle strength. Regulation of daily living habits to avoid fatigue and provide rest must be planned according to the patient's life-style as much as possible. The patient should know that minor infection or illness may precipitate an acute attack.

POST-THYMECTOMY NURSING INTERVENTIONS

Routine post-surgical care is needed plus:

1. Post-thoracic surgery procedures (e.g., chest tubes)
2. Ventilatory support with frequent suctioning
3. Anticholinesterase and steroid drugs started slowly
4. Reassurance that positive effects of a thymectomy occur over long periods (even years)
5. Protection from infections (i.e., sterile technique for suctioning, intermittent urinary catheterization rather than an indwelling catheter, etc.)

COMPLICATIONS: MYASTHENIC OR CHOLINERGIC CRISIS?

Myasthenic and cholinergic crises both have extreme weakness as the predominant symptom. Myasthenic crisis is caused by insufficient drug dose. Cholinergic crisis is due to an overdose of drugs and the patient has increased salivation and sweating. An impending cholinergic crisis can be detected by constricting pupils. Two millimeters is the maximum constriction that should be allowed before intervention. To distinguish between these crises, a Tensilon® test is used with a ventilator on standby. If the patient becomes weaker, a cholinergic (overdose) crisis exists. Treatment is to discontinue anticholinesterase drugs. After 72 hours, drug therapy is usually restarted in small increments. Atropine (an anticholinergic drug) may control symptoms but may also block important symptoms of anticholinesterase overdose. Monitoring ventilatory function with arterial blood gases is imperative.

Myasthenic crisis is established by muscular improvement with the Tensilon® test. Anticholinesterase drugs are given and repeated as needed. Steroids are usually avoided during a crisis. Monitoring, assessing, and documenting muscular strength and arterial blood gases are continued throughout the crisis. Identification of the precipitating etiology is important to treat and/or correct the cause. Communication with the patient throughout treatment, by whatever means possible, facilitates rest and trust in the nurse.

Meningitis

DEFINITION

Meningitis is an acute infection of the pia and arachnoid membrane surrounding the brain *and* the spinal cord. Therefore, meningitis is always a cerebrospinal infection.

PATHOPHYSIOLOGY

A pathogenic organism gains access to the pia-arachnoid space and causes an inflammatory reaction in the pia and arachnoid, in the cerebrospinal fluid, and in the ventricles of the brain since these are all communicating structures. The first response is a hyperemia of the meningeal vessels followed by the infiltration of neutrophils into the subarachnoid space. An exudate forms and very quickly enlarges covering the base of the brain and extending through the subarachnoid space and into the sheaths of cranial and spinal nerves. Polymorphonuclear leukocytes attempt to control the invading pathogen. Within a few days, leukocytes and histiocytes increase in number in an attempt to "wall off" the exudate from the pathogen or its toxins. Towards the end of the second week, the cellular exudate has formed two layers. The outer layer is composed of polymorphonuclear leukocytes and fibrin directly under the arachnoid membrane. The inner layer is composed of lymphocytes, plasma cells, and macrophages and is next to the pia.

With appropriate drug therapy destroying the pathogen, these two layers begin to resolve. The outer cellular layer against the arachnoid disappears. If the infection was arrested quickly enough, the inner layer will also disappear. However, if the infection lasts for several weeks, the inner layer which contains fibrin forms a permanent fibrous structure over the meninges. This produces a thickened, often cloudy, arachnoid membrane and causes adhesions between the pia and arachnoid membranes.

The adhesions and prior inflammation results in congestion of tissues and blood vessels. A degeneration of nerve cells follows, eventually resulting in congestion of adjacent brain tissue. This congestion causes cortical irritation and increased intracranial pressure. Cerebral edema may lead to hydrocephalus. If uninterrupted, a progression of vasculitis with cortical necrosis, petechial hemorrhage within the brain, hydrocephalus, and cranial nerve damage occurs.

ETIOLOGY

Organisms obtain access to the subarachnoid space through penetrating head injuries, basal skull fractures with a torn dura mater, ICP monitoring, cranial surgery, mastoiditis, acute otitis media, lumbar punctures, injury to the paranasal sinuses, and sepsis. The organism may be viral or bacterial. The most common bacteria is meningococcus. In children, it is *Hemophilus influenzae*. Other bacteria include *Streptococcus*, *Staphylococcus*, *Pneumococcus*, and occasionally the tuberculous organism.

CLINICAL SIGNS AND SYMPTOMS

Suspect meningitis if a fever, severe headache, and nuchal rigidity (resistance to flexion of the neck) exist. Positive Kernig and Brudzinski signs, photophobia, decreased sensorium, and signs of increased intracranial pressure are common. Kernig's sign is the inability to fully extend the leg when the thigh is flexed to the abdomen. Brudzinski's sign is the involuntary adduction and flexion of the legs with attempts to flex the neck. With meningitis, a headache becomes progressively worse and is accompanied by nausea, vomiting, irritability, confusion, and seizures. If the causative organism is meningococcus, a skin rash is common.

DIAGNOSIS

A major diagnostic tool is examination of the cerebrospinal fluid (CSF). Variations of the CSF depend upon the causative organism. CSF protein levels are usually elevated and higher in bacterial than in viral cases. A decreased CSF sugar is common to bacterial meningitis and may be normal in viral meningitis. Appearance of the CSF is purulent and turbid in bacterial meningitis. It may be the same or clear in viral meningitis. The most predominant cell in the CSF is the polymorphonuclear leukocyte.

Cultures of blood, sputum, and nasopharyngeal secretions are performed to identify the causative organism.

X-rays of the skull may demonstrate infected sinuses. CAT scans are usually normal in uncomplicated meningitis. In other cases, CAT scan may reveal evidence of increased intracranial pressure.

COMPLICATIONS

The most common complication of meningitis is residual neurologic dysfunction. Cranial nerve dysfunction often occurs with cranial nerves III, IV, VI, or VII in bacterial meningitis. Usually the dysfunction disappears within a few weeks. Hearing loss may be permanent after bacterial meningitis but is not a complication of viral meningitis.

Cranial nerve irritation can have serious sequelae. Cranial nerve II is compressed by increased intracranial pressure. Papilledema is often present and blindness may occur. When cranial nerves III, IV, and VI are irritated, ocular movements are affected. Ptosis, unequal pupils, and diplopia are common. Irritation of cranial nerve V is evidenced by sensory and corneal changes and cranial nerve VII results in facial paresis. Irritation of cranial nerve VIII causes tinnitus, vertigo, and deafness.

Hemiparesis, dysphasia, and hemianopsia may occur. These signs usually resolve within several hours. If resolution does not occur, it suggests a cerebral abcess, subdural empyema, subdural effusion, or cortical venous thrombophlebitis.

Acute cerebral edema may occur with bacterial meningitis causing seizures, third nerve palsy, bradycardia, hypertension, coma, and death.

A non-communicating hydrocephalus may occur if the inner layer of the exudate has caused adhesions which prevent the normal flow of the cerebospinal fluid from the ventricles. Surgical implantation of a shunt is the only treatment.

NURSING INTERVENTIONS

Administration of antibiotics at scheduled times maintains a therapeutic blood level. Isolation precautions will protect the staff and visitors but need not be continued past 48 hours after the institution of antibiotic therapy.

Body temperature can be controlled by use of antipyretic drugs as indicated and a hypothermia blanket.

Headache is usually treated with analgesics, and a darkened, quiet room will help both the headache and photophobia.

If seizures occur, anticonvulsant medication is indicated. Documentation, progression, limb involvement, and duration of the seizures will help determine an effective medication regimen.

Dyspnea and respiratory distress require standard treatment.

A central venous pressure line or a pulmonary artery catheter may be inserted to monitor fluid balance and the cardiovascular status. Standard nursing procedures for these types of complications are followed.

Guillain-Barré Syndrome

Synonyms for Guillain-Barré syndrome include Landry-Guillain-Barré disease, acute inflammatory polyradiculoneuropathy, and infectious polyneuritis.

DEFINITION

Guillain-Barré syndrome is an acute inflammatory disease, thought to be autoimmune or viral, that affects peripheral nerves, spinal nerves, and sometimes cranial nerves, first with edema and then demyelination.

PATHOPHYSIOLOGY

In the normal course of the disease, the patient usually has an upper respiratory or gastrointestinal infection 1–2 weeks prior to the development of the Guillain-Barré syndrome. The predominant pattern is weakness starting in the lower extremities and advancing (often very rapidly) to motor paralysis and progressing up the body. The progression may stop at any point. The first pathological sign of the syndrome is a perivascular lymphocytic infiltration. Following this, characteristic infiltration occurs in the myelin, breaking it down but not damaging the axon. This is called segmental demyelination. If the syndrome progresses, the infiltration becomes more intense and affects the axon, resulting in muscle denervation and atrophy. If the infiltration occurs in the distal segment of the axon, regeneration will occur because the nerve cell body has been spared. If the infiltration occurs at the proximal end of the axon, the nerve cell body may die and regeneration cannot occur. This is known as Wallerian degeneration. Collateral motor fibers may re-innervate the destroyed muscle, restoring the lost function partially or completely. As the infiltration process ends, recovery of motor function begins proximally and progresses distally.

DIAGNOSIS

Examination of the CSF is done to determine if the CSF protein is elevated (up to 700 mg %) with only a few cells present. This represents albuminocytologic dissociation (high protein/few cells) which is specific for Guillain-Barré syndrome.

ETIOLOGY

Specific etiologic agents are unknown. The most currently popular theory is that a slow acting measles virus is the causative agent. Guillain-Barré occurs at any age with a peak incidence between 30 and 40 years old. Both sexes are equally affected.

CLINICAL PRESENTATION

Symptoms usually develop 1–3 weeks after an upper respiratory infection and occasionally after a gastrointestinal infection. Infrequently, polyneuritis may occur after surgery or after lymphomatous disease immunizations such as rabies and Swine flu.

Weakness of the lower extremities evolving more or less symmetrically occurs over a period of hours to days to weeks, usually peaking by the fourteenth day. Distal muscles are the more severely affected. Paresthesia (numbness and tingling) is frequent but pain is rare. Paralysis usually follows paresthesia in the extremities. Hypotonia and areflexia are common, persistent symptoms. Objective sensory loss is variable with deep sensibility more affected than superficial sensations.

Autonomic nervous function is rarely altered. Sinus tachycardia, hypertension, and anhydrosis (absence of sweating) are uncommon findings. Urinary retention occurs occasionally, but catheterization is seldom needed for more than a few days.

If cranial nerve involvement occurs, it is most frequent in cranial nerve VII, and then in cranial nerves VI, III, XII, V, and X (most to least frequent). Consequently, dysphasia is common if the paresthesia and paralysis extend to the cranial nerves.

VARIATIONS IN CLINICAL PRESENTATION

Landry's ascending paralysis moves from legs to trunk to arms to head. It usually peaks in 10–14 days.

Fisher's variant is complete ophthalmoplegia (paralysis of the eye muscles), ataxia, and areflexia.

Cases with a steady or stepwise progression over weeks or months may be asymmetrical. Some body parts will be recovering while others are getting worse. There may be relapses, but these are uncommon.

COMPLICATIONS

The most serious complication is respiratory failure as the paralysis advances upward. Constant monitoring will provide for immediate intervention if failure occurs.

Infection, either respiratory or urinary, may occur and intervention begun if fever develops.

Due to muscle atony and immobility, ileus development, venous thrombophlebitis, and pulmonary emboli may occur.

TREATMENT AND NURSING INTERVENTIONS

The objective of therapy is to support body systems until recovery occurs. Respiratory failure and infection are serious threats to recovery. Monitoring the vital capacity and ABGs is essential. If the vital capacity drops to less than 800 cc or if the ABGs deteriorate, a tracheostomy may be done so that the patient can be mechanically ventilated. Strict sterile suctioning is needed to prevent infection whether the patient has an endotracheal tube or a tracheostomy. Excellent bronchial hygiene and chest physiotherapy will help clear secretions and prevent respiratory deterioration. If fever develops, sputum cultures should be obtained to identify a specific pathogen (if one is present in the respiratory tract) so that appropriate antibiotic therapy may be instituted.

A communication system MUST be established with the patient using whatever muscle action is possible. This is extremely difficult if the disease progresses to involvement of the cranial nerves. At the peak of a severe syndrome, communication from the patient may be impossible. The nurse must explain all procedures *before* doing them and reassure the patient that shortly muscle function will return to some part of the body so they may then communicate their needs and desires to the nurses.

Monitoring blood pressure, cardiac rate, and cardiac rhythm is important since some transient cardiac dysrhythmias have been reported. Hypotension, secondary to the muscular atony, may occur in severe cases or at the peak of the attack. Vasopressor agents may be required. Otherwise, vasoactive drugs are seldom used because the patient's sensitivity to drugs is altered.

Urinary retention is not uncommon for a few days. Intermittent catheterization may be preferred to a Foley catheter in an effort to avoid urinary tract infection.

Physiotherapy is indicated very early to help counter the hazards of immobility. Passive range of motion and attention to body extremity position help maintain function and prevent contractures.

Nutritional needs must be met with consideration of gastric dilatation, ileus development, and aspiration potential if the gag reflex is lost. Initially, tube feedings may be used to ensure adequate caloric intake or in some centers hyperalimentation may be started.

Fluid and electrolytes are monitored carefully to prevent electrolyte imbalances and possible occurrence of ADH secretion dysfunction.

Steroid therapy is controversial as is anticoagulant therapy unless signs of a phlebitis or pulmonary embolism develop.

PROGNOSIS

In a good critical care area, less than 5% of all cases will experience permanent neurologic dysfunction. Without critical care medical treatment and nursing, approximately 25% will die.[1]

---

[1] Adams, RD, Maurice V: Principles of Neurology. New York: McGraw-Hill, pp. 420–421, 1977

Neurologic Bibliography

*Adams RD, Victor M (eds): Principles of Neurology. New York: McGraw-Hill, 1977

Balla JI: Pathways in Neurological Diagnosis. Chicago: Yearbook Medical Publishers, 1980

Barr ML: The Human Nervous System: An Anatomic Viewpoint, 3rd ed. Hagerstown, MD: Harper & Row, 1979

Borg N, Mikas DL, Stark J, Williams SM (eds): Core Curriculum for Critical Care Nursing, 2nd ed. American Association of Critical-Care Nurses. Philadelphia: W. B. Saunders, pp. 177–254, 1981

Bruce DA: The pathophysiology of increased intracranial pressure. In Current Concepts, A Scope Publication. Kalamazoo, MI: The Upjohn Co., 1978

*Carini E, Owens G, Conway-Rutkowski BL (eds): Neurological and Neurosurgical Nursing, 8th ed. St. Louis, MO: C.V. Mosby, 1978

Cloward RB: Acute cervical spine injuries. In Clinical Symposia, Vol. 32, No. 1. Summit, NJ: Ciba-Geigy Corporation, 1980

Coping with Neurologic Disorders: Nursing Photobook. Springhouse, PA: Intermed Communications, 1982

*Curtis BA, Jacobson S, Marcus EM (eds): An Introduction to the Neurosciences. Philadelphia: W. B. Saunders, 1972

*Davis JE, Mason CB: Neurological Critical Care. New York: Van Nostrand Reinhold Company, 1979

Dejong RN, Sahas AL, Aldrich CK, Milligan JO: Essentials of the Neurological Examination. Philadelphia: Smith Kline Corporation, 1974

*Diamond E: The Nervous System: Disease, Diagnosis, Treatment. Bowie, MD: Robert J. Brady Co., 1976

Fields WS: Aortocranial occlusive vascular disease (stroke). In Clinical Symposia, Vol. 26, No. 4. Summit, NJ: Ciba-Geigy Corporation, 1974

Goldberg S: Clinical Nueroanatomy Made Ridiculously Simple. Miami, FL: Medmaster, Inc., 1979

*Guyton AC: Textbook of Medical Physiology, 6th ed. Philadelphia: W. B. Saunders, pp. 560–721, 1981

Hudak CM, Lohr TS, Gallo BM (eds): Critical Care Nursing, 3rd ed. Philadelphia: J. B. Lippincott, pp. 321–405, 1982

*Jackson FE: The pathophysiology of head injuries. In Clinical Symposia, Vol. 18, No. 3. Summit, NJ: Ciba-Geigy Corporation, 1966

*A Programmed Approach to Anatomy and Physiology: The Nervous System, 2nd ed. Bowie, MD: Robert J. Brady Co., 1974

*Pryse-Phillips W, Murray TJ: Essential Neurology, 2nd ed. Garden City, NY: Medical Examination Publishing Co., 1982

*Redelman K (ed): Neurological injuries. *In* Critical Care Quarterly, Vol. 2, No. 1. Germantown, MD: Aspen Systems Corporation, 1979

Rhoton AL, Jackson FE, Gleave J, Rumbaugh CT: Congenital and traumatic intracranial aneurysms. *In* Clinical Symposia, Vol. 29, No. 4. Summit, NJ: Ciba-Geigy Corporation, 1977

*Schmidt R (ed): Fundamentals of Neurophysiology, 2nd ed. New York: Springer-Verlag, 1978

*Snyder M, Jackle M: Neurologic Problems: A Critical Care Nursing Focus. Bowie, MD: Robert J. Brady Co., 1981

*Sundt TM: Blood flow regulation in normal and ischemic brain: *In* Current Concepts, a Scope Publication. Kalamazoo, MI: The Upjohn Co., 1979

Taylor JW, Ballenger S: Neurological Dysfunctions and Nursing Intervention. New York: McGraw-Hill, 1980

IV

The Renal System

24

Anatomy of the Renal System

Learning Objectives

By the end of this chapter, the nurse will be able to:

1. Identify the location of the kidneys in the body.
2. List three protective coverings of the kidneys.
3. Identify the characteristics of each one of these three protective coverings of the kidneys.
4. Identify the shape and size of the kidneys.
5. Locate the cortex and percentage of kidney tissue which comprises the cortex.
6. Identify the component structures in the medulla of the kidney.
7. Explain why there is no symmetry in renal anatomy.
8. Identify the basic functioning unit of the kidneys.
9. Distinguish between cortical nephrons and juxtamedullary nephrons.
10. List the component parts of the nephrons starting with the glomerulus.
11. Name the membrane surrounding the glomerulus.
12. Describe the proximal convoluted tubules.
13. Describe the three portions of the loop of Henle.
14. Describe the distal convoluted tubule, the collecting tubule, and the collecting duct and their relationship.
15. Identify the portions of the juxtaglomerular apparatus (JGA): Include the macula densa, the polkissen cells, and the specialized afferent arteriolar cells.
16. Briefly describe the arterial vascular system of the kidney.
17. Identify the arterial blood circulation to the peritubular capillary network.
18. Explain the sympathetic nervous system control over constriction of renal arteries.
19. Explain the parasympathetic nervous system innervation of the kidney.
20. Identify four congenital abnormalities in the anatomy of the urinary system.

The Kidney

Perhaps it is more accurate to title this chapter "Anatomy of the Kidney." Discussion of the kidney anatomy is very detailed; however, there are only passing comments on the ureters, bladder, and the urethra. With a conceptualization of the anatomy of the kidney ingrained in our minds, it is far easier to understand the physiology of the kidney and its effect on our entire body.

LOCATION

The kidneys lie in the retroperitoneal space on each side of the vertebrae. The right kidney is a little lower than the left because the liver impinges on it. Even so, the tops of the kidneys are about at the level of the eleventh or twelfth thoracic vertebra and the bottom edges of the kidneys are about at the level of the second lumbar vertebra. The posterior surfaces are protected by the last two ribs.

The coverings of the kidneys help to protect them posteriorly and to prevent massive blood loss from trauma. The outermost protective covering is pararenal fat which completely surrounds the three coverings of the kidneys.

THREE PROTECTIVE COVERINGS

There are three protective coverings of the kidneys. The outermost layer is the *renal fascia*. This is a membrane sheet which surrounds a layer of *perirenal fat*. (Note that this is different from pararenal fat.) This perirenal fat is actually a very dense layer of adipose tissue. It is very compact and surrounds the innermost covering of the kidney, the *fibrous renal capsule*. This fibrous renal capsule is a thin, resistant membrane which is contiguous with the kidney tissue itself.

SHAPE AND SIZE

The kidneys are bean shaped organs with an indentation on their medial surfaces. The indented area is called the hilum. The hilum is the area in the renal pelvis at which the renal artery and vein enter and leave the kidney. The average kidney is 10–12 cm long, 5–6 cm wide (from the hilum to the outer cortex), and 3–4 cm thick. Its average weight is about 160–180 gm. (For comparison, 2.5 cm = 1 in. and 160–180 gm = about 4.5 oz.)

Gross Anatomy of the Kidney

The *cortex* is the outer one-third of the kidney tissue (Figure 24-1). It is composed of the glomeruli of all of the nephrons and the convoluted portions of the distal and proximal tubules. The cortex extends into the medulla between structures called pyramids. These extensions are the renal columns. The cortex itself extends inward from the renal capsule to the *base* of the pyramids.

The *medulla* is the inner portion of the kidney. The medulla contains the loops of Henle, the vasa recta, and the collecting ducts. These loops and ducts are arranged in triangles or pyramids. The tips of the pyramids are called papillae. Groups of papillae merge to form into a single papilla to enter the calyx (singular) which collects urine flow from the collecting duct. Calyces (plural) channel the urine into the renal pelvis. Eventually, the urine will flow from the renal pelvis into the ureter.

The number of calyces varies from 8 to 16

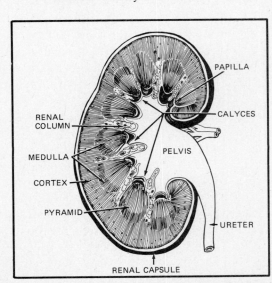

Figure 24-1. Gross anatomy of the kidney.

per kidney. Therefore, there is no symmetry in renal anatomy.

The Nephron

The nephron is the functional unit of the kidney. Each kidney has more than one million nephrons. Up to 75% of the kidneys' nephrons can be destroyed before the remaining nephrons are unable to compensate. While compensation is occurring, the functioning nephrons filter a higher solute load. Due to this increased workload, the functioning nephrons hypertrophy.

There are two types of nephrons: the cortical nephron and the juxtamedullary nephron.

THE CORTICAL NEPHRONS

These nephrons (Figure 24-2) have glomeruli that lie close to the cortical surface and have thin, *short* segments of the loops of Henle. The loops of Henle do enter the medulla but *do not* go past the outer medulla. Since the loops of Henle in the cortical nephrons are short and do not extend into the inner medulla, they do not participate in the *concentration* of urine. About 70% of the kidneys' nephrons are cortical nephrons with short or nonexistent loops of Henle.

JUXTAMEDULLARY NEPHRONS

These nephrons (Figure 24-3) are found in the inner one-third of the cortex. They have long loops of Henle that dip deep into the medulla and are surrounded by the peritubular network (the vasa recta). The lowest part of each loop of Henle has a thin wall in contrast to the sides of the loops as they dip into the medulla. This portion is called the thin descending segment of the loop. This segment is physiologically permeable to water and is probably impermeable to solutes. The thin ascending segment of the loop of Henle returns to the distal tubule. It is impermeable to water and is solute permeable. After the loop dips deeply into the medulla and then returns to the distal tubule, the fluid flows into the collecting ducts and down to the renal pelvis. These nephrons have a great capacity to concentrate urine. They are sodium-retaining nephrons due to their long loops of Henle.

In hypovolemic and hypotensive situations, a large portion of the renal blood flow is shunted from the cortical nephrons to the

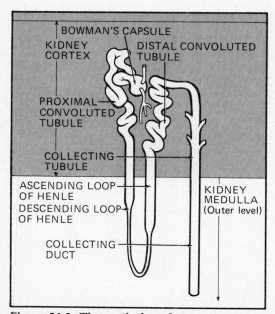

Figure 24-2. The cortical nephron.

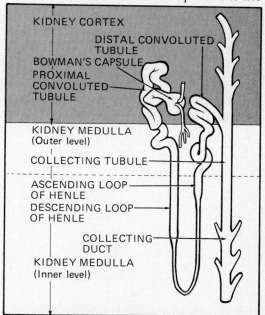

Figure 24-3. The juxtaglomerular nephron.

juxtamedullary nephrons to maintain urine formation.

Structural Anatomy of the Nephron

The nephron, as the functional unit of the kidney, is composed of the glomerulus, the proximal convoluted tubule, the loop of Henle, the distal convoluted tubule, the collecting ducts, a juxtaglomerular apparatus (JGA), a peritubular capillary network, and the vasa recta (found only in juxtamedullary nephrons which comprise a specialized division of the peritubular capillary network).

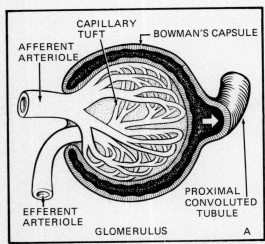

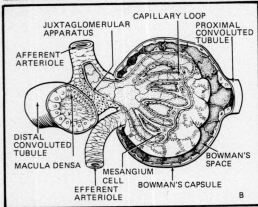

Figure 24-4. The glomerulus (A = schematic view; B = detailed view).

THE GLOMERULUS

This is a network of capillaries (Figure 24-4) that are spherical in shape and are formed by the afferent arterioles dividing into between two and eight subdivisions. These subdivisions branch to form as many as 50 capillary loops. These loops are supported by tissue called mesangium. This spherical unit, the glomerulus, is enclosed by an epithelial-lined membrane. This membrane is called *Bowman's capsule*. The efferent arteriole carries the blood out of the glomerulus.

THE PROXIMAL CONVOLUTED TUBULE

This is twisted around itself and thus its name (Figure 24-5). It is about 14 mm in length and about 55 mm in diameter. It is next to the glomerulus, and the end towards the glomerulus (proximal end) has tiny threadlike projections which form tiny tufts of a brushlike border on the inner lumen of the tubule to help resorb the

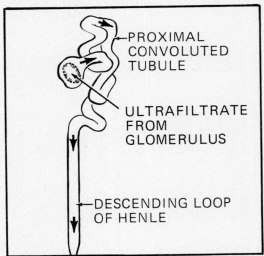

Figure 24-5. The proximal convoluted tubule.

glomerular filtrate. The brush border increases the resorptive surface area per unit length of the tubule. The proximal convoluted tubule ends in the medulla of the kidney and there it becomes the descending limb of the loop of Henle.

THE LOOP OF HENLE

This has three distinct portions (Figure 24-6): a thick descending limb, a thin segment which is the actual loop, and a thick ascending limb. The loops of Henle in the cortical nephron reach just to the inside of the kidney medulla. The loops of Henle in the juxtamedullary nephron reach almost to the tips of the pyramids (the papillae) and then start ascending to become the ascending limb of the loop of Henle. The peritubular capillary network surrounds the loop portion of the juxtamedullary nephron. As the long loop of Henle dips deep into the medulla, it is surrounded by the vasa recta, which are straight capillary loops (Figure 24-6).

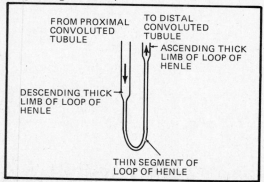

Figure 24-6. The Loop of Henle.

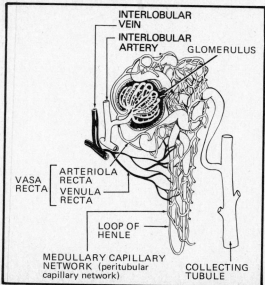

Figure 24-7. The vasa recta and peritubular capillary network.

Thirty percent of the nephrons in each kidney are juxtamedullary nephrons that have long loops of Henle which are surrounded by the *vasa recta* (Figure 24-7).

THE DISTAL CONVOLUTED TUBULE

This begins where the ascending limb of the loop of Henle starts twisting (Figure 24-8). The distal convoluted tubule closely passes its own glomerulus and may even touch it. The distal convoluted tubule continues without convolutions to become the collecting tubule.

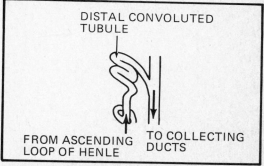

Figure 24-8. The distal convoluted tubule.

THE COLLECTING TUBULE

This extends to become the *collecting duct* which itself empties into a common collecting duct which in turn empties into the renal pelvis (Figure 24-9).

THE JUXTAGLOMERULAR APPARATUS (JGA)

All nephrons have a juxtaglomerular apparatus (JGA). The JGA has three specific components. As the distal convoluted tubule passes between the afferent and efferent arterioles, there are some specialized cells (Figure 24-10). These cells and their nuclei are very tightly packed together. These packed cells are called the *macula densa*, one of the components.

There are also specialized cells on the outside of the afferent and efferent arterioles at this point that are referred to as polkissen cells or juxtaglomerular cells (depending upon the text being read). These cells are a second component of the JGA. It

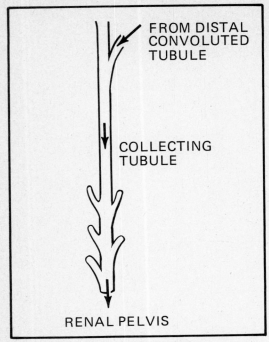

Figure 24-9. The collecting tubule.

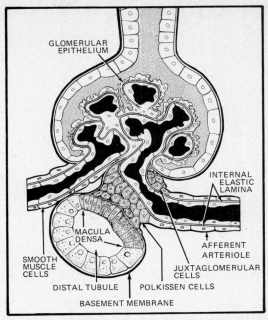

Figure 24-10. The juxtaglomerular apparatus.

is thought that the macula densa or these specialized cells secrete an unidentified substance, possibly uncleaved renin granules.

An area where the distal convoluted tubule passes by or touches the efferent arterioles is the third component of the JGA. The JGA and its actions are covered in Chapter 25 on renal physiology.

Vascular System of the Kidney

One renal artery arises from the aorta and enters the kidney (Figure 24-11). It is uncommon, but there may be more than one renal artery. The renal artery enters in front of the midline of the kidney at the hilum and bifurcates immediately at the kidney pelvis.

After this first splitting at the kidney pelvis, the renal arteries develop many branches called interlobar arteries. These interlobar arteries, as their name implies, travel between lobes of the renal parenchyma inside the renal columns towards the point where the cortex and medulla meet.

At the interface of the cortex and medulla, the interlobar arteries branch to form the arcuate arteries. These arteries form arcs between the lobes of the parenchyma.

From each arcuate artery, multiple interlobular arteries spread into the cortex. These interlobular arteries form short muscular afferent arterioles that supply the glomeruli. Efferent arterioles drain the blood from the glomerulus and most of this flows through the peritubular capillary network that surrounds the cortical portions of the tubules. The small amount of remaining arterial blood flows into straight capil-

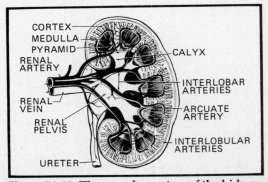

Figure 24-11. The vascular system of the kidney.

lary loops called *vasa recta*. These extend down into the medulla to provide arterial blood to the lower parts of the thin segments of the loop of Henle before looping upward to enter the interlobular veins. From the interlobular veins, the blood enters the arcuate veins, then the interlobar veins, then the renal veins, and then the inferior vena cava.

Nerve Supply of the Kidney

The sympathetic nervous system controls constriction of renal arteries. These nerves follow the same course as the arterioles in order to maintain vasoactive tone of the arterioles.

The parasympathetic nervous system innervates the kidney through the vagus nerve fibers arising from the celiac plexus.

Ureter, Urinary Bladder, and Urethra

The ureter averages 10 inches in length (Figure 24-12). The urine leaves the kidney pelvis entering the ureter. The ureter moves the urine along by peristaltic action to the urinary bladder. The bladder is a hollow, muscular organ. It has a normal capacity of one-half to one pint. At the bottom of the bladder is the urethra. It is about six to eight inches long in males, one to one and one-fourth inches in females.

Congenital Abnormalities in the Anatomy of the Urinary System

The most common abnormality of the urinary tract is bifid ureters (Figure 24-13). In

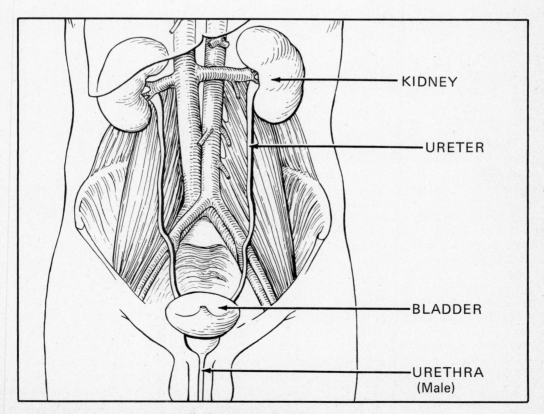

KIDNEY

URETER

BLADDER

URETHRA
(Male)

Figure 24-12. The ureter, urinary bladder, and urethra.

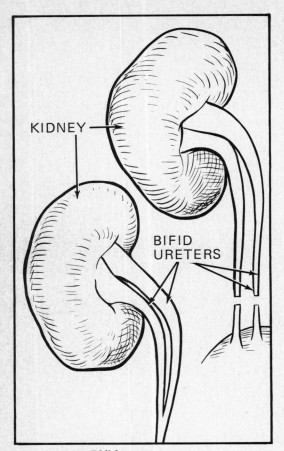

Figure 24-13. Bifid ureters.

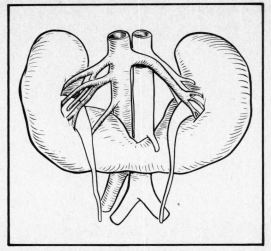

Figure 24-14. Fused kidneys.

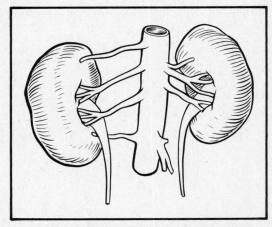

Figure 24-15. Multiple arteries entering the kidneys.

this condition, two ureters leave the renal pelvis and may continue as two ureters into the bladder. Commonly, the two ureters fuse into one before entering the bladder. If the ureters do not fuse, one may enter the bladder and the other may enter elsewhere (floor of urethra, roof of vagina, or such).

One in 700 people have fused kidneys (Figure 24-14). The fusion is usually at the inferior poles producing a "horseshoe" kidney. This is a problem only if the person has frequent infections or if the kidney compresses some abdominal organs. Infections are treated medically. If compression of organs occurs, surgery may be indicated.

About 3% of the kidneys have two or more arteries entering the kidney (Figure 24-15). This is significant if the kidney is a proposed transplant organ. It is difficult, if

not impossible, to maintain adequate perfusion of a kidney with multiple arteries. Most of the time, such a kidney is rejected as a potential donor.

Occasionally, an ectopic kidney (Figure 24-16) is present. One or both kidneys may be involved. More commonly, the left kidney is located deep in the pelvis and the right kidney is located in its normal position. This may present no problems, or it may cause infections. If pressure on other organs occurs, clinical treatment may be required.

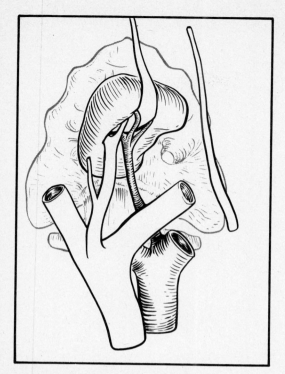

Figure 24-16. An ectopic kidney.

25

Physiology of the Renal System

Learning Objectives

By the end of this chapter, the nurse will be able to:

1. List the seven functions of the kidney.
2. Identify the three processes involved in the formation of urine.
3. Describe the autoregulatory system of the glomerulus when filtration pressures are high and low.
4. List five factors that affect the glomerular filtration rate.
5. Explain the effect of each of the five factors that affect glomerular filtration rate.
6. Define diffusion, osmosis, secretion, and absorption in relation to kidney function.
7. Explain pinocytosis.
8. Trace the formation of urine starting with the ultrafiltrate of the glomerulus and ending with urine entering the renal pelvis. Include the movement of ions in each portion of the nephron.
9. List the three mechanisms of body water regulation.
10. Describe the release and action of antidiuretic hormone.
11. Explain the countercurrent multiplier system.
12. Differentiate between threshold and nonthreshold substances.
13. Elucidate the use and significance of the BUN, creatinine, and creatinine clearance tests.
14. Identify the three mechanisms for excretion of acids by the kidney including an example of each and the amount of acid excreted by each mechanism.
15. Explain the renin-angiotensin mechanism for renal control of blood pressure.
16. Draw the renin cascade starting with the stimulation of the JGA.
17. Discuss the *major* effect of prostaglandins.
18. Describe the kidney's role in red blood cell synthesis.

Physiological processes of the kidney include the formation of urine, the regulation of body water, the regulation of electrolytes, the excretion of metabolic waste products, the regulation of acid-base balance in the body, the regulation of blood pressure, and erythropoietin secretion.

In this chapter, each aspect will be covered individually, except for the regulation of electrolytes which will be covered in Chapter 26. It is important, however, to remember that all processes are continuous and concurrent.

Formation of Urine

Three processes are involved in the formation of urine: glomerular filtration, tubular reabsorption, and tubular secretion.

Glomerular Filtration

The kidneys receive 20–25% of the cardiac output. Ninety-five percent of this quantity of blood will go through the glomerulus where some solutes will be filtered out. An autoregulatory system exists to protect the vitally important glomerulus. The afferent and efferent renal arterioles constrict or dilate in response to systemic blood pressure. If systemic blood pressure increases, the afferent arteriole will constrict. This effectively reduces the pressure of the blood entering the glomerulus. In the same way, if systemic blood pressure decreases, the afferent arteriole will dilate to allow more blood to enter the glomerulus.

When the afferent arteriole constricts to reduce the pressure of blood in the glomerulus, the efferent arteriole relaxes (dilates) to allow the blood to leave more rapidly. This helps the control of glomerular pressure. Conversely, when systemic pressure drops, the afferent arteriole dilates to let more blood into the glomerulus and the efferent arteriole constricts to help maintain the glomerular pressure. Below a mean systolic blood pressure of about 75 mm Hg, this autoregulatory system fails and the glomerulus suffers the effects of hypotension.

Glomerular filtration is influenced by two factors: filtration pressure and glomerular permeability.

1. *Filtration pressure* is determined in part by the anatomical blood flow through the nephron. Each nephron is actually perfused by two capillary beds (Figure 25-1). The glomerular capillary bed is perfused by the afferent arteriole with an average hydrostatic pressure of about 60 mm Hg. The peritubular capillary bed is perfused by the efferent arteriole, which resists blood flow. Because of this, the glomerular capillary bed has a high pressure (which may be termed glomerular hydrostatic pressure). The peritubular capillary bed has a low pressure of about 13 mm Hg.

   The high pressure in the glomerulus tends to filter fluid out of the glomerulus and into the Bowman's capsule. At the same time and following the same principles, the low pressure in the peritubular capillary bed tends to draw fluid from the interstitial spaces into the peritubular capillaries. The high pressures in the glomerulus cause a rapid filtration of fluid. The low pressure of the capillary bed of the peritubular system facilitates rapid uptake of the excreted tubular fluids by the peritubular capillaries. This diminishes backleak and increases *net* reabsorption.

   Blood is brought into the glomerulus by the afferent arteriole. The pressure is close to 60 mm Hg, so fluid is forced from the glomerular capillaries into the Bowman's capsule. This fluid is now called the glomerular ultrafiltrate. It is called an ultrafiltrate because protein size molecules (and larger) cannot filter out of the glomerular capillaries. Those proteins remain in the blood entering the peritubular capillaries from the efferent arteriole. The retained protein molecules cause an increase in the plasma osmotic pressure. This causes the rapid reabsorption of fluid from the peritubular interstitial spaces.

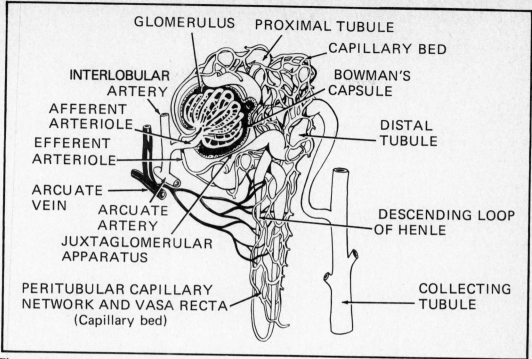

Figure 25-1. The capillary beds of a nephron.

2. *Glomerular permeability* is the second influence on glomerular filtration. The glomerular membrane is different from other capillary membranes in the body. The glomerular membrane has three layers: the endothelial layer of the capillary, a basement membrane, and a layer of epithelial cells on the *outer* surface of the capillary (Figure 25-2). In spite of three layers, the glomerular membrane is 100 to 1,000 times *more* permeable than the usual capillary. Obviously, it is not the three layers that increase the permeability. The endothelial cells lining the glomerular capillary are full of thousands of tiny holes called fenestrae. Outside the capillary endothelium is a basement membrane which is like a mesh of fibers. The outer layer of epithelial cells is different in that they are not touching each other and the space between each epithelial cell is called a slit-pore. Any particle greater than seven millimicrons cannot penetrate the slit-pore.

COMPOSITION OF GLOMERULAR ULTRAFILTRATE

Normally, the ultrafiltrate is free of protein and red blood cells since they are too large

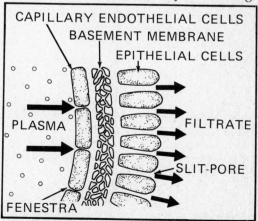

Figure 25-2. The three layers of the glomerular membrane.

to pass through the slit-pores. The semi-permeable membrane of the glomerular capillary allows water, nutrients, electrolytes, and wastes to filter into Bowman's capsule.

GLOMERULAR FILTRATION RATE (GFR)

In the healthy kidney, there is a *combined* average GFR of 125 ml/minute. The total quantity of glomerular filtrate per day is about 180 liters. More than 99% of this filtrate is reabsorbed in the tubules. The equation for calculating the GFR is the urine concentration of a substance times the urine flow rate divided by the plasma concentration of the same substance. The substance must be freely filtered and not affected by the tubules (Figure 25-3). The normal adult urine volume per 24 hours is about one to one and one-half liters.

$$GFR = \frac{(U_x \cdot V)}{P_x}$$

$$GFR = \frac{\text{URINE CONCENTRATION OF A FREELY FILTERED SUBSTANCE} \quad X \quad \text{URINE FLOW RATE}}{\text{PLASMA CONCENTRATION OF SUBSTANCE IN } U_x}$$

Figure 25-3. The equation for calculating the glomerular filtration rate.

FACTORS AFFECTING THE GFR

Any change in the glomerular hydrostatic pressure will alter the GFR. The most common cause of change in the hydrostatic pressure is change in the systemic blood pressure. This changes the actual *flow of blood* into the glomerulus. Alterations in the afferent and efferent arteriole tone (constriction-dilatation) will also affect the glomerular pressure and hence the GFR.

Any alteration in the composition of the plasma, such as an increase in oncotic pressure (the osmotic pressure due to the presence of colloids in a solution), will alter the GFR. Such conditions as hyperproteinemia, hypoproteinemia, hypovolemia, or hypervolemia will also alter the composition of plasma due to alterations in the extracellulur fluid (ECF) and intracellular fluid (ICF). Thus, these states will alter the GFR.

The GFR will automatically be altered by any abnormality of structure, presence of disease, or ingestion of nephrotoxic substances.

Tubular Absorption and Secretion

The glomeruli filter a total of 180 liters per day and normal urine output is one to one and one-half liters per day. The nephrons' tubular function is responsible (in part) for determining urinary output.

The nephron uses two processes to convert this 180 liters of ultrafiltrate to just one to one and one-half liters of urine. The two processes are absorption and secretion. These processes may be active or passive and are influenced by hormones, electrochemical gradients, and Starling's law.

Let us now define some terms necessary to our discussion:

Diffusion is the movement of *solutes* from an area of high concentration to an area of low concentration.

Osmosis is the movement of *water* from an area of high water concentration to an area of low water concentration.

Absorption, as discussed here, is the movement of solutes and water from the tubule *into the peritubular network* (i.e., from the filtrate back into the bloodstream).

Secretion, as discussed here, is the movement of solutes and water from the peritubular network *into the tubule* (i.e., from the bloodstream back into the filtrate).

Passive transport is the movement of solutes by diffusion following concentration gradients and electrical gradients.

Active transport is the movement of any substance against an electrical or concentration gradient. This requires energy. The energy is usually supplied by ATP.

A mnemonic may help unravel the maze of the movement of solutes in the various tubules. Cations are carried by active transport, CAT—carried active transport. Is it hard to remember what cations are and what anions are? ANI stands for a negative ion and therefore, anions are passively transported. Na$^+$, K$^+$, H$^+$ are the most common cations in our body. Cl$^-$ and HCO$_3^-$ are the most common anions in our body.

As with most "rules," there is always an exception. In the collecting duct, chloride (anion) is actively absorbed and the cations are passively absorbed. Table 25-1 traces the formation of urine starting with the ultrafiltrate and finishing with urine after passing through both convoluted tubules, the loop of Henle, and the collecting ducts.

Protein is absorbed in the *opening border* of the proximal convoluted tubule. The protein attaches itself to the membrane (Figure 25-4). The membrane then invaginates (i.e., surrounds) the protein. Once inside the cell, the cell membrane returns to normal and the protein is digested to its basic parts and then is absorbed into the peritubular fluids. This process of absorption is called pinocytosis.

The major function of the loop of Henle is to concentrate or dilute urine as necessary. This is accomplished by the countercurrent mechanism which maintains the hyperosmolar concentration in the renal medulla. (This is covered under body water regulation.)

Table 25-1. Urine formation.

Start: *Ultra-filtrate*

Proximal Convoluted Tubule	Loop of Henle (3 parts)	Distal Convoluted Tubule	Collecting Duct
60–80% ultrafiltrate absorbed	I. *Descending Limb*	*Absorbed*	*Absorbed*
Absorbed	H$_2$O absorbed—this portion very permeable to H$_2$O	HCO$_3^-$ H$_2$O if ADH is present	Na$^+$
Na$^+$ Cl$^-$ glucose amino acids ALL K$^+$		Na$^+$ actively if aldosterone adequate	*Secreted*
HCO$_3^-$	Na$^+$ secreted; fluid becomes increasingly hypertonic		H$^+$ K$^+$ NH$_3$
Secreted		*Secreted*	H$_2$O if ADH is present
H$^+$ urea drugs organic acids	II. *Actual Thin Segment Loop*	K$^+$ H$^+$ urate ion	Aldosterone also has an effect here
HCO$_3^-$ and H$^+$ regulates acid-base balance	permeable to H$_2$O	Fluid is hypotonic	FINISH: URINE
H$_2$O passively ABSORBED	III. *Ascending Limb*		Flows into renal pelvis, ureters, bladder
Fluid leaves isotonic to plasma	Na$^+$ absorbed Cl$^-$ absorbed actively; relatively impermeable to H$_2$O		

Notes:

1. Sulfates, nitrates, and phosphates are absorbed only enough to maintain the ECF concentration.
2. ALL K$^+$ from the filtrate is absorbed in the proximal tubule.
3. The K$^+$ secreted in the distal convoluted tubule equals about 12% of the K$^+$ in the original filtrate. Under certain circumstances, secretion may *exceed* the original filtered load.

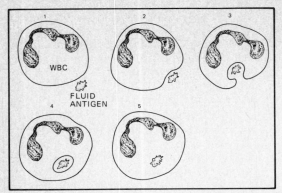

Figure 25-4. Protein absorption by pinocytosis.

Body Water Regulation

Throughout the discussion of body regulation, the terms osmolar and osmolal will be used interchangeably. This is common in both clinical practice and in writing. Osmolarity is the concentration of particles in solution. Osmolality is the amount of solvent in relation to the particles. In actuality, the terms are used interchangeably.

The volume and concentration of body water content is maintained by the thirst-neurohypophyseal-renal axis. Approximately 60% of ideal body weight is water in males and 50–55% in women. Figure 25-5 shows the distribution of this water throughout the body. There are three mechanisms that help regulate body fluid: thirst, ADH, and the countercurrent mechanism of the kidney.

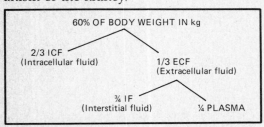

Figure 25-5. Distribution of water throughout the body.

THIRST

This is the major force in our awareness of a need for water. The thirst center is located in the hyothalamus near the antidiuretic hormone area and the supraoptic nuclei of the brain. Intracellular dehydration, due to any reason, causes the sensation of thirst. The most common cause of intracellular dehydration is an increase in osmolar concentration of the ECF. Increased sodium concentration of the ECF causes osmosis of fluid from the neuronal cells of the thirst center. Other important and frequent causes of thirst are excessive angiotensin II in the blood, hemorrhage, and low cardiac output.

The role of the thirst center is to maintain a conscious desire to drink the exact amount of fluid needed to maintain a normal body hydrated state or return a dehydrated state to the normal state of hydration.

ANTIDIURETIC HORMONE (ADH)

This is the second regulator of body water and it works closely with the thirst mechanism. The plasma protein and extracellular fluid sodium concentrations determine the osmolality of the extracellular fluid. Normal serum osmolality is 280–300 mOsm/liter. Acid-base control mechanisms of the kidney adjust the negative ion in relation to the extracellular concentration (osmolality) to equal the positive ions in the body. Sodium is the most plentiful positive ion, so it controls the osmolality. Antidiuretic hormone is synthesized in the supraoptic nuclei of the hypothalamus. Antidiuretic hormone then drips down the supraoptical-hypophyseal tracts to the posterior pituitary (neurohypophysis) where it is stored. The supraoptic area of the hypothalamus is so close to the thirst center that there is an integration of the thirst mechanism, osmolality detection, and antidiuretic hormone release.

The osmosodium receptors respond to changes in osmolality (sodium concentration) in the extracellular fluid compartment. The osmosodium receptors are located in the supraoptic nuclei of the brain. An increase in osmolality excites the osmoreceptors. They signal the neurohypophyseal tract that antidiuretic hormone is needed. The posterior pituitary (neurohypophysis) releases the antidiuretic hormone it has stored. In the presence of antidiuretic hormone and aldosterone, the distal convoluted tubules and the collecting ducts reabsorb water. The reabsorption of the water leaves a hypertonic urine. To review this important cycle of responses: Increased osmolality leads to exciting the neurons, which leads to release of antidiuretic hormone, which leads to increased reabsorption of water in the distal convoluted tubule and the collecting ducts. This cycle will continue until the concentration of the extracellular fluid compartment and fluid homeostasis are returned to normal.

On the reverse of this cycle, if osmolality of the extracellular fluid compartment decreases, antidiuretic hormone release is inhibited because the osmoreceptors are not stimulated. Without antidiuretic hormone, the distal tubules and collecting ducts are impermeable to water. Urine will be very dilute because the water cannot be reabsorbed. This will continue until the loss of water has raised the concentration of the extracellular fluid compartment solutes to normal.

THE COUNTERCURRENT MECHANISMS

The kidney provides the third regulator of body fluid. This method is used to concentrate urine and excrete excessive solutes. Excreting dilute urine is no problem for the kidney unless there is a neurological dysfunction, an endocrine dysfunction, or traumatic injuries. These conditions may result in an inappropriate release and effect upon normal kidney function of antidiuretic hormone, aldosterone, and/or cortisol. Concentrating urine to rid the body of waste solutes is a complex interaction between the long loops of Henle, the peritubular capillaries, and the vasa recta.

The countercurrent multiplier mechanism functions constantly in a loop cycle with fresh filtrate continuously entering the loop of Henle. At the entry to the loop, the filtrate has a concentration of 300 mOsm/liter. The medulla increases this concentration so that at the tips of the papillae in the pelvic tip of the medulla the concentration of the filtrate is 1,200–1,400 mOsm/liter.

It is essential for the medullary interstitium to be hyperosmolar. There are four steps in concentrating the solutes to produce this hyperosmolality (Figure 25-6).

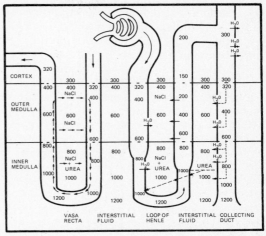

Figure 25-6. The countercurrent multiplier mechanism for maintaining medullary interstitial hyperosmolality and concentrating urine.

In step one, chloride ions are actively transported from the thick portion of the ascending limb of the loop of Henle into the upper medullary interstitial fluid. The active transport of chloride pulls sodium and some potassium, magnesium, and calcium along also.

In step two, the collecting ducts actively transport sodium into the medullary interstitial fluid. Chloride follows along passively. Steps one and two increase medullary interstitial fluid hyperosmolality by about 500 milliosmoles.

In step three, the collecting duct yields urea to the lower medullary interstitial fluid if antidiuretic hormone is present. The hormone makes the collecting duct mildly permeable to urea and very permeable to water. So water leaves the collecting duct to enter the medullary interstitium resulting in a strongly urea concentrated collecting duct. Urea, following concentration gradients, then diffuses out into the medullary interstitial fluid also. This increases the medullary osmolarity by about another 200–400 milliosmoles.

In step four, water osmosis occurs from

the thin segment of the loop of Henle because of the high urea concentration in the lower medullary interstitial fluid. As the water moves from the loop of Henle, sodium ion concentration in the thin limb increases. Due to the high concentration, sodium and chloride passively diffuse out of the collecting duct into the lower medullary interstitium. This increases the osmolarity of the medullary interstitial fluid to between 1,000 and 1,200 milliosmoles.

Now that excess solutes are concentrated in the medullary interstitium, they must not be allowed to re-enter the bloodstream via the peritubular capillary network which completely wraps around the loop of Henle. This is prevented by a very sluggish blood flow in these capillaries and a very small amount of blood being present—less than 2% of the total renal blood supply— keeping ion movement to a minimum. Throughout the countercurrent multiplier activity, ion movement from the loop of Henle into the medullary interstitium has been ionic *secretion* (ions moving *from* the tubule lumen) either actively or passively and by diffusion or osmosis.

It is now necessary to remove the ion solutes from the medullary interstitial fluid into the ascending limb of the loop of Henle so they may be excreted with the urine water. This is accomplished by the *countercurrent exchange mechanism*. The vasa recta is this mechanism, but it receives help from the poor blood perfusion of the medullary interstitium just discussed. The vasa recta are essentially straight tubes forming a long, slender U-shaped blood vessel. Each side of the slender U is very close to each other and the central portion of the U contains medullary interstitial fluid. Both sides of the U are highly permeable so fluids and solutes readily exchange places in the high concentration gradients of the lower medullary interstitium.

As the blood in the vasa recta flows back up the ascending loop of Henle, excess sodium and urea diffuse out of the blood in exchange for water diffusing into the blood. The *blood* leaves the medulla with almost the same osmolarity as when it entered the descending loop.

The fluid in the loop of Henle becomes more concentrated in the presence of antidiuretic hormone since water has diffused out. In the ascending thick limb of the loop of Henle and the diluting segment of the distal convoluted tubule, the osmolarity of the filtrate drops somewhat. In the distal convoluted tubules and the collecting ducts, the osmolarity depends upon the presence of antidiuretic hormone and aldosterone. If these hormones are present, sodium and water will be absorbed and the tubule fluid will remain concentrated as it passes through the collecting ducts to the renal pelvis to enter the ureter. If the hormones are not present, water will *not* be secreted and a more dilute urine will enter the ureter. NOTE: Since *only* juxtamedullary nephrons have long loops of Henle, these are the nephron units responsible for concentrating and diluting the filtrate as urine is formed. The cortical nephron units do not participate in these processes.

The countercurrent mechanisms are the ways in which slight changes in concentration in one part of the system have a major effect across the kidney medulla and make the task of controlling electrolytes far more easy and far more efficient.

Excretion of Metabolic Waste Products

The metabolic waste products (estimated to be in excess of 200 different substances) handled by the kidneys are classified as threshold substances, nonthreshold substances, and electrolytes, water, and other substances that may be reabsorbed or excreted by the kidneys according to individual fluctuating needs.

Threshold substances are those that are entirely reabsorbed by the kidneys *unless* the substances are present in excessive concentration in the blood. Glucose is the most commonly known threshold substance. Amino acids are also threshold substances.

Nonthreshold substances are *not* reabsorbed by the kidney tubules. Creatinine is the most abundant. Urea is included in this category even though urea passively diffuses back into the kidney bloodstream.

Proteins and acids of disease processes (lactic acid, ketones, etc.) are nonthreshold substances.

Water and most electrolytes will be absorbed or secreted acccording to individual needs.

There are two commonly used tests to determine efficiency of kidney function in handling waste products: BUN and creatinine.

1. *The blood urea nitrogen (BUN)* measures the level of urea, a nitrogen waste product of protein metabolism. The BUN is an *unreliable* test of renal function because the BUN level is affected by many factors. In the presence of liver disease, the BUN will remain low because the liver cannot synthesize urea at a normal rate. Conversely, with normal kidney function, dehydration, GI bleeding, sepsis, trauma, drugs, diet, and changes in catabolism may elevate the BUN markedly (increasing as much as 50 mg/100 ml). Food in the digestive tract may also falsely elevate the BUN. Therefore, the BUN should be drawn fasting.

2. *Serum creatinine* is a more reliable index of kidney function. Creatinine is a waste product of muscle metabolism and is freely filtered. This means that the nephron tubules neither reabsorb nor secrete creatinine. The normally functioning kidney filters creatinine from the blood at a rate equal to the GFR. Since the amount of creatinine produced each day is constant and is proportional to the body's muscle mass, serial serum creatinines are valuable indices of kidney function EXCEPT in septic patients and patients with muscle wasting diseases.

Normally, a BUN to creatinine ratio of 10:1 is present in serum. A ratio of 20:1 or more is indicative of prerenal insufficiency (water and salt depletion), a high protein catabolism, or low renal perfusion pressures.

An elevation of *both* BUN and creatinine above the normal ratio indicates renal disease. In these patients, a creatinine clearance is usually performed. *Creatinine clearance is probably the most reliable index of kidney function available.* Normal creatinine clearance value is 125 ml/min; however, 80 ml/min is accepted as the lowest satisfactory value for considering kidney function normal. Urine is collected for 12–24 hours and a blood serum sample is drawn half way through the urine collection. The formula for calculating creatinine clearance is found in Appendix I. If the BUN, creatinine, and creatinine clearance tests are normal, the kidneys are functioning adequately in excreting metabolic waste products from the body.

Regulation of Acid-Base Balance

The body acid-base balance is maintained by the lungs, blood buffers, and the kidneys. The lungs and blood buffer systems were covered in the pulmonary unit. The kidneys regulate acid-base balance by controlling the bicarbonate ion (HCO_3^-) and in much lesser quantity, the hydrogen ion (H^+).

The normal diet contains some acids (phosphates and sulfates) that must be excreted. In addition, protein catabolism is markedly increased in the critically ill. Protein catabolism adds to the acid load of the body. Products of protein catabolism are eliminated by the kidneys.

Four mechanisms provide for the excretion of acid and regulation of acid-base balance by the kidneys:

1. *Direct excretion of hydrogen ions:* This is a very minute amount (less than 1 mEq of hydrogen ion per day) and it has only a minor role in acid-base control. A passive secretion of hydrogen ion occurs in the proximal tubules. An active secretion of hydrogen ion occurs in the distal tubules.

2. *Excretion of hydrogen (H^+) with urine buffers:* Nonvolatile acids are excreted in this process. The glomerulus filters these acids and bicarbonate. The phosphate acids filtered are an example of the process for excreting hydrogen ion with a urine buffer.

$$H_2CO_3 + Na_2HPO_4 \rightarrow NaHCO_3 + NaH_2PO_4$$

| Carbonic acid | Disodium phosphate | Sodium bicarbonate | Sodium biphosphate |

The carbonic acid will combine with disodium phosphate and will yield sodium bicarbonate and sodium biphosphate. The sodium bicarbonate will break down into sodium and bicarbonate and be reabsorbed as needed. The sodium biphosphate added a hydrogen ion to become a molecule and will be excreted in urine. The net result of the phosphate and sulfate wastes filtered by the glomerulus is the addition of a hydrogen ion per molecule excreted. Up to 20 mEq/day may be excreted with these buffers.

3. *Utilizing ammonia (NH₃):* The third mechanism of acid-base control by the kidneys is excretion of acids. Chemically, ammonia is produced in renal tubular cells and diffuses into tubular fluid where carbonic acid combines with ammonia and actually produces two factors that benefit acid-base control.

$$NH_3 \; + \; H_2CO_3 \; \rightarrow \quad NH_4^+ \; + \quad HCO_3^-$$

ammonia	carbonic acid	ammonium ion	bicarbonate ion

Ammonium (ammonia with one additional hydrogen ion) combines with anions.

$$\overset{\text{CA}}{2NH_4HCO_3 + Na_2SO_4 \rightarrow 2NaHCO_3 + (NH_4)_2SO_4}$$

ammonium bicarbonate	sodium sulfate	sodium bicarbonate	ammonium sulfate

The ammonium sulfate (which now has two hydrogen ions) is excreted in the urine. The sodium bicarbonate is available to buffer in the body as needed. This system provides a very large influence on acid-base balance. Up to 50 mEq of acid per day may be excreted by utilizing ammonia.

4. *Production of and reabsorption of bicarbonate* is the fourth control mechanism of acid-base balance by the kidney. This is sometimes referred to as the titration of bicarbonate ion against the hydrogen ion.

New bicarbonate ion is actually manufactured in the distal convoluted tubule if needed. The formula is

$$H_2O \; + \quad CO_2 \; \overset{\text{CA}}{\rightleftharpoons} \; H_2CO_3 \; \overset{\text{CA}}{\rightleftharpoons} \; H^+ \; + \quad HCO_3^-$$

water	carbon dioxide	carbonic acid	hydrogen ion	bicarbonate ion

CA is carbonic anhydrase, a catalyst. It speeds up the chemical reaction without actually entering into the chemical reaction. The brush border of the proximal convoluted tubule contains a great deal of carbonic anhydrase. The distal convoluted tubule does not. The formation of carbonic acid is very rapid in the proximal tubule. The carbonic acid thus produced ionizes more slowly in the distal tubule. As it ionizes, hydrogen ion is excreted into the urine. The ionized bicarbonate is absorbed into the ECF (in the interstitium) along with sodium (reabsorption of bicarbonate).

This entire chemical reaction can start in the distal tubule (formation of new bicarbonate). In this instance, carbon dioxide comes from cellular metabolism or from dissolved carbon dioxide in the renal venous blood. The carbon dioxide combines with water present in the distal tubule to form carbonic acid. This is termed the hydration of carbon dioxide (with the catalyst carbonic anhydrase [CA]). In formula form:

$$H_2O \; + \quad CO_2 \; \overset{\text{CA}}{\rightleftharpoons} \; H_2CO_3 \; \overset{\text{CA}}{\rightleftharpoons} \; H^+ \; + \quad HCO_3^-$$

water	carbon dioxide	carbonic acid	hydrogen ion	bicarbonate ion

The carbonic acid then dissociates into hydrogen ion and bicarbonate ion to buffer as needed. If the body is in acid-base balance, the carbonic acid dissociates into water and carbon dioxide. The water joins the urine. The carbon dioxide rapidly diffuses into the ECF (in the interstitium). The bicarbonate in the distal tubule is mainly new bicarbonate formed there. The original bicarbonate filtered by the glomerulus was reabsorbed in the proximal tubule.

In acidotic states, there is an increase in hydrogen ion secretion in the distal tubule which accompanies an increased excretion of acid buffers (phosphates and sulfates). The four acid-base regulators of the kidneys come into play with ammonia transformation into ammonium as the predominant control. Because more acid is being excreted in the urine, urine pH may be as low as 4.4.

In alkalotic states, there is a decrease in hydrogen ion secretion in the distal tubules. This is accompanied by an excess bicarbonate excretion in the urine resulting in urine which is alkaline (i.e., pH > 7.0).

Regulation of Blood Pressure

The kidneys participate in regulation of blood pressure through four different mechanisms.

1. MAINTAINING ECF VOLUME AND COMPOSITION

The functions of the glomerular autoregulatory system of the afferent and efferent arterioles were covered earlier. Once this autoregulatory system fails, plasma flow will be increased a little (by the remaining three mechanisms). Vasoconstriction will maintain or elevate the blood pressure for a short while only. If no more defense mechanisms exist, then only intravenous fluids, plasmanate, albumin and such will alter the volume flow and/or composition of the plasma and the ECF. As the flow of plasma decreases, the patient becomes hypotensive, hypoxic, and hypoperfused. As the plasma flow deficit and the extracellular deficits are corrected, the patient becomes more closely normotensive.

2. ALDOSTERONE EFFECT ON BLOOD PRESSURE

Aldosterone's main effect is in maintaining normal sodium concentration in the extracellular fluid compartment. Sodium is the most abundant cation in the extracellular fluid. All other cations and anions will be present in varying ratios to the sodium. Aldosterone promotes reabsorption of sodium in both the proximal convoluted tubule and the collecting ducts of the kidneys. Sodium will "drag along" water, bicarbonate, chloride, and other ions as it is reabsorbed. This mechanism will help restore extracellular and intracellular fluid volumes, alter the composition of the compartments as needed, and subsequently, in a normal, healthy kidney maintain the blood pressure.

3. RENIN-ANGIOTENSIN MECHANISM

This mechanism has the most potent effect upon systemic blood pressure once angiotensin II is released into the vascular system because of its vasoconstricting properties. Any and all factors which decrease glomerular filtration rate may activate this system.

THE RENIN-ANGIOTENSIN CASCADE

Once activated, the juxtaglomerular apparatus (JGA), located adjacent to the glomeruli, releases inactive renin (that has presumably been stored in the JGA). Then the renin-angiotensin cascade is:

Angiotengenisin (renin granules)
    ←Renin enzyme (inactive renin)
    ↘Angiotensin I
    ←Converting enzyme in the lungs
    ↘Angiotensin II

Angiotensin II is the most potent vasoconstricting agent known. Angiotensin II in the circulatory system causes a severe constriction of peripheral arterioles and a milder constriction in the venous system. It also causes a constriction of renal arterioles. This results in the kidneys reabsorbing sodium and water. This reabsorption expands the extracellular fluid volume.

Angiotensin II stimulates the release of aldosterone, in addition to constricting the renal arterioles, to enhance sodium and water reabsorption supporting an increase in circulating volume (mechanism II). This increase in sodium stimulates the thirst mechanism (mechanism I) in an effort to help re-establish circulating volume.

On rare occasion, some factors initiate the release of renin and the release is *never* turned off. The continuous presence of renin *may* maintain an active system known as malignant hypertension. The key to treating malignant hypertension is to cut off the release of renin.

4. PROSTAGLANDINS

These are the last mechanism the kidney has to affect systemic blood pressure. The role prostaglandins play in blood pressure control is still hypothetical. It was once thought that prostaglandins were originally located in the seminal vesicles and produced by the prostate gland (thus their name). It is now known that prostaglandins are lipids found in most cells, but highly concentrated in the kidneys, the brain, and the gonads. It is also known that prostaglandins or their precursors are synthesized in the medullary interstitial cells and the collecting tubules of the kidneys.

Theoretically, prostaglandins promote a *vasodilation* of the renal medulla to maintain renal perfusion.

Prostaglandins may have a systemic effect upon blood pressure, but it is more likely that prostaglandins' *major* effect is intrarenal—to maintain renal perfusion in the face of severe or prolonged systemic hypoperfusion.

Red Blood Cell Synthesis and Maturation

Renal erythropoietic factor is an enzyme that is currently thought to be released by a hypoxic kidney (decreased renal oxygen). After being released into the bloodstream, the erythropoietic factor reacts with a glycoprotein to break away as erythropoietin. Erythropoietin circulates in the blood for about 24 hours. During this time, it stimulates red blood cell production by the bone marrow. After five or more days, a maximum rate of red blood cell production is achieved. The life of the RBC is approximately 120 days.

Either the kidney itself synthesizes the erythropoietic factor by releasing an enzyme called renal erythropoietin factor, or some other factor which is the precursor of erythropoietin. Bone marrow, by itself, does not respond to hypoxia by producing new red blood cells.

Patients with chronic renal failure walk around with hemoglobins of five and six grams. Because the kidneys are not functioning, they do not respond to hypoxia and they cannot produce erythropoietin factor. It is believed that possibly 10% of erythropoietin is formed in some place other than the kidney.

26

Renal Control of Electrolytes and Electrolyte Imbalances

Learning Objectives

By the end of this chapter, the nurse will be able to:

1. List the major electrolytes of the body and the normal serum levels of each.
2. Explain the body's regulating mechanisms for sodium.
3. Compare the symptoms and treatment of hypernatremia and hyponatremia.
4. List the major causes of hypernatremia and hyponatremia.
5. Describe the body's regulating mechanisms for potassium.
6. Compare the symptoms and treatment of hyperkalemia and hypokalemia.
7. List the major causes of hyperkalemia and hypokalemia.
8. Explain the body's regulating mechanisms for calcium.
9. Compare the symptoms and treatment of hypercalcemia and hypocalcemia.
10. List the major causes of hypercalcemia and hypocalcemia.
11. Describe the body's regulating mechanisms for phosphate.
12. Compare the symptoms and treatment for hyperphosphatemia and hypophosphatemia.
13. List the major causes of hyperphosphatemia and hypophosphatemia.
14. Explain the body's regulating mechanisms for magnesium.
15. Compare the symptoms and treatment for hypermagnesemia and hypomagnesemia.
16. List the major causes of hypermagnesemia and hypomagnesemia.
17. Explain the body's regulating mechanisms for chloride.
18. Compare the symptoms and treatment of hyperchloremia and hypochloremia.

Within one hour of cessation of kidney function, physiologic deterioration of the body begins due to a lack of electrolyte regulation. Electrolytes are in a precarious balance in the critically ill patient. Continuous monitoring is essential to correct imbalances early, to retard generalized deterioration, and to provide assistance to the kidneys in re-establishing homeostasis.

The electrolytes of major concern are sodium, potassium, calcium, chloride, phosphate, and magnesium. All electrolyte imbalances are a result of either ingestion of or reabsorption of too much of the electrolyte or lack of ingestion or excretion of too much of the electrolyte. Most body fluid imbalances are caused by a dysfunction in the regulation of electrolytes and water by the kidney. The kidneys even attempt to compensate for vomiting and diarrhea.

Sodium (Na+)

SODIUM REGULATION

Sodium is the most prevalent cation in our bodies' *extracellular fluid* compartment and it directly influences the fluid (water) load of the body. It is the second most important intracellular fluid cation. It exists in the body in combination with an anion, usually chloride. Sodium is important in maintaining extracellular fluid osmotic pressure. It is also responsible for some of the water exchange between intracellular (ICF) and extracellular (ECF) compartments.

REABSORPTION OF SODIUM

Normal serum sodium level (which is nearly identical to extracellular fluid sodium level) is 135–145 mEq/L. To maintain this level, sodium is reabsorbed from four parts of the kidney. The majority of filtered sodium is reabsorbed in the proximal convoluted tubules, and lesser amounts in the loop of Henle, in the distal convoluted tubule, and in the collecting ducts.

Effects of the glomerular filtration rate on sodium reabsorption were discussed in Chapter 25 in the discussion on urine formation.

EXCRETION OF SODIUM

Sodium may be excreted to maintain its level in the normal serum range of 135–145 mEq/L. Aldosterone has the greatest influence on sodium excretion.

Aldosterone is a mineralocorticoid secreted by the adrenal cortex. It is the most potent natural inhibitor of sodium excretion. Aldosterone production and release is stimulated by high potassium levels, steroids (ACTH), and angiotensin II. Aldosterone acts on the distal convoluted tubule and the collecting duct to promote reabsorption of sodium and excretion of potassium. Without aldosterone present, the distal tubule and the collecting ducts cannot "fine tune" the amount of sodium reabsorbed. The increased reabsorption of sodium in the presence of aldosterone also results in reabsorption of water.

A *Third Factor* influences sodium excretion by the tubules. What the Third Factor actually is is still unknown. Some researchers feel it is an unidentified hormone. The point of origin for the Third Factor is also unknown. It is known that the Third Factor increases tubular *excretion* of sodium. If the Third Factor is blocked, sodium is reabsorbed.

Diuretic therapy is usually thought of in relation to potassium. However, furosemide (Lasix®) blocks the chloride pump in the thick portion of the ascending limb of the loop of Henle. This effectively blocks reabsorption of sodium. Ethacrynic acid plays a similar role. All of the loop diuretics may block sodium reabsorption.

An increased glomerular filtration rate increases sodium excretion. Decreased aldosterone and increased antidiuretic hormone levels increase sodium excretion also.

Sodium Imbalance— Hypernatremia

A serum sodium level above 145 mEq/L is termed hypernatremia. If there is a pure water loss or decreased intake, the hematocrit (HCT) will also be elevated, serum chloride will be above 106 mEq/L, urine specific gravity will be greater than 1.025, and urine sodium levels will be low. Hypernatremia is one of the most dangerous electrolyte disturbances due chiefly to neurologic and endocrine side effects. Hypernatremia may cause some depression of cardiac function. In clinical practice, hypernatremia sufficient to cause appreciable electrocardiographic abnormalities is incompatible with life.[1]

PATHOPHYSIOLOGY

Hypernatremia is simply too much sodium ingested or too little sodium excreted by the kidneys. It is almost always related to a decreased intake or an increased output of water.

ETIOLOGY

Hypernatremia has two categories: (1) that in which kidney function is normal and (2) that in which kidney function is abnormal.

1. **With normal kidney function**: A lack or insufficiency of antidiuretic hormone (ADH) is the most common cause of hypernatremia. Without ADH, excessive water is excreted (e.g., diabetes insipidus). The presence of aldosterone conserves the sodium. Any condition leading to polyuria with conservation of sodium results in hypernatremic dehydration (but conservation of sodium is not required to cause hypernatremia in all situations). Potassium depletion, hypercalcemia, and uncontrolled diabetes mellitus and diabetes insipidus are the most common causes of this form of hypernatremia. However, the mechanisms of the hypernatremia are different in each condition.

The comatose patient is a high-risk patient for hypernatremia since the thirst mechanism cannot be recognized or expressed.

Drug therapy may cause iatrogenic hypernatremia. Osmotic diuretics and administration of sodium bicarbonate are drug causes of hypernatremia.

Endocrine imbalances may precipitate hypernatremia. Excessive secretion of adrenocorticotropic hormone (ACTH) is a major cause, as is the presence of aldosterone in the absence of ADH.

---

[1]Chung EK: Electrolytes and the heart. *In* Electrolytes and the Body's Systems. New York: Intermed Communications, Inc., p. 6, 1977

2. **In abnormal kidney function**: There are two basic causes of hypernatremia. One is represented by nephrogenic diabetes insipidus, an inability of the kidney tubules to respond to ADH (antidiuretic hormone) and conserve water (which would dilute the sodium concentration). A second cause is that the kidneys may be too damaged to filter and excrete sodium.

CLINICAL PRESENTATION

Hypernatremia may occur with fluid retention or with dehydration. With fluid retention, edema, weight gain, and hypertension may be present. The more severe the fluid retention, the more severe the symptoms which may progress to dyspnea, agitation increasing to manic activity and convulsions, and a firm, rubbery skin turgor.

In hypernatremia with dehydration, signs include dry, sticky mucous membranes, oliguria, fever, tachycardia, and agitation progressing to manic activity, convulsions, coma, and death.

COMPLICATIONS OF HYPERNATREMIA

In hypernatremia with fluid retention, the excess fluid causes hypertension (which may become irreversible), a high cardiac output, and, eventually, pulmonary edema.

In hypernatremia without fluid retention, dehydration leads to hypotension, hypovolemia, decreased cardiac output, hypoxia, and respiratory arrest.

TREATMENT OF HYPERNATREMIA

Fluid administration in a dehydrated patient is the key to diluting the sodium and halting the progression towards respiratory arrest. Identifying and treating the underlying cause is the key to successful treatment of hypernatremia with fluid retention. The challenge is to stabilize the patient's hypertension, prevent pulmonary edema, and maintain neurologic stability.

Monitoring serum sodium is the guide to efficacy of treatment.

Sodium Imbalance— Hyponatremia

Hyponatremia is present when the serum sodium level is less than 130 mEq/L. Usually, the plasma chloride will be less than 98 mEq/L. Hematocrit (HCT) may be decreased due to water excess. Urine specific gravity is from normal to less than 1.010.

PATHOPHYSIOLOGY

Either too much water is ingested or retained by the kidneys, too little sodium is ingested (rare except in actual starvation) or too little sodium is reabsorbed by the kidneys, or too much sodium is excreted by the kidneys in hyponatremia.

ETIOLOGY

Hyponatremia is due to either (a) an excessive amount of water or (b) sodium depletion.

(a) Excessive amounts of water can occur in many situations. The postgastric or postintestinal surgery patient who has nasogastric suction in use and who is receiving intravenous D_5W may become hyponatremic in only two or three days. Repeated tap water enemas may result in hyponatremia. Occasionally, there are patients who simply drink far too much plain water.

Volume depletion (hypovolemia) is the main noniatrogenic, physiologic cause of hyponatremia. The most common cause is the syndrome of inappropriate ADH (SIADH) release. In this case the blood supply of ADH (antidiuretic hormone) never cuts off because there is no feedback mechanism or a neoplasm is present. The presence of ADH results in the kidneys reabsorbing water continuously and so diluting the body's sodium levels. This could be classified as isovolemic hyponatremia secondary to increased water intake and/or increased production of ADH (SIADH).

(b) Sodium depletion may occur with water retention or with dehydration.

The most common cause of hypovolemic hyponatremia is overuse of the thiazide diuretics and furosemide (Lasix®) resulting in a dilutional hyponatremia. Diarrhea is probably the second most common cause of hypovolemic hyponatremia. Addison's disease presents the same situation. Nasogastric suctioning and extreme diaphoresis without I.V. replacement of sodium cause hypovolemic hyponatremia. Diuresis, which can be due to exertion, hyperglycemia, and other factors, is also a cause of hypovolemic hyponatremia. Certain renal diseases such as interstitial nephritis may cause a hypovolemic hyponatremia as well as an aldosterone deficiency.

Hypervolemic hyponatremia often occurs in congestive heart failure (CHF) patients and patients with cirrhosis of the liver or the nephrotic syndrome due to water retention by the kidneys secondary to low cardiac output.

In isovolemic hyponatremia, the decreased sodium is dilutional.

In hypovolemic hyponatremia, sodium is lost and water follows. Proportionately more sodium is lost.

In hypervolemic hyponatremia, both sodium and water increase with a greater proportional increase in water.

CLINICAL PRESENTATION

Hyponatremia with Dehydration

If the hyponatremia is associated with decreased extracellular fluid, the symptoms are essentially the same as heat prostration. Apprehension and anxiety are followed by a feeling of impending doom. The patient is weak, confused or stuporous, and may have abdominal cramps and muscle twitching. In some cases, convulsions follow the muscle twitching rather quickly. Mucous membranes are dry. Azotemia develops and progresses to oliguria, then anuria. In severe cases, vasomotor collapse occurs with hypotension, tachycardia, and shock.

An interesting clinical presentation exists in cases of hyponatremia associated with dehydration. As dehydration progresses, fluid moves from the extracellular to the intracellular compartments. This transfer of fluid leaves the tissue more "plastic." In these instances, if you press a finger over the sternum, the fingerprint remains due to plasticity. At this point, the patient is very critically ill. This "finger printing of the sternum" indicates that much extracellular fluid has been excreted and plasma fluid has moved into the intracellular spaces from the vascular system. Without emergency treatment, the patient may die very quickly. In less severe cases, symptoms may include lassitude, apathy, headache, anorexia, nausea, vomiting, diarrhea, muscle spasms, and cramps.

Hyponatremia with Water Retention

In hyponatremia with water excess, signs of water intoxication are usually present. These are essentially signs of central nervous system involvement. They include apathy, coma, confusion, headache, generalized weakness, convulsions, and death.

Severe hyponatremia with water retention *or* dehydration generally leads to shock, convulsions/coma, and death.

TREATMENT OF HYPONATREMIA

The goal of treatment is to re-establish normal serum sodium levels as rapidly as possible while avoiding a fluid overload. In every instance except SIADH, replacement of sodium with normal or hypertonic saline is indicated. Close monitoring of all systems is essential along with serial serum sodium levels during this period.

In SIADH, the treatment is to restrict *ALL* water intake while attempting to aid the kidneys in excreting water normally. In susceptible SIADH patients, hypertonic saline administration may induce congestive heart failure.

Potassium (K$^+$)

POTASSIUM REGULATION

Potassium is the most prevalent intracellular cation in the body. Normal serum level is 3.5–5.0 mEq/L. Potassium maintains osmolarity and electrical neutrality inside the cell. Intracellular homeostasis is needed for converting carbohydrates into energy and for reassembling amino acids into proteins.

Transmission of nerve impulses are dependent upon potassium. The muscles of the heart, lungs, intestines, and skeletal muscles cannot function normally without potassium.

ALL of the potassium filtered by the glomeruli is reabsorbed in the proximal convoluted tubule. Potassium that is excreted is secreted from the interstitial medullary space into the distal convoluted tubules. It amounts to about 10–12% of the original potassium volume of the ultrafiltrate in the proximal convoluted tubules. The amount of potassium excreted depends largely upon the *volume* of urine. About 85% of the potassium is excreted in the urine and about 15% in the intestines. Even in hypokalemia (decreased potassium), a large urine volume will excrete potassium, further compounding problems. Sodium and potassium will compete against each other for reabsorption, and sodium normally wins. The normal ratio of potassium to sodium ion reabsorption is 1:35.

Sodium and potassium are intimately related, and factors which affect sodium reabsorption and excretion also affect the potassium. Potassium levels are commonly raised by intravenous fluids containing potassium chloride. Although the kidneys act readily to conserve sodium, potassium is poorly conserved, especially in patients who are critically ill and therefore under physiologic stress.

Factors that enhance excretion of potassium include an elevated intracellular potassium level (which may be caused by an acute metabolic or respiratory alkalosis that forces potassium into the cells). Diuretics and other factors resulting in high volume flow rates in the distal convoluted tubule result in increased excretion of potassium. Aldosterone functions as a feedback mechanism on the distal convoluted tubule and collecting ducts to reabsorb sodium and excrete potassium when the extracellular fluid potassium level is increased. This is aldosterone's normal action. The enhancement of sodium reabsorption may force potassium excretion.

Potassium maintains an extracellular to intracellular fluid gradient. This gradient is affected by the adrenal steroids, hypo-natremia, glycogen formation, testoster-one, and pH changes. The most significant of these influences is the pH. Serum potassium moves inversely to the pH. If the pH falls, potassium concentration increases. If the pH rises, potassium concentration decreases due in part to the ionic charge of potassium and hydrogen. The exact change is 0.6 mEq/L of potassium for every 0.1 unit change in pH. Serum potassium must be evaluated with the arterial blood gases to avoid compounding problems of potassium therapy.

Potassium Imbalance— Hyperkalemia

Hyperkalemia is a potassium level greater than 5.5 mEq/L. It is a common occurrence in burns and crush injuries of tissue which release potassium from the cells into the extracellular and plasma fluid compartments.

PATHOPHYSIOLOGY

Hyperkalemia is due to an inability of the kidney tubules to excrete potassium ions. Tubular damage or increased potassium load that exceeds the kidney's ability to handle the quantity of potassium results in hyperkalemia.

ETIOLOGY

Hyperkalemia can be due to acute and chronic renal disease, low cardiac output, or sodium depletion. Any factor that destroys the cells will release the intracellular potassium, thus causing hyperkalemia. Such factors would include burns, trauma, and crush injuries of the tissues increasing serum potassium levels. Excessive ingestion by the patient of potassium chloride, found in antacids and salt substitutes, is by no means a rare cause of hyperkalemia. Excessive administration of potassium chloride is a more rare cause of hyperkalemia (iatrogenic induced) but it occurs, especially in the treatment of acidosis. Hypoaldosteronism (adrenal cortical insufficiency) is a less common cause.

CLINICAL PRESENTATION

Hyperkalemia causes a dilated and flaccid heart accompanied by a bradycardia. Generalized muscle irritability or flaccidity, which may be severe enough to be a flaccid paralysis, and numbness of extremities are present. Often, oliguria is present. There may be abdominal cramping and diarrhea. Generally, the patient is apathetic and may be confused.

EKG tracings show a tall, peaked or tent-shaped T wave with potassium levels of 5.5–7.5 mEq/L. In marked hyperkalemia (potassium of 7.5–9 mEq/L), there is a flattening and widening of the P wave, a prolonged P-R interval, and, usually, depression of the S-T segment. In severely advanced hyperkalemia (potassium of 8–9 mEq/L and often more than 10 mEq/L), the P waves disappear and intraventricular conduction disturbances occur producing intraventricular and supraventricular dysrhythmias progressing to ventricular tachycardia, ventricular standstill or fibrillation, and death.

TREATMENT OF HYPERKALEMIA

A serum potassium level above 7.5 mEq/L is considered an emergency. Treatment is initiated to prevent increasing bradycardia and cardiac arrest. The objective of treatment is to reduce the serum potassium to a "safe" level as rapidly as possible.

Intravenous 10% glucose with regular insulin will induce a cellular deposition of potassium with glycogen. Intravenous sodium bicarbonate will buffer cellular hydrogen and allow potassium to move intracellularly. Calcium chloride, calcium gluconate, or calcium gluceptate will oppose the cardiotoxic effects of hyperkalemia. (Calcium therapy is contraindicated in patients on digoxin.) Kayexalate® is given orally or via the rectum to rid the body of potassium. (Kayexalate® forces a one-for-one exchange of sodium for potassium in the intestinal cell wall.) *Caution*: Monitoring for sodium retention and gastrointestinal bleeding is imperative. Sorbitol® is used to induce semi-liquid stools (an osmotic diarrhea).

These measures are all emergency steps

to buy time in evaluating the underlying cause of the hyperkalemia. If the cause is physiologic or if the hyperkalemia is refractory, dialysis is indicated. If the cause is overingestion, the emergency treatments may be sufficient and the patient may need only additional conservative treatment, close monitoring, and teaching to prevent recurrences.

Potassium Imbalance— Hypokalemia

Hypokalemia is a serum potassium level of less than 3.5 mEq/L. It is almost always accompanied by other electrolyte and fluid imbalances.

PATHOPHYSIOLOGY

Hypokalemia is simply a potassium loss greater than potassium intake.

ETIOLOGY

Hypokalemia may be due to alkalosis, which stimulates secretion of potassium in the distal convoluted tubules of the kidney. Diuretic therapy, without potassium replacement, is a common cause. Endocrine dysfunction (increased ACTH, thyroid storm) and renal dysfunction (tubular acidosis) may all cause hypokalemia.

Gastric and intestinal surgery, nasogastric suctioning, and intestinal diseases predispose the patient to hypokalemia unless replacement therapy is maintained.

CLINICAL PRESENTATION

Hypokalemia has many of the same signs as hyperkalemia. There is a general malaise and muscle weakness which may progress to a flaccid paralysis. Anorexia, nausea, and vomiting may accompany a paralytic ileus. Mental status may range from drowsiness to coma. Hypotension may be present and may lead to cardiac arrest. If the patient is on digitalis, signs of digitalis toxicity may be present because hypokalemia potentiates the effect of digitalis.

Cardiac dysrhythmias are most commonly atrial unless the hypokalemia is pro-

found, in which case premature ventricular beats are found. Other ventricular dysrhythmias are rare, unless digitalis toxicity complicates the picture. EKG tracings most commonly show a prominent U wave. Depression or flattening of the S-T segment or inversion of the T wave may be apparent. An inverted T wave may fuse with the U wave, giving a *false* appearance of a prolonged Q-T interval. The Q-T interval is *NOT* altered by hypokalemia.[2] There is a generalized irritability of the heart in hypokalemic states.

Weakness of the muscles result in shallow respiration which may progress to apnea. In hypokalemia, death may be due to respiratory arrest.

TREATMENT OF HYPOKALEMIA

Emergency treatment of *severe* hypokalemia is the *slow* (*NEVER* rapid) intravenous administration of potassium chloride *while* monitoring the patient's EKG patterns for dysrhythmias due to hyperkalemia. Monitoring patient symptoms, serum potassium levels, and arterial blood gases is imperative to prevent an iatrogenic hyperkalemia.

Nonemergency treatment is to replace potassium with intravenous fluids with potassium chloride added or with oral potassium supplements. (Oral supplements should be diluted to prevent gastrointestinal irritation and to facilitate absorption.) Monitor (and record) the patient's intake and output, cardiac status, potassium levels, and signs of alkalosis or impending digitalis toxicity.

Calcium (Ca++)

CALCIUM REGULATION

Normal serum calcium concentration is 8.5–10.5 mg/dl. Calcium, with phosphorous, makes bones and teeth rigid and

---

[2]Dunn MJ: Importance of sodium and potassium in arterial hypertension. *In* Electrolytes and the Body's Systems. New York: Intermed Communications, Inc., p.9, 1977

stong. Calcium is an integral part of cell cement, holding cells together and maintaining strength and thickness (thus permeability) of the cell membranes. Calcium exerts a quieting action on nerve cells thus maintaining normal transmission of nerve impulses. Calcium also activates specific enzymes of the blood clotting process and those involved in the contraction of the myocardium.

Ninety-eight percent of calcium filtered by the kidneys is reabsorbed along the same pathways as sodium. There are four major factors influencing calcium reabsorption: (1) parathyroid hormone, (2) vitamin D, (3) corticosteroids, and (4) diuretics.

1. *Parathyroid hormone (PTH)*: If the serum PTH level is increased, one result is stimulation of tubular reabsorption of ionized calcium from renal tubules. Reciprocally, the PTH increases phosphate excretion and there is an increase in calcium absorption from the gastrointestinal tract. PTH will mobilize calcium from the bones when the kidneys cannot/do not reabsorb sufficient calcium.

2. *Vitamin D* must be present in an activated form to promote absorption of calcium from the small intestines. Vitamin D is ingested in food, especially milk and vitamin pills. The vitamin must then be activated by ultraviolet (sun) light changing a chemical in the skin. This vitamin is additionally changed in the liver and, finally, the kidneys convert the vitamin to 1,25-dihydroxycholecalciferol which is known as activated vitamin D. The activated vitamin D promotes absorption of calcium from the small intestines. PTH stimulates this activation process since a low serum level of calcium precludes an increase of calcium absorption in the kidney without PTH.

3. *Corticosteroids* are suspected of interfering with the activation of vitamin D, possibly in the liver, and decreasing the amount of calcium absorbed from the small intestines.

4. *Diuretics* can cause increased excretion of calcium and the other electrolytes. If a fluid volume loss results in a decreased total body fluid volume, there will be a decreased glomerular filtration rate (GFR) resulting in *reduced* calcium excretion.

Calcium Imbalance— Hypercalcemia

Hypercalcemia exists when the serum calcium level is above 10.5 mg/dl.

PATHOPHYSIOLOGY

Increased renal reabsorption of calcium may cause hypercalcemia. It may also be the result of increased intestinal absorption of calcium due to excessive dietary calcium intake. (In this instance, there must also be an excessive vitamin D ingestion.) There will be an increased calcium mobilization out of bone in primary hyperparathyroidism, prolonged immobilization, and thyrotoxicosis.

ETIOLOGY

Hyperparathyroidism caused by parathyroid adenoma will cause hypercalcemia mainly by increasing bone resorption but also by continuously stimulating the kidneys to reabsorb calcium. This also occurs in carcinoma of the parathyroid glands but is quite rare.

Multiple myelomas and metastatic carcinoma of the bone ("osteolytic [bone] lesions") cause hypercalcemia secondary to the release of calcium from the bone into the serum.

Prolonged bedrest or immobilization potentiates the movement of calcium from the bones, teeth, and intestines. Frequently, the calcium is deposited in joints, muscle tissue close to joints, and in the kidneys as calcium "stones."

Drugs, especially thiazide diuretics, *inhibit* calcium excretion leading to hypercalcemia in susceptible patients. Excessive doses of vitamin D cause hypercalcemia because such an excess increases calcium reabsorption in the intestines.

Renal tubular acidosis, thyrotoxicosis, and hypophosphatemia may all cause hypercalcemia in susceptible patients.

CLINICAL PRESENTATION

Hypercalcemia has an effect on almost every body system. Neurologic changes are subtle personality changes in early and mild hypercalcemia progressing to lethargy, confusion, and coma as the severity of the hypercalcemia increases. Neuromuscular changes progress from weakness and hypotonicity to flaccidness.

The renal system may be affected by the formation of calcium calculi with varying amounts of urine output dependent upon the location of the calculi, which may cause thigh or flank pain. Polyuria and polydipsia are often present because the increased calcium inhibits the action of ADH on the distal tubules and the collecting ducts.

Gastrointestinal symptoms include anorexia, nausea, vomiting, and constipation. Hypercalcemia stimulates gastric acid secretion and may lead to peptic ulcers. The hypotonicity caused by hypercalcemia results in decreased intestinal motility, and thus, constipation.

Cardiac changes are less common in hypercalcemia than hyperkalemia. The earliest EKG change is a shortening of the Q-T interval due to shortening of the S-T segment. It is *extremely* important to remember that digitalis and calcium are synergistic. Sudden death in hypercalcemia is often attributed to ventricular fibrillation due to this synergism.

An interesting ocular abnormality known as band keratopathy occurs on occasion due to deposition of calcium crystals in the cornea. This is called a metastatic calcification. Calcium is deposited at the lateral borders of the cornea in the shape of parentheses. If the calcification is extensive, calcium will be deposited in semi-lunar bands across the cornea connecting the parentheses. This band keratopathy may be seen by the naked eye.

COMPLICATIONS OF HYPERCALCEMIA

Three major complications of hyper-calcemia are the development of renal calculi (due to high urine calcium levels), neuropathies (due to the depressant action of calcium on the central and peripheral nervous systems), and cardiac dysrhythmias (due to stimulation of the myocardium).

TREATMENT OF HYPERCALCEMIA

The objective of treatment is to reduce the serum calcium level. Normal saline I.V.s and diuretics will increase the GFR and thus excretion of calcium, providing there are no obstructive calculi. These treatments require accurate intake and output monitoring.

Drug therapy includes corticosteroids (which will decrease gastrointestinal absorption of calcium), mithramycin (which actually depresses mobilization of calcium *from* the bones), and phosphates (which will bind to calcium in the intestines and precipitate calcium when administered intravenously).

Neurologic and cardiac monitoring are essential in assessing the efficacy of treatment. Some underlying causes (such as multiple myeloma) will tend to make hypercalcemia refractory to treatment. In such cases, the goal of therapy becomes keeping the calcium level as low as possible.

Calcium Imbalance— Hypocalcemia

Hypocalcemia is a clinical condition in which the serum calcium level is less than 8.5 mg/dl.

PATHOPHYSIOLOGY

Hypocalcemia usually develops from an excessive loss of calcium (e.g., diarrhea, diuretics, hyperlipoproteinemia, malabsorption syndromes, or from hypoparathyroidism).

ETIOLOGY

Chronic renal failure is probably the most common cause of hypocalcemia. If calcium is lost in peritoneal dialysis and/or hemo-dialysis, a hyperphosphatemia may occur. This enhances a peripheral deposition of calcium. Calcium deposits keep calcium from being available to raise serum levels. There is also an inability of the patient with chronic renal failure to absorb calcium from the intestines secondary to a lack of activated vitamin D.

Alkalosis can cause a hypocalcemia because the calcium becomes bound to a protein and thus remains inactive in the serum.

Chronic malabsorption syndromes are probably the second most common cause of hypocalcemia. These syndromes are found in gastrectomy patients, patients with small bowel diseases, patients who eat a high fat diet (fat impairs calcium absorption), and patients with a magnesium deficiency (magnesium inhibits PTH).

Malignancies are not infrequent causes of hypocalcemia. These include osteoblastic metastases (whereby calcium is used for abnormal bone synthesis) and medullary carcinoma of the thyroid (causing an increased secretion of thyrocalcitonin which in turn stimulates osteoblasts and prevents calcium from entering the serum).

Hypoparathyroidism of any etiology causes hypocalcemia since there is a decreased secretion of PTH. The most common causes are surgical removal of the parathyroids, adenoma of the parathyroids, depleted magnesium levels (inhibits PTH), and idiopathic hypoparathyroidism.

Vitamin D deficient states (or nonactivated vitamin D) is often seen in chronic renal failure, liver failure, and rickets. Without activated vitamin D, calcium is not absorbed from the intestines.

Acute pancreatitis causes a precipitation of calcium in the inflamed pancreas and in intra-abdominal lipids.

In hyperphosphatemia, phosphates and calcium bind together and precipitate in tissues. This is commonly found in chronic renal failure due to decreased excretion of phosphates. Increased oral intake of phosphates almost never causes hyperphosphatemia *if* renal function is normal.

CLINICAL PRESENTATION

Neuromuscular irritability is the overwhelming symptom present and the most dangerous. Muscle tremors and cramps are present in mild hypocalcemia. As the calcium level drops, tetany and generalized tonic-clonic seizures occur. Neuromuscular irritability causes labored, shallow respirations. Wheezing will be present if bronchospasms have occurred. Bronchospasms may lead to laryngospasm and tetany of the respiratory muscles resulting in respiratory arrest. Monitoring the neurologic status by Chvostek's sign and by Trousseau's sign is important.

To test Chvostek's sign, tap your finger over the supramandibular portion of the parotid gland which is located in the subcutaneous tissue of the cheek. If the upper lip twitches on the side of stimulation, the test is positive.

To test Trousseau's sign, apply a blood pressure cuff to the arm and inflate it until a carpopedal spasm occurs. If no spasm appears in three minutes, the test is negative. To test this result, remove the blood pressure cuff and have the patient hyperventilate (>30 breaths/minute). The respiratory alkalosis that develops may produce the carpopedal spasm. This indicates a positive test.

The neuromuscular irritability frequently causes a decreased cardiac contractility leading to a cardiac arrest. The earliest EKG change is a lengthening of the Q-T interval due to a lengthening of the S-T segment. Significant dysrhythmias *due to hypocalcemia* are extremely rare. The neuromuscular irritability may also cause biliary colic and paralytic ileus.

Occasionally, the main symptom first noticed is an alteration in blood clotting. Calcium is necessary for normal blood clotting, so hypocalcemia is often accompanied by bleeding dyscrasias.

TREATMENT OF HYPOCALCEMIA

The aim of treatment is to raise the calcium level to normal as rapidly as possible to halt or prevent tetany.

If phosphate deficiency is present, phosphates should be administered before calcium (prevents precipitation). In cases of tetany or impending tetany, intravenous 10% calcium gluconate, calcium gluceptate, or calcium chloride is administered. The patient must be on a cardiac monitor because a rapid infusion may enhance digitalis *and* because hypocalcemic patients are often also hyperkalemic.

Vitamin D supplements are administered if a deficiency is present.

Monitoring serum calcium, phosphate, and potassium levels along with EKG monitoring and neurologic monitoring (using Chvostek's and Trousseau's signs) will evaluate the efficacy of patient treatment.

Phosphate ($PO_4^{\equiv}$)

The normal serum level is 3.0–4.5 mg/dl. The phosphate ion is found in bones and is a major factor in intracellular production of ATP (energy). It combines with proteins and lipids to form important intracellular molecules. Intracellular phosphate ions may react with the genetic DNA and RNA molecules.

PHOSPHATE REGULATION

Phosphate levels are influenced by two major factors. Parathyroid hormone increases renal excretion of phosphate ions. The concentration of calcium is the second factor in regulating phosphate. Calcium and phosphate have a reciprocal relationship. If calcium levels increase, phosphate levels decrease and, conversely, if calcium levels decrease, phosphate levels increase.

Reabsorption of phosphates occurs actively in the proximal convoluted tubule in the presence of sodium. (Without sodium, phosphates will not be reabsorbed.)

Excretion of phosphates is regulated by PTH and the GFR. PTH inhibits reabsorption of phosphates in the proximal tubule, so phosphates will be excreted. The GFR regulates phosphates in the same manner as for most of the electrolytes.

Phosphate Imbalance— Hyperphosphatemia

A serum level above 5.5 mg/dl constitutes hyperphosphatemia.

PATHOPHYSIOLOGY

Inability to excrete phosphates or excessive ingestion of phosphates are the two pathologic processes of hyperphosphatemia. The inability to excrete phosphates may be due to a decreased GFR (of one-tenth the normal) or to renal failure.

Excessive ingestion of phosphates may be due to diet, excessive laxative use, or use of cytotoxic drugs.

ETIOLOGY

The most common cause is acute and chronic renal failure. Routine use (or abuse) of phosphate-containing laxatives and enemas is probably the second most common cause. Treatment of leukemias and lymphomas is most often with a cytotoxic agent. Hypoparathyroidism causes hyperphosphatemia secondary to the effects of PTH on the kidney. Occasionally, overadministration of intravenous or oral phosphates will induce a hyperphosphatemia.

CLINICAL PRESENTATION

Clinical presentation for hyperphosphatemia is the same as for hypocalcemia. Elevated phosphate levels enhance the movement of calcium into bone.

If seizures occur, they are due to hypocalcemia caused by hyperphosphatemia. Remember that calcium and phosphate have a reciprocal relationship.

Metastatic calcification occurs when calcium and phosphates chemically combine to form calcium phosphate. This then precipitates in arteries, soft tissue, and joints.

TREATMENT

The object of therapy is to decrease the serum phosphate level. Effective therapy is giving aluminum hydroxide gels which combine with phosphate, limiting the amount of phosphate available for absorption in the intestines. It is important NOT to confuse gels with antacid preparations. Patients need to be taught the difference to help prevent recurrences.

Phosphate Imbalance— Hypophosphatemia

Hypophosphatemia is a serum phosphate level of less than 3.5 mg/dl.

PATHOPHYSIOLOGY

Any factor that increases the cellular uptake to form sugar phosphates will decrease serum levels of phosphate. A decreased phosphate absorption from the intestines (malabsorption syndromes) is another process causing hypophosphatemia. Loss of proximal convoluted tubular function (renal phosphate wasting) resulting in hypophosphatemia is seen in Fanconi's syndrome and in cases of rickets that are vitamin D resistant.

ETIOLOGY

Chronic alcoholism results in a dietary deficiency of phosphates and may interfere with the absorption of any phosphates present.

Abuse (including overuse) of phosphate binding gels such as Amphojel® causes hypophosphatemia.

Hyperparathyroidism (causing renal phosphaturia) and malabsorption syndromes are causative factors.

Long-term hyperalimentation may contribute to hypophosphatemia if phosphates are not included in the solution in adequate amounts. (Utilization of the high glucose content in hyperalimentation solutions requires phosphates.) This is no longer a common etiology.

Chronic phosphate depletion occurs in Fanconi's syndrome. This syndrome exhibits a loss of phosphates in the urine leading to osteomalacia in adults and rickets in children. Osteomalacia is a softening of the bones due to demineralization and accompanying chronic hypocalcemia.

CLINICAL PRESENTATION

Complaints of general malaise, anorexia, and vague muscle weakness may be of chronic or acute onset. With chronic onset, muscle wasting is apparent. With an acute onset, rhabdomyolysis (a diffuse muscle-wasting necrosis) is due to a depletion of intracellular ATP and a concurrent decrease in all ATP-mediated processes. (This is commonly seen in heroin addicts and others who "shoot-up" with their kness propped over the wooden arms or backs of chairs or their extemities bent at close to 90-degree angles for prolonged periods of time. This decreases arterial circulation and results in an acute nontraumatic rhabdomyolysis.)

Hypercalcemia and hypercalciuria, with associated symptoms, are indices of acute phosphate depletion due to hyperparathyroidism (PTH increases serum calcium by removing it from bone and decreases serum phosphate by excretion in the urine).

Hypoxia occurs because of a decrease in dissociation of oxygen and hemoglobin. Hypoxia causes mental confusion.

Complicating hypophosphatemia may be osteomalacia (defined earlier) and Zieve's syndrome. This syndrome is rare and usually seen in chronic alcoholism. It is a severe intravascular hemolysis caused by a phosphate depletion that results in a decrease of 2,3-DPG in RBCs.

TREATMENT

The objective of therapy is to replace the phosphates, first by intravenous administration, and then orally. Use of phosphate-binding gels is discontinued and then treatment of the underlying cause of hypophosphatemia is started.

Magnesium (Mg++)

The normal serum level is 1.5–2.5 mEq/L. The magnesium ion is the second major *intracellular* cation. It is involved in the cellular enzyme activity and many biochemical reactions. Almost half of the body's magnesium is in the heart, liver, and skeletal muscles.

MAGNESIUM REGULATION

Renal reabsorption of magnesium is essentially the same as calcium. The presence of sodium directly affects the reabsorption in the proximal tubules. Without sodium, there is no reabsorption. PTH appears to have a minimal effect on reabsorption. Reabsorption processes of calcium and magnesium are mutually suppressive.

Magnesium Imbalance— Hypermagnesemia

Hypermagnesemia is a serum level above 2.5 mEq/L. This is extremely rare.

PATHOPHYSIOLOGY

Reabsorption is similar to the calcium process. The presence of excessive sodium (due to any cause) being absorbed in the renal tubules may "drag" an excessive amount of magnesium back into the blood, also.

ETIOLOGY

Chronic renal disease and untreated diabetic acidosis are the usual causes. Addison's disease, hyperparathyroidism, and excessive magnesium administration are other causes.

CLINICAL PRESENTATION

Lethargy, coma, and impaired respirations are the usual symptoms. All of the symptoms of hyperkalemia may be present. EKG changes consist first of prolonged P-R intervals, followed by widening of the QRS complex as the magnesium concentration rises. Death usually occurs with a concentration of 6 mEq/L or more.

TREATMENT

Attempts to lower magnesium levels by hemodialysis with a hypomagnesium dialysate have been successful.

Magnesium Imbalance— Hypomagnesemia

A magnesium level of less than 1.5 mEq/L is a state of hypomagnesemia.

PATHOPHYSIOLOGY

Any inhibition of absorption of magnesium from the gastrointestinal tract or of reabsorption from the renal system may account for hypomagnesemia.

ETIOLOGY

Severe malabsorption syndromes, acute pancreatitis, chronic alcoholism, primary aldosteronism, and diabetic acidosis during DKA treatment are the usual causes.

CLINICAL PRESENTATION

Neuromuscular and central nervous system hyperirritability characterize hypomagnesemia. Muscle tremors, delerium, convulsion, and coma are seen. Hypomagnesemia may result in digitalis-induced dysrhythmias.

TREATMENT

The objective of treatment is simply to provide sufficient magnesium to raise the serum level. This can be achieved by intravenous administration of fluids with this ion added or orally by a diet high in magnesium.

Chloride (Cl^-)

Normal serum chloride level is 98–106 mg/dl. Chloride was the first electrolyte that could be easily measured. The "chloride shift" (Chapter 2) was the index to treatment.

REGULATION OF CHLORIDE

Chloride is reabsorbed by the kidney at all of the sites for sodium reabsorption. Chloride moves freely with the gastric and intestinal fluids and is reabsorbed accordingly.

Excretion of chloride is influenced by the acid-base balance. In acidosis, chloride is excreted while bicarbonate is reabsorbed. This helps maintain electrochemical balance. In alkalosis, chloride is reabsorbed while bicarbonate is excreted.

Chloride Imbalance— Hyperchloremia

Hyperchloremia is a serum chloride level above 106 mg/dl.

An excessive ingestion of chloride or an excessive kidney reabsorption of chloride ions are the pathophysiologic changes in hyperchloremia.

ETIOLOGY

Excessive ingestion of chloride is the usual cause of hyperchloremia.

CLINICAL PRESENTATION

The symptoms are the same (or very similar) to hypokalemia.

TREATMENT

The objectives of treatment are to reduce the chloride level, which is most often achieved by the treatment for metabolic acidosis (Chapter 3).

Chloride Imbalance— Hypochloremia

Hypochloremia is a serum chloride level of less than 98 mg/dl.

PATHOPHYSIOLOGY

Chloride ions are lost through excessive vomiting or gastric suction without replacement of electrolytes. This results in a physiologic metabolic alkalosis. The bicarbonate ion and chloride ion normally balance each other in kidney function.

ETIOLOGY

Prolonged loss of gastric juices, either by vomiting or gastric suction without electrolyte replacement, is the predominant cause.

CLINICAL PRESENTATION

Symptoms of hypochloremia include changes in sensorium, possible neuromuscular irritability, and usually slow, shallow respirations.

TREATMENT

The objective of treatment is to replace the lost chloride ions either orally or intravenously and to treat the metabolic alkalosis to re-establish acid-base balance.

— 27

Acute Renal Failure

Learning Objectives

By the end of this chapter, the nurse will be able to:

1. Define acute renal failure.
2. Explain the pathophysiology of prerenal failure.
3. List the common causes of prerenal failure.
4. Differentiate between intrarenal cortical and intrarenal medullary failure.
5. List the common causes of intrarenal cortical and medullary failure.
6. Define the pathophysiology of postrenal failure.
7. List the common causes of postrenal failure.
8. Explain the three phases of acute renal failure.
9. List the four major problems in renal failure.
10. State at least one nursing intervention for each of the four major problems in renal failure.

Definition

Acute renal failure (ARF) is a sudden reduction in the glomerular filtration rate that may produce oliguria or anuria with a concurrent increase in plasma creatinine and blood urea nitrogen (BUN). Oliguria is present if less than 300–400 cc of urine are produced per day. This is an obligatory water loss—the minimum amount of urine needed to rid the body of its daily wastes.

There is a disagreement regarding terminology. Some texts refer to acute renal failure as acute vasoactive nephropathy. Other specialists use acute renal failure interchangeably with acute tubular necrosis (ATN). Still other nephrologists use the term acute tubular necrosis in its purest sense: when there is cortical and/or medul-

lary involvement of the kidney. In this text, the term acute renal failure will be used as a general term and acute tubular necrosis as a specific term when renal cortical and/or medullary involvement is present.

Pathophysiology

Acute renal failure (ARF) is classified into three categories: (1) prerenal, (2) intrarenal, and (3) postrenal.

1. *Prerenal ARF* is usually a decreased renal perfusion secondary to a circulatory inadequacy. A decreased renal perfusion means a decrease in renal artery pressure leading to a reduced afferent arteriole pressure. Afferent arteriole pressures of less than 100

mm Hg may decrease glomerular filtration. The end result is decreased GFR resulting in oliguria and/or anuria.

Hypovolemia is the most common cause of acute renal failure in the critically ill patient.

2. *Intrarenal ARF* is caused by disease or injuries of the nephron from the glomerulus to the collecting duct. Subsequently, these intrarenal conditions can be cortical or medullary in nature.

Cortical conditions involve swelling of the renal capillaries and cellular proliferation. Infectious, vascular, and/or immunologic processes cause edema and some resultant cellular debris which obstruct the glomeruli, resulting in a fall in urine output.

Medullary involvement specifically affects the tubular portions of the nephron causing necrosis. The extent of medullary damage differs depending upon nephrotoxic injury or ischemic injury. Tubular necrosis, which occurs in a local, patchy pattern, is the result of nephrotoxic injury. Nephrotoxic injury affects the epithelial cells which *can* regenerate after the nephrotoxic injury is resolved. Ischemic injury extends to involve the tubular basement membrane and may involve peritubular capillaries and other parts of the nephron. Ischemic injury is more serious since the tubular basement membrane *cannot* regenerate.

3. *Postrenal ARF* usually indicates an obstruction is at or below the level of the collecting ducts. The obstruction may be partial or complete. If the obstruction is complete, the blockage and subsequent back up of urine flow involves both kidneys. Partial obstruction increases renal interstitial pressure. Glomerular filtration pressure is opposed to an increasing renal interstitial pressure force as urine backs up due to the obstruction. Eventually, urine output decreases due to decreased glomerular filtration.

Etiology

Prerenal failure has many causes. The MAJOR cause is hemorrhage resulting in hypovolemia with fluid and electrolyte imbalance. Other causes include decreased glomerular perfusion after an acute myocardial infarction and/or congestive heart failure. Excessive use of diuretics may also cause prerenal failure. Occasionally, following anesthesia and surgery, increased renal vascular resistance and/or the hepatorenal syndrome occur(s). Septicemia progressing to gram negative septic shock results in vasodilation and a resultant hypovolemia. Marked peripheral vasodilation, known as the third space phenomena, may occur and so decrease glomerular perfusion. Embolism or thrombosis may cause a bilateral renal vascular obstruction, resulting in decreased or no perfusion.

Intrarenal failure etiologies can be fairly well categorized as either of cortical etiology or medullary etiology. Table 27-1 summarizes the multiple causes of cortical and medullary intrarenal failure.

Table 27-1. Causes of intrarenal failure.

Cortical Nephron Failure
  Infections:
      Acute Glomerulonephritis
      Acute Pyelonephritis
  Goodpasture's Syndrome
  Severe Hypercalcemia
  Systemic Lupus Erythematosus (SLE)
  Malignant Hypertension

Medullary Nephron Failure
  Acute Tubular Necrosis (major cause)

  Nephrotoxic Causes:
      Exotoxins including:
        Heavy Metals
        Pesticides
        Fungicides
        X-ray Contrast Media
        Antibiotics:
            Aminoglycosides
            Cephalosporins
            Tetracyclines
            Penicillins

  Ischemic Causes:
      Endotoxins
      Crush Injuries
      Burns
      Overdoses
      Sepsis
      Cardiogenic Shock
      Postsurgical hypotension
      Hemorrhage with Multiple Trauma
      Hemolysis of Blood Transfusion
      Reaction

Postrenal ARF causes are obstructive in nature. Some causes are prostatic hypertrophy; bladder, pelvic, or retroperitoneal tumors; renal calculi; ureteral blockage (after surgery or instrumentation); urethral obstruction; bladder infections; or a neurogenic bladder.

If arterial blood perfusion drops below 60 mm Hg for over 40 minutes, the development of ARF is very high. If ARF is a postsurgical complication, the mortality rate approaches 60%. Overall, the mortality rate of ARF ranges from 40% to 70%.

Phases of ARF

There are three phases in the cycle of ARF: (1) an oliguric phase, (2) a diuretic phase, and (3) a recovery phase.

1. *The oliguric phase* reflects the obstruction of tubules from edema, tubular casts, and cellular debris. Damage to the tubules makes absorption and secretion of solutes variable. If the obstruction and damage is severe enough, a backleak of filtrate though the epithelium may occur, returning the filtrate into the circulation.

During the oliguric phase, laboratory reports will indicate rising levels of urea, creatinine, and potassium. The fluid and electrolyte imbalances caused by retaining the metabolic waste products are the greatest dangers to the patient.

2. *The diuretic phase* indicates the beginning of the return of tubular function. The diuretic phase occurs anytime in the first 30 days of ARF; but usually, it occurs between days 10 and 17. The greatest danger to the patient in this phase is excessive loss of water and electrolytes. Extreme diuresis is due to the osmotic diuretic effect produced by the elevated BUN and the inability of the tubules to conserve sodium and water resulting in an output of 3,000 cc or more of urine per 24 hours.

3. *The recovery phase* begins when the diuresis is no longer excessive. There is a gradual improvement in kidney function. This improvement may continue for 3–12 months. The end result may be a permanent reduction in the glomerular filtration rate which may or may not be sufficient to maintain adequate renal function without dialysis.

Acute renal failure may progress to chronic renal failure but is uncommon unless the patient has an underlying kidney disease or is of advanced age.

Clinical Presentation of ARF and ATN

Clinical signs and symptoms may be overlooked during the first few days due to the primary illness. Oliguria may be present or not. Fifty percent of ARF patients are nonoliguric. Most ATN patients are anuric. So, urine volume alone is not an adequate guide to renal function. Progressive azotemia (an excess of urea or other nitrogenous bodies in the blood) occurs as a result of decreased GFR in spite of apparently adequate urine output. ARF or ATN should be diagnosed before uremic signs are present.

Table 27-2 summarizes the uremic signs of ARF and ATN.

Table 27-2. Uremic signs of acute renal failure (ARF) and acute tubular necrosis (ATN).

Respiratory:
  Deep or Rapid Respiratory Rate
    (Metabolic Acidosis)
  Bilateral Rales
  Pulmonary Edema

Cardiovascular:
  Tachycardia
  Dysrhythmias
  Pericarditis
  Friction Rub

Neurologic:
  Decreased LOC
  Confusion
  Lethargy
  Stupor

Gastrointestinal:
  Nausea
  Vomiting
  Anorexia
  Constipation or Diarrhea

Diagnosis

Diagnosing ARF or ATN maybe a difficult task, especially in the non-oliguric patient. Factors which must be considered in a diagnosis include urinary volume, urinary sediment, BUN levels, serial serum creatinines, creatinine clearance, arterial blood gases, trauma, postsurgical status, and possibly a kidney biopsy. Usually, an intravenous pyelogram (IVP) is done before a kidney biopsy.

URINARY VOLUME

Complete anuria suggests obstruction or cortical necrosis. It may occur in acute glomerulonephritis and complete postrenal obstruction but is very rare otherwise. Daily urine output may be constant or may gradually increase in acute renal parenchymal disease. Different degrees of obstruction are suggested by large and irregular daily urine volumes. Partial obstruction can cause progressive azotemia, even though there may be normal or increased urine volume.

URINARY SEDIMENTS

In *prerenal failure* there are moderate numbers of hyaline and finely granular casts seen. Urinary Na+ is less than 10 mEq/L. Specific gravity is greater than 1.020. There is minimal or no proteinuria.

In *intrarenal failure* there are usually numerous renal tubular cells, tubular cell casts, coarse granular casts, red cells, red cell casts, hemoglobin casts, and hematuria.

In *postrenal failure* there is scanty sediment, rare white cells, red cells, hyaline casts, and finely granular casts.

URINE SODIUM, SPECIFIC GRAVITY, BUN, CREATININE

In *prerenal failure* the Na+ is less than 15 mEq/L. The specific gravity is more than 1.018. The BUN is greater than the creatinine (normal ratio 10:1).

In *postrenal failure* the Na+ is elevated. Specific gravity varies. The BUN and creatinine are elevated due to the complete obstruction.

KIDNEY BIOPSY

Ninety percent of all kidney biopsies have a significant but subclinical bleeding that averages 75–200 ml of blood. Ten percent of all biopsies will have gross hematuria. One percent of all biopsies will have a retroperitoneal bleed that requires blood transfusion. Of all biopsies, 0.5% bleed sufficiently to require surgery to control the bleeding; 0.01% of biopsies bleed to the extent of requiring a nephrectomy. Biopsies are not performed on polycystic kidneys. IVPs are almost always a preliminary test (prior to biopsies).

Management of Patient Care in ARF

There are four major problems of patient care in renal failure: (1) an increase in the products of catabolism, (2) severe electrolyte imbalance with associated acidosis, (3) fluid overload, and (4) infection. Let us look at these problems individually, even though in the clinical setting these problems normally occur concomitantly.

1. *Increase in the products of catabolism:* Caloric requirements of the patient must be met mainly through an adequate *carbohydrate* diet intake. Protein catabolism increases in the critically ill and stressed patient. A decrease in proteins available for catabolism will retard the rate of azotemia, decrease the incidence and severity of acidosis, and decrease the occurrence and levels of hyperkalemia in the serum.

2. *Serum electrolyte imbalance and acidosis:* Sodium intake is restricted unless there is a serum sodium deficit. No salt substitutes are used because of their potassium content. CAREFUL management of fluids and sodium intake will prevent overhydration, congestive heart failure, hyponatremia, and water intoxification.

Hyperkalemia—Each patient's tolerance to potassium is different. However, concentrations above 6.0 mEq/L cause abnormalities in the electrocardiogram and require emergency treatment. Potassium intoxication results from ingestion of potassium salt associated with diuretic therapy, and/or intake of large quantities of low sodium milk which is high in potassium. Potassium intoxication can occur as the result of catabolism associated with fever. It also occurs as a result of decreased potassium excretion caused by volume depletion or drugs. Metabolic acidosis can also cause hyperkalemia. The fall of the pH forces hydrogen ions into the cells and potassium into the extracellular fluid.

The goal of emergency treatment was covered in Chapter 26. The reader is referred to this chapter for review.

3. *Fluid overload:* It is essential to determine the patient's state of hydration and to continually assess this state.

Indicators of overhydration include weight gain, edema, anasarca, ascites, increased B/P, JVD (jugular vein distention), and dyspnea. Indicators for dehydration include weight loss, decreased B/P, poor skin turgor, no evidence of JVD, and decreased central venous pressure (less than 5 cm H_2O).

Fluids are restricted to amounts equal to urine output plus 400 cc for insensible fluid loss. It is vitally important that *accurate daily* weights are taken using the *same* scales. It is also important to remember that 1,000 cc of fluid weighs about 2.2 lb or 1.0 kg.

4. *Infection:* Since proper kidney function affects ALL body systems, the chance of infection is greatly increased in renal failure patients. The body defense systems do not function properly and the patient is predisposed to urinary tract infections, septicemia, pneumonia, and wound/skin infections due to the severe pruritis some patients experience. A good nutritional intake for the patient and proper hygiene will help prevent infections. If fever develops, culture and sensitivities of blood, urine, sputum, or any sore should be performed to identify the invading organism. Once identified, appropriate antibiotic therapy is started with antibiotic doses adjusted to renal function (since most antibiotics are excreted by the kidneys).

28

Peritoneal Dialysis

Learning Objectives

By the end of this chapter, the nurse will be able to:

1. Define peritoneal dialysis.
2. Define osmosis, diffusion, and filtration in relation to peritoneal dialysis.
3. List at least eight indications for peritoneal dialysis.
4. List four contraindications for peritoneal dialysis.
5. List two relative uses for peritoneal dialysis.
6. Describe four factors that increase the effectiveness of peritoneal dialysis.
7. Explain at least three advantages and three disadvantages of peritoneal dialysis.
8. List at least five complications of peritoneal dialysis.
9. Identify three signs of impending complications of peritoneal dialysis.
10. Define nursing interventions *before* peritoneal dialysis is instituted.
11. Identify the normal and abnormal color characteristics of the dialysate. State the significance of each.
12. Explain the intake-output records that must be kept on the peritoneal dialysis patient.

When the patient in acute renal failure has an increase in catabolism, or a rapid clinical or chemical deterioration, a decision must be made for either peritoneal dialysis or hemodialysis. Many clinical factors about the patient will influence the choice of dialysis.

Peritoneal dialysis has been used since the 1940s to treat renal failure. The objectives of dialysis are to drain off metabolic waste products and to re-establish fluid and electrolyte balance.

Principles Employed

Three principles are utilized in peritoneal dialysis. They are osmosis, diffusion, and filtration.

1. *Osmosis* is the movement of *fluid* aross a semipermeable membrane, from a less concentrated solution to a more concentrated solution. To increase osmotic strength, one increases osmolarity. This is accomplished by increasing the glucose

concentration in the dialysate. The higher concentration will "drag" more solutes out with the water. Stated differently, the amount of water drawn from the patient depends on the amount of glucose put in the dialysate.

2. *Diffusion* is the movement of *particles* (or solutes) across a semipermeable membrane, from a more concentrated solution to a less concentrated solution. Diffusion is facilitated by the higher concentration of solutes in the blood than in the dialysis solution (the dialysate).

3. *Filtration* is the process of hydrostatic pressure pushing body fluids out through the body's membranes. The peritoneum's filtering surface is about 22,000 cm^2. This is about the same amount of surface availability of the kidneys.

The peritoneum is a strong, smooth, colorless, serous membrane that lines the abdominal cavity with a parietal layer and wraps the abdominal organs with a visceral layer (Figure 28-1).

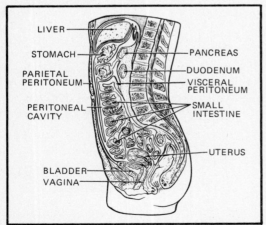

Figure 28-1. The peritoneal space (female).

The dialysate is instilled into the abdominal cavity between these two layers of peritoneum. The visceral peritoneum is contiguous with the intestinal wall and the capillary beds of the intestines. The dialysate is instilled into the peritoneal space, bathing the intestines. Thus, osmosis, diffusion, and filtration occur readily. The dialysate is usually left in the abdomen 20–30 minutes. This is called dwell time and is the common time, but it is not a universally standard time.

Indications for Peritoneal Dialysis

There are many instances in which peritoneal dialysis *may* be used. In acute renal failure, peritoneal dialysis may be used simply to treat the failure; or it may be used to prevent uremia while ascertaining an underlying cause, and/or while stabilizing a patient for surgery.

If a chronic renal failure patient has had a recent infection, he or she may undergo peritoneal dialysis to prevent localization of the infection at the fistula site. Patients who have an "arteriovenous access crisis," that is, an unavailability of the vascular access route for hemodialysis, may undergo peritoneal dialysis until an access route is available.

Circulatory overload from renal impairment with congestive heart failure is amenable to peritoneal dialysis. Refractory hyperkalemia and/or metabolic acidosis when alkali cannot be given are both indicators for peritoneal dialysis. Sometimes poisonings and drug overdoses are treated by peritoneal dialysis, but hemodialysis is more common because it removes the toxins more rapidly.

In chronic renal failure, peritoneal dialysis may postpone the need for chronic hemodialysis. In patients with diabetes, chronic hemodialysis may cause blindness associated with diabetic retinopathy. These patients may be candidates for peritoneal dialysis.

Often, a renal failure patient is at high risk of developing seizures due to rapid changes in electrolyte status. This is known as the "disequilibrium syndrome." To decrease the risk of seizures during *hemodialysis*, the patient may undergo peritoneal dialysis first; then, when seizures are less likely, a change to hemodialysis may be made.

Peritonitis is a controversial topic. Some nephrologists believe in adding antibiotics to the dialysate in addition to oral or intravenous antibiotics. The rationale is to bathe the infected area itself with antibiotics. Other nephrologists believe that peritonitis is justification for stopping peritoneal dialysis. The rationale here is to treat the patient with intravenous antibiotics to prevent septic shock from developing or weakening (to the actual point of rupture) an inflamed, infected visceral peritoneum and the intestinal wall contiguous with the peritoneum.

Contraindications for Peritoneal Dialysis

Any patient with blood clotting dyscrasias should not undergo peritoneal dialysis until (or if) the blood clotting problems have been resolved.

Patients with fresh postoperative vascular prostheses, such as a fresh femoral-popliteal bypass, are not candidates for peritoneal dialysis. The procedure may result in graft failure at the site of anastomosis resulting in exsanguination.

Obviously, anyone having had recent peritoneal surgery or anyone with postoperative abdominal drains is not able to undergo peritoneal dialysis. In the first instance, the peritoneum may not be strong enough to hold the dialysate without rupture or tearing of the peritoneum; and in the second case, abdominal drains preclude any dwell time since the dialysate would flow out the drains.

Abdominal adhesions or any other condition where a danger of puncturing viscera exists is a contraindication to peritoneal dialysis.

Relative Use for Peritoneal Dialysis

Occasionally, cases of acute necrotizing pancreatitis with renal failure may be treated with peritoneal dialysis.

The acute myocardial infarction patient with renal failure may be treated with peritoneal dialysis instead of hemodialysis to avoid the adverse effects of hemodynamic imbalance of hemodialysis. (In hemodialysis, a certain volume of the patient's blood is in the "kidney machine" and not in the patient during the entire procedure time.)

Increasing Effectiveness of Peritoneal Dialysis

There are four main factors that increase the effectiveness of peritoneal dialysis. They are concentration, temperature, time, and volume.

Increasing glucose concentration increases the clearance of water and solutes by osmosis, the "drag effect." When concentrations of glucose are high, osmosis occurs more rapidly and "drags" some other solutes with it.

The temperature of the dialysate influences effectiveness of peritoneal dialysis. Urea clearance is 35% *greater* at body temperature (98.6°F) than at room temperature (75°F). For both patient comfort and effectiveness of dialysis, the dialysate should be warmed to 98°F.

Time is an influence on the effectiveness of dialysis. The more rapid the exchange, the more efficient. Rapid means no more than one hour for instilling, dwelling, and draining (i.e., one complete exchange).

The volume of the dialysate influences effectiveness. An exchange volume of three liters of dialysate in one hour almost doubles the urea clearance achieved with one liter per hour. Most adults are tolerably comfortable with two liters per exchange and few can tolerate three liters, so we settle for the two-liter volume.

Advantages of Peritoneal Dialysis

Peritoneal dialysis can be done in almost any hospital. It can be initiated quickly. There is no need for systemic anticoagulation. There is a decreased chance of seizures and a decreased risk of hypotension. Elaborate expensive equipment requiring highly trained personnel is avoided.

Disadvantages of Peritoneal Dialysis

Respiratory insufficiency is common with peritoneal dialysis. As 2,000 cc of fluids are infused into the abdomen, both the fluid and abdominal viscera will push against the diaphragm, decreasing the depth of respirations. There is an increased chance of atelectasis and pneumonia. Two liters of fluid in the abdomen are uncomfortable to many patients. Xylocaine added to the infusion may relieve this discomfort.

Peritoneal dialysis is slower to rid the body of waste products than hemodialysis. It takes 48–72 hours to complete peritoneal dialysis, as opposed to 3–4 hours for hemodialysis. Prolonged peritoneal dialysis results in a protein depletion. There is a greater protein loss in peritoneal dialysis than hemodialysis. Often the protein loss is as high as 0.5 gm/L. This leads to acites, poor wound healing, and decreased resistance to infection.

If peritonitis sets in, it is usually due to staphylococcus or gram negative organisms. With peritonitis, some physicians will stop the peritoneal dialysis and others will continue it.

There may be difficulty in retrieving the dialysate in peritoneal dialysis, although by turning the patient side to side this is often resolved.

Perforation of the bladder and/or bowel can occur with insertion of the trocar. For this reason, the first dialysate infused is NOT allowed to dwell in the abdomen but is drained immediately so that one may observe the color and characteristics of the outflow fluid.

Shock may develop if the dialysate is hypertonic (4.25% glucose instead of the usual 1.5% glucose concentration). The *very* first sign of shock is usually an increase in the heart rate.

Complications of Peritoneal Dialysis

Infection is one of the most common complications of peritoneal dialysis. Insertion of the catheter under sterile technique and closed sterile instillation and drainage of dialysate will help reduce infection. Nursing intervention of daily (or more often) sterile changes of the dressing over the tube insertion site helps decrease the chance of infection. Perhaps the most effective prevention of infection is to keep the procedure time to 36 hours or less.

Volume depletion occurs if the dialysis is effective and removes several hundred milliliters of fluid per exchange. This will result in volume hypotension. Water removal may cause *hypernatremia*, if the 4.25% glucose dialysate (which is hypertonic) is used. Nursing intervention includes monitoring for signs of increasing sodium retention.

Volume overload may be a problem. When the patient is severely hyponatremic, sodium and water move into the third space. As third spacing resolves by sodium and water returning to the intravascular bed, cardiovascular overload may occur. Shortening dwell time and repositioning the patient may help. If not, the patient will need to go to hemodialysis.

Hyperglycemia may be severe if hypertonic fluid is used in the diabetic. Hyperosmolar coma and death have occurred. If hyperglycemia develops, the dialysis *MUST BE STOPPED* until the blood sugar is controlled. Suspect hyperglycemia if the patient complains of thirst or if there is a deterioration in the mental sensorium.

Metabolic alkalosis may occur if dialysis is continued for a long time. Dialysate fluid contains sodium lactate or acetate (45 mEq/L) which will be converted to sodium bicarbonate in the body. (The acetate or lactate would precipitate if added to the dialysate fluid.)

Digitalis intoxication is a frequent, serious complication. It is a result of lowering the serum potassium and at the same time correcting hypocalcemia, hyponatremia, and acidosis. The dose of the digitalis must be reduced in uremic patients. Serum levels of cardiac glycosides are not affected by routine dialysis.

Disequilibrium syndrome occurs more often in hemodialysis and will be covered in Chapter 29.

Perforation of viscera may occur when inserting the trocar. The trocar used to insert the catheter may perforate the bowel. If this has occurred, the dialysate will return brownish and fecal appearing. If the trocar perforates the bladder, either the patient has a sudden urge to void *or* the dialysate fluid may flow from the urethra. In either instance, *stop* the procedure and the physician will determine what action is warranted.

Signs of Impending Trouble

Severe pain at the end of inflow or outflow is not normal. This may be caused by the temperature of the dialysate, incomplete draining of the previous exchange, early stage development of peritonitis, or instillation of too much dialysate.

Bleeding is common in *small* amounts, especially where the catheter was inserted. The first exchange may be *slightly* blood-tinged. A large amount of blood indicates a ruptured viscera. Stop the dialysis. If the patient develops diarrhea, the bowel is probably ruptured. The presence of urine indicates rupture of the bladder. In *all* cases, stop the exchange and notify the physician.

Impending shock is the third sign of trouble. If the patient's systolic blood pressure drops 10 mm Hg or more, call the physician stat. This small drop in blood pressure indicates impending shock.

Nursing Interventions for the Patient on Peritoneal Dialysis

To help obtain the patient's cooperation, the nurse should explain the procedure, making the patient aware of the discomforts of, limited mobility during, and duration of the procedure. The patient should be weighed before the procedure and either daily or after the last exchange (using the same scales).

The physician will order the amount of heparin to be added to the dialysate (to prevent fibrin or blood from clotting the catheter). The amount of potassium chloride added depends on the patient's serum potassium level *and* the state of digitalization of the patient and the arterial blood gases.

Some physicians add lidocaine (usually 50 mg/2 liters of dialysate) for generalized abdominal discomfort. Some physicians also add antibiotics if peritonitis is present or suspected.

Peritoneal Procedure

Have the patient void or catheterize the patient immediately before the physician inserts the catheter. Figure 28-2 shows areas of catheter insertion and the catheter.

The physician numbs the insertion site with lidocaine, preps the skin to decrease germs, and introduces the trocar through a stab wound. The catheter is inserted and usually sutured or taped in place (Figure 28-3). The dialysate, which has been warmed, and the tubing setup is now connected to the catheter.

The first dialysate solution must be drained *as soon as it is instilled* to insure patency of the catheter. Outflow should drain in a steady stream.

If the catheter is patent, warmed dialysate should be infused, allowed to "dwell" (stay) in the abdomen, usually for 20–30 minutes, and then allowed to drain as completely as possible. One exchange should take about an hour.

The dialysate drained from the abdomen has certain characteristics. If it is normal, it will be clear, pale yellow. If the drainage is cloudy, suspect infection or peritonitis. If it is brownish, suspect bowel perforation. If it is amber, suspect bladder perforation. If it is *slightly* bloody during the first four exchanges, it may be normal. After four exchanges, if the dialysate is still bloody, stop and notify the physician. The patient may have abdominal bleeding or a uremic coagulopathy.

Periodic cultures are obtained of the dialysate drainage, and usually, the tip of the catheter is cultured when it is removed.

Monitoring of vital signs every 15 minutes the first hour and then every one to two hours is the usual procedure *if* the vital signs are stable. The *outflow period is the most likely time for abnormal or changing vital signs.* Signs of impending shock, fluid overload, and pulmonary edema will be most apparent in this outflow period.

Intake and Output Record

One of the most critical aspects of peritoneal dialysis is the intake-output record. It must be kept meticulously. Hospital policies vary in the format for recording peritoneal dialysis intake and output. The basic pattern is quite standard. Information needed is the time the exchange was started, the number of the exchange, the amount of fluid infused, the "dwell" time, the amount of fluid drained, and the fluid balance.

Fluid balance is crucial. If 2,000 cc were instilled and only 1,750 cc drained out, the patient fluid balance is +250 cc. If the next exchange instills 2,000 cc and drains 1,900 cc, the patient fluid balance for the exchange is +100 cc. The present balance would now be +350 cc. Assume the third exchange is with a 4.5% dialysate (hypertonic solution). The amount instilled was

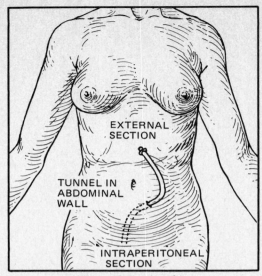

Figure 28-3. The catheter in place.

2,000 cc. The output drainage was 2,275 cc. The patient balance for *this* exchange is −275 cc. The patient gave back more fluid than instilled in this exchange. However, in the continuous fluid balance columns, the patient is still at a fluid balance of +75 cc. Intake and output records are maintained for each exchange and overall for total exchanges. When the peritoneal catheter is removed, there is a final total fluid balance for the dialysis session. (A sample flow sheet record is included here.)

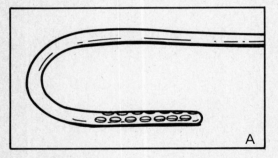

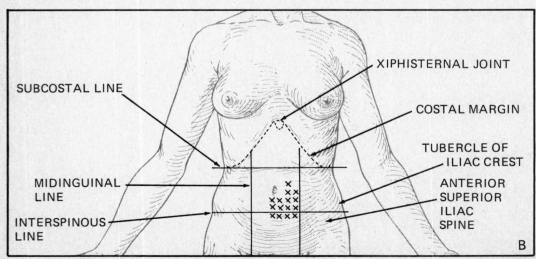

Figure 28-2. Peritoneal dialysis catheter (A) and areas of catheter insertion (B).

Sample Peritoneal Dialysis Flow Sheet

Exchange Number	Percent Solution	Medication Added	Solution In		Amount Infused	Dwell Time (Min.)	Solution Out		Fluid Out This Exchange	Balance This Exchange	Cumulative Fluid Balance
			Time Start	Time Ended			Time Start	Time Ended			
1	1.5	None	10:00 AM	10:15 AM	2,000 cc	0	10:15 AM	10:35 AM	1,750 cc	+250 cc	+250 cc
2	1.5	50 mg Xylocaine	10:40 AM	11:00 AM	2,000 cc	30	11:30 AM	11:50 AM	1,900 cc	+100 cc	+350 cc
3	4.5	None	11:55 AM	12:20 PM	2,000 cc	20	12:40 PM	1:00 PM	2,275 cc	−275 cc	+75 cc
4											
5											
6											
7											
8											
9											
10											
11											
12											
13											
14											
15											
16											

Comments:

29

Hemodialysis

Learning Objectives

By the end of this chapter, the nurse will be able to:

1. Define hemodialysis.
2. State at least one contraindication to hemodialysis.
3. Differentiate between "regional" and systemic (or general) heparinization.
4. Explain the difference between a shunt and a fistula.
5. Explain cannulation.
6. Define thrill and bruit.
7. List five nursing interventions for the patient on hemodialysis.
8. Explain disequilibrium syndrome and its treatment.
9. List at least four of the most common complications of hemodialysis and what treatment is needed.
10. Differentiate between venous and arterial air embolism, explaining the appropriate treatment.

Hemodialysis is a process of removing metabolic waste products of the body by use of extracorporeal circulation (the artificial kidney). This means the patient's blood is transferred by tubing to a machine that functions like a kidney to filter out the wastes and then returns the filtered blood to the patient by another tube. Hemodialysis uses the same principles of osmosis, diffusion, and filtration that are used in peritoneal dialysis.

Reasons for Hemodialysis

All of the reasons for performing peritoneal dialysis are the same as those for hemodialysis (except in patients with myocardial infarction). Other reasons for performing hemodialysis include acute renal failure due to trauma or infection, chronic renal failure no longer controlled by medication and diet, and cases where rapid removal of toxins, poisons, drugs, and such is essential.

Contraindications for Hemodialysis

Labile cardiovascular states that would deteriorate with rapid changes in intravascular fluid volume are the major contraindications to hemodialysis.

In past years, patients who could not tolerate systemic heparinization could not be hemodialyzed. Today, however, the kidney machine has a heparin pump to keep blood anticoagulated within the hemodialysis machine. Before the blood is returned to the patient, a protamine pump (Figure 29-1) neutralizes the heparin and the blood is returned to the patient. This process is called *regional heparinization*.

For the patient without a condition that would be worsened by heparin, general heparinization is used. In these cases, 2,000—5,000 units of heparin are injected into the arterial line at the start of hemodialysis and 1,000—2,000 units of heparin are added for each hour that the patient is on the machine. As is true with any patient on an anticoagulant, these patients must be monitored closely for signs of bleeding.

Access to Circulation

In order to hemodialyze someone, there must be a way of taking the patient's blood, running it through the artificial kidney, and returning it to the patient in a continuous cycle for several hours.

There are two types of access: One is external, the other internal. An arteriovenous shunt is external and an arteriovenous fistula is internal.

The Arteriovenous Shunt

The arteriovenous shunt (Figure 29-2) is the oldest technique for access. It is a semipermanent appliance that channels blood from an artery, through a kidney machine, and back into a vein. Part of the shunt lies subcutaneously and part outside the skin.

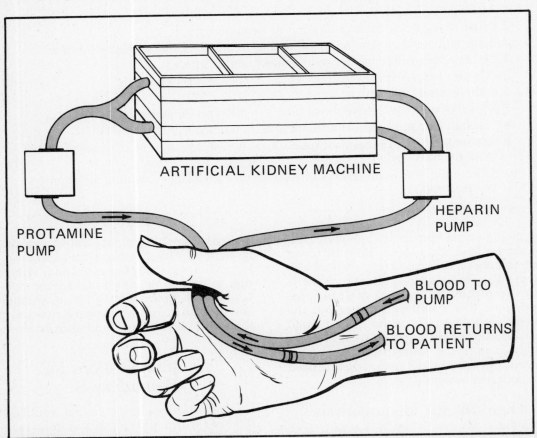

Figure 29-1. The kidney machine with a heparin and protamine pump.

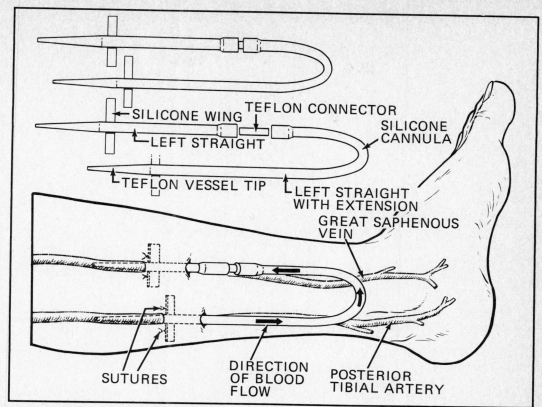

Figure 29-2. An arteriovenous shunt.

When the patient is not undergoing hemodialysis, blood flows directly from the artery, through the shunt, and into the vein. Shunts are inserted under local anesthesia. The favored sites are the patient's arm, wrist, legs, and ankles. In the upper extremity, the preferred vessels are from the radial artery to the cephalic vein. In the lower extremity, the preferred vessels are from the posterior tibial artery to the great saphenous vein. Most patients are dialyzed two or three times a week.

Cannulation is a special permanent external arteriovenous shunt which is only occasionally used. A cannulation is similar to a cut down and allows the physician to suture teflon-tipped, Silastic tubes into an artery and a vein. The tubes are then brought to the skin surface through a stab wound and joined by a special connector. The cannulation procedure is more stressful than the other shunts. There is usually some bleeding and swelling. After the local anes-

thetic has worn off, the patient tends to have a fair amount of discomfort. Unrelieved or severe pain due to vessel spasms needs to be reported immediately. Clotting of the cannula tends to occur with unrelieved spasms.

Nursing interventions are to notify the doctor; to medicate as ordered; to apply warm, moist packs; and to elevate the cannulated arm on two or three pillows. Signs and symptoms of a clotted cannula are the same as for arteriovenous shunts.

Shaldon catheters (Figure 29-3) are short-term shunts. They can be placed in the femoral vein with one catheter in the vena cava above the renal artery. The "venous" catheter is above the renal artery (higher in the vena cava). One Shaldon catheter can be inserted in the femoral vein and the second catheter can be placed in an arm vein. The use of an arteriovenous shunt in an extremity can be remembered by a mnemonic: shunt–see–short-term. (The shunt can

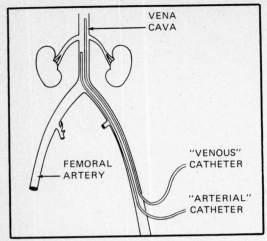

Figure 29-3. Shaldon catheters.

be seen and is for short-term use.) Shaldon catheters are also short-term shunts.

Arteriovenous Fistula

The internal arteriovenous fistula is permanent. The mnemonic is fistula–feel–forever. (A fistula one can feel and is for permanent use.) The fistula may be made by anastomosis of a vein and an artery in almost any direction. The anastomsis or fistula (Figure 29-4) allows for blood to flow directly from the artery into the vein. When the fistula matures, the vein (called an ar-

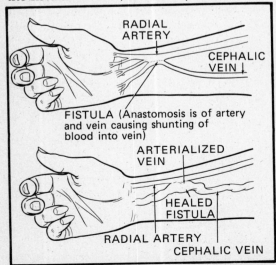

Figure 29-4. Anastomosis to form arteriovenous fistula.

terialized vein) will have thickened, elastic, self-sealing walls to withstand the insertion of large bore needles (14–16 gauge).

If bovine grafts are used, they are tunneled under the skin in a U-shape (Figure 29-5).

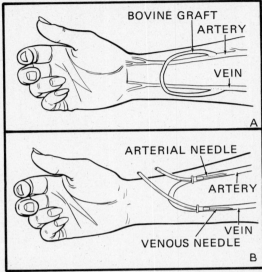

Figure 29-5. A bovine graft in place (A) and placement of needles in bovine graft for hemodialysis (B).

ADVANTAGES OF AN ARTERIOVENOUS FISTULA

There are fewer infections with a fistula than a shunt, and infections are more easily treated. There is less chance of thrombus formation. Fistulas have a longer life than shunts, thus they require fewer revisions. The patient has a greater degree of independence with a fistula: The patient can bathe, swim, participate in sports and so on. There is minimal home care required with a fistula, whereas a shunt requires daily cleaning and such.

DISADVANTAGES OF AN ARTERIOVENOUS FISTULA

Venous hypertension and the "steal syndrome" are the major disadvantages. In venous hypertension, there is too much blood in the extremity distal to the fistula. This may cause ulcerations and may necessitate a fistula revision. In the "steal syndrome" there is insufficient blood to the extremity due to excessive diversion of arterial blood to the vein at the anastomosis. Symptoms of this include coldness and poor function of the extremity. In severe cases, gangrene may develop with necrosis of the extremity tips. The "steal syndrome" is corrected by revising the fistula.

Once an access site is available, an evaluation of the patient's most recent electrolytes is made to determine what adjustments in the dialysate bath are to be made. An accurate predialysis weight of the patient must be made each day; an estimate must also be made of the patient's dry weight. By calculating the difference between predialysis weight and dry weight, it is possible to know how much fluid should be removed from the patient. By weighing the patient postdialysis, it is possible to calculate exactly how much fluid was removed or added to the patient.

Nursing Interventions for Hemodialysis

A major problem is to prevent infection. This is attempted by cleaning the shunt site daily using sterile technique and also by cleaning the fistula site until the incision is healed. If the shunt or fistula become infected, culture and sensitivity is done to identify the infecting organism. Once identified, intravenous antibiotics are started. If the shunt or fistula remains infected, it is removed and a new shunt or fistula is created.

The prevention of thrombosis is always a challenge. *Anything* that decreases blood flow increases the chance of thrombosis. Some examples are hypotension, hypovolemia, tourniquets, B/P cuffs, tight clothing and jewelry, heavy handbags and packages, and dehydration.

If the shunt is patent, one can see blood flowing freely through it—and it feels warm. Looking at the shunt, one should see that the blood is rather bright red. There should *not* be any layering of the blood components—like cells at the bottom, clear sera at the top. Proximal to the insertion site, one should feel a "thrill"—the turbulence of the arterial blood. With a stethoscope, one should hear a "bruit" (pronounced bru-ee)—arterial blood turbulence. If either the thrill or bruit is absent, notify the physician immediately.

If the shunt becomes clotted, the physician may insert a catheter to remove the clot. CAUTION! Unless you have *experience* and *finesse, DO NOT* try to remove the clot. After patency has been established, routine use of heparin will maintain patency.

To prevent hemorrhage due to shunt disconnection, clamps are attached to the dressing to ensure immediate availability. If the catheter becomes unconnected, clamp the arterial cannula *first* to control excessive blood loss from the arterial system and then clamp the venous cannula. If you are going to attach the shunt to the kidney machine, unclamp the *venous cannula first* and then the arterial cannula.

The same precautions taken for shunts are also taken for fistulas. A thrill and bruit should be present. *Do not* use the arm with a fistula for intravenous fluids, B/P, venipuncture, or injections. Clean the fistula daily using sterile technique and report bleeding, skin discoloration, drainage (which should be cultured), and such.

Complications of Hemodialysis

There are nine fairly common complications of hemodialysis.

1. *Hypotension* is caused by dehydration, sepsis, and/or blood loss. The patients may already be hypotensive or may rapidly become hypotensive when dialysis is initiated. This is treated by reducing the blood flow, discontinuing ultrafiltration, and giving fluids. If the patient does not respond to this method of treatment, dialysis is discontinued.

2. *Cardiac dysrhythmias* may be caused by potassium intoxication but, most often, no specific electrolyte derangement can be identified. In some instances, dysrhythmias may be related to the development of transient myocardial ischemia. Premature ventricular contractions (PVCs) are the most common abnormality. Treatment consists of decreasing the blood flow and using appropriate medication as indicated and as necessary. The dialysis procedure must be

stopped if the dysrhythmia is severe and/or does not respond to treatment.

3. *Congestive heart failure* in most instances is secondary to fluid overload, which can be reversed by ultrafiltration.

4. *Coagulation* problems occur due to an abnormal coagulation mechanism, which is an occurrence in renal failure. It is believed that platelet dysfunction is the principle abnormality.

5. *Heparin rebound* develops in some patients. The mechanism responsible is a *relative* heparin excess due to the rapid degradation of protamine. Regional heparinization resolves this problem.

6. *Hemolysis* is the destruction of red blood cells (RBCs). Hemoglobin in the RBC is released into the surrounding fluid. This may occur in an improper or inadequate dialysate bath mixture if the arterial pump is too tightly occluded or if a transfusion reaction occurs.

7. *Convulsions* may be caused by hypertension, water intoxication, dialysis disequilibrium syndrome, and cerebral vascular accidents. These complications may occur at any time.

8. *Disequilibrium syndrome* is characterized by cerebral symptoms in patients with severe renal failure at the beginning, during, or immediately following hemodialysis. These disturbances are more common in the early phase of treatment. Agitation, twitching, confusion, and frank grand-mal seizures are seen.

The cause of this dysfunction is thought to be related to a rapid, efficient dialysis. With a rapid decline in the level of blood urea, time is insufficient for an equal lowering of urea across the "blood-brain barrier." This is thought to cause an osmotic gradient diuresis of water from the cerebral blood and extracellular fluid in the central nervous system, resulting in cerebral edema and increased intracranial pressure.

Treatment of this syndrome should be aimed at prevention. Ten percent mannitol is used for the first few dialyses. Peritoneal dialysis may also be used for several exchanges *before* hemodialysis.

9. In *acidosis*, a lower pH and a lower-than-normal blood P_{CO_2} does not change appreciably after dialysis. A state of metabolic acidosis may be transformed into one of a mild respiratory alkalosis. Acid-base changes in the cerebrospinal fluid with dialysis can vary markedly. These changes should be considered as contributing factors in the disequilibrium syndrome.

Two other complications occur more rarely in hemodialysis. They are air embolism and hepatitis. Hepatitis will be covered in the gastrointestinal section of the text.

Air Embolism

There are two types and they may occur at any time during dialysis.

1. *Systemic arterial air embolism:* When air enters the pulmonary vein (through a leak in the tubing, a loose connection, or the disconnection of tubing), it reaches the left side of the heart and systemic arterial circulation. Arterial air emboli cause serious symptoms by occluding arterioles or capillaries of the brain or coronary arteries. The latter may be responsible for ventricular fibrillation and sudden death. The former may result in convulsions, coma, and death.

2. *Systemic venous air embolism:* An *AVERAGE* lethal dose is suspected to range from 5 to 7.5 cc per kilogram of weight when the rate of intravenous injection is very rapid (1–5 seconds). The quantity of venous air required to cause symptoms is dependent upon the speed of air infusion and the state of health of the patient.

PATHOPHYSIOLOGY OF AIR EMBOLISM

Air introduced into the bloodstream follows the physical laws of air-fluid mixture. The air rises to the highest point to be on top of the fluid. If the patient is sitting up or reclining at 30 degrees, the air travels up the venous system to the head where it will enter small vessels of the brain. The small vessels will either fill completely or some of the blood will settle under the air. The air is "locked in" with no place to go. Absorption of air is an *extremely* slow process, except in the lungs. The patient usually shouts and holds his or her ears from the sound of air rushing up the venous system. This is rapidly followed by tonic-clonic convulsions. Muscular twitching occurs. The end result is rapid brain cell damage. Death will occur if critical areas of brain are destroyed.

In the sitting patient with dialysis access in the lower extremities, air enters the venous system of the leg and travels to the inferior vena cava, then up through the right atrium to the superior vena cava, and then finally to the head.

The patient who is lying flat when air is introduced has a different pathophysiological course. The air enters the right atrium and moves into the right ventricle. The pumping action of the heart forms a blood-air foam. Essentially, the air is trapped in the right ventricle and cannot be propelled from the heart. Additional blood cannot enter the right side of the heart since blood is already there. Blood cannot enter the pulmonary system. The lack of pulmonary blood return to the left atrium quickly stops the pumping of blood into the systemic circulation.

The symptoms are deep respiration, coughing, cyanosis, unconsciousness, and then cessation of breathing. Auscultation over the heart reveals a "mill wheel" sound during both phases of contraction. This is the sound of air turbulence in the heart.

A patient in Trendelenburg's position when air enters will show unusual signs because the air will travel to the patient's legs since the air *must* follow the physical air-fluid laws. Cyanosis of the legs and patchy areas that are pale will be noted on the toes and feet.

TREATMENT OF AIR EMBOLISM

Once air embolism has occurred, rapid corrective action is imperative. There are several important differences in the resuscitation of a patient with an air embolism as compared with the usual cardiopulmonary resuscitation. The patient *must* be placed in Trendelenburg's position and turned on his or her left side. Once the patient has been resuscitated, he or she *must be kept* in the Trendelenburg's left side position until the air is absorbed. This will prevent movement of the air into the cerebral tissues and heart and promote movement towards the feet (air will be higher than fluid). The absorption time will vary, but it usually takes a long time, from days to weeks, and there is an extremely high mortality rate.

Renal Bibliography

Borg N, Mikas DL, Stark J, Williams SM (eds): Core Curriculum for Critical Care Nursing, 2nd ed. American Association of Critical-Care Nurses. Philadelphia: W. B. Saunders, pp. 261–312, 1981

Chung EK: Electrolytes and the heart. *In* Electrolytes and the Body's Systems. New York: InterMed Communications, Inc., p. 6, 1977

Dunn MJ: Importance of sodium and potassium in arterial hypertension. *In* Electrolytes and the Body's Systems. New York: InterMed Communications, Inc., p. 9, 1977

Ellis PD (ed): Renal failure. *In* Critical Care Quarterly, Vol. 1, No. 2. Rockville, MD: Aspen Systems Corporation, 1978

Freidman HH (ed): Renal, electrolyte, and blood-gas and acid-base problems. *In* Problem-Oriented Medical Diagnosis, 2nd ed. Boston, MA: Little, Brown and Co., 1979

Freitag JJ, Miller LW (eds): Fluid and electrolyte disturbances, and renal disease. *In* Manual of Medical Therapeutics, 23rd ed. Boston, MA: Little, Brown and Co., 1980

Grant JCB, Basmajian JV: Grant's Method of Anatomy by Regions, 7th ed. Baltimore, MD: Williams and Wilkins, pp. 59–66, 267–275, 1965

*Guyton AC: Textbook of Medical Physiology, 6th ed. Philadelphia: W. B. Saunders, pp. 391–455, 453–457, 463–473, 1981

*Harrington AR, Zinnerman SW: Renal Pathophysiology. New York: John Wiley and Sons, 1982

*Jackle M, Rasmussen C: Renal Problems: A Critical Nursing Focus. Bowie, MD: Robert J. Brady Co., 1980

Kinney MR, Dear CB, Packa DR, Voorman DMN (eds): The renal system; and Regulation and assessment of water and electrolyte balance; and Dialysis therapy. *In* AACN'S Clinical Reference for Critical Care Nursing. New York: McGraw-Hill, 1981

*McLeod DG, Mittemeyer BT: The urinary system: Disease, diagnosis, treatment. Bowie, MD: Robert J. Brady Co., 1973

*Metheny N, Snively WD: Nurses' Handbook of Fluid Balance, 2nd ed. Philadelphia: J.B. Lippincott, pp. 18–86, 205–216, 1974

Muir BL: Mineral/electrolyte imbalance. *In* Pathophysiology: An Introduction to the Mechanisms of Disease. New York: John Wiley and Sons, 1980

*A Programmed Approach to Anatomy and Physiology: The Urinary System, 2nd ed. Bowie, MD: Robert J. Brady Co., 1972

Reichlin S: Neural control of the pituitary gland: Normal physiology and pathophysiologic implications. *In* Current Concepts, A Scope Publication. Kalamazoo, MI: The Upjohn Co., 1978

Renal and urologic disorders. *In* Diseases (causes and diagnosis, current therapy, nursing management, patient education). Nursing 82 books, The nurse's reference library. Springhouse, PA: Intermed Communications, Inc., 1982

Roberts SL: Behavioral Concepts and the Critically Ill Patient: Englewood Cliffs, NJ: Prentice-Hall, 1976

*Wilson RF (ed): Principles and techniques of critical care. *In* Critical Care Manual, Vol. 1, Sec. I through Sec. L. Kalamazoo, MI: The Upjohn Co., 1977

V

The Endocrine System

— 30 ——————————————————

Classification of Hormones and the Negative Feedback System

Learning Objectives

By the end of this chapter, the nurse will be able to:

1. Identify the primary function of the endocrine system.
2. List the major endocrine glands.
3. Explain the way hormones reach their target organs.
4. Differentiate between local and general hormones.
5. Identify the most significant hormone(s) of the:
   a. Anterior pituitary gland
   b. Posterior pituitary gland
   c. Thyroid gland
   d. Parathyroid gland
   e. Adrenal medulla
   f. Adrenal cortex
6. Explain the negative feedback system in relation to hormones and endocrine glands.
7. Explain the action of the four types of hormones (amines, peptides, proteins, and steroids).
8. Explain *cyclic* AMP (cAMP) and genetic activation.

The primary function of the endocrine system is to regulate metabolic functioning of the body. Metabolic functioning includes chemical reactions and the rates of these reactions, growth, transportation of chemicals, secretions, and cellular metabolism.

A close interrelationship exists between the nervous system (responsible for integration of body processes) and the endocrine system (responsible for appropriate metabolic activity). Neuronal stimulation is required for some specific hormones to be secreted and/or to be secreted in adequate amounts.

The endocrine system is composed of specific glands (Figure 30-1) which secrete their chemical substances directly into the bloodstream.

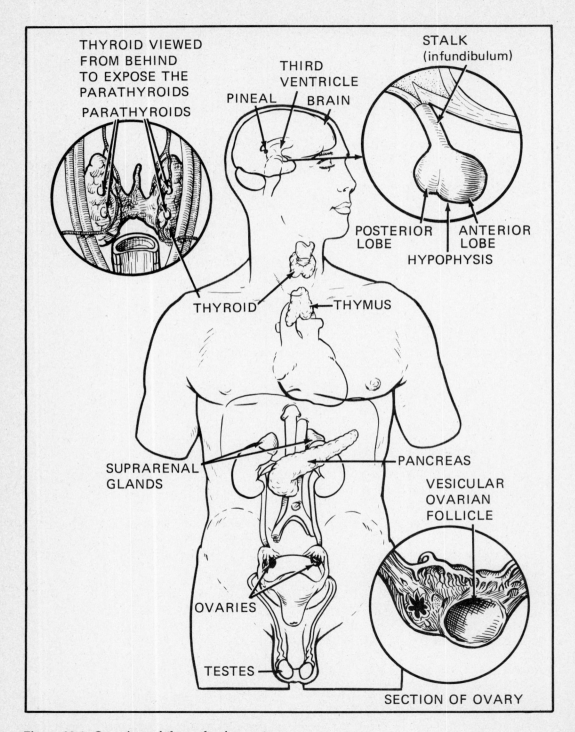

Figure 30-1. Overview of the endocrine system.

The major single endocrine glands are the pituitary (also called the hypophysis) and the thyroid. The parathyroids are usually four glands, not two sets of paired glands. The adrenals are the *one pair* of endocrine glands. Other glands exist that contain endocrine components and function in both the endocrine system and another system. These glands are the ovaries and testes (collectively termed the gonads) and the pancreas. The thymus gland has a major role in immunology but is sometimes included in the endocrine system.

All endocrine glands are very vascular. The endocrine glands function by extracting substances from the blood to synthesize into complex hormones. Hormones are released from the specific endocrine glands into the veins that drain the glands themselves. The circulatory system is used to transport endocrine substances to target glands and tissues throughout the body.

Classification of Hormones

The substances secreted by endocrine glands are chemicals called hormones. Hormones exert a physiological control on body cells. *Local* hormones are those released in specific areas (or tissues) and they exert a limited, local effect. Acetylcholine is an example of a local hormone having physiologic control at some synapses in the nervous system. *General* hormones are secreted by a specific endocrine gland and transported by the vascular system to a specific, predetermined site.

TYPES OF HORMONES

Hormones may be amines, peptides, proteins (or protein derivatives), or steroids. Prostaglandins are often considered tissue hormones. The first three types of hormones are water soluble and do not require a carrier molecule for transportation throughout the body. Steroids and thyroxine are not water soluble and must have a carrier substance to transport them to their site of action, known as the target cell.

Prostaglandins are unsaturated fatty acids of which three types have been identified according to their chemical structure. They are synthesized in the seminal vesi-

cles, brain, liver, iris, kidneys, lungs, and other areas. Prostaglandins have a potent effect but are considered local hormones, not general hormones.

IMPORTANT GENERAL HORMONES

All of the general hormones are important for regulatory action on functions in the body. However, dysfunction of certain hormones would rarely, if ever, be a reason for admission to a critical care area. These include oxytocin, follicle-stimulating hormone (FSH), luteinizing hormone (LH), prolactin, melanocyte-stimulating hormone (MSH), corticosterone, deoxycorticosterone, and androgens (including estrogens, progesterone, and testosterone). These hormones will not be detailed in this text.

The general hormones which may precipitate an admission to a critical care area because of dysfunction are listed in Table 30-1 and will be covered in the following three chapters.

Action of Hormones

AMINE, PROTEIN, AND PEPTIDE HORMONES

These hormones include growth hormone, ACTH, TSH, PTH, calcitonin, insulin, the catecholamines, glucagon, ADH, FSH, LH, and prolactin. Since these hormones do not require a carrier substance because they are water soluble, their concentrations may fluctuate rapidly and widely. These hormones are thought to react with specific surface receptors on the target cell membrane. This alters the membrane enzymes and leads to a change in the *intracellular* concentration of an enzyme. The hormone is called the "first" messenger and the intracellular enzyme is called the "second" messenger. This second messenger is *cAMP* (cyclic 3',5' adenosine mono phosphate). cAMP (within the cell) activates enzymes, causes protein synthesis, alters cell permeability, causes muscle relaxation/contraction, and causes secretion. It is by the action of cAMP that many hormones exert control over the cells.

Table 30-1. Endocrine glands and hormones of significant importance.

Glands	Hormones
Adenohypophysis (Anterior pituitary)	Adrenocorticotropin (ACTH), somatotropin or growth hormone (GH), thyroid-stimulating hormone (TSH)
Neurohypophysis (Posterior pituitary)	Antidiuretic hormone (ADH), oxytocin
Thyroid	Thyroxine, triiodothyronine, calcitonin
Parathyroid	Parathyroid hormone (PTH, parathormone)
Adrenal medulla	Epinephrine, norepinephrine
Adrenal cortex	Glucocorticoids (cortisol), mineralocorticoids (aldosterone)
Pancreas	Insulin, glucagon

STEROIDS AND THYROXINE

These hormones include the sex hormones, aldosterone, cortisol, and thyroxine. These hormones are able to cross the cell membrane easily and then bind with an intracellular receptor. The hormone-receptor complex reacts with chromatin in the cell nucleus to synthesize specific proteins. Because these hormones are lipid chemicals, the reactions take longer to occur, but are no less potent than the amine, protein, and peptide hormone reactions.

The Negative Feedback System

Some hormones are needed in very minute amounts in the body for variable amounts of time; some have prolonged action periods; and some affect and interact with other hormones, producing a very complex, intricate system to control. A control system must exist to maintain this complex system.

Most control systems, including the endocrine system, act by a negative feedback mechanism. When there is an increased hormone concentration, physiological control is increased and a stimulus is received in the hypothalamus. This results in an inhibition of hormone releasing factors which is negative in relation to the stimulus. In the same manner, when there is deficient or absent hormone concentrations, a stimulus is received in the hypothalamus which results in an increased release of hormone stimulating factors. This again is a negative (or opposite) response to the stimulus sent to the hypothalamus.

The greater the need for the hormone, the greater the intensity of the stimulus, and similarly, the greater the concentration of the hormone, the lesser the intensity of the stimulus.

When a hormone concentration is deficient, as more hormone is produced and/or secreted, the physiological control of the body cells increase. With an increase in physiological control, the feedback stimulus relayed to the endocrine gland decreases in intensity and release of the hormone decreases as homeostasis is achieved. The reverse process applies when the hormone concentration is excessive.

It is known that the hypothalamus produces releasing and inhibiting hormones (or factors) whose single target is the anterior pituitary gland, the so-called "master gland." It is believed that all hormones have releasing and inhibiting factors produced by the hypothalamus, but only eight are known at this time (Table 30-2).

The principles of achieving regulatory control are similar with all the hormones listed in Table 30-1, with the exception of the hormones of the adrenal medulla.

The hormones of the adrenal medulla—epinephrine and norepinephrine—are under control of the autonomic nervous system. The hormones of the neurohypophysis (the posterior pituitary) are under control of the sympathetic nervous system and other factors.

Tropic hormones, secreted only by the adenohypophysis (anterior pituitary), cause an increase in size and secretion rates of other endocrine glands and are controlled by the negative feedback system as well as other factors.

All adenohypophysial hormone releasing and inhibitory factors (except the adrenal medulla) are carried by the hypothalamo-

hypophysial tract from the hypothalamus into the median eminence (Figure 30-2) and then into the pituitary stalk. In the stalk, the hypophysial portal system carries the releasing and inhibitory factors into the adenohypophysis for storage until needed.

The two neurohypophysial hormone releasing and inhibiting factors are formed in the paraventricular nucleus and supra-optic nucleus in the hypothalamus (Figure 30-2). They are then carried by nerve fibers into the neurohypophysis for storage. The transport of the pituitary hormones is covered in more detail in Chapter 31.

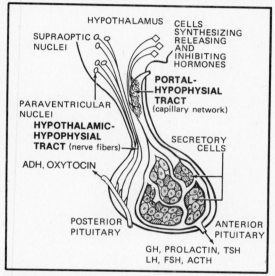

Figure 30-2. The paraventricular nucleus and supra-optic nucleus of the hypothalamus.

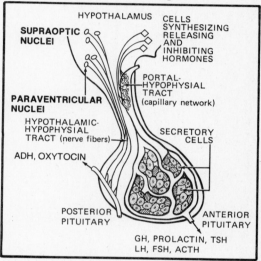

Figure 30-3. The portal-hypophysial tract and the hypothalamic-hypophysial tract of the hypothalamus.

Table 30-2. Releasing and inhibiting factors produced by the hypothalamus.

Hypothalamic Hormones		
Releasing	Inhibiting	Peripheral Hormone
Growth hormone-releasing hormone (GRH)	Growth hormone-inhibiting hormone (GIF)	Growth hormone
Prolactin-releasing hormone (PRH)	Prolactin-inhibiting hormone (PIH)	Prolactin
Corticotropin-releasing hormone (CRF)	—	Adrenal steroids
Follicle-stimulating hormone-releasing hormone (FRH)	—	Gonadal steroids
Luteinizing hormone-releasing hormone (LRF)	—	Gonadal hormones
Thyrotropin-releasing hormone (TRH)	—	Thyroid hormones

— 31

Anatomy, Physiology, and Dysfunction of the Pituitary Gland

Learning Objectives

By the end of this chapter, the nurse will be able to:

1. List the three parts of the pituitary gland.
2. Identify the origin of the adenohypophysis.
3. Identify the origin of the neurohypophysis.
4. Explain the hypothalamic-hypophysial portal vessel system.
5. Define exocytosis.
6. List six major hormones of the adenohypophysis.
7. Explain two disorders resulting from excessive growth hormone.
8. Describe a disorder resulting from insufficient growth hormone.
9. List two major hormones of the neurohypophysis.
10. Explain the action of antidiuretic hormone.
11. Identify the control mechanism of antidiuretic hormone.
12. Define diabetes insipidus and list etiological factors.
13. Explain the treatment of diabetes insipidus.
14. Explain the pathophysiology of the syndrome of inappropriate antidiuretic hormone (SIADH).
15. List common causes and presenting signs and symptoms of SIADH.
16. Explain the objectives of therapy of SIADH.

The pituitary gland is often referred to as the "master gland" of the body since its hormones control and regulate many other endocrine glands. The pituitary gland is now often called the hypophysis. It has two lobes: the anterior pituitary, known as the adenohypophysis, and the posterior pituitary, known as the neurohypophysis. A mnemonic may help keep these names straight. The anterior pituitary starts with an "A" as does the adenohypophysis (anterior = adeno).

Anatomy of the Hypophysis

The hypophysis develops from two types of tissues. The adenohypophysis is an outgrowth of the pharyngeal tissue, which grows upward toward the brain in the embryo. The neurohypophysis is an outgrowth of the hypothalamus, which grows downward in the embryo.

LOCATION AND SIZE

The hypophysis is located in the sella turcica which is a hollow depression in the sphenoid bone (Figure 31-1) of the brain. It is a small gland weighing one-half to one gram and is about one centimeter in diameter. The hypophysis is attached to the hypothalamus by the hypophysial stalk.

LOBES OF THE HYPOPHYSIS

The two lobes of the hypophysis are separated by the pars intermedia (Figure 31-2). The pars intermedia is almost avascular and is a small band of fibers between the hypophysial lobes. The function of the pars intermedia, other than to separate the anterior lobe of the hypophysis from the posterior lobe, is unknown.

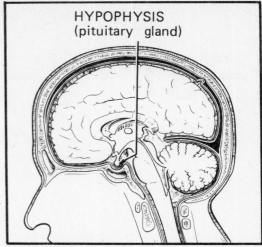

Figure 31-1. Location of the hypophysis (pituitary gland).

Structure of the Adenohypophysis

The adenohypophysis is composed of epithelial type cells (embryologic extension of pharyngeal tissue). Many different types of these epithelial cells have been identified for each hormone formed.

In the adenohypophysis are microscopic blood vessels composing the hypothalam-

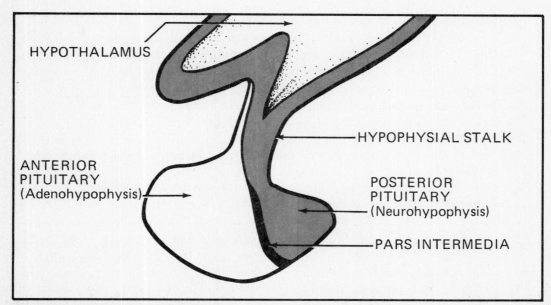

Figure 31-2. Lobes of the hypophysis.

ic-hypophysial portal vessels (Figure 31-3). These vessels connect the hypothalamus and the adenohypophysis (by passage through the pituitary stalk) and terminate in the anterior pituitary sinuses.

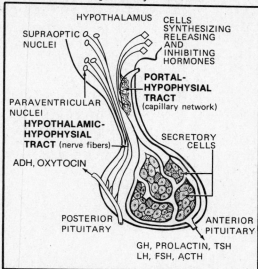

Figure 31-3. The hypothalamic-hypophysial portal vessels.

Substances carried in the hypothalamic-hypophysial vessels are actually hormone factors and not hormones per se. These factors are releasing and inhibiting factors (see Table 30-2). For *each* adenohypophysial hormone, there is an associated releasing factor. For *some* adenohypophysial hormones, there are inhibitory factors.

Structure of the Neurohypophysis

Many cells of the neurohypophysis (posterior pituitary) are called pituicytes. Pituicytes are like the glial cells of the nervous system. The pituicytes provide supporting tissue for nerve tracts that arise from the supraoptic nuclei and paraventricular nuclei of the hypothalamus. The supraoptic nuclei and the paraventricular nuclei form the neurohypophysis hormones. These hormones are carried by the nerve tracts through the hypophysial stalk and terminate in bulbous knobs in the neurohypophysis. The knobs lie *on* the surface of capillaries. As hor-mones that were formed in the hypothalamus and stored in the bulbous knobs are needed, exocytosis occurs. "Exocytosis" is the discharge of substances from a cell that are too large to diffuse through the cell membrane. The hormone is thus secreted from the bulbous knobs onto the capillaries and is absorbed into the vascular system.

The adenohypophysis has a vascular relationship to the hypothalamus, whereas the neurohypophysis has a neural relationship.

Physiology of the Pituitary Gland

The action of the various hormones is to control the activity of the target glands and target tissues. There are two basic mechanisms of hormone action: cyclic AMP and genetic activation; these were covered in Chapter 30. Cyclic AMP (cAMP) initiates actions characteristic of the target cell. For example, parathyroid hormone cells activated by cyclic AMP form and secrete parathyroid hormone (parathormone); specific cells in the pancreas activated by cyclic AMP form and secrete glucagon. Known hormones affected by cyclic AMP include secretin, glucagon, parathormone, vasopressin, catecholamines, adrenocorticotropin, follicle-stimulating hormone, thyroid-stimulating hormone, and hypothalamic releasing factors.

Hormones of the Adenohypophysis

Six major hormone factors, all formed in the hypothalamus, are secreted by the adenohypophysis.

1. The thyrotropin-releasing hormone (TRH) causes the release of thyroid-stimulating hormone (TSH).
2. The growth hormone-releasing hormone (GRH) causes release of the growth hormone (GH) or somatotropin (STH). The growth hormone-inhibiting hormone (GIF) or somatostatin inhibits the release of growth hormone.

3. Corticotropin-releasing hormone (CRH) causes release of adrenocorticotropin (ACTH).
4. Follicle-stimulating hormone-releasing hormone (FRH) causes release of follicle-stimulating hormone (FSH).
5. Luteinizing hormone-releasing hormone (LRF) causes release of luteinizing hormone (LH).
6. Prolactin-inhibiting hormone (PIH) causes inhibition of prolactin secretion.

Action of Adenohypophysial Hormones

All of the major adenohypophysial hor- mones have an effect upon a target gland *except* growth hormone. Thyroid and parathyroid hormonal action is discussed in Chapter 32. Hormonal action of the adrenal gland is discussed in Chapter 33. Hormonal action of the pancreas is discussed in Chapter 34.

Growth Hormone and Metabolism

Growth hormone is also called somatotropin. Somatotropin has a general effect upon bones, organs, and soft tissues; and it is, therefore, considered a peripheral hormone. It influences the growth of body tissues.

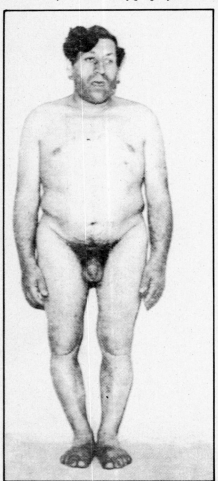

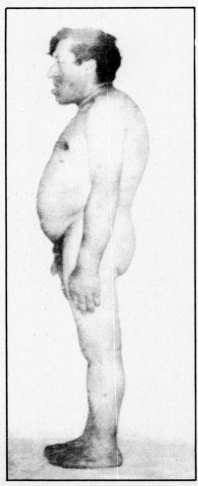

Figure 31-4. Acromegaly.

Growth hormone has an important role in all aspects of metabolism. Growth hormone increases the rate of intracellular protein synthesis throughout the body. It is a factor in the mobilization of fatty acids from adipose tissue and in the conversion of these fats into energy. Growth hormone conserves carbohydrates by decreasing glucose utilization in the body.

GROWTH HORMONE FACTORS

There are specific factors which stimulate or inhibit the release of growth hormone.

The most common factors inhibiting the release of GH include hyperglycemia, sustained corticosteroid therapy at high levels, and the release of growth hormone-inhibiting factor (GIF) from the hypothalamus.

Common factors promoting release of the growth hormone include pituitary tumors, hypoglycemia, exercise, decreased amino acid levels, and the release of growth hormone-releasing hormone (GRH) from the hypothalamus.

Growth hormone secretion follows a diurnal pattern with most release occurring in the first 2 hours of *deep* sleep. This follows the non-REM stage of sleep pattern.

Dysfunction of the Hypophysis (Pituitary)

GROWTH HORMONE AND BONES

Once the epiphyses of the long bones have united with the bone shafts, there can be no increase in the *length* of the bones. The *thickness* of the bones can still increase, however.

If there is oversecretion of growth hormone (commonly tumor-related) *prior* to adolescence, *all* body tissues grow rapidly, including bones. The result is *gigantism* in which a height of 8–9 feet is not uncommon. Most giants are hyperglycemic and 10% will develop diabetes mellitus. Giants who do not receive treatment usually die in early adulthood due to deterioration of the hypophysis. Since most gigantism is due to a tumor in the adenohypophysis, treatment is surgical removal of the tumor if possible. Radiation therapy may be tried if surgery is not feasible.

If there is oversecretion of growth hormone after adolescence, the result is *acromegaly* (Figure 31-4). In acromegaly, soft tissues (especially the tongue, lips, liver,

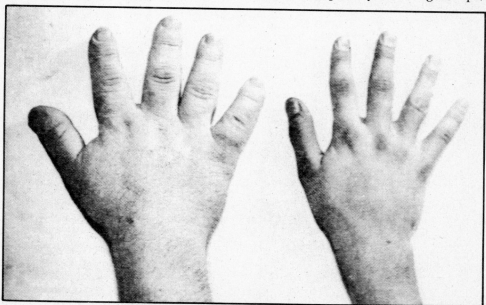

ACROMEGALIC HAND   NORMAL HAND

Figure 31-4. Continued.

and kidneys) become greatly enlarged. Bones grow in thickness. The most affected bones are the membranous bones—the cranium, nose, lower jawbone, forehead, and small bones of the hands and feet. Overgrowth of vertebrae may cause a kyphosis (hunchback). Treatment of acromegaly is directed towards arrest of the disease process by excising a pituitary tumor if possible. Reversal of the process in not usual.

Inadequate secretion of growth hormone results in *dwarfism* (growth retardation). In most cases, body growth is proportional but markedly decreased (Figure 31-5). Mental retardation is not usual. If growth hormone is the only pituitary deficiency (true in 10% of the cases), the dwarf will experience puberty and may reproduce.

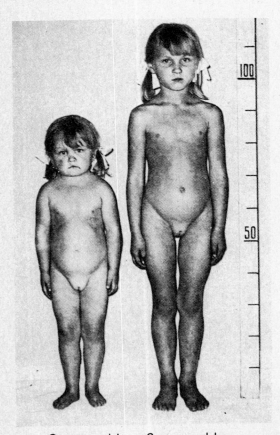

8 years old   6 years old

Figure 31-5. Dwarfism—two sisters.

Hormones of the Neurohypophysis

There are two hormones released by the neurohypophysis: antidiuretic hormone (ADH), also called vasopressin, and oxytocin. Oxytocin will not be discussed in this text.

Antidiuretic hormone (ADH) is formed mainly in the supraoptic nuclei of the hypothalamus. (The paraventricular nuclei mainly form oxytocin. The ratio of ADH to oxytocin formed in the supraoptic nuclei is 6:1, whereas the ratio is 1:6 in the paraventricular nuclei.) ADH is transported from the supraoptic nuclei by neurophysins. Neurophysins are protein carriers that bind very loosely with ADH and oxytocin to transport these hormones to the neurohypophysis for storage until needed.

ACTION OF ANTIDIURETIC HORMONE (ADH)

ADH works on the distal convoluted tubules and the collecting ducts of the kidney. ADH alters the permeability of these tubules and ducts. Without ADH, the tubules and ducts are impermeable to water. In the presence of ADH, these tubules and ducts become permeable to water thus allowing large quantities of water to leave the tubules and collecting ducts and to re-enter the hypertonic medullary interstitial fluid. This helps to conserve and balance the fluid content of the body.

CONTROL OF ANTIDIURETIC HORMONE

Serum sodium levels and extracellular fluid osmolality exert a major influence on ADH. Osmoreceptors shrink when hypertonicity of the extracellular fluid exists. The osmoreceptors emit impulses to the hypothalamus and ADH is released from the neurohypophysis to reabsorb water from the kidneys and to re-establish homeostasis. When body fluids become diluted, stimulated osmoreceptors result in the inhibition of ADH, and water is NOT reabsorbed from the kidneys. Many factors control ADH in addition to the serum sodium and extracellular osmolality. Inadequate blood volume stimulates volume receptors in the periphery, the carotid sinus, the left atrium of the heart, and the aortic arch, stimulating release of ADH. ADH response is much greater in hemorrhagic states than in altered osmolality states.[1] Trauma, anxiety, pain, and specific drugs enhance ADH release.

ADH release is inhibited by a decreased serum osmolality and pituitary surgery.

Neurohypophysial Dysfunction

There are two main neurohypophysial disorders: diabetes insipidus and the syndrome of inappropriate ADH (SIADH).

DIABETES INSIPIDUS

When there are decreased levels of ADH, diuresis and dehydration occur. Decreased levels of ADH occur when there is damage or destruction of the ADH neurons in the supraoptic and paraventricular neurons of the hypothalamus. Diabetes insipidus results.

Symptoms

Diabetes insipidus symptoms include dilute urine (until *severe* dehydration occurs) with a specific gravity between 1.001 and 1.005. Urinary output varies from 4 to 15 liters per day. Polyuria is often of sudden onset. Polyuria may not occur until 1–3 days post injury due to the utilization of stored ADH in the neurohypophysis. Polydipsia will occur unless the thirst center has been damaged. There is an increased serum osmolality and a decreased urine osmolality. A relative diabetes insipidus may occur in cases of high dose, lengthy steroid therapy with a specific gravity of the urine ranging from 1.000 to 1.009 and urinary volume about 6–9 liters per day.

---

[1] Reichlin S: Neural control of the pituitary gland: Normal physiology and pathophysiologic implications. *In* Current Concepts, A Scope Publication. Kalamazoo, MI: Upjohn Co., p. 22, 1978

Etiologies

The two leading etiologies of diabetes insipidus are hypothalamic or pituitary tumor and closed head injuries with damage to the supraoptic nuclei and/or hypothalamus. Postoperative diabetes insipidus is usually transient. Other causes include inflammatory and degenerative systemic conditions, but these are not common.

Treatment

The objective of therapy is *first* to prevent dehydration and electrolyte imbalances while determining and treating the underlying cause. Injections of vasopressin tannate (oil base for slow release) every other day will control diabetes insipidus. Intramuscular injections of vasopressin must be warmed and vigorously shaken to mix well and to decrease the pain of injection. D-amino-D-arginine vasopressin (DDAVP) is a nasal spray with minimal side effects and prolonged antidiuretic effects. Following head trauma or neurosurgery, an aqueous vasopressin of 5–10 units subcutaneously may be used to decrease the risk of water intoxication. Diabetes insipidus may resolve in only a few days in these conditions.

Nursing Interventions

Of prime importance is the ACCURATE intake and output record of the patient. Monitoring body weight, electrolytes, urine specific gravities, blood urea nitrogen, and signs of dehydration and shock will allow for early intervention in cases prone to deterioration.

THE SYNDROME OF INAPPROPRIATE SECRETION OF ADH (SIADH)

SIADH is the second dysfunction of ADH. In SIADH there is either increased secretion or increased production of ADH. This increase is unrelated to osmolality and causes a slight increase in total body water. There is a severely decreased sodium ion concentration in extracellular fluid and serum (hyponatremia).

Etiologies

SIADH is occasionally caused by pituitary tumor, but much more commonly by a bronchogenic (oat cell) or pancreatic carcinoma. Head injuries, other endocrine disorders (Addison's disease and hypopituitarism), pulmonary disease (such as pneumonia, lung abcesses), central nervous system infections (and tumors), and drugs such as tricyclics, oral hypoglycemic agents, diuretics, and cytotoxic agents are all possible etiologies.

Symptoms and Complications

The most common symptoms of SIADH are personality changes, headache, decreased mentation, lethargy, nausea, vomiting, diarrhea, anorexia, decreased tendon reflexes, seizures, and coma. Complications of SIADH include seizures, coma, and death.

Treatment

The FIRST step in treating SIADH is to restrict fluid intake to prevent water intoxication. Then, the objective of therapy is to correct electrolyte imbalances. In severe cases, 3% hypertonic saline and intravenous furosemide (Lasix®) are used. Supplemental potassium is necessary. Demeclocycline (less than 2,400 mg/day) and lithium carbonate (up to 900 mg/day) have proven useful by interfering with the normal ADH effect of increasing cAMP in the distal tubules and collecting ducts.

Nursing Interventions

With SIADH it is necessary to maintain strict fluid restrictions and to monitor the patient for electrolyte imbalances as indicated by confusion, weakness, lethargy, vomiting, and/or seizures. If the patient is comatose, turning, suctioning as needed, and standard nursing care procedures are required. Cardiac monitoring will allow for early identification of impending hyperkalemia and its associated cardiac problems. Nutritional needs of the patient must be met without increasing fluid intake. Emotional support of the alert patient by stating that this condition CAN be treated successfully will help to obtain cooperation from the patient unless there is an untreated psychological problem.

32

Anatomy, Physiology, and Dysfunctions of the Thyroid and Parathyroid Glands

Learning Objectives

By the end of this chapter, the nurse will be able to:

1. Describe the shape, location, and structure of the thyroid gland, including the follicular sacs and colloid.
2. List three hormones secreted by the thyroid and list their actions.
3. Explain the "iodide pump."
4. Explain "organification of thyroglobulin."
5. Describe the release mechanism for thyroxine and triiodothyronine.
6. Describe the shape and location of the parathyroid glands.
7. Identify two types of cells in the parathyroid glands, state the function of each, and name the hormone secreted by the parathyroid glands.
8. List the actions of the parathyroid hormone, and identify a vitamin essential to promoting the normal function of the parathyroid hormone.
9. Explain the pathophysiology of myxedema and myxedema coma.
10. List presenting symptoms of myxedema, three drugs used to treat myxedema, and three complications of myxedema.
11. Explain the pathophysiology of Graves' disease.
12. List six common signs and symptoms of hyperthyroidism and four complications of hyperthyroidism.
13. Define thyrotoxic crisis and identify its etiologic factors.
14. Explain four objectives of treating thyroid storm and four complications of the storm.
15. Identify three nursing interventions in thyroid storm.
16. List three etiologies of hypoparathyroidism and explain the result of a deficiency of the parathyroid hormone.
17. Identify gastrointestinal, respiratory, and neurological symptoms of hypoparathyroidism.
18. Explain Trousseau's and Chvostek's signs.
19. Identify the objective of treatment and four complications of hypoparathyroidism.
20. List two precautions of calcium replacement therapy.

Anatomy of the Thyroid Gland

LOCATION AND SHAPE

The thyroid gland is in the anterior portion of the neck at the lower part of the larynx and the upper part of the trachea (Figure 32-1). The thyroid has two lobes which, with a little imagination, resemble a butterfly's wings. The lobes lie on either side of the trachea and are connected by a narrow band of tissue called the isthmus, which lies across the second and third tracheal rings.

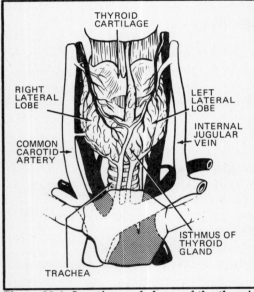

Figure 32-1. Location and shape of the thyroid gland.

INTERNAL STRUCTURE

Each lobe of the thyroid is divided into lobules by dense connective tissue. Each lobule (Figure 32-2) is composed of sac-like structures called follicles. The follicles are lined with cuboidal epithelium.

The follicular sacs are filled with a thick, viscous material called colloid. Colloid is actually thyroglobulin, which will be converted to thyroxine as needed. Storage, synthesis, and release of thyroxine is controlled by the hypothalamic-releasing hormone (factor) and the thyroid-stimulating hormone of the adenohypophysis.

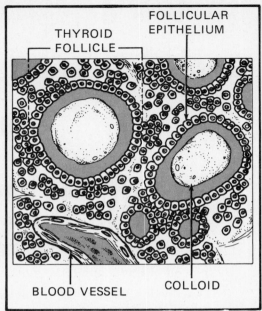

Figure 32-2. Internal structure of the thyroid follicles.

Physiology of the Thyroid Gland

The thyroid gland secretes three important hormones: thyroxine, triiodothyronine, and calcitonin. Approximately 90% of the hormone is thyroxine and 10% is triiodothyronine. In peripheral tissues, thyroxine is converted to triiodothyronine. The function of these two hormones are essentially the same. Intensity, speed of action, and formation of these hormones are different.

IODIDE TRAPPING (THE IODIDE PUMP)

To form thyroid hormones, iodides must be removed from blood and extracellular fluids and transported *into* the thyroid gland follicles. The basal membrane of the thyroid gland has the ability to transfer iodide into the thyroid cells. The iodide then diffuses throughout the thyroid cells and follicular sacs. This process in known as iodide trapping. The iodide is stored until thyroglobulin in needed. It then becomes ionized by the enzyme peroxidase and hydrogen peroxide, converting the iodide into iodine at the point where thyroglobulin is released intracellularly. If the peroxidase system is blocked, thyroid hormone production ceases.

ORGANIFICATION OF THYROGLOBULIN

Thyroglobulin is the major component reacting with iodide to form thyroxine. Thyroid cells synthesize the glycoprotein thyroglobulin, which is the colloid filling the follicular sacs. The binding of iodide with the glycoprotein is termed the organification of thyroglobulin, and the iodide is then an oxidized iodine. The oxidized iodine will slowly bond with tyrosine (an amino acid). In the presence of enzymes, this bonding is very rapid. Chemical reactions progress to yield thyroxine and triiodothyronine. The thyroid hormones are stored in an amount that is equal to the normal body requirements for 1–3 months.

RELEASE OF THYROXINE AND TRIIODOTHYRONINE

These two thyroid hormones separate from the thyroglobulin molecule. Separation is a multistep process involving several intermediate chemicals. The end result is that thyroxine and triiodothyronine are lysed from the glucoprotein. Once freed, these thyroid hormones enter the venous circulatory system of the thyroid gland itself and are carried into the systemic circulation. The strongest stimulation to release these hormones is cold temperature. Thyrotropin-releasing hormone factors (TRH) will stimulate release of thyroid-stimulating hormone (TSH), and thyroxine and triiodothyronine will be released from the thyroid gland (but not in as rapid a response as to cold).

The release of these hormones is inhibited by heat, insufficient hypothalamic releasing factors (which result in insufficient thyroid-stimulating hormones [TSH]), and/or increases in plasma glucocorticoids.

ACTION OF THYROXINE AND TRIIODOTHYRONINE

An interesting "rule of four" exists. Once these two hormones are in the peripheral tissues, triiodothyronine is four times as strong in initiating metabolic activities as thyroxine. Thyroxine's effect upon the tissues will last four times as long as triiodothyronine's effect. So these two hormones balance each other very well.

THYROXINE FUNCTION

Approximately *one milligram* of iodine *per week* is needed for normal thyroxine formation. Iodides are absorbed from the gastrointestinal tract. Two-thirds of ingested iodides are excreted in the urine and the remaining one-third is used by the thyroid gland to form the glycoprotein thyroglobulin.

The major effect of the thyroid hormones is to increase all the metabolic activities of the body, excluding the brain, spleen, lungs, retina, and testes. In children, the thyroid hormones also promote growth.

PRODUCTION, RELEASE, AND ACTION OF CALCITONIN

Calcitonin is manufactured in special thyroid cells called parafollicular cells or C cells. These cells are found in the interstitial tissue between the follicles of the thyroid gland.

An increase in plasma concentration of calcium stimulates the release of calcitonin as will the ingestion or administration of magnesium and/or glucagon.

Calcitonin functions in a relationship with parathyroid hormone more so than with the thyroid hormones. Calcitonin's major effect is on bones. Calcitonin reduces plasma calcium levels by immediate decrease in osteoclast activity, a transient increase in osteoblastic activity, and a prolonged prevention of new osteoclast formation. Calcitonin also interacts with parathormone in the urinary excretion of calcium, magnesium, phosphates, and other electrolytes.

Anatomy of the Parathyroid Glands

SIZE AND LOCATION

Four small, flat, roundish glands are located on the posterior surface of the lateral lobes of the thyroid (Figure 32-3). Usually one parathyroid gland is located at the superior end of each thyroid lobe, and another gland is located at the inferior end of each lateral lobe of the thyroid. This location may vary considerably. It is normal to have four glands; however, there may be fewer or more than four glands.

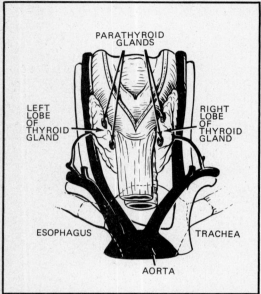

Figure 32-3. Location of the parathyroid glands (posterior view).

INTERNAL STRUCTURE

Two types of cells have been identified in the adult parathyroid glands. *Chief cells* (Figure 32-4) are the main cells in the adult. *Oxyphil cells* (Figure 32-4) are present in adults but are frequently absent in children. The function of oxyphil cells is unknown. There is the possibility that oxyphil cells are modified chief cells.

Physiology of the Parathyroid Glands

HORMONE SECRETION

The parathyroid glands secrete a hormone termed parathormone (PTH). If two of the glands are inadvertently removed during a subtotal thyroidectomy, the remaining

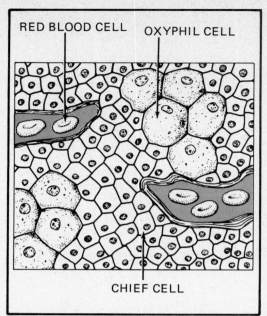

Figure 32-4. Chief cells and oxyphil cells of a parathyroid gland.

glands will produce sufficient parathormone for the body's needs. Some parathyroid tissue should be preserved. This tissue will hypertrophy and continue to secrete parathormone. Chief cells in the parathyroid gland are responsible for the secretion of parathormone. Oxyphil cells may also secrete some hormones.

When hypothalamic releasing factors are stimulated by a decreased serum calcium level or an increased serum magnesium/phosphate concentration, a series of reactions occur resulting in the secretion of parathormone.

Parathormone release is also inhibited by hypothalamic factors (PIH) when serum calcium is increased or when there is an excessive concentration of vitamin D.

ACTION OF PARATHYROID HORMONE

The main action of parathormone and calcitonin is conservation of normal blood calcium levels. Parathormone decreases renal tubular reabsorption of phosphates, sodium, potassium, and amino acids. It increases reabsorption of calcium, magnesium, and hydrogen ions.

Activated vitamin D (discussed in Chapter 26) is essential for parathormone to function appropriately. The release of parathyroid hormone is controlled by a negative feedback mechanism between the blood calcium levels, the hypothalamus, and the parathyroid glands.

Target cells of the parathyroid glands include all bones (in a reciprocal relationship with calcium), kidney cells, and the gastrointestinal tract, if there is sufficient ingestion of vitamin D.

Thyroid Dysfunction

Common thyroid disorders result from too little (hypothyroidism) or too much (hyperthyroidism) of the thyroid hormone secretions.

Hypothyroidism, also called myxedema, results from a lack of thyroid hormones. Myxedema coma is the result of *severe* deficiency or total absence of thyroid hormones.

Hyperthyroidism is also called Graves' disease. The fulminant form of hyperthyroidism is called thyroid storm or thyrotoxic crisis. Storm or crisis may occur at any time.

Hypothyroidism (Myxedema)

Hypothyroidism is present when there is insufficient secretion of thyroid hormone. In hypothyroidism, the thyroid gland is usually small and consists of large amounts of fibrous tissue. Some 60% of all cases have autoantibodies present, caused by an autoimmune process.

Hypothyroidism is a chronic disease that is 10 times more common in females than in males and occurs in all age groups, but most commonly after the age of 50.

Physiological signs and symptoms of hypothyroidism are the same regardless of the etiologic basis.

ETIOLOGY

Thyroidectomy is a major factor if a hyperthyroid state existed. More common etiologies include inadequate dosage of thyroid medications in the known hypothyroid patient and post-thyroidectomy patient. Lack of compliance with the prescribed medical regimen, cessation of medication, pituitary tumors, autoimmune processes, and idiopathic factors are other causes of hypothyroidism.

SIGNS AND SYMPTOMS OF HYPOTHYROIDISM (MYXEDEMA)

A common symptom is edema of the face and a puffiness of the eyelids (Figure 32-5). Bloating of the face produces a broad, round shape. Lips become thickened and develop a cyanotic hue. Weakness, fatigability, exertional dyspnea, sensation of cold, paresthesia of the fingers, and loss of hearing are frequent symptoms. Lethargy, lack of concentration, failing memory, and alteration in mentation occur. Skin and hair changes are often early signs of hypothyroidism. The skin becomes dry and scaly and the hair becomes friable, dry, and falls out. Total body hair may be involved. These signs increase as the condition progresses to myxedema coma.

COMPLICATIONS OF HYPOTHYROIDISM (MYXEDEMA)

The most serious complication of hypothyroidism is its progression to myxedema coma and death if untreated. Hypothyroidism is associated with an increased incidence of early, severe arteriosclerosis. Anemia and increased sensitivity to hypnotic and sedative drugs may become serious problems. Resistance to infection is suppressed and response to treatment of infection is poor. Angina and myocardial infarction are especially common *after* starting replacement thyroid therapy. The therapy improves and increases myocardial action, but the arteriosclerosis prevents increased delivery of oxygen to the myocardium. Commonly, this results in ischemia and infarction.

TREATMENT OF HYPOTHYROIDISM (MYXEDEMA)

The optimum treatment for hypothyroidism is *early* intervention. The only possibility for prevention of complications is the

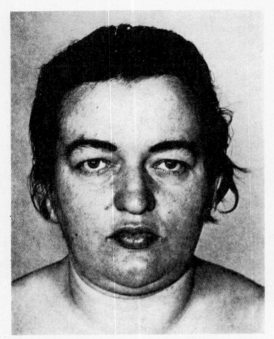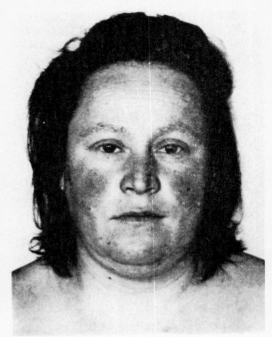

Figure 32-5. Facial appearance of two patients with myxedema.

early recognition of hypothyroidism and close monitoring of medication therapy for the remainder of the patient's life. This, of course, necessitates the patient's compliance with the medical regimen.

Usual **thyroid hormone replacement** may be accomplished with: (a) desiccated thyroid extract (Thyroid USP®) in daily doses of 60 mg P.O. with an increase every 15–30 days to a daily maximum of 180 mg P.O.; (b) levothyroxine sodium or L-thyroxine sodium (Synthroid®) in doses of 0.025–0.1 mg P.O daily with an increase of 0.05–0.1 mg every 1–4 weeks until stable. A maintenance dose is 0.1–0.4 mg daily P.O.; or (c) liothyronine sodium (T_3), known as (Cytomel®), in 25 mcg daily P.O. Increase dose 12.5–25 mcg daily every 1–2 weeks until stable. Usual maintenance dose is 25–75 mcg daily P.O.

Myxedema Coma

Myxedema coma is a life-threatening emergency that is fatal without treatment.

CLINICAL PRESENTATION

Myxedma coma is characterized by hypothermia, hypoventilation, hyponatremia, hypotension, and a bradycardia. The crisis occurs more commonly in winter than in summer due to exposure to cold. Myxedema crisis also occurs frequently following trauma, infection, and central nervous system depression.

The most frequent complication not already mentioned is seizures, which may be almost continous as death becomes imminent.

TREATMENT OF MYXEDEMA COMA

A multiple systems approach must be used in treating this emergency. Mechanical ventilation is used to control hypoventilation, carbon dioxide narcosis, and respiratory arrest. Intravenous hypertonic normal saline and glucose will correct the dilutional hyponatremia and hypoglycemia. Hydrocortisone (100 mg daily) may be used to treat a possible adrenocortical insufficiency (commonly associated problem). Thyroid therapy is started immediately without waiting for laboratory confirmation of the diagnosis. Levothyroxine sodium (L-thyroxine sodium) is the most commonly used drug in this emergency. Intravenous doses of 0.2–0.5 mg during the first 24 hours may be followed by an additional 0.1–0.3 mg I.V. if required after 24 hours. Oral doses may then be tolerated. Vasoactive drugs may be used to support blood pressure. Bradycardia may require treatment with drugs or with a temporary pacemaker.

Hyperthyroidism

Toxic goiter and thyrotoxicosis are synonyms for hyperthyroidism. Hyperthyroidism due to Graves' disease is thought to be an autoimmune process, although the terms are used interchangeably.

ETIOLOGY

In hyperthyroidism, the thyroid gland enlarges, usually to two or more times the normal size. This releases excess thyroid hormones into the body increasing the systemic adrenergic activity. Hyperthyroidism is thought to be caused by a failure of the negative feedback system. Some cases are due to thyroid adenomas, goiters, or familial traits.

CLINICAL PRESENTATION OF HYPERTHYROIDISM

Exophthalmos (protruding eyeballs) is a clinical sign of hyperthyroidism or Graves' disease (Figure 32-6). The common signs and symptoms are marked fatigue accompanied by insomnia, tachycardia, heat intolerance, emotional lability, irritability, nervousness, and weight loss (often extreme).

DIAGNOSIS AND TREATMENT

The diagnosis is confirmed by T_3 and T_4 test results and an increased ^{131}I uptake by the thyroid. Some physicians feel that the ^{131}I test is the only reliable index, along with the patient's symptoms, to establish a diagnosis of hypo- or hyperthyroidism. Treatment may be medical or surgical. Propylthiouracil or methimazole is given orally

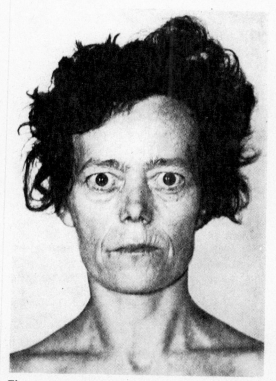
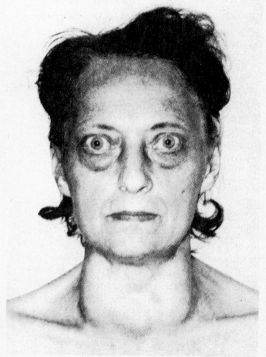

Figure 32-6. Facial appearance of two patients with hyperthyroidism.

for 6 weeks to decrease synthesis and secretions of hormones from the thyroid. After the patient is euthyroid, ^{131}I or a subtotal thyroidectomy may be used as definitive therapy. The patient usually requires daily thyroid medication (for life) after surgery.

COMPLICATIONS OF HYPERTHYROIDISM

Heart failure, malnutrition, and ventilatory failure (due to exhaustion) are common. A more life-threatening complication is thyroid storm.

Thyrotoxic Crisis (Thyroid Storm)

Thyrotoxic crisis is a metabolic emergency and has a greater than 20% mortality rate.

PATHOPHYSIOLOGY

This is the same as for hyperthyroidism.

ETIOLOGIES

Any factor that increases synthesis and secretion of thyroid hormones may cause a storm. Etiologic factors include subtotal thyroidectomy (due to release of thyroid hormones during the surgery), ketoacidotic states, abruptly stopping antithyroid drugs or overdosing on thyroid medications (intentional or otherwise). Trauma, stress, and/or infection may precipitate a crisis.

CLINICAL PRESENTATION

The thyroid storm syndrome characteristically includes hyperthermia, tachydysrhythmias, diarrhea, dehydration, and altered neurologic status including agitation, tremors, hyperkinesia, delirium, and stupor/coma. Nausea and vomiting with weight loss is common.

TREATMENT

Treatment of the thyroid storm is of an emergency nature. Treatment is started *without* waiting for laboratory confirmation of the diagnosis. The FIRST objective is to support vital functions, which necessitates respiratory, cardiac, and renal monitoring.

Second, a reversal of peripheral effects of excessive thyroid hormone is achieved by intravenous propranolol hydrochloride (Inderal®) to decrease the hypermetabolic activity. Propranolol is a beta-adrenergic blocker used to control tachycardias which are often resistant to digitalis therapy. Propranolol is changed to oral doses as soon as possible since effects may last 4–8 hours. Reserpine in doses of 0.5–1 mg I.M., then 2.4 mg I.M. every 2 hours helps reverse peripheral effects, provides sedation, decreases anxiety, and may help reduce the tachycardia. Maximum dose is 4 mg. When tolerated, P.O. dose is 0.1–0.5 mg daily for maintenance.

Third, the reduction of the available and circulating thyroid hormones must be achieved. Iodine solutions may slow the release of thyroid hormones. The two most commonly used are Lugol's solution and sodium iodide. Lugol's solution is 30 drops of iodine mixed in milk or juice and given orally through a straw to prevent staining of the teeth. If Lugol's solution cannot be used, *slow* intravenous sodium iodide from 1 to 2 gm may achieve the desired results. Propylthiouracil in doses of 900–1,200 mg orally will reduce synthesis of thyroid hormones.

Fourth, high doses of hydrocortisone will help support body functions in this extreme stress situation. Doses as high as 300 mg per day may be needed.

Fifth, large amounts of vitamin B complex are required, along with glucose, protein, and carbohydrates, to provide the body with necessary nutrients for the extreme catabolic state it is in.

Sixth, identification and treatment of the underlying cause is essential to prevent recurrence.

NURSING INTERVENTIONS

General symptomatic supportive care is appropriate. A quiet environment with limited visitors helps decrease external stress. Physiologic stress is often treated with hydrocortisone daily.

Cooling blankets are useful in hyperpyrexia. Cooling to the extent of shivering and piloerection (hair on arms standing up, such as with goose bumps) may have a rebound effect of raising the temperature even higher and increasing metabolic activity. Aspirin is *avoided* because it increases free thyroxine levels.

Fluids, electrolytes, and glucose are given to prevent dehydration and imbalances, and provide energy to meet metabolic needs.

Iodine may be given by nasogastric tube or intravenously to prevent release of thyroid hormones.

COMPLICATIONS OF THYROTOXIC CRISIS

If untreated, thyroid storm results in heart failure, exhaustion, coma, and death. With treatment, the sequence is frequently the same. Thyroid storm is most often seen in the summer in undiagnosed or inadequately treated hyperthyroid persons. The presence of stress, infection, nonthyroid surgery, diabetic ketoacidosis, and trauma may result in thyroid storm so intense that it is not amenable to reversal.

Parathyroid Dysfunction

A major parathyroid dysfunction is hypoparathyroidism. This state is a metabolic crisis. Hypoparathyroidism is often seen with hypocalcemia.

PATHOPHYSIOLOGY

A deficiency of the parathormone causes a hypocalcemic state resulting in abnormal neuromuscular activity (calcium level less than 8.5 mg/dl). It is thought that this deficiency occurs secondary to a dysfunction in the calcium and in the phosphate concentration feedback loops control systems.

ETIOLOGY

Acute hypocalcemia is usually secondary to ischemia or damage of the parathyroid gland during a thyroidectomy. Very rarely, radiation therapy (^{131}I) of the thyroid may cause a hypoparathyroidism, as can acute pancreatitis. It may also be idiopathic.

CLINICAL PRESENTATION

Nausea, vomiting, and abdominal cramps are common. Dyspnea may be accompanied by a laryngeal stridor and cyanosis. Neurological signs and symptoms are prominent. There may be confusion, emotional lability, paresthesias of fingers and toes, and muscular twitching progressing to tetany and convulsions.

DIAGNOSIS

Laboratory blood work will show a hypocalcemia. Urine tests will reveal a hypophosphaturia and perhaps a hypocalcuria. Two signs are a positive Trousseau and a positive Chvostek sign; both were explained in Chapter 27. These signs are not always present.

TREATMENT

The objective of treatment is to raise serum calcium levels to normal. If seizures and tetany have not developed, oral calcium supplements are indicated with additional vitamin D to promote calcium absorption. (Calcium may be given with food but not with milk since milk products will decrease calcium absorption.)

Some types of calcium chloride should only be given through a central line, as infiltration in a peripheral line will result in tissue necrosis and sloughing. Calcium cannot be infused in saline due to precipitation formation with sodium bicarbonate, forcing calcium ion excretion in the kidneys.

Cardiac status must be monitored *especially* if the patient is on digitalis. Digitalis and calcium have a synergistic action.

COMPLICATIONS

Complications include seizures, tetany, shock, and death. A quiet environment with supportive equipment (ventilator, pacemaker) on standby may be useful in preventing death.

NURSING INTERVENTIONS

Preventive nursing care in hypoparathyroidism may avoid the complications of seizures and tetany. The environment should be modified to be as quiet as possible including the limiting of visitors until the patient is well stabilized.

A respirator on standby will provide for immediate intervention in the advent of hypoventilation or deteriorating respiratory status as shown by serial arterial blood gases. Emotional and physical stress often cause hyperventilation. In turn, hyperventilation causes alkalosis, which may precipitate tetany.

Cardiac monitoring is essential since calcium therapy may alter cardiac conduction times with resultant dysrhythmias.

Standard monitoring of intake/output, response to medication therapy, neurological status, and such are applicable to these patients as the medication therapy will cause a change in the patient's electrolytes and fluid balance.

Administration of calcium as ordered, with special attention to possible infiltration and precipitation if being given intravenously, and AVOIDING milk products if being given orally will help ensure maximum benefit with minimal side effects of the drugs.

Trousseau's sign is elicited by occluding circulation to the arm. This is done by maintaining a B/P cuff pressure just above the systolic level. If positive, the patient's hand will develop a carpopedal spasm within 3 minutes. A carpopedal spasm results in a hollow palm position and fingers rigid and flexed at the metacarpophalangeal joints.

Chvostek's sign is elicited by lightly tapping the facial nerve in front of the ear. If positive, there is a unilateral contraction of the facial muscles.

— 33 —

Anatomy, Physiology, and Dysfunction of the Adrenal Glands

Learning Objectives

By the end of this chapter, the nurse will be able to:

1. Identify the location and the two parts of the adrenal glands.
2. List three zones of tissue in the adrenal cortex.
3. List the three classes of hormones secreted by the adrenal cortex and identify the most important hormone in each class.
4. Define corticosteroids and catecholamines.
5. Identify the major factors resulting in the secretion of corticosteroid and catecholamine hormones.
6. List two hormones secreted by the adrenal medulla.
7. Explain the action and site of action of the catecholamines.
8. Identify factors resulting in the release of catecholamines.
9. Identify the two life-threatening dysfunctions of the adrenal gland.
10. List at least four effects of a mineralocorticoid deficiency.
11. List at least four effects of a glucocorticoid deficiency.
12. Identify four etiologic factors in Addison's disease and explain the treatment of Addison's disease.
13. Differentiate the pathophysiology of Addison's disease and acute adrenal crisis.
14. List at least four causes of adrenal crisis.
15. Identify six presenting symptoms of acute adrenal crisis.
16. List five complications of acute adrenal insufficiency.
17. Explain the rationale of treatment for acute adrenal insufficiency.

Anatomy of the Adrenal Glands

The adrenal glands are a pair of glands located on the top of each kidney (Figure 33-1). Each of the pair of adrenal glands is identical to the other.

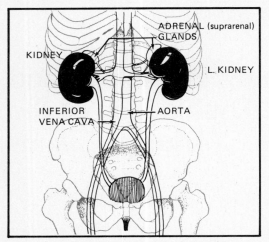

Figure 33-1. The location of the adrenal glands.

The adrenal gland is composed of two separate parts (Figure 33-2). The adrenal cortex is the outer two-thirds of the gland. The adrenal medulla is the inner one-third of the gland. A mnemonic for remembering where each part lies is the letter "M". "M" stands for the **m**edulla and the **m**iddle.

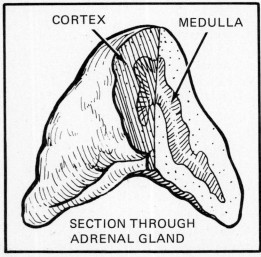

Figure 33-2. Section showing cortex and medulla of the adrenal gland.

THE ADRENAL CORTEX

The adrenal cortex is composed of three distinct regions or zones (Figure 33-3). The outermost zone is the zona glomerulosa. The middle zone is the zona fasciculata. The innermost zone is the zona reticularis. The zona glomerulosa functions by itself. The zona fasciculata and zona reticularis function together as a unit.

The zona glomerulosa is a thin zone located on the outer part of the cortex, directly under the capsular covering. The cells in this zone are arranged in clumps. The regulation of the hormone (aldosterone) secreted in the zona glomerulosa is completely independent of the regulatory controls over the zona fasciculata and the zona reticularis. The regulatory control of the zona

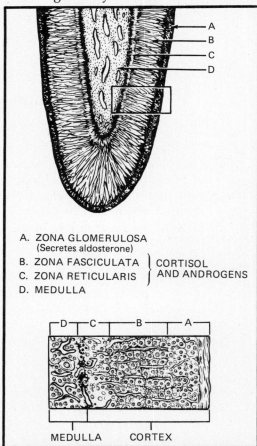

A. ZONA GLOMERULOSA
   (Secretes aldosterone)
B. ZONA FASCICULATA ⎫ CORTISOL
C. ZONA RETICULARIS ⎬ AND ANDROGENS
D. MEDULLA

Figure 33-3. The zones and the medulla of the adrenal gland.

glomerulosa is the release of ACTH releasing factors from the hypothalamus and ACTH stimulating factors from the adenohypophysis.

The zona fasciculata is the largest of the three zones. Its cells are arranged in straight rows. *The zona reticularis* is composed of an anastomosing network of cells. These two zones function together to regulate cortisol and androgen hormones and are controlled by the same regulatory mechanisms of the adenohypophysis.

THE ADRENAL MEDULLA

Cells of the adrenal medulla (Figure 33-2) develop from the same embryological source as the sympathetic neurons. The cells are also called chromaffin cells because of their histiologic staining characteristics. Because of their origin, the adrenal medulla cells are related functionally to the sympathetic nervous system.

Physiology of the Adrenal Glands

Functionally, the adrenal cortex and the adrenal medulla are totally different. Without adrenal cortex hormones or replacement therapy, death occurs in 3–14 days.

Adrenal Cortex Hormones

The hormones secreted by the adrenal cortex are classified as corticosteroids since they are synthesized from the steroid cholesterol. (As a group, the more than 30 corticosteroids may be referred to as corticoids.)

The adrenal cortex secretes three classes of hormones: the glucocorticoids, mineralocorticoids, and the androgenic hormones.

THE GLUCOCORTICOIDS

Originally, the glucocorticoids were thought to control the blood glucose level in the body. It has since been discovered that glucocorticoids play a major role in utilization of carbohydrates, proteins, and fats.

Cortisol

This glucocorticoid is responsible for 95% of the adrenocortical secretory actions. Cortisol is the most important hormone of this class of steroid hormones. Cortisol affects all body cells (especially the liver). It is secreted by the zona fasciculata and the zona reticularis in response to stress (both physical and psychogenic), trauma, and infection.

Cortisol is active in all metabolic processes. These include the ability of the body to stimulate gluconeogenesis by the liver up to 10 times its normal rate. (It does this by increasing the migration of amino acids from the extracellular fluids to the liver, by increasing the migration of amino acids from muscles into the liver, and by increasing all of the enzymes needed to convert the amino acids into glucose in the liver.) Cortisol decreases the cellular uptake of glucose to a mild extent and inhibits cellular utilization of glucose to a moderate degree.

Cortisol decreases protein storage in all body cells except the liver, resulting in muscle weakness and decreased functions of immunity in the lymphoid tissues. The proteins stored in tissues are shifted to the liver (called mobilization of amino acids) and this shift results in decreased protein synthesis.

Cortisol promotes fatty acid mobilization weakly, but that mobilization is sufficient to provide some fat for body energy in the absence of the normal glucose.

Cortisol has a strong anti-inflammatory effect and, in sufficient amounts, may block and/or reverse the inflammatory process.

The hypothalamus provides the negative feedback mechanism responsible for corticotropin-releasing factors (CRF) and corticotropin-inhibitory factors (such as exogenous intake of corticosteroids).

THE MINERALOCORTICOIDS

Mineralocorticoids are named as such since their action is chiefly with the extracellular fluid electrolytes (minerals) of sodium and potassium. The most important mineralocorticoid is aldosterone, which is secreted in the zona glomerulosa.

Aldosterone

This mineralocorticoid's most important function is regulation of sodium and potassium movement through renal tubule walls. It also plays a minor part in hydrogen ion transport.

Aldosterone exerts its action on the distal convoluted tubules and the collecting ducts. There is a slight effect upon sweat glands (to conserve salt in hot conditions). The *primary* aldosterone action causes an increase in sodium reabsorption and potassium excretion by the kidney. Since water follows sodium, aldosterone secretion tends to change the extracellular fluid *volume* in proportion to its secretion.

Aldosterone excess may rapidly cause a severe hypokalemia, including a muscle weakness, and muscle paralysis if the potassium level is reduced to half its normal value. Hypertension may occur due to the increase in the extracellular fluid volume.

The release of aldosterone is stimulated by an increased serum potassium level, the renin-angiotensin cascade, decreased serum sodium levels, and adrenocorticotropic hormone (ACTH).

Decreased levels of aldosterone allow the extracellular level of potassium to rise to double the normal potassium level, resulting in severe hyperkalemia and cardiac toxicity as evidenced by weakness of contractions. A concurrent decrease in serum sodium and increase in water loss occurs. A potassium level only slightly higher will cause a cardiac death.

THE ANDROGENS

Several androgens are secreted by the adrenal cortex, but their alterations are not usually a primary cause for treatment in a critical care area and will not be covered in this text except to mention that they are secreted by the zona fasciculata and the zona reticularis.

Adrenal Medulla Hormones

The hormones secreted by the adrenal medulla are classified as **catecholamines** and have very far-reaching effects. Catecholamines are synthesized in the adrenal medulla as well as by sympathetic nerve fiber endings, the brain, and some peripheral tissues. Both of the catecholamines secreted by the adrenal medulla have an effect on the adrenergic (sympathetic) receptor sites. There are three sites termed alpha, $beta_1$, and $beta_2$. Table 33-1 lists the adrenergic receptors and their functions.

Table 33-1. Adrenergic receptors and their functions.

Alpha Receptor	Beta Receptor
Vasoconstriction	Vasodilatation (B_2)
Iris dilatation	Cardioacceleration (B_1)
Intestinal relaxation	Increased myocardial strength (B_1)
Intestinal sphincter contraction	Intestinal relaxation (B_2)
Pilomotor contraction	Uterus relaxation (B_2)
Bladder sphincter contraction	Bronchodilatation (B_2)
	Calorigenesis (B_2)
	Glycogenolysis (B_2)
	Lipolysis (B_1)
	Bladder relaxation (B_2)

EPINEPHRINE (ADRENALIN)

Epinephrine (Adrenalin) accounts for 80% of the total catecholamine secreted by the adrenal medulla and excites both alpha and beta adrenergic receptor sites equally.

A major action of epinephrine is the "fear, fight, flight" body response to stress. These actions would include positive effects on the cardiac muscle, shifting blood to certain muscles, decreasing gastrointestinal function, bronchiole dilatation accompanied by hyperpnea and tachypnea, and a serum glucose level increase.

Epinephrine is released by sympathetic nervous system stimulation and other hormones such as insulin and histamine.

NOREPINEPHRINE

Norepinephrine accounts for 20% of catecholamines secreted by the adrenal medulla. Norepinephrine excites mainly alpha receptors and to a slight degree beta receptors. Norepinephrine action is similar to adrenalin with two notable exceptions. The effect of norepinephrine is not as intense as adrenalin on cardiac and metabolic functions. Also, norepinephrine has a *more* intense action than adrenalin on skeletal muscle vasculature. This increases peripheral vascular resistance due to the increased vasoconstriction.

The sites of action for norepinephrine are body cells and vascular beds, and releasing factors for norepinephrine are the same as for epinephrine.

Adrenal Gland Dysfunction

Adrenal insufficiency is a major life-threatening dysfunction of the adrenal cortex. It is also known as hypoadrenalism and/or hypocorticism.

Addison's Disease

Addison's disease is a chronic dysfunction of the adrenal glands resulting in an *inadequate* adrenal secretion of cortisol and aldosterone (adrenal insufficiency).

PATHOPHYSIOLOGY

The adrenal cortex dysfunction results in a deficiency of mineralocorticoids and glucocorticoids.

Mineralocorticoid decrease results in an aldosterone deficiency. Without aldosterone, there is an increased excretion of sodium. The depletion of sodium leads to dehydration and hypotension. At the same time, there is a retention of potassium. If the potassium concentration increases sufficiently, there is first a flaccidity of the cardiac myocardium followed by cardiac cell paralysis as the potassium level rises. Hemoconcentration, acidosis, decreased cardiac output, shock, and death due to the cardiac paralysis occurs.

A decrease in glucocorticoids results in a cortisol deficiency which affects major body systems. Anorexia, nausea, vomiting, and abdominal pain result in a weight loss. The neurological effects of cortisol deficiency include fatigue, lethargy, apathy, confusion, and psychoses. Cardiovascular effects include an impaired response to the vasoactive catecholamines. Energy-producing mechanisms are altered, for example, decreased glucogenesis (causes hypo-glycemia) and fat mobilization. The decreased cortisol level stimulates the pituitary to secrete ACTH unrestrained. There is a decreased resistance to both physical and psychogenic stress.

Melanin pigmentation (Figure 33-4) is increased in most cases of Addison's disease. The increased pigmentation is unevenly distributed and is probably due to increased secretion of MSH with ACTH from the adenohypophysis.

ETIOLOGY

The most frequent cause is a primary atrophy of the adrenal cortex. This may be an autoimmune process. Often tubercular destruction of the cortex or a cancerous tumor causes Addison's disease. Stress may be a factor.

TREATMENT

If untreated, the patient dies within a period of a few days to a few weeks. Replacement therapy of small amounts of mineralocorticoids and glucocorticoids may prolong life for years.

Strict adherence to a diet low in potassium and high in sodium will help prevent complications.

If a tumor is the etiological factor, surgery is performed.

COMPLICATIONS

Addisonian crisis may be fatal. A crisis may occur anytime there is an increase in stress since the adrenal cortex CANNOT increase its production of cortisol. Steroids should be increased in patients with Addison's disease who are under stress. Even a slight cold necessitates increased steroid hormone levels. The only successful treatment of Addisonian crisis is *massive* doses of glucocorticoids. Often as much as 10 or more times the *normal* dose must be used to prevent death.

Acute Adrenal Insufficiency

Adrenal crisis and Addisonian crisis are synonyms for acute adrenal insufficiency and may be used interchangeably.

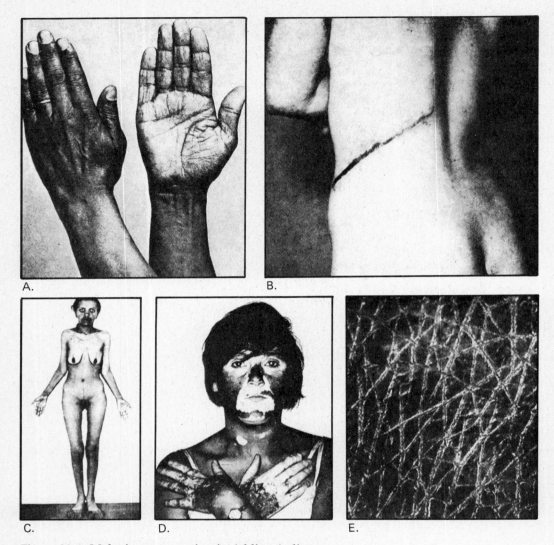

A.

B.

C.

D.

E.

Figure 33-4. Melanin oversecretion in Addison's disease.

ETIOLOGY

Usually an underlying chronic condition (Addison's disease) is present before a crisis. In addition to this chronic disease, an infection, trauma, a surgical procedure or some extra stress occurs and the patient develops acute adrenal insufficiency. Less common causes of acute adrenal insufficiency are adrenalectomy, Waterhouse-Friderichsen syndrome, abrupt cessation of steroid therapy, chemotherapy, and hypothalamic diseases. An autoimmune response may be a factor.

CLINICAL PRESENTATION

Anorexia, nausea, vomiting, diarrhea, and abdominal pain lead to increased fluid and electrolyte disturbances. Fever may lead to alterations in consciousness. Hypotension precedes shock and coma.

DIAGNOSIS

Patient history, physical examination, and presenting symptoms are usually sufficient to provide a tentative diagnosis and to indicate the need for immediate treatment. Definitive laboratory studies are those evaluating endocrine function and identifying resultant system dysfunction or imbalances in the electrolytes.

COMPLICATIONS

Death is the common complication, although it is usually preceded by dysrhythmias, hypovolemia, shock, and coma.

TREATMENT

Adequate circulatory volume is vital. Continuous monitoring of vital signs to identify developing dysfunction provides for early intervention. Glucocorticoids must be replaced. An intravenous glucocorticoid such as hydrocortisone should be given. Physical and psychological stress should be avoided.

NURSING INTERVENTIONS

Continuous monitoring of the respiratory system with a ventilator on standby is indicated. If serial arterial blood gases show deteriorating respiratory status, the patient may be intubated and placed on the respirator. Standard nursing procedures for ALL artificially ventilated patients should be instituted.

Cardiac and hemodynamic monitoring will reveal early signs of impending dysrhythmias and shock providing an opportunity for early intervention.

Intake and output records will indicate renal function.

Emotional support of the patient and family is of utmost importance in an attempt to decrease exogenous stress as much as possible.

Hypercorticism—Cushing's Syndrome

Hypercorticism is a marked increase in the production of mineralocorticoids, gluco-corticoids, and androgen steroids resulting in the condition known as Cushing's syndrome (NOT to be confused with Cushing's triad).

ETIOLOGY

Cushing's syndrome is usually due to adrenal tumors or a pituitary tumor. A pituitary tumor causes increased release of ACTH which results in hyperplasia of the adrenal cortex.

CLINICAL PRESENTATION

Increased glucocorticoids (cortisol) causes increased glucogenesis resulting in hyperglycemia. It causes increased protein tissue wasting. It also causes increased fat resulting in the typical "moon face" and increased trunk fat (Figure 33-5). The increased cortisol causes mood swings ranging from euphoria to depression.

Increased mineralocorticoids (aldosterone) result in increased potassium excretion causing dysrhythmias, renal disorders, and muscle weakness. The increased aldosterone causes a decrease in sodium secretion. The increased sodium causes an increase in fluid retention resulting in edema and usually an increase in blood pressure. (Eighty percent of patients with Cushing's syndrome have hypertension.)

Increased sex hormones (androgens) cause increased facial hair and acne.

DIAGNOSIS

Patient history, physical examination, and presenting symptoms are usually sufficient to provide a tentative diagnosis. Definitive laboratory studies are those evaluating endocrine function and identifying resultant system dysfunction or imbalance.

TREATMENT

Treatment consists of removing the tumor, if possible, which will necessitate steroid replacement. A diet low in sodium and high in potassium is required.

NURSING INTERVENTIONS

Routine postsurgical nursing care is required. In addition, the patient must be

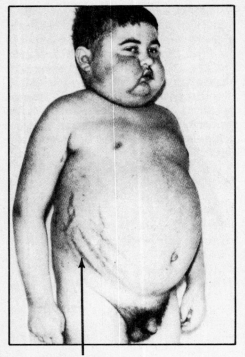
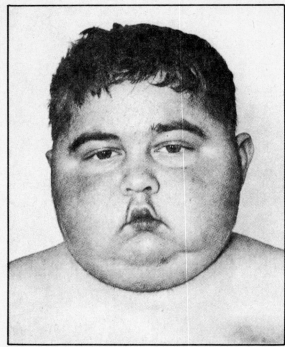

PURPLE STRIAE

Figure 33-5. Cushing's syndrome showing "moon face," trunk fat, and purple striae.

assessed for endocrine imbalance indicating a need for replacement therapy. The patient's immune system will have been depressed because of the increased steroid levels prior to surgery, so signs of infection must be closely monitored. Education relating to diet therapy and medication regimens is essential to prevent endocrine crises in the future.

NOTE: The increase in mineralocorticoids may also cause Conn's syndrome (increased blood pressure and decreased potassium levels due to a benign aldosterone secreting tumor).

Hypofunction of the Adrenal Medulla

Hypofunction of the adrenal medulla does NOT cause systemic problems because the sympathetic nervous system will compensate for decreases in epinephrine and norepinephrine.

Hyperfunction of the Adrenal Medulla

Hyperfunction of the adrenal medulla can be life-threatening primarily due to the possibility of CVAs and CHF. In hyperfunction, epinephrine increases blood pressure, cardiac output, pulse, and metabolism. Norepinephrine increases the blood pressure more than epinephrine does. Hyperfunction may be precipitated by stress and/or exertion.

Pheochromocytoma

Hyperfunction of the adrenal medulla is the most common cause of pheochromocytoma. Pheochromocytoma is an encapsulated, vascular tumor of chromaffin tissue of the adrenal medulla.

DIAGNOSIS

Signs and symptoms are the major diagnostic clues. However, hyperfunction of the adrenal medulla often resembles other disorders which must be ruled out. These include diabetes mellitus, essential hypertension, and psychoneurosis.

CLINICAL PRESENTATION

The outstanding symptom is the extremely high blood pressure secondary to the excessive medulla hormones. Other signs and symptoms include increased sympathetic nervous activity, sweating, headache, palpitations, apprehension, nausea/vomiting, tremor, pallor or flushing of the face, abdominal and/or chest pain, and hyperglycemia.

TREATMENT

Treatment is surgical removal of the pheochromocytoma. A preoperative diet low in sodium and carbohydrates is usual.

NURSING INTERVENTIONS

Preoperatively the nurse should promote rest and decrease patient apprehension. Postoperative routine procedures are instituted; in addition, the patient must be closely monitored for shock, hypotension (due to decreased levels of epinephrine and norepinephrine), hypoglycemia, and hemorrhage (the adrenal glands are VERY vascular).

34

Anatomy, Physiology, and Dysfunction of the Pancreas Gland

Learning Objectives

By the end of this chapter, the nurse will be able to:

1. List the two major types of tissue composing the pancreas.
2. Define acini.
3. List three types of cells found in the islets of Langerhans and identify the hormone secreted by each type of cell.
4. Explain the primary function of glucagon.
5. List two mechanisms of altering glucose metabolism by glucagon.
6. List the target cells for glucagon and for insulin.
7. Identify two factors that stimulate insulin secretion.
8. List four actions of insulin.
9. Define diabetic ketoacidosis (DKA) and list four etiologies.
10. Define the diagnostic criterion for DKA.
11. Explain the effect of insulin on hyperglycemia.
12. Explain the action of acetyl-CoA.
13. Identify at least nine signs and symptoms of DKA.
14. List six objectives of the treatment of DKA.
15. Identify eight complications of DKA.
16. Differentiate between DKA and HHNK (hyperosmolar coma).
17. Explain the pathophysiology of HHNK and list at least three diagnostic criteria of HHNK.
18. List nine common symptoms and signs of HHNK.
19. Explain the need for hypotonic fluids in treating HHNK.
20. Define hypoglycemia and list common exogenous and endogenous etiologies of hypoglycemia.
21. Describe the clinical presentation of hypoglycemia.
22. Explain immediate treatment of hypoglycemia and identify the complications of hypoglycemia.
23. Describe the Somogyi effect.

The pancreas has a dual classification. It is considered an accessory digestive gland since it produces many enzymes essential to digestion. These enzymes are released through exocrine glands (glands that release substances through ducts).

The pancreas (Figure 34-1) is also classified as an endocrine gland because it releases two hormones directly into the bloodstream.

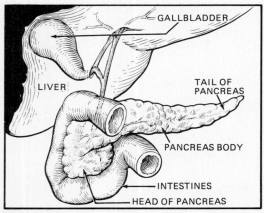

Figure 34-1. The pancreas.

Anatomy of the Pancreas Gland

There are two major types of tissues found in the pancreas: the acini and the islets of Langerhans. *The acini* secrete digestive enzymes into the duodenum by exocrine glands. These will be discussed in Chapter 43 (Accessory Digestive Organs). *The islets of Langerhans* cells are scattered throughout the pancreas and may be called pancreatic islets by some texts.

THE ISLETS OF LANGERHANS

Three structurally and functionally different cells comprise the islets of Langerhans: alpha, beta, and delta cells (Figure 34-2).

1. *Alpha* cells are located within the clusters of islet cells. Alpha cells secrete the hormone glucagon, which is often called the hyperglycemic factor. Alpha cells secrete directly into the venous system of the pancreas.
2. *Beta* cells are located within the clusters of islet cells and are slightly smaller than alpha cells. Beta cells secrete insulin. The insulin molecules are very complex amino acid structures.

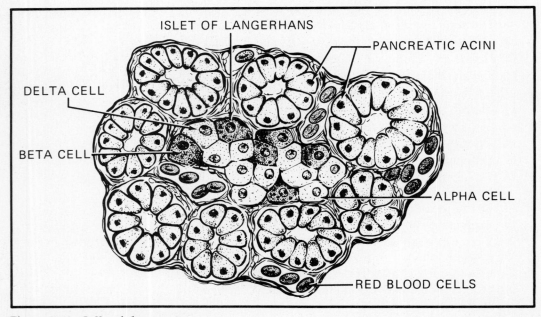

Figure 34-2. Cells of the pancreas.

3. *Delta* cells are located within the clusters of the islet cells. Delta cells secrete a recently identified hormone called somatostatin. Somatostatin is the same as the growth hormone-inhibiting hormone secreted by the hypothalamus. Somatostatin has an effect upon glucagon and insulin secretion.

Physiology of the Pancreas

GLUCAGON

The alpha cells of the islets of Langerhans secrete the hormone glucagon which affects many body cells, especially the liver cells. Glucagon is secreted when blood amino acid levels rise and in the presence of a decreased blood glucose level.

The primary action of glucagon is an antagonist to insulin and its primary functioning site is the liver. The most important aspect of this action is to increase blood glucose levels. Glucose metabolism is altered by two important actions of glucagon: *Glycogenolysis* (the breakdown of liver glycogen stores) releases glucose for use in the body. *Gluconeogenesis* (the formation of glucose from other substances) provides new glucose for the body. There is also an increase in fatty acid oxidation and in urea formation as a natural response to glucagon.

INSULIN

This is a small protein of two amino acid chains. If the chains become separated, insulin loses its effectiveness. Once secreted into the circulatory system, insulin is removed by the liver and degraded. Most insulin only circulates for about 10 minutes before the degradation process occurs. This allows control and rapid initiation or cessation of insulin action when being administered intravenously.

The target cells for insulin action are all body cells and especially liver cells. Factors which facilitate secretion of insulin are an increase in blood glucose levels and the growth hormone levels. A decreased insulin level results in hyperglycemia, ketosis, and acidosis.

Insulin action includes transporting glucose across cell membranes, increasing fatty acid storage, enhancing protein synthesis, and decreasing the breakdown of triglycerides in cells.

Glucose Metabolism Dysfunction

Dysfunction of glucose metabolism treated in critical care areas include diabetic ketoacidosis, hyperosmolar coma, and insulin shock.

Diabetic Ketoacidosis

The digestion of carbohydrates raises the blood glucose level, which stimulates the pancreas to secrete insulin. If insulin cannot be secreted, or secreted in sufficient amounts, hyperglycemia develops.

PATHOPHYSIOLOGY

A lack of insulin prevents peripheral cell utilization of available blood glucose. The liver inhibits the production of glycogen, and glycogen which is available is rapidly degraded. This releases free glucose into the blood, further raising the blood sugar level.

Since the cells cannot utilize the free glucose, protein stores release amino acids, and adipose tissue releases fatty acids. The amino acids and free fatty acids are synthesized by the liver, which is producing excessive amounts of acetyl-CoA. The acetyl-CoA is rapidly degraded into keto, acetoacetic, and beta-hydroxybutyric acids. These acids are produced faster than the kidneys and lungs are able to dispose of them, causing a metabolic acidosis. Ketones (keto acids or ketoanions) are excreted by the kidneys producing a positive urine acetone test. Acetoacetic acid and beta-hydroxybutyric acid are oxidized into acetone. The acetone is exhaled and is responsible for the sweet, fruity smell of the breath. (It is the acetone of the acetoacetic acid that has the odor; beta-hydroxybutyric acid is odorless.)

ETIOLOGY

The most common causes of diabetic keto-acidosis (DKA) are failure to take insulin, increased stress due to illness, trauma, surgery, cardiac conditions, and occasionally psychogenic trauma. Pregnancy and pancreatitis may also precipitate a diabetic keto-acidotic state.

CLINICAL PRESENTATION

The most common symptoms are polydipsia, polyuria, polyphagia (usually with weight loss), dyspnea, and a generalized malaise. Nausea, vomiting, anorexia, and abdominal pain may be present. Signs of dehydration, tachycardia, orthostatic hypotension, and weakness are usually present. Respirations are Kussmaul in character and may have an acetone smell. Mentation ranges from lethargy to coma.

DIAGNOSIS

Serum glucose levels are above 300 mg/100 ml. Urine tests reveal glycosuria and acetone. DKA should be ruled out in any patient who is comatose, dehydrated, and having deep, labored respirations.

TREATMENT

The objectives of treatment are to correct acidemia, hyperglycemia, hypovolemia, hyperosmolality, potassium deficit (if present), and ketonemia. Underlying conditions responsible for the diabetic ketoacidosis such as infections must be treated concurrently.

Resolving the DKA is the most effective method of restoring normal acid-base balance.

Hypovolemia is corrected by rapid infusions of 0.9% normal saline or 0.45% normal saline. Isotonic or hypotonic fluids are administered to counter the hyperosmolality which accompanies DKA. CAUTION! When the serum glucose level is decreased to 250 mg/dl, the fluids should be changed from saline to 5% glucose in 0.5% normal saline. This change will help avoid hypoglycemia, hypokalemia, and cerebral edema caused by the glucose di-uresis. Correcting the hypovolemia usually corrects the hyperosmolality and, over a period of hours, the ketonemia. Patients may move from DKA coma to insulin shock without regaining consciousness. The addition of glucose by intravenous fluids helps prevent this.

Hyperglycemia is corrected by insulin administration. Normally, an intravenous bolus of insulin is administered followed by *slow* continuous intravenous infusion. Insulin may be administered by subcutaneous injections of 10–100 units per hour. Intramuscular injection is not advocated in the crisis stage of DKA due to poor peripheral absorption.

Potassium deficits and other electrolyte imbalances may precipitate cardiac and/or neurological disturbances. Potassium is usually added to intravenous fluids as the insulin forces potassium from the plasma back into the cells producing a hypokalemia. However, the patient's potassium levels may be normal or high. Continuous monitoring and gradual changes to effect a correction over a 24-hour period are safer than massive, rapid changes. The exception to this is the patient whose life is threatened by extremes of hypo-hyperkalemia.

COMPLICATIONS OF DIABETIC KETOACIDOSIS

Acidosis, electrolyte imbalances, acute renal failure, pulmonary edema, cerebral edema, seizures, CSF acidosis, shock, and coma are the major complications of DKA.

NURSING INTERVENTIONS

Maintaining a patent airway and suctioning as required to prevent aspiration is essential. Monitoring respiratory status by observation and arterial blood gases will identify impending hypoxia.

Cardiac monitoring due to electrolyte imbalances will reveal early dysrhythmias. With *hypo*kalemia, U waves are normally present. In *hyper*kalemia peaked or tented T waves are present. There may be a tachycardia which converts to a bradycardia if the hyperkalemia increases.

Monitor urinary output and listen to lung sounds frequently to identify pulmonary edema, especially in the presence of underlying cardiac diseases. Check urine hourly for acetone and sugar. The objective is to achieve a 1+ glycosuria (assuring the patient is NOT going into insulin shock). Once adequate urinary output is present, electrolytes are often added to the intravenous fluids to correct imbalances.

Blood sugar may be monitored hourly by Dextrostix and confirmed by laboratory results every 2–3 hours to guide in the administration of regular insulin. Long-acting insulin is NOT used in DKA crisis.

Potassium is checked frequently since initially it moves from the cells into the blood and much is excreted in the urine. When insulin is given, potassium shifts back into the cells. In addition to the laboratory results, the cardiac monitor will show if the patient's serum potassium is low, normal, or high.

Neurologic status is assessed hourly. Hyperglycemia does not have a deleterious effect upon brain cells, but other elctrolyte imbalances and cerebral edema will affect the cells.

Controversy exists over the use of bicarbonate to correct the acidosis present in DKA. Bicarbonate given intravenously does not cross the blood/brain barrier. It causes a shift in the bicarbonate-carbonic acid ratio which releases carbon dioxide. Carbon dioxide crosses the blood/brain barrier dissolving in the spinal fluid. This raises the carbonic acid level and increases cerebral acidosis which may prolong diabetic coma.

Hyperosmolar Coma—HHNK

HHNK stands for hyperosmolar, hyperglycemic, nonketotic coma. In this condition, there is enough insulin being released in the body to prevent ketosis, but there is not enough insulin to prevent hyperglycemia.

PATHOPHYSIOLOGY

Hyperglycemia increases the solutes in the extracellular fluid causing a hyperosmolality. Cellular dehydration occurs because of the hyperosmolality which is also the cause of diuresis. Without treatment, an osmotic gradient develops between the brain and the plasma resulting in dehydration and central nervous system dysfunction. The end result of dehydration is a decreased glomerular filtration rate and the development of azotemia.

Typically, the HHNK patient is over 50 years old, becomes ill, and has a general malaise. Due to this, the patient is anorexic and eats and drinks poorly, which leads to dehydration. Since the patient is not eating, the body uses protein and fat for energy to maintain body processes. Almost the same pathophysiologic pattern of DKA appears in HHNK. The *difference* is that in HHNK, a sufficient amount of insulin is released to prevent the development of ketosis. The patient may be stuporous or comatose before being seen by a physician.

ETIOLOGY

One of the common causes of HHNK is the undiagnosed or untreated diabetic. Frequently, a mild diabetic state exists without any problems until the diabetic is under stress. Iatrogenic causes account for some cases of HHNK due to hyperalimentation, the administration of hypertonic intravenous fluids, and the administration of steroids.

CLINICAL PRESENTATION

Usually the patient is over 50 years old. The patient is lethargic or comatose. Symptoms include polyuria, polydipsia, nausea, vomiting, weight loss, and decreasing urinary output. Dehydration is apparent with dry skin and mucous membranes. A tachypnea is present. Tachycardia, hypotension, and glycosuria are present.

DIAGNOSIS

The three most outstanding symptoms may well be the blood sugar level (commonly over 1,000 mg), the plasma hyperosmolarity (as high as 450 mOsm/kg), and an extremely elevated hematocrit. Urine and plasma are both negative for acetone.

The BUN is elevated and there is a marked leukocytosis.

COMPLICATIONS

Shock, coma, acute tubular necrosis, and vascular thrombosis are common complications. Approximately 50% of HHNK patients will die.

TREATMENT

Correcting the fluid balance is one of the first objectives of treatment. It is ESSENTIAL that fluids be administered, and as many as 10–20 liters may be administered during the first 24 hours. The hypoinsulinemia may be corrected by the use of insulin, usually not exceeding more than 100 units in the first 24 hours. Hyperglycemia is not known to have deleterious effects upon the brain, but hyperosmolar dehydration may cause seizures. If metabolic acidosis is present, it is usually corrected by the administration of sodium bicarbonate. This is controversial for the same reasons as in DKA. Electrolyte imbalances are corrected. As much as 200–400 mEq of potassium during the first 24–48 hours to correct the potassium imbalance may be required. Close and continuous monitoring is necessary to identify further changes or deterioration in the patient's electrolyte status. Cardiac monitoring and hourly neurological checks will provide clues to changing status.

NURSING INTERVENTIONS

The primary nursing responsibility is the administration of intravenous fluids to correct both the dehydration and hyperosmolality without putting the patient into pulmonary edema. As much as 20 liters of isotonic or hypotonic (controversial) fluids are given over the first 48 hours. The nurse must monitor breath sounds hourly to determine if pulmonary edema is developing.

Cardiac monitoring is continous to identify dysrhythmias due to electrolyte imbalances—especially hypo/hyperkalemia. Also, one must monitor the patient to detect early signs of congestive heart failure.

Administration of insulin to correct hyperglycemia is usually accomplished by a loading intravenous dose of insulin followed by repeated doses as indicated by the blood glucose level. The nurse may monitor the patient's glucose level by Dextrostix hourly and have it confirmed by laboratory results every 2–4 hours.

Neurologic status should be evaluated hourly to provide information on the efficacy of treatment.

Skin and mouth care are important aspects of preventing infection and keeping the patient comfortable.

Hypoglycemic Reaction (Insulin Shock)

PATHOPHYSIOLOGY

A decreased blood level of glucose is the criterion for the label of hypoglycemic reaction or insulin shock. The decrease may be due to a defect in the process of forming glucose, either glyconeogenesis or glycogenolysis, or by the removal of glucose by the use of adipose, muscle, or liver tissues.

ETIOLOGY

Causes of hypoglycemia include an intolerance of fructose, galactose, or amino acids. Postgastrectomy patients may have hypoglycemia. A broad range of drugs such as alcohol, insulin, and sulfonylurea drugs may be the origin. Endocrine dysfunctions, liver disease, severe CHF, and pregnancy may cause hypoglycemia. In diabetic patients, overdoses of insulin or exercising without adjustment of insulin dosage are the common causes of insulin shock.

CLINICAL PRESENTATION

The early signs and symptoms are restlessness, diaphoresis, tachycardia, and hunger. (Propranolol hydrocloride [Inderal®] may hide these signs and symptoms.) If the hypoglycemia progresses to less than 50 mg/dl, the central nervous system is affected and the patient may exhibit behavior which may be from bizarre to a coma. Headache, weakness, tremors, nausea, and personality changes are common signs and symptoms.

DIAGNOSIS AND TREATMENT

A glucose level of less than 45 mg/dl with a Dextrostix is sufficient to infuse 50 mg of 50% dextrose intravenously. The patient will usually respond within 1–2 minutes. A sample of blood should be drawn prior to giving the glucose to confirm the diagnosis by laboratory tests. If hypoglycemia is present in a NON-diabetic, additional tests must be performed to rule out endocrine disorders or tumors. If hypoglycemia is present in a known diabetic, the underlying cause of the insulin shock must be identified and corrected.

COMPLICATIONS

The brain obtains almost all of its energy from glucose metabolism. If the glucose level is maintained below 45–50 mg/dl, cerebral ischemia, edema, and neuronal hyperexcitability occurs. If the blood glucose level drops to 20–40 mg/dl, clonic convulsions may occur. If the blood glucose level drops below 20 mg/dl, coma develops. If not promptly reversed, the low blood glucose levels may cause irreversible brain damage, myocardial ischemia, infarction, and death.

THE SOMOGYI EFFECT

When too much insulin is administered, hypoglycemia occurs. The hypoglycemia alerts the body's defense systems, which overreact. With hypoglycemia, certain anti-insulin hormones are secreted. These include epinephrine, glucagon, glucocorticoids, and growth hormones. Because of these hormones, hyperglycemia occurs.

Most often a cycle occurs. Hypoglycemia one day may be followed by one or more days of hyperglycemia. In some patients, the cycle is so short that periods alternate within the same day. Symptoms of hypoglycemia in a hyperglycemic patient may indicate a Somogyi effect. Blood sugar levels may reach dangerously high levels because of this rebound effect.

Endocrine Bibliography

Borg N, Mikas DL, Stark J, Williams SM (eds): Core Curriculum for Critical Care Nursing, 2nd ed. American Association of Critical-Care Nurses. Philadelphia: W. B. Saunders, pp. 314–343, 1981

Ezrin C: The pituitary gland. In Clinical Symposia, Vol. 15, No. 3. Summit, NJ: Ciba-Geigy Corporation, 1963

Freitag JJ, Miller LW (eds): Thyroid disease. In Manual of Medical Therapeutics, 23rd ed. Boston, MA: Little, Brown and Co., pp. 323–374, 1979

*Guyton AC: Textbook of Medical Physiology, 6th ed. Philadelphia: W. B. Saunders, pp. 916–991, 1981

Huttner WA: Endocrine and metabolic problems. In Problem-Oriented Medical Diagnosis, 2nd ed. Freidman H H (ed): Boston, MA: Little, Brown and Co., pp. 276–314, 1979

Kinney MR, Dear CB, Vorrman DMN (eds): AACN's Clinical Reference for Critical-Care Nursing. New York: McGraw-Hill, pp. 641–677, 1981

*Kosowicz J: Atlas of Endocrine Diseases. Bowie, MD: Charles Press, 1978

Muir BL: Endocrine imbalance. In Pathophysiology: An Introduction to the Mechanisms of Disease. New York: John Wiley and Sons, pp. 340–363, 1980

Perry MO: Metabolic response to trauma. In Care of the Trauma Patient, 2nd ed. Shires GT (ed): New York: McGraw-Hill, pp. 62–74, 1979

*A Programmed Approach to Anatomy and Physiology: The Endocrine System. Bowie, MD: Robert J. Brady Co., 1972

Reller LB, Schalch DS, Ruldolph C: Endocrinology. In Reller LB, Sahn SA, Schrier RW (eds): Clinical Internal Medicine. Boston, MA: Little, Brown and Co., pp. 377–405, 1979

VI

The Hematologic System

35

Anatomy and Physiology of the Organs Forming Blood Elements and the Development of These Elements

Learning Objectives

By the end of this chapter, the nurse will be able to:

1. List the organs associated with forming blood elements.
2. Explain the hematologic functions of the spleen and the liver.
3. Identify the components of the lymphatic system and describe lymphatic capillaries, lymphatic vessels, lymph nodes, and lymph fluid.
4. Differentiate between the thoracic outlet and the right lymphatic duct.
5. Describe the anatomical composition of erythrocytes.
6. Explain the life cycle of an erythrocyte.
7. Explain the production of hemoglobin.
8. Identify six leukocytes, differentiating granular and agranular.
9. Explain the difference between fixed and free histiocytes.
10. Contrast the following differential shifts:
    a. Shift to the left
    b. Shift to the right
    c. Regenerative shift
    d. Degenerative shift
11. Compare monocytes and lymphocytes.
12. Compare eosinophils and basophils.
13. Compare thrombocytes and plasma cells.
14. Compare neutrophils and megakaryocytes.
15. Explain the primary function of RBCs.

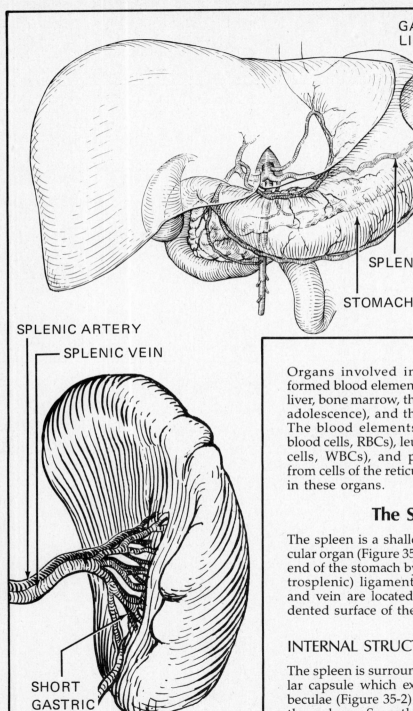

GASTROSPLENIC
LIGAMENT

SPLEEN

SPLENIC ARTERY

STOMACH

SPLENIC ARTERY

SPLENIC VEIN

SHORT
GASTRIC
ARTERY

Figure 35-1. The spleen showing gastrosplenic ligament.

Organs involved in the production of formed blood elements include the spleen, liver, bone marrow, the thymus gland (until adolescence), and the lymphatic system. The blood elements, erythrocytes (red blood cells, RBCs), leukocytes (white blood cells, WBCs), and platelets, are formed from cells of the reticuloendothelial system in these organs.

The Spleen

The spleen is a shallow, bowl-shaped vascular organ (Figure 35-1) attached to the left end of the stomach by the mesenteric (gastrosplenic) ligament. The splenic artery and vein are located in the hilus, the indented surface of the spleen.

INTERNAL STRUCTURE

The spleen is surrounded by a fibromuscular capsule which extends inward as trabeculae (Figure 35-2) forming partitions in the spleen. Smooth muscle in the surrounding capsule and in the trabeculae provides for contraction which can pump blood into the circulation.

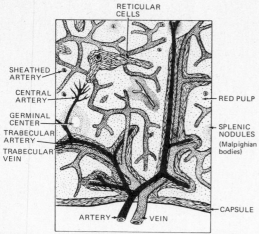

Figure 35-2. Trabeculae forming partitions in the spleen.

The spleen is composed of two types of spongy tissue known as the white pulp and the red pulp (Figure 35-3). The white pulp is randomly located throughout the spleen and contains typical loose lymphatic nodules and lymphatic strands of tissue. The red pulp comprises most of the spleen and consists of an abundance of reticular tissue and reticular cells lining the blood-filled venous sinuses.

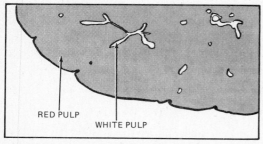

Figure 35-3. Red and white pulp of the spleen.

PHYSIOLOGY OF THE SPLEEN

An artery enters the splenic capsule to reach the splenic pulp where the artery bifurcates to connect through many small capillaries to large venous sinuses. Some of the small capillaries are very porous so that RBCs and foreign matter pass through the capillary walls into the red pulp. The strands of reticular tissue comprising the red pulp filter foreign material, cellular debris, and infectious organisms. Gradually,

the whole blood cells permeate the pulp and reach the venous sinuses. Any foreign matter not phagocytized by the red pulp is phagocytized by the phagocytic cells lining the venous sinuses. The lymphatic nodes and strands of the white pulp and the reticular strands of the red pulp effectively filter foreign matter, cellular debris (both abnormal cells and aged, deteriorating cells), and invading organisms from the circulating blood.

FUNCTIONS OF THE SPLEEN

The spleen provides a number of functions; however, it is not essential to life. If removed, some of its functions are carried on by other lymphatic organs.

The primary function of the spleen is that of a filtering system which has just been discussed.

The spleen functions as a reservoir for blood. If removed, no other organ assumes this role. The spleen usually has 150–250 milliliters of blood it can pump out if needed. In some extreme cases this volume may approach several hundred milliliters.

Other functions of the spleen include the production of antibodies and removal of the iron from disintegrating erythrocytes. The iron is eventually transported to the red bone marrow for re-use. The spleen also produces some leukocytes, primarily lymphocytes and monocytes.

The Liver

EXTERNAL ANATOMY AND LOCATION

The liver is divided into two lobes with the left lobe much smaller than the right (Figure 35-4). The lobes are divided by the falciform ligament. The liver is the largest organ in the body. It is attached to the right diaphragm and moves rhythmically with respirations. It is partially protected by the lower portion of the thoracic cage.

INTERNAL ANATOMY AND PHYSIOLOGY

When the common hepatic artery reaches the liver, it bifurcates to form the arteries for

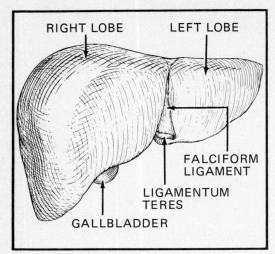

Figure 35-4. The liver.

the right and left lobes. Once inside the liver, the arteries branch to form interlobular segments. The lobule is fairly concentric in shape (Figure 35-5) and forms the functioning unit of the liver. Each lobule consists of interconnected cords of hepatic cells.

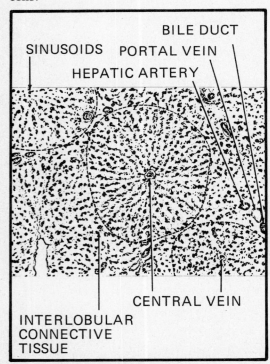

Figure 35-5. A liver lobule.

Around each lobule are several portal triads consisting of a hepatic artery, a hepatic vein, and a branch of the biliary duct. The artery and vein empty into randomly spaced vessels known as sinusoids. The sinusoids, lined with Küpffer cells, transport the blood into the central vein of each lobule (Figure 35-6).

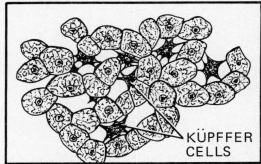

Figure 35-6. Küpffer cells which line the sinusoids.

The Küpffer cells phagocytize bacteria in the blood. There are more phagocytic cells in the liver than any other body tissue. All blood from the gastrointestinal tract (portal circulation) **must** pass through the liver before re-entering the general circulation. Because of this anatomical fact, the liver plays a major role in defense against infection. The Küpffer cells are from the reticuloendothelial system.

The liver is also the major area for the formation of the plasma clotting factors, except factor VIII.

Bone Marrow

Specialized cells in the red bone marrow (Figure 35-7) are more efficient in removing **very small particulate matter** (protein toxins) than the phagocytizing cells of the liver and spleen.

The bone marrow is also the site of primary importance in the production of precursors of red and white blood cells.

The Thymus

LOCATION AND GROSS ANATOMY

The thymus gland is located behind the sternum in the superior portion of the ster-

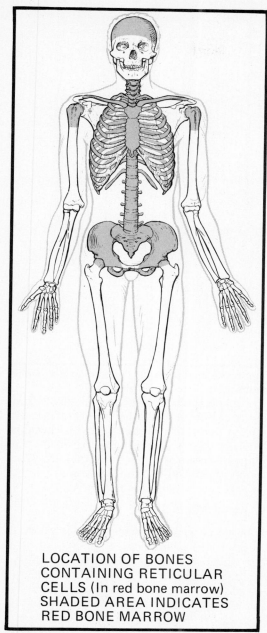

LOCATION OF BONES
CONTAINING RETICULAR
CELLS (In red bone marrow)
SHADED AREA INDICATES
RED BONE MARROW

Figure 35-7. Location of bones containing reticular cells (in red bone marrow). Shaded area indicates red bone marrow.

num (Figure 35-8). It is a large, two-lobed organ in the infant and very important to immunity.

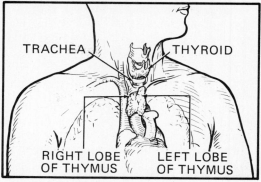

TRACHEA   THYROID

RIGHT LOBE   LEFT LOBE
OF THYMUS   OF THYMUS

Figure 35-8. Thymus gland.

By adolescence, the thymus gland tissue begins to be replaced by fibrous connective tissue and fat. This change is completed by adulthood and the gland is no longer considered an essential part of the immune defense system.

INTERNAL ANATOMY AND PHYSIOLOGY

The thymus lobes are divided into lobules by connective tissue with each lobule having a cortex and a medulla (Figure 35-9).

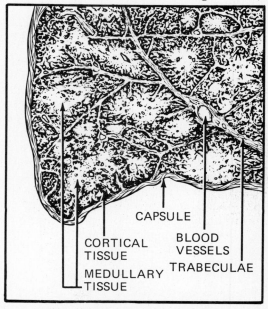

CAPSULE

CORTICAL
TISSUE

BLOOD
VESSELS

MEDULLARY
TISSUE

TRABECULAE

Figure 35-9. Cortex (dark outer portion) and medulla (light inner portion) of a section of a thymus lobule.

The cortex contains clusters of lymphocytes (sometimes called thymocytes) but no lymphatic nodules. A special substance stimulates production of lymphocytes.

The medulla is composed of loose thymocytes and thymic (Hassall's) corpuscles whose function is unknown.

Certain cells in both the cortex and medulla are thought to be special reticular cells that produce a thymic hormone which is involved in the bodies' immune capabilities.

The Lymphatic System

The lymphatic system is composed of lymph, lymphatic capillaries, lymphatic vessels, and lymph nodes.

LYMPH FLUID

Lymph fluid has a composition similar to that of plasma. It contains large quantities of leukocytes (mainly in the form of lymphocytes), a few erythrocytes, and a few platelets. Lymph fluid can clot, but it does so much more slowly than blood since lymph composition has fewer erythrocytes, platelets, and fibrinogen than blood. Lymph fluid has glucose, amino acids, urea, and creatinine in the same concentration as plasma has.

Lymph fluid does not circulate in the lymphatic capillaries and lymphatic vessels due to compression forces upon the capillaries. Although the capillaries and vessels do not have a specialized pump, the flow of lymph toward the heart is continuous due to (a) the formation of new lymph, (b) the compression of the capillaries and vessels by arteries which pushes the lymph toward the heart through unidirectional valves in the lymph vessels, (c) the contraction of skeletal and smooth muscles which squeezes the lymphatic vessels like the arteries, and (d) the thoracic pressures "pulling" the lymph toward the heart.

LYMPH CAPILLARIES

Lymph capillaries are small dead-end vessels which merge to form lymph vessels. The vessels have thinner walls than veins,

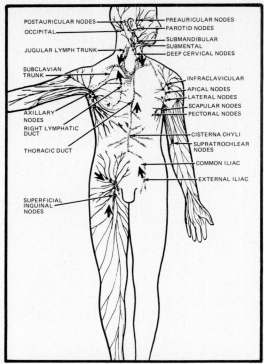

Figure 35-10. Location of lymph nodes in the body.

more valves than veins, and are larger than vein capillaries. Nodes are strategically spaced throughout the body. The location of these nodes is seen in Figure 35-10. The lymph vessels merge to form the right lymphatic duct and the thoracic duct.

LYMPH VESSELS

Lymph vessels are more permeable than veins to large molecules such as plasma proteins. The vessels filter the intercellular fluids of water and blood. *Only* the lymphatic system can return proteins from intercellular fluids to the blood because of the size of the proteins.

The lymph vessels which merge to form the right lymphatic duct drain lymph from the upper right quadrant of the body and the head (Figure 35-11) to the venous system via the right subclavian vein. The thoracic duct drains lymph from the entire remaining portions of the body (Figure 35-11) and returns it to the blood via the left subclavian vein.

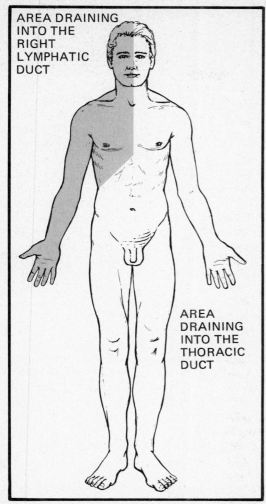

Figure 35-11. Lymph drainage of the upper right quadrant (shaded area). Lymph drainage of the remainder of the body (thoracic duct).

LYMPH NODES

Lymph nodes are placed in specific locations among the lymph vessels, especially the cervical, axillary, and inguinal regions. Clusters of nodes are also found in the lungs, along the aorta, and in the intestinal mesentary (Figure 35-12).

STRUCTURES AND PHYSIOLOGY OF LYMPH NODES

Lymph nodes are oval bodies of lymphatic tissue encapsulated by fibrous tissue. The interior of the lymph node is a matrix of connective tissue forming compartments

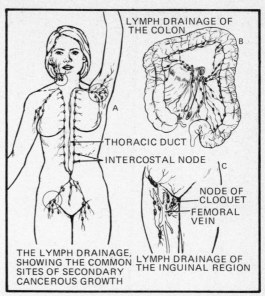

Figure 35-12. Locations of major lymph nodes: (A) aorta and lungs, (B) intestines, (C) inguinal region.

which contain lymphocytes (white blood cells). Each lymph node receives several different afferent lymph vessels (Figure 35-13) and usually has a single efferent vessel to drain the node.

The lymph nodes produce lymphocytes and plasma cells. As the lymph fluid makes its way through the node, the node filters and removes any foreign material, degenerating cells, and microorganisms. The lymph node develops a globulin from the disintegration of lymphocytes. This globulin is a blood protein containing antibodies and other immune bodies (e.g., antitoxins, agglutins, and bacteriolysins). As the lymph flows through this matrix of lymphocytes (the lymph node medulla), it eventually reaches efferent vessels which exit the node cortex at the hilus (indentation) of the node. The lymph nodes usually become tender and swollen if they are fighting an infection.

Development and Differentiation of the Formed Blood Elements

There are three cellular elements in the blood formed from the organs that have

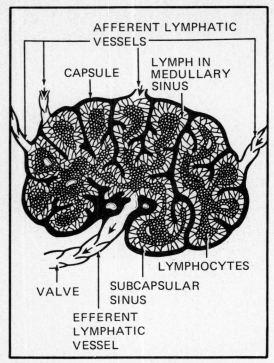

AFFERENT LYMPHATIC
VESSELS
CAPSULE
LYMPH IN
MEDULLARY
SINUS
LYMPHOCYTES
VALVE
SUBCAPSULAR
SINUS
EFFERENT
LYMPHATIC
VESSEL

Figure 35-13. A typical lymph node.

just been reviewed. These formed blood elements are called the erythrocytes (red blood cells, RBCs), leukocytes (white blood cells, WBCs), and the thrombocytes (platelets).

HEMATOPOIESIS

Hematopoiesis is a term used to signify the production of blood cells. The red blood cells and most of the white blood cells are formed in the red bone marrow. A commonly accepted theory of the origin of blood cells is that there is a common primitive cell, the reticuloendothelial cell. It is believed that from this reticuloendothelial cell the other blood cells develop through specific steps and stages.

MATURATION OF THE NORMAL CELL

Blood cells go through several stages of development during the maturation process including changes in the cytoplasm, the nucleus, and the size of the cell.

The Cytoplasmic Maturation

The immature cytoplasm matures by a gradual loss of the cytoplasmic RNA. In some cells, the cytoplasm develops fine granules as the cells mature. The cell granules are first few and nonspecific. As the cell matures, the granules become numerous and assume a specific function. The amount of cytoplasm in relation to the size of the cell will increase as the cell matures.

Nuclear Maturation

The nucleus of the cell is round or oval and is very large in proportion to the rest of the cell. As the cell matures, the nucleus become smaller in size and may take on varied shapes. The chromatin of the nucleus changes from a very fine, delicate pattern to a coarse, clumped form in the mature cell. Nucleoli, which are present in the early stages of cell development, gradually disappear as the cell matures.

The Cell Size

During the natural process of cell maturation, the cell becomes smaller. The size of the mature red blood cell or small lymphocyte is the size that most of the mature cells finally achieve.

Red Blood Cell Production (Erythropoiesis)

A hormone, erythropoietin, is produced by the kidney in response to insufficient oxygen from whatever cause. The erythropoietin stimulates stem cells in the red bone marrow to begin the differentiating and maturing process, producing more red blood cells. The cell in the reticulocyte stage stays in the bone marrow about 2 days and is then released into the general circulation with a life expectancy of 120 days, plus or minus 20 days.

The erythropoientin released by the kidneys during hypoxemia is thought to be acted upon by various humoral and endocrine controls. It is also thought that erythropoientin may be produced in small amounts somewhere in the body other than in the kidneys. This would explain why chronic renal failure patients produce RBCs even in small amounts with low hemoglobin levels.

HEMOGLOBIN PRODUCTION

Synthesis of hemoglobin requires the same nutrients as RBC production—namely iron, vitamin B_{12}, and folic acid. The heme molecule is formed from iron in the ferrous state combining with a specific porphyrin. This heme molecule combines with a protein globulin in the bone marrow. Four of these specific hemoglobin molecules unite by specific alpha and beta chains of amino acids forming the tetramer of hemoglobin. An insufficient amount of nutrients or iron in the ferric state decreases and/or stops hemoglobin production. It is difficult for the body to use iron in its ferric state because ferric iron cannot carry oxygen. (Ranges of hemoglobin are found in Appendix II.)

Erythroid Series

The erythroid series is the process of maturation of the red blood cells through several stages. The cell progresses from the undifferentiated reticuloendothelial cell through each stage of maturation and finally becomes the mature red blood cell.

STAGES OF CELL MATURATION

There are basically six changes that the red blood cell goes through in order for a cell to become a mature red blood cell. The normal erythropoiesis starts with the pronormoblast (rubriblast), then the basophilic normoblast (prorubricyte), the polychromatic normoblast (rubricyte), the orthochromic normoblast (metarubricyte), reticulocyte, and the mature red blood cell.

During normal erythropoiesis, the cytoplasm becomes progressively larger, while at the same time any nucleoli disappear and the nucleus changes from a loose pronormoblast to a solid mass in the orthochromic normoblast stage. By the mature RBC stage, the nucleus is extruded from the cytoplasm completely. The cell size declines. The pronormoblast is usually 14–18 microns in diameter and the mature RBC is 6.7–7.7 microns in diameter. Figure 35-14 depicts the changes in the cytoplasm, the nucleus, and the size of the cell during the cell's maturation through the erythroid series.

The mature RBC is released into the circulation when the storage capacity of the red bone marrow is exceeded. The primary function of the RBC is to transport oxygen to the body tissues. RBCs also participate, to a degree, in the maintenance of acid-base balance because the hemoglobin inside the RBC functions as a buffer. The hemoglobin in the normal adult contains polypeptide chains to which the heme molecule can attach. The development of hemoglobin occurs throughout maturation of the blood cell during each stage of the erythroid series.

STRUCTURE OF THE RED BLOOD CELL

The red blood cell is a nonnucleated, round, biconcave cell. The RBC has an outer membrane composed primarily of lipoproteins. These lipoproteins are thin and pliable forming a surface upon which the antigen determining blood type attaches.

The inner part of the red cells is called the stroma. It is composed primarily of lipids and proteins. It is a thick and spongelike material to which hemoglobin can attach. The stroma contains antigenic material that determines whether the person's blood type is A, B, AB, or O. Although the red blood cell membrane has two layers to it— the outside membrane and the stroma—it is highly permeable to hydrogen, chloride, water, and bicarbonate ions. It is less permeable to sodium and potassium ions but it maintains a stable intracellular concentration through the active transport produced by the sodium and potassium pumps.

Red Blood Cell Destruction

During the life span of the mature RBC, specific factors occur to precipitate destruction of the RBC.

Some time between 100–120 days, the cytoplasmic enzymes that produce ATP for

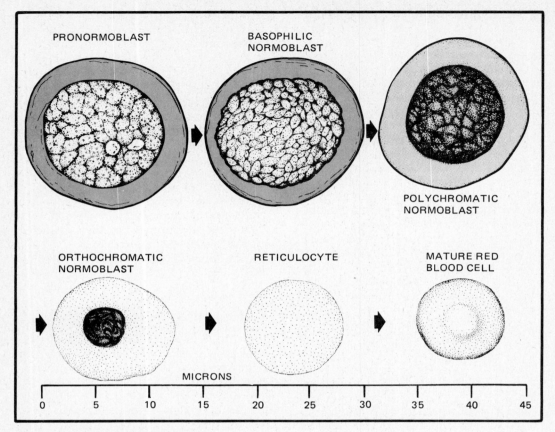

Figure 35-14. Normal erythropoiesis.

metabolic activity become used up. Loss of ATP results in the RBC membrane becoming nonpliant and fragile resulting in rupture of the RBC. With the loss of membrane patency, intracellular ion concentration cannot be maintained. ATP cannot maintain iron in its ferous state. Subsequently, the iron converts to a ferric state that cannot transport oxygen. Lack of ATP also prevents oxidation of intracellular proteins.

With a slowing down or loss of ATP concentration, the RBC's membrane becomes so fragile that it disintegrates. Many RBCs rupture in the spleen because the RBC, which is 8 microns in diameter, is forced through the red pulp, which is only 3 microns wide.

After the RBC ruptures, hemoglobin is released and is phagocytized by reticuloendothelial cells. These cells separate the iron from the hemoglobin molecule. The iron is returned to the bone marrow by transferrin for re-use. The heme part of the hemoglobin is converted into the bile pigment bilirubin by the reticuloendothelial cell and then transported in the blood to the liver. The liver will eventually secrete the bilirubin in the form of bile.

Hemolysis (destruction of the RBC) may occur before the normal life span if the RBC membrane or hemoglobin are abnormal. Glycolytic and enzyme defects will result in early destruction of the RBC. The most common defects are insufficient glucose-6-phosphate dehydrogenase (G6PD) and insufficient hexokinase.

Trauma cases result in a destruction of RBCs secondary to gross damage as occurs in crushing injuries and such.

The spleen and liver remove the aged or abnormal red cell, while immature RBCs are destroyed by reticuloendothelial organs such as the bone marrow itself, the blood, lungs, lymph nodes, and to some extent by the spleen and liver.

White Bood Cell Production (Leukopoiesis)

Leukocytes (white blood cells, WBCs) are the body's main defense system due solely to the WBC's ability to move to and from an infection site. Leukocytes are able to reproduce rapidly and alter their characteristics according to the situation. There are five basic white cells: three types which contain granules that are formed in bone marrow and two types without granules, the monocytes and lymphocytes. The three granular cells may be classified as granulocytes. Monocytes (agranular) are formed in the bone marrow and migrate to lymphoid tissues for storage. A few lymphocytes are formed in the lymph nodes and do not contain granules.

The Myeloid (Granulocytic) Series

THE GRANULOCYTES

The mature forms of the granulocytes are called neutrophils, eosinophils, and basophils. They are formed in the red bone marrow and may be stored in the marrow until needed. Granulocytes usually circulate in the blood for 6–8 hours after release from the bone marrow and another 2–3 days in the tissues. If a serious infection exists, it may be only several hours before the granulocytes have phagocytized as many invaders as possible and are themselves destroyed.

DEVELOPMENT OF THE GRANULOCYTES

The granulocytes progress through various steps in the myelogenous series (Figure 35-15) to become mature granulocytes by changes in the cytoplasm and nucleus of each cell stage. The granulocyte begins as a myeloblast and continues through the stages of the leukoblast, the promyelocyte, the myelocyte, the metamyelocyte, and the band cell, to mature into the segmented neutrophil, the eosinophil, and the basophil.

CYTOPLASMIC AND NUCLEUS DIFFERENTIATION

In the developing granulocyte, the cytoplasm of the myeloblast is without granules. The cytoplasm is smaller than the nucleus of the cell in this stage and the nucleus is round or slightly oval. Normally, two or three nucleoli are present.

The leukoblast is about the same size as the myeloblast. It usually has at least a few nonspecific granules in the cytoplasm. The nucleus is round or oval and comprises more than one-half of the cell. The chromatin of the nucleus is often a little coarser than in the myeloblast. Two or three nucleoli are present.

The promyelocyte cytoplasm contains many granules that begin to differentiate with specific granules appearing in this stage. The neutrophilic promyelocyte, the eosinophilic promyelocyte, and the basophilic promyelocyte have granules which differ in size, shape, and function.

From the myelocyte stage on, the cells are incapable of division and will continue to develop into the specific mature granulocyte of this stage as determined by the specific granules in the cytoplasm.

The band cell has the same cytoplasm as the metamyelocyte and a nucleus which is a thin rod or band shape with a coarse chromatin pattern.

The segmented neutrophil is a mature granulocyte which is metabolically active, utilizes both aerobic and anaerobic glycolysis, moves by pseudopods to areas of infection, and phagocytizes the invading bacteria.

The eosinophil is the second mature granulocyte and it has the ability to move and phagocytize parasites. It is active in antigen-antibody reactions, allergic reactions, and with parasitic infections.

The basophil contains heparin and histamine. Roughly one-half of the histamine content in the body is contained in the basophil granules. It functions in allergic reactions.

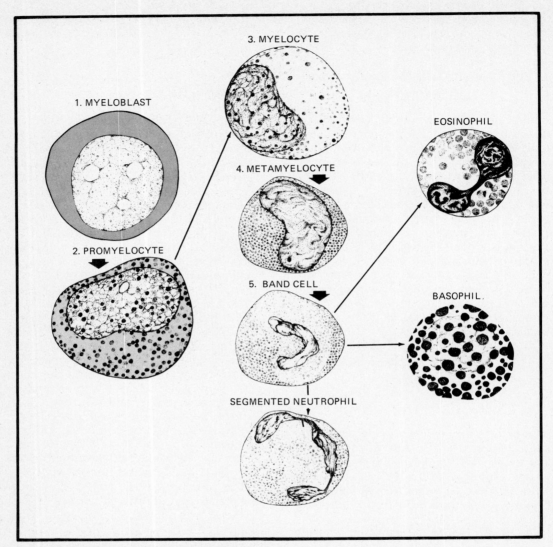

Figure 35-15. Maturation of granulocytic cells.

The mature granulocytes are stored in the red bone marrow until needed. These three mature granulocytes are sometimes referred to as polymorphonuclear lymphocytes, PMNs, or polys.

The Development of the Lymphocytic Series

There are no really well-defined stages of lymphocyte maturation so they must be identified by morphology, size, and staining properties (Figure 35-16). Staining properties are beyond the scope of this text and the reader is referred to specific hematologic texts for more in-depth study.

The lymphocyte progresses through various stages to become a mature lymphocyte by changes in the cytoplasm and the nucleus of each cell stage. The lymphocyte begins as a lymphoblast (reticular lymphocyte or nonleukemic lymphoblast), progresses to the prolymphocyte, and then to the mature lymphocyte as either a small

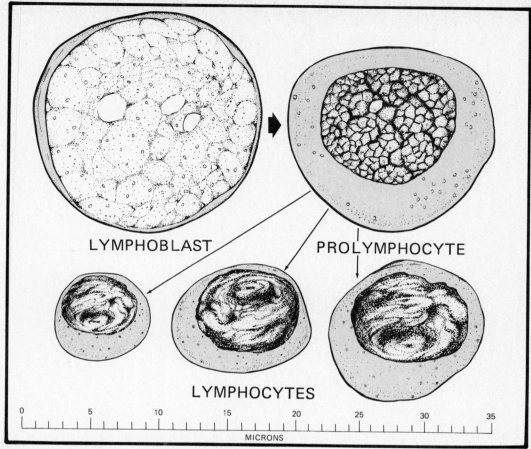

Figure 35-16. Maturation of the lymphocyte.

lymphocyte, a medium lymphocyte, or a large lymphocyte.

CYTOPLASMIC AND NUCLEUS DIFFERENTIATION

The lymphoblast is composed mainly of a large round or oval nucleus. The nuclear chromatin is formed of strands or granules which result in a reticular appearance. There are usually one or two nucleoli present. The cytoplasm that is present is non-granular.

MATURE LYMPHOCYTES

In the mature form, the lymphocyte occurs in three different sizes: small, medium, and large. The larger the lymphocyte, the greater the amount of cytoplasm in the cell. The

nucleus is round, oval, or slightly indented. The nucleus of both the small and medium size lymphocytes has a centrally located position, whereas the large lymphocyte has an eccentric nucleus.

LYMPHOCYTE PHYSIOLOGY

The lymphatic system was covered in the first portion of this chapter. Suffice it to add that small lymphocytes move quite freely between the peripheral circulatory system and lymphatic tissues and organs. The life span of a lymphocyte may approach 2 years unless needed to fight infections. A lymphocyte's main function is related to immunity in the body by synthesizing antibodies. This results in an increase in cell size and the lymphocyte being able to subdivide to produce new T cells or B cells. B cells may subdivide to form plasma cells. (T cells and B cells are extremely important in cellular immunity and immunological reactions, which are discussed in Chapter 36.)

PLASMA CELLS

If mitosis of the lymphocyte results in the formation of plasma cells, there are three stages in the formation: the plasmablast, the proplasmacyte, and the plasmacyte (Figure 35-17).

CYTOPLASMIC AND NUCLEUS DIFFERENTIATION

The plasmacyte, or plasma cell, usually has less nongranular cytoplasm than the cells of the previous two stages. The plasma cell has a round or oval eccentric nucleus with no identifiable nucleoli.

The plasma cell is produced predominantly in lymph nodes and the spleen. The plasma cell plays a role in humoral immunity by synthesizing and releasing immunoglobulins (antibodies) into the plasma.

The Monocytic Series

Monocytes are formed mainly in the bone marrow and migrate to the spleen and other lymphoid tissue for maturation. The monocyte progresses through the stages of monoblast, promonocyte, and the mature monocyte (Figure 35-18).

CYTOPLASMIC AND NUCLEUS DIFFERENTIATION

The mature monocyte is usually larger than other peripheral blood cells. The cytoplasm is abundant, often contains fine granules and vacuoles, and may be irregular in shape. The nucleus has dense, stringy chromatin.

MONOCYTIC FUNCTION

Monocytes are very mobile and phagocytic due to an abundance of internal enzymes and lipases. The life span of a monocyte is approximately 80 hours. Phagocytosis is accomplished by the monocyte extending pseudopods (extensions) which surround foreign substances. Once the pseudopods have enclosed the foreign substance, phagocytosis and digestion of the substance occur. The monocyte also destroys foreign substances by pinocytosis, which is the process of attracting and attaching foreign substances, especially fluids, to the cell membrane. The cell then invaginates pulling the foreign substance into its inte-

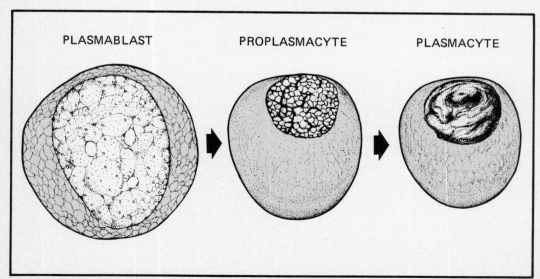

Figure 35-17. Maturation of the plasma cell.

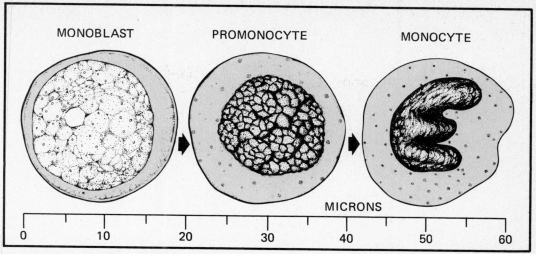

Figure 35-18. Maturation of the monocyte.

rior where it commences to digest the substance.

Monocytes which act by phagocytizing foreign substances are referred to as macrophages or histiocytes. There are two types of histiocytes: fixed histiocytes and free histiocytes.

Fixed histiocytes are located within specific body organs including Küpffer cells lining the sinusoids of the liver, pulmonary alveoli, the spleen, and various body fluids.

Free histiocytes are those monocytes that have become macrophages and have the ability to pass through vascular membranes to trap and maintain foreign substances in the body tissues at inflamed areas.

The Thrombocytic Series

The thrombocyte is thought to originate from the primitive reticuloendothelial cell as the megakaryoblast. It then progresses through three stages: promegakaryocyte, megakaryocyte, and, finally, the mature thrombocyte. The thrombocyte is sometimes referred to as a blood platelet (Figure 35-19).

CYTOPLASMIC AND NUCLEUS DIFFERENTIATION

The cytoplasm of platelets contains numerous granules and has no nuclei. The num-

ber of platelets produced is related to the amount of cytoplasm in the cell.

The new platelet in the bloodstream has a 10-day life span.

THROMBOCYTIC FUNCTION

The platelets contain numerous proteins, carbohydrates, lipids, and enzymes which make the platelets very active metabolically. The primary function of the platelet is to maintain hemostasis and capillary integrity. The role of the platelet in hemostasis is covered in Chapter 37.

Leukocyte Concentration

The normal adult white blood cell count is between 6 thousand and 10 thousand cells per cubic millimeter of blood. Children have more leukocytes (in the form of lymphocytes) than adults. There are also 250 thousand to 500 thousand platelets per cubic millimeter of blood.

A differential count is done to aid in diagnosis. The normal adult differential count per 100 cells is neutrophils—62.0; eosinophils—2.3; basophils—0.4; monocytes—5.3; and lymphocytes—30.0.

SHIFTS OF THE DIFFERENTIAL

A few bands (immature neutrophils) are normally found in the peripheral circulation. In a differential, a significant number

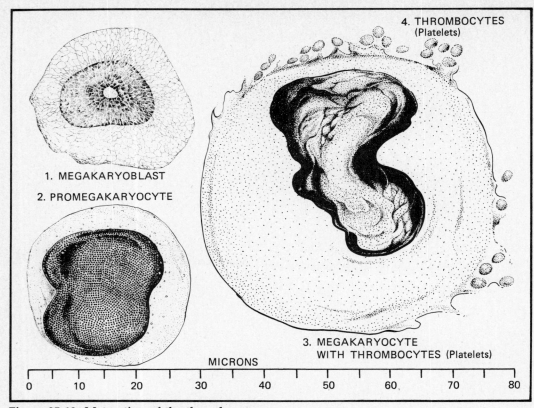

Figure 35-19. Maturation of the thrombocyte.

of bands indicates an infection and is termed a "shift to the left." The presence of mature, hypersegmented neutrophils (more segmented nuclei) is termed a "shift to the right." This usually indicates pernicious anemia and/or hepatic disease. A "degenerative shift" occurs with an increase in band cells and a low leukocyte (WBC) count which indicates bone marrow depression. A "regenerative shift" indicates a stimulation of the bone marrow. It is indicated by an increased number of band cells, metamyelocytes and myelocytes, and an elevated WBC count. This occurs in such cases as pneumonia and appendicitis.

Properties of White Blood Cells

Specific characteristics of WBCs explain their efficiency in defending the body against infectious agents. There are four specific characteristics: diapedesis, ameboid motion, chemotaxis, and phagocytosis.

Diapedesis. This is the movement of a small portion of the cell progressively squeezing through a capillary pore which is much smaller than the overall white blood cell (Figure 35-20). While a portion of the cell is squeezing through the capillary pore, it is markedly constricted and reexpands to its normal size on the other side of the capillary pore.

Ameboid Motion. White blood cells, especially the granulocytes, move through the tissue by ameboid motion (Figure 35-21). In this motion a portion of the cell is extended in one direction and the remainder of the cell is pulled up to join it (similar to the movement of an inch worm).

Chemotaxis. This is the characteristic of a specific chemical to release a substance (attracting or repelling) which affects the WBCs to respond in the appropriate manner to the particular substance (Figure 35-22).

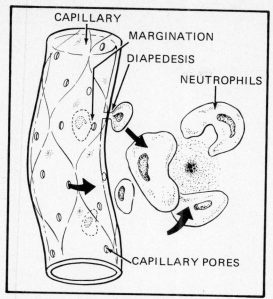

Figure 35-20. Diapedesis of the WBCs.

Phagocytosis. This is the process of white blood cells invaginating foreign substances and destroying them internally (Figure 35-23).

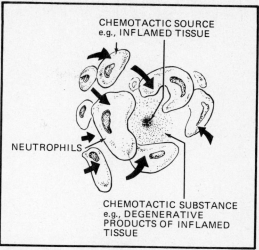

Figure 35-22. Chemotactic movement of neutrophils toward area of tissue damage. Chemotactic substances attract neutrophils from throughout the body.

Specific factors of white blood cells are summarized in Table 35-1. The table includes the type, source, characteristics, function, and significance of increased counts of the leukocytes.

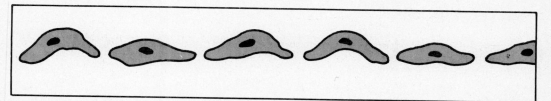

Figure 35-21. Ameboid movement of WBCs.

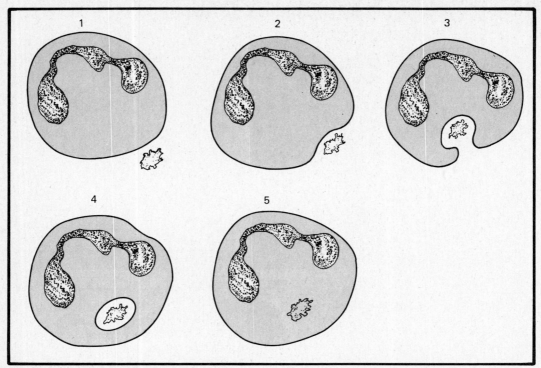

Figure 35-23. Phagocytosis of WBCs.

Table 35-1. Leukocytes.

Type	Source	Characteristics	Function	Increased Count
Neutrophil	Red bone marrow	Granular cytoplasm, 3- to 5-lobed nucleus	Phagocytosis	Leukemia, pyogenic infections
Eosinophil	Red bone marrow	Granular cytoplasm, 2-lobed nucleus	Non-phagocytic, little known of exact function	Parasitic infections, allergy, leukemia
Basophil	Red bone marrow	Granular cytoplasm, irregular nucleus, may be S-shaped	Exact function unknown	Leukemia
Lymphocyte	Lymphoid tissue	Thin layer of nongranular cytoplasm, large nucleus	Production of antibodies, non-phagocytic	Chronic infections, viral infections, leukemia
Monocyte	Lymphoid tissue	Thick layer of nongranular cytoplasm; large, kidney-shaped nucleus	As a macrophage	Tuberculosis, protozoal infection, leukemia

Immunity and Inflammation

Learning Objectives

By the end of this chapter, the nurse will be able to:

1. Define immunity and list the types of immunity possible.
2. Describe the process of initiating clone activity and explain the clones of lymphocytes.
3. Distinguish between T-lymphocytes and B-lymphocytes.
4. Contrast humoral immunity and cellular immunity.
5. Identify the functions of cellular immunity.
6. Explain the formation of antibodies and the secondary plasma cell response.
7. Identify and explain the function of each of the five immunoglobulins.
8. Explain the antigen-antibody and agglutination characteristics of O, A, B, and AB type blood.
9. Describe the formation of sensitization in Rh negative persons.
10. Explain the two types of Coomb's tests and the significance of each test.
11. Explain cold agglutinin's and the treatment.
12. Explain the structure, function, and initiation of the complement cascade.
13. Explain cytotoxic reactions, subacute hypersensitivity reactions, and delayed hypersensitivity reactions.
14. Define inflammation.
15. Explain the immediate inflammation reaction to injury.
16. Explain the leukocyte activity reaction to injury.

Immunity

The ability of the body to resist or combat invading organisms is termed immunity. There are three types of immunity: innate, passive, and acquired immunity. Acquired immunity is further divided into humoral immunity and cellular immunity.

INNATE IMMUNITY

Innate immunity is the natural body factors that help prevent infection. This form of immunity includes the resistance of the skin to invading microorganisms. Acid secretions of the stomach and enzymes of the intestines help to protect against injested microorganisms. Phagocytosis by blood cells protects us from some bacteria. Chemical compounds of the blood including lysosomes, basic polypeptides, properdin, and some natural antibodies provide additional innate immunity.

PASSIVE IMMUNITY

Passive immunity is only a temporary form of immunity acquired by the injection of antibodies or sensitized lymphocytes into a person. This person then has this specific passive immunity for 2–3 weeks. An example of passive immunity is the use of gamma globulin for a pregnant woman in the first trimester who has been exposed to measles and has not previously had them or the vaccine.

ACQUIRED IMMUNITIES

There are two types of acquired immunity: humoral immunity and cellular immunity. Humoral immunity is acquired by the body developing specific antibodies (B-lymphocytes) made of globulin molecules that attack invading agents. These specific antibodies are called immunoglobulins. Cellular immunity is acquired by special lymphocytes becoming sensitized against specific invading agents. These lymphocytes are called sensitized T-lymphocytes.

Although humoral and cellular immunity are different, they have a similar basic development and to some extent a synergistic action. Both humoral and cellular immunity are the result of development of lymphocytes in response to specific foreign bodies called antigens.

The lymphocytes destined to provide humoral immunity by the production of antibodies are produced in some unknown spot in the body, probably the fetal liver and possibly Peyer's patches (in the intestines) and the appendix. These special lymphocytes have been discovered to develop in the bursa of Fabricius found in birds and thus are termed B-lymphocytes.

Some of the lymphocytes will migrate to the thymus gland for maturation into T-lymphocytes and are responsible for cellular immunity. Once these T-lymphocytes

have been acted upon in the thymus gland by a hormone, thymopoietin (or thymosin), they circulate through body fluids and migrate into lymphoid tissue. Thymopoietin stimulates the activity of the T-lymphocytes both in the blood and in the lymphoid tissue by causing increased proliferation.

Monocytes which are trapped in the lymphoid tissue at the time of stimulation are believed to play a major role in the sensitizing process. These trapped monocytes enlarge to become tissue macrophages known as reticulum cells and are found in the spleen, lymph nodes, liver, and the lymphoid tissue. These reticulum cells phagocytize invading microorganisms causing a release of antigenetic products from the microorganisms. The antigenetic products are believed to pass directly from the macrophages to the lymphocytes (because of their internal positioning) stimulating the specific lymphocyte clone.

CLONES FROM LYMPHOCYTES

Lymphocytes that have been sensitized to a specific foreign agent (antigen) continue to produce protection through the process of lymphatic clones. A specific type of sensitized lymphocyte will form only that one specific type of antibody or sensitized lymphocyte. Each lymphocyte in the lymphoid tissue can form 10,000–100,000 different types of T-lymphocytes or antibodies (B-lymphocytes). Once stimulated, the sensitized lymphocyte will form more lymphocytes or antibodies for the specific antigen. Stimulated lymphocytes *always* produce the lymphocyte or antibody for a *specific* antigen. This process is called a clone of lymphocytes. Lymphocytes are cloned by the thymus becoming T-lymphocytes and migrating to lymph nodes throughout the body for storage until needed. Clones are excited by their specific antigen and may react in two ways: (1) If the clone is a T-lymphocyte, a large number of T-lymphocytes will be formed (cloned) and (2) if the clone is a B-lymphocyte, large numbers of plasma cells will form producing antibodies (immunoglobulins). Immunoglobulins have five groups known by various abbreviations, such as IgE, IgG. Some authorities think that it is probable for T-lymphocytes which are excited to excite B-lymphocytes against the same antigen to aid in immunity.

Once a sensitized T-lymphocyte or an antibody (B-lymphocyte) has been formed against a specific antigen, the T-lymphocytes and B-lymphocytes respond to future antigens anamnestically (antigen memory). The first exposure to an antigen requires some time for T-lymphocytes or B-lymphocytes or plasma cells to be formed. This is a primary (first-exposure) response. A second exposure to the same antigen elicits a rapid, strong reaction due to the memory cells of the lymphocytes. This is known as the secondary response or the anamnestic response and will occur repeatedly every time an antigen invades the body.

Some T-lymphocytes are located in the deep cortical areas of the lymph nodes; however, most of the T-lymphocytes are in the blood and a few are present in bone marrow. T-lymphocytes continuously circulate in the blood and lymph fluid where they function as an immune surveillance system against antigens.

HUMORAL IMMUNITY

Humoral immunity involves the production of immunoglobulins and the antigens that determine blood type and Rh factors. At the initiation of humoral immunity, B-lymphocytes attach to or identify antigens which are then collected by groups of macrophages. The B-lymphocytes form plasma cells which produce antibodies against the antigen and have a maximal effect within minutes to hours. Plasma cells divide about once every 10 hours for nine divisions. Thus, about 500 plasma cells are produced in 5 days. The mature plasma cell produces gamma globulin antibodies and releases them at the rate of about 2,000 molecules per *second* per plasma cell. The antibodies migrate from the lymphoid tissues to the circulating blood with a survival rate of days or weeks. The antibodies produced by the B-lymphocytes are immunoglobulins. Once B-lymphocytes have developed antibodies against a specific antigen, they also are anamnestic.

MECHANISM OF ANTIBODY ACTION

Antibodies have the ability to react in three different ways to protect the body against antigens. Antibodies may attack the antigen directly. Antibodies may activate the complement system so that it can destroy the antigen. Antibodies can change the environment by activating the anaphylactic system to release specific chemicals that will alter the potency of the antigen.

Antibodies attack the antigen by causing many antigens to clump together, destroying their activity. This is termed *agglutination*.

Antibodies may attach to the soluble antigen complex causing the antigen to become insoluble and inactive. This is termed *precipitation* since the insoluble complex is an aggregation of antibodies and antigens forming a visible mass.

Antibodies may not be able to remove the antigen. In these cases, the antibodies may attach to the toxic portions of the antigen. This is termed *neutralization*.

Some antibodies are very potent and are able to attack the antigen membrane resulting in rupture of the antigen cell.

Usually the antibodies are not potent enough to destroy the antigens by themselves and require the assistance of the complement, properdin, and the anaphylactic system.

The Complement System

The complement system consists of nine enzyme precursors. These are called C1 through C9. When an antibody attaches to the reactive site of the antigen, a "cascade" is activated and the enzyme precursor forms molecules which attack the antigen in several different ways. The complement system also protects the body against the antigen by initiating local tissue reactions. Once activated, the complement cascade continues its reactions through the entire system.

The more important actions of the complement cascade are: (1) Proteolytic enzymes digest portions of the cell membrane, resulting in lysis of the antigen and

(2) Complement enzymes attach to the surface of the antigens making them extremely vulnerable to phagocytosis by neutrophils and macrophages. This process is termed *opsonization* and provides for an increased number of antigens to be destroyed.

Some of the complement factors have a chemotactic effect upon neutrophils and macrophages, increasing phagocytosis of antigens in the infected area.

Agglutination and neutralization of viruses inactivate the antigens.

Local inflammation from the complement products causes hyperemia, coagulation of proteins in the tissues, vasodilatation of blood vessels supplying increased leukocytes, and such.

Properdin

Properdin is a high molecular weight serum protein. It functions as an integral part of the humoral immunity system. The properdin system functions only in the presence of the complement system and magnesium. Properdin helps destroy bacteria, neutralizes viruses, and plays a role in the hemolysis of RBCs.

The Anaphylactic System

The IgE antibodies attach to antigen cell membranes in the blood and tissues. The most important cells in this system are basophils in the blood and mast cells in tissue adjacent to blood vessels.

As soon as an antibody attaches to the antigen cell membrane there is an immediate rupturing which releases specific factors in the involved area. One of these factors is lysosomal enzymes which produce local inflammation. Another factor is histamine release resulting in vasodilatation and increased permeability of the capillaries. Another factor is the chemotactic substance attracting eosinophils which help phagocytize antibody-antigen complexes. There is another factor called slow-reacting substance of anaphylaxis. This substance results in prolonged contraction of specific smooth muscle such as found in the bronchi.

Reactions of the anaphylactic system may be very harmful and even fatal to the body as a result of allergic type responses.

IMMUNOGLOBULINS

Antibodies from B-lymphocytes are proteins that are called immunoglobulins and are abbreviated as Ig. Five major classes of immunoglobulins are known: IgG, IgM, IgA, IgD, and IgE. The third letter in each class merely differentiates the classes according to the amino acid sequences and polypeptide chains that form the immunoglobulin molecule. The sequence of amino acids on the polypeptide chains provides antigen receptor sites (due to the variability of the amino acids) at one end of the polypeptide chain.

IgG is the most abundant immunoglobulin circulating in the blood and various other body fluids. It is the most common antibody and the *only* one that can cross the placenta. IgG functions mainly against bacterial antigens but also, to a lesser extent, against viruses.

IgA exists in exocrine secretions (polymeric units) and in the blood (monomeric units). The secretory polymeric units are found in tears, saliva, and membranes of the respiratory and intestinal tracts. Most of the exocrine secretion antibodies are IgA but also contain small amounts of IgG and IgM antibodies. IgA protects our bodies against infection on mucosal surfaces by preventing the microorganism from attaching to the epithelial surfaces. Some pathogenic microorganisms contain enzymes to produce IgA proteases which break down the IgA molecule.

IgM antibodies are the largest of the immunoglobulins and are found mainly in the blood. IgM functions in much the same way as IgG; however, IgM concentration decreases as IgG antibodies increase. IgM antibodies are more efficient in activating complement and are more efficient in binding antibodies than IgG. Since IgM does not cross the placental barrier, an increased IgM level in neonates indicates a viral or bacterial intrauterine infection or an ABO incompatibility.

IgD antibodies are only a fraction of the total immunoglobulins in the body and are poorly understood. IgD antibodies are present on the B-lymphocytes of fetuses and neonates (implying some active protection or development and maturation of the immune system during intrauterine and neonatal periods).

IgE is found in trace amounts and is thought to be produced by cells in respiratory and intestinal mucosa. IgE antibodies include reagins which produce allergic type reactions (wheal-flare reactions) releasing histamine. Necrosin is one reagin which promotes histamine release.

BLOOD GROUP PHENOTYPES

Blood groups are determined genetically by the *antigen* on the surface of the erythrocytes. Although more than 30 common antigens are known to react with the erythrocyte, only four antigens are involved in determining a person's blood type. Table 36-1 summarizes the characteristics of the ABO blood types.

The type of antigen (agglutinogens) present in the erythrocyte and the type of antibodies (agglutinins) in the serum determine blood types. No person ever has both an antigen and its antagonistic antibody present in his or her blood. An example would be an individual with A type blood, which indicates the presence of A antigens. This person cannot have anti-A antibodies in the serum because the blood cells would be totally destroyed by the interaction of the antigens and the antibodies.

A type blood means that the person has A type agglutinogens in the erythrocyte and anti-B agglutinins in the plasma. Consequently, this person cannot receive type B or type AB blood but may receive type A or type 0 blood safely.

B type blood means that the person has B type agglutinogens in the erythrocyte and anti-A agglutinins in the plasma.

AB type blood means that the person has both A and B agglutinogens in the erythrocyte and no agglutinins in the plasma. This person is known as the "universal recipient" since no antibodies are present in the plasma.

O type blood means that there are no agglutinogens in the erythrocyte but there are both anti-A and anti-B agglutinins in the plasma. This person is known as the "universal donor" because his or her erythrocytes contain no antigens that could be destroyed by antibodies within the recipient's blood in a transfusion.

AGGLUTINATION

When blood is mismatched in the laboratory so that blood containing the same agglutinins are mixed with cells containing the antagonist agglutinogens, clumping or agglutination results. The process of agglutination takes only several minutes. Donor blood is diluted about 50 times with saline to prevent clotting before testing. Two separate drops of this blood suspension are placed on slides and a drop of anti-A agglutinin is mixed with one drop. Anti-B agglutinin is mixed with the second drop. If after several minutes the cells of one drop have clumped together, an immune reaction has occurred. This specific unit of blood cannot be used for transfusion in the specific patient tested with this agglutination without resulting in a hemolytic transfusion reaction.

RH BLOOD TYPES

A number of systems have been identified that will result in hemolytic reactions. Of these systems, the Rh factor is the most

Table 36-1. Characteristics of ABO blood types.

Blood Group	Agglutinogens	Agglutinins
	(Antigens in Red Cells)	(Antibodies in Serum)
A	A	anti-B
B	B	anti-A
AB	A and B	None
O	None	anti-A and anti-B

common and the Rh D is the most potent reaction. The major difference between the ABO and the Rh reactions is that the ABO reactions occur by spontaneous agglutinin reaction, whereas the Rh reaction occurs only after sensitization. Rh factors are inherited and typing the blood for Rh factors is achieved in a manner similar to the agglutination tests.

Persons who are Rh positive have erythrocytes which carry an Rh or D antigen and never have anti-Rh or anti-D antibodies in their serum. Persons who are Rh negative develop anti-Rh or anti-D antibodies in their serum after exposure to Rh positive blood. Possible methods of exposure include an accidental transfusion of Rh positive blood into a person with Rh negative blood. If this is a first exposure, no reaction will occur since it takes time to sensitize and develop antibodies. A second exposure will result in a hemolytic reaction. Equally as common as the transfusion reaction (or possibly more common) is the Rh negative mother who is carrying an Rh positive fetus. Rh negative mothers usually become sensitized during the first few days *following* delivery of the baby, not during the pregnancy. Degenerative products of the placenta release antigens into the blood of the mother supplying her with a large dose of the baby's Rh positive antigen. If the Rh positive antigen can be destroyed before it can initiate antibodies, the mother will not become sensitized. This is commonly accomplished today by innoculating the Rh negative mother with serum from another Rh negative person who has already formed anti-Rh agglutinogens. These injected anti-Rh agglutinogens circulate for as much as 8 weeks in the mother's blood destroying all the Rh positive factors from the placenta. Once anti-Rh positive antibodies have been formed by the mother, the process cannot be reversed and subsequent pregnancies increasingly produce erythroblastosis fetalis.

AGGLUTININS

These are antibodies that adhere to the erythrocyte membrane and cause coagulation of RBCs if the blood plasma temperature is below normal body temperature. For this reason, a person with cold agglutinins must receive blood that is warmed but NOT overheated. Overheating the blood would cause a degradation of proteins. This condition is seen predominantly in blacks and in patients with chronic diseases, anemia (severe or hemolytic), and cirrhosis of the liver.

Nursing responsibilities include all the monitoring for normal blood transfusions **and** close observation for signs of incompatibility of recipient and donor cold agglutinins.

COOMBS' TEST

A Coombs' test is used to determine the presence of hemolyzing antibodies in either a direct or indirect test. The direct Coombs' test detects IgG immunoglobulins attached to erythrocytes whereas the indirect Coombs' test detects IgG immunoglobulins in the plasma. This test is used predominantly to determine sensitization of pregnant women to indicate possible neonatal problems.

CELLULAR IMMUNITY

This form of acquired immunity is the result of sensitization of T-lymphocytes to a specific antigen. Cellular immunity does not involve immunoglobulins. The major difference between cellular and humoral immunity is that antibodies are released in humoral immunity and whole sensitized lymphocytes are released in cellular immunity.

Cellular (T-lymphocyte) immunity is formed from memory cells in the same manner as antibodies are formed in humoral immunity. T-lymphocytes originally are sensitized by an antigen which attaches directly to the T-lymphocyte cell membrane. If more T cells are needed, there is an overall increase in the total WBCs due to increased neutrophils, bands, and immature blast forms.

The life span of T-lymphocytes in cellular immunity is known to be much longer (perhaps 10 years or more) than in humoral immunity (usually a few months, rarely 2 years). Thus, cellular immunity is far more persistent than humoral immunity.

The cellular immunity system is far more potent in destruction of the slow developing bacteria than the humoral system. Cellular immunity is active against some types of cancer cells, some viruses, fungi, protozoa, and the graft rejection reaction in transplants. Once stimulated, the cellular immune system can "attack" the invading antigen directly or indirectly.

Direct Attack: Sensitized lymphocytes adhere to the antigens in the cell membrane of the invader such as a cancer cell. The sensitized lymphocytes immediately swell at the point of attachment releasing cytotoxic lysosomal enzymes. This direct attack is weaker than the indirect effects of cellular immunity.

Indirect attack: Three substances are involved in the indirect attack. First, the release of lysosomal enzymes initiates a sequence of reactions much more potent than the original attack. One of the substances released is *transfer factor*. This factor affects nonsensitized small lymphocytes enabling them to assume the characteristics of the original lymphocyte, thus increasing the number and effect of the sensitized lymphocytes. A second substance is the *macrophage chemotactic factor* which attracts the macrophages to enter the area of the sensitized lymphocyte. A third substance keeps the macrophages in the vicinity of the sensitized lymphocyte. This factor is called the *migration inhibition factor*. Finally, B-lymphocytes (especially IgM) arrive and assist in neutralizing the antigen for removal by the macrophage.

AUTOIMMUNITY

Unfortunately, the immune tolerance to ones own tissues is lost in some instances. This loss has multiple etiologies, but usually this loss is the result of destruction of some of the body's tissues. This destruction releases some antigens which presumably combine with proteins from bacteria or viruses forming new types of antigens. The result is an autoimmunity. One type of autoimmunity develops in myasthenia gravis in which the immunity is against the muscle portion of the neuromuscular junction, causing paralysis. In rheumatic fever, autoimmunity occurs in the heart tissue and joints following a specific streptococcal toxin. Autoimmunity may be generalized and systemic such as occurs in lupus erythematosus with different body tissues being affected at the same time. The mere presence of autoantibodies is not pathognomonic for an autoimmune disease.

RESPONSES TO CELLULAR IMMUNITY

There are four possible reactions in the cellular immunity system, all hypersensitive reactions. There is an immediate hypersensitivity reaction, an anaphylactic reaction, a subacute hypersensitivity reaction, and delayed hypersensitivity reaction.

An immediate hypersensitivity reaction is the acute hemolytic transfusion reaction. This is cytotoxic and results in damage to a specific cell because of complement-fixing antibody attacks against the cell's surface antigen.

An anaphylactic reaction is a systemic chemical reaction especially directed towards smooth muscle and vascular tissue. The intensity and speed of the anaphylactic reaction is often lethal.

The subacute hypersensitivity reaction may be local or systemic and is dependent upon the presence of immune complexes and activation of the complement system with an infiltration of polymorphonuclear leukocytes. A systemic reaction occurs in serum sickness and a local reaction is the arthus lesions.

A delayed hypersensitivity reaction occurs in 48–72 hours in a tuberculin skin test, for example, and longer in host-graft rejection.

Inflammation

Inflammation is a series of changes in the tissues in response to injury. As soon as tissue injury occurs, regardless of the cause, many substances are freed by the damaged tissue and move into surrounding fluids. Some of these substances are histamine, bradykinin, serotonin, and other less important chemicals.

PROCESS OF INFLAMMATION

With the occurrence of damaged tissue there is an immediate vasoconstriction of the small blood vessels in the injured area. The brief vasoconstriction is followed by vasodilatation due to neural response and chemical response. The vasodilatation of arteries and arterioles results in blood flow increasing the area. This results in an increased hydrostatic pressure in the capillaries causing an increased amount of fluid to leave the vessel and enter the tissue spaces. Due to this, lymph flow is increased during the initial stages of inflammation; but, later lymph flow is impeded by fibrin clots filling the lymphatic vessels.

Concurrent with the vasodilatation, vascular permeability increases primarily in the venules and later in the capillaries. During inflammation, endothelial cells swell and gaps develop between the cells. These gaps provide a route for plasma proteins and fluid to move from the venules into the tissue space. Consequently blood remaining in the vascular system becomes concentrated. Blood flow slows down as blood viscosity increases. If severe enough, blood flow may actually stop and stasis occurs. As stasis develops, red cells begin to clump together. This allows the leukocytes to adhere to the endothelium. Within one hour, leukocytes have formed a layer covering the entire endothelium of the venules. This layering is called *margination* (or pavementing).

Shortly after margination occurs, leukocytes enter the tissue spaces by emigration. Emigration is an active process of pseudopods extending from the leukocytes and passing between the endothelial cells by ameboid movement.

RBCs cannot move by ameboid motion, but hydrostatic pressure forces red cells through the gaps in the endothelium following the path of the leukocytes and their movement by *diapedesis.*

Chemotactic attraction pulls the leukocytes from the venules to the site of injury. As soon as the leukocytes arrive at the site of injury, they become actively phagocytic, ingesting cellular debris, foreign material, and microorganisms that are present.

The initial leukocyte response to inflammation is primarily achieved by neutrophils. An increased production of neutrophils (neutrophilia) starts in 30–45 minutes after injury and has a peak phagocytic activity in 6–8 hours. After the neutrophilia, monocytes migrate to the injured area and change into macrophages. This begins approximately 4 hours after injury and the peak phagocytic activity occurs in 16–24 hours. While the macrophages are phagocytizing the injured site, antibodies are formed. Leukocytosis, which is a result of the neutrophilia, may occur and result in an increased sedimentation rate. When tissue injury occurs, damage is usually greater in the lymphatic vessels (due to their fragility) than in the blood vessels. Fluid that escapes from the venules contains fibrinogen and other clotting factors which form a fibrin clot in the damaged lymphatic vessels. The clot prevents drainage from the injured area and the inflammatory reaction is localized. The localization of the inflammatory process limits the spread of microorganisms and may lead to abscess formation. The abscess is filled with pus that contains bacteria, enzymes, and dead tissue.

In summary, tissue injury occurs releasing histamine, bradykinin, and serotonin into the area. An initial vasoconstriction gives way to vasodilatation and increased permeability of the venus capillaries. This results in large amounts of fluid, protein, and fibrinogen leaking into the tissues causing local (brawny) edema. The injured area is blocked by fibrinogen clots which effectively "wall off" the inflammation. Tissue macrophages form the line of defense after the initial invasion of neutrophils into the inflamed area which becomes the second line of defense. Leukocytosis occurs as macrophages and monocytes form the third line of defense. The phagocytizing macrophages result in the formation of pus. Pus formation usually continues until all infection is supressed. Occasionally, an abscess full of pus forms and either ruptures spontaneously or is surgically drained.

— 37 ——————————————

Hemostatic Mechanisms and Hypovolemic Shock

Learning Objectives

By the end of this chapter, the nurse will be able to:

1. Define hemostasis.
2. Identify normal factors causing vasoconstriction.
3. Explain the process of platelet aggregation.
4. List five acquired defects in hemostatic disorders of blood vessels.
5. List at least two congenital defects in hemostatic disorders of blood vessels.
6. Define thrombocytopenia and its significance.
7. Define thrombocytosis and its significance.
8. Define hypovolemic shock.
9. List at least five common etiologies of hypovolemic shock.
10. Explain the pathophysiology of hypovolemic shock.
11. List the presenting signs and symptoms of hypovolemic shock.
12. List at least five nursing interventions for hypovolemic shock.
13. List eight complications of hypovolemic shock.

Hemostatic Mechanisms

Hemostasis is the process by which the body protects itself from excessive blood loss. The major processes are vasoconstriction, platelet aggregation, and coagulation. (Coagulation mechanisms will be covered in Chapter 39 along with disseminated intravascular coagulation.) When the hemostatic mechanisms for preventing blood loss become inadequate to contain the loss, hypovolemic shock occurs.

VASOCONSTRICTION

Immediately after the severing of a blood vessel, constriction and myogenic spasm of the vessel occur from neural, endocrine, and metabolic mechanisms. The greater the degree of injury and the more that the vessel is traumatized, the greater the vasospasm response. Localized vascular spasm may continue for up to 30 minutes. This allows time for the process of platelet plugging and blood coagulation to occur.

Tissue damage has an effect upon the neural and constricting forces. Neural reflexes include stimulation of the sympathetic nervous system, release of epinephrine, norepinephrine, serotonin, and lipoproteins. In a crushed vessel injury, neural control and vasoconstriction control bleeding more effectively than in a clean cut because of the greater release of these substances into the surrounding tissues.

PLATELET AGGREGATION

Platelets that are circulating in the blood migrate to the wound. Platelets are round or oval fragments of the megakaryocytes formed in the bone marrow and number from 200,000 to 400,000 in the normal, healthy human. At the wound site, the platelets contact collagen in the vessel endothelium and/or the damaged endothelial cell, resulting in spontaneous swelling of the platelet. The platelets become irregular in shape with an adhesive substance on the surface which causes them to adhere to the damaged endothelium and to secrete enzymes and ADP. The enzymes are responsible for the formation of *thromboxane A* in the plasma.

ADP and thromboxane A stimulate nearby platelets to form an irregular, sticky surface which adheres to the original platelets. This cycle continues until there is an accumulation of platelets forming a loose plug in the damaged endothelium. This plug temporarily controls bleeding until a blood clot has had time to form. The platelets in the loose plug undergo autolysis and during the 24–48 hours in which this occurs, the platelet plug has been changed into a dense fibrin mass. Eventually this mass is gradually digested by fibrolytic enzymes.

A prolonged bleeding time may be indicative of a disorder of the vascular mechanisms for control of bleeding.

ABNORMALITIES IN VASOCONSTRICTION AND PLATELET AGGREGATION

Defects in the vascular system may be congenital or acquired anomalies which prevent vasoconstriction.

Congenital defects include Ehlers-Danlos syndrome (hyperextensibility of joints, hyperelasticity and fragility of the skin, poor wound healing, and hyperfragility of capillaries) and collagen deficient disorders.

Acquired anomalies are usually related to septicemia but are often associated with drugs (purpura secondary to vascular fragility) and more rarely are related to an allergic vasculitis. Vitamin C deficiences result in an abnormal vascular permeability.

Platelet disorders are classified as congenital, acquired, quantitative, or qualitative. Congenital causes include hereditary capillary fragility, hereditary hemorrhagic telangiectasia, and the Elhers-Danlos disease previously mentioned.

Acquired platelet disorders are usually secondary to drug ingestion, anorexia nervosa, and malnutrition especially in the heavy alcohol consumer. Acquired disorders may also occur from systemic disorders such as collagen diseases, polyarteritis nodosa, amyloidosis, and allergies.

Thrombocytopenia is a decreased number of platelets (quantitative and/or qualitative) and may be the primary or secondary condition. Idiopathic thrombocytopenic purpura is a primary cause of uncontrollable bleeding secondary to failure of platelets to aggregate for unknown reasons. Secondary thrombocytopenia is most commonly caused by drugs and chemicals, leukemia, aplastic anemia, bone marrow infiltration, malignant lymphomas, and systemic lupus erythematosus. Less common causes include infection, alcoholism, and massive blood transfusion.

Thrombocytosis is an increased number of platelets (quantitative and/or qualitative) usually defined as more than one million per cubic milliliter. Because of the increased number of platelets, the viscosity of the blood is increased and may lead to "sludging" of the blood. Blood clot formation in small vessels is common and may cause tissue necrosis distal to the clot and/or bleeding secondary to leakage from the damaged vessels. Thyrombocytosis is usually seen with inflammatory responses, iron deficiency anemia, and post splenectomy. It also occurs in polycythemia vera, myelofibrosis, and chronic granulocytic leukemia.

Hypersplenism is usually caused by portal hypertension and results in an increased (quantitative) accumulation of platelets in the spleen.

Hypovolemic Shock

Hypovolemic shock is the loss of blood and plasma sufficient to prevent adequate tissue oxygenation throughout the body. The loss is, therefore, great enough to result in decreased circulating blood volume, decreased venous return to the heart, and reduced cardiac output.

ETIOLOGIES

Multiple causes of hypovolemic shock exist. Hemorrhage, trauma, burns, surgery, peritonitis, pancreatitis, hemothorax, hemoperitoneum, gastrointestinal bleeding, and esophageal varices are some causes.

Other causes that precipitate hypovolemic shock include diabetes mellitus, diabetes insipidus, dehydration, intestinal obstruction, and diuretic therapy.

PATHOPHYSIOLOGY

The microcirculation is a group of blood vessels that act as an independent organic unit to regulate blood supply to the tissues. The microcirculation (Figure 37-1) is comprised of vessels having a unique function. Each functioning unit is interactive with the others to maintain the balance between blood flow and tissue demand. The microcirculation is capable of adjusting blood flow in relation to tissue metabolic needs. It also plays a significant role in maintaining oncotic balance, in facilitating the movement of large molecules through the interstitium, and in regulating total blood volume.

The components of the microcirculation are the vascular system between arterioles and venules, namely the capillaries. The arterioles bifurcate at 90° angles at points called metarterioles or precapillary arterioles. Smooth muscle cells cover the metarterioles at the bifurcation but disappear as each metarteriole becomes a true capillary.

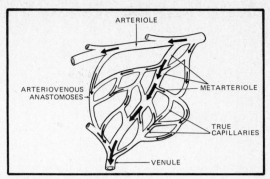

Figure 37-1. Microcirculation.

At the point of metarteriole bifurcation into true capillaries, there is a muscle sphincter. This precapillary sphincter acts as an autoregulatory system dilating to allow increased perfusion when blood pressure is low or constricting when blood pressure is increased to adjust to the metabolic needs of the tissues in normal states.

The precapillary sphincter constricts in cases of shock and sympathetic nervous system stimulation to maintain perfusion of the vital organs. This constriction directs the available blood from nonessential tissues such as the stomach to vital organs, especially the heart and brain. This is the first compensatory mechanism with the development of shock.

Many chemical and humoral factors alter the regulation in the microcirculatory system. These are listed in Table 37-1. This mechanism is a negative feedback resulting in adaptive responses. If the shock is mild and/or slow in developing, the negative feedback of the microcirculatory system will reverse the shock state. If the shock is severe and/or rapid in developing, this negative compensatory feedback is inadequate to reverse the shock state. Failure to restore a hemostatic state allows a positive feedback system to develop. In this vicious cycle of positive feedback, an inadequate tissue perfusion leads to a deterioration in cardiovascular function which decreases tissue perfusion even more. Consequently, in these instances, the shock state precipitates an even more severe shock state leading to death if not reversed.

The release of catecholamines (epinephrine and norepinephrine) in early

Table 37-1. Regulation of the microcirculatory system.

Chemical	C	D	Humoral	C	D
Hypoxemia		+	Catecholamines		
Hydrogen		+	Epinephrine	+	+
Potassium		+	Norepinephrine	+	
Hypercapnea		+	Dopamine	+	+
Hyperosmolarity		+			
			Amines		
			Serotonin	+	+
			Acetylcholine		+
			Histamine		+
			Polypeptides		
			Angiotensin	+	
			Kinins	+	
			Vasopressin		+

C = Vasoconstriction   D = Vasodilatation

shock results in vasoconstriction of the microcirculatory vessels at the precapillary sphincter level. The precapillary sphincter constriction is an attempt to increase venous return to the heart (by prevention of blood flow in unnecessary tissues) which in turn improves cardiac output and tissue perfusion.

The hemodynamic mechanism to resolve shock is movement of fluid from the interstitial space into the vascular tree, causing an increase in plasma volume. This fluid shift occurs because change in the hydrostatic pressure in the capillaries alters fluid exchange across the capillary membrane. With increased fluid shifting into the vascular tree, the plasma is diluted, decreasing plasma oncotic pressure and fostering more fluid movement into capillary beds. After hemorrhage, the liver synthesizes new proteins immediately to replace the lost plasma proteins in an attempt to force the fluid shift from the interstitium to the vascular tree maintaining adequate intravascular volume.

The renin-angiotensin-aldosterone cascade is activated by decreased renal blood flow. The renin is acted upon in several stages to convert it to angiotensin II. Angiotensin II is the most potent vasoconstrictor known. It augments the blood pressure, increasing blood flow. Angiotensin II and the catecholamines (epinephrine and nor-epinephrine) increase vasoconstriction in all organs EXCEPT the brain and heart. At the same time, aldosterone secretion is stimulated by angiotensin II. Aldosterone increases sodium retention by kidneys thereby increasing water reabsorption through the "drag" effect. This additional retention of water helps increase intravascular volume.

A low cardiac output, secondary to hypovolemia, stimulates the neurohypophysis to increase release of the antidiuretic hormone (ADH). ADH promotes water reabsorption through its actions on the convoluted tubules and collecting ducts of the kidneys. ADH also has a vasoconstricting effect further increasing arterial pressure. ADH is sometimes called vasopressin because of this action.

Hypovolemia and a low cardiac output stimulate the hypothalamic thirst center. If the patient is alert, he or she will be very thirsty and drink as much water as possible. This will help replace lost fluids. Figure 37-2 depicts the vicious cycle of decompensated hypovolemic shock.

Cerebral ischemia develops when the arterial pressure drops $\frac{60 \pm 10}{40}$ resulting in a hypercarbia. The hypercarbic state stimulates the cerebral vasomotor center. This results in the most extreme sympathetic constriction of the vascular tree. If sustained for long, small vessels in the periphery may become completely blocked.

Failure of Compensatory Mechanisms

CELLULAR EFFECTS

Cell function becomes based on anaerobic metabolism rather than aerobic metabolism, causing lactic acid production and depletion of ATP (a high energy phosphate).

The mitochondrial function of maintaining intracellular transport fails and the mitochondria are unable to maintain a patent cell membrane. Thus, sodium and potassium balance across the cell membrane is altered, decreasing the resting membrane potential and the cell's action potential.

As the cell membranes in the microcir-

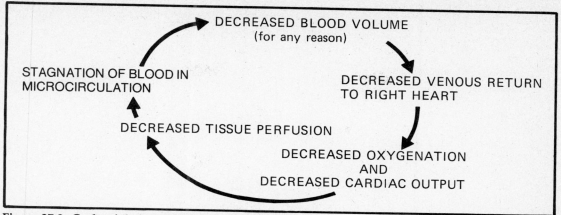

Figure 37-2. Cycle of decompensation of hypovolemic shock.

culation deteriorate, organelles, especially lysosomes, are released into surrounding tissues and begin damaging the surrounding cells. The gastrointestinal tract is the primary site of lysosomal enzyme release.

METABOLIC EFFECTS

Endocrine and metabolic changes occur in hypovolemic shock. The sympathetic nervous system and release of epinephrine and norepinephrine have been discussed. They are the cause of the tachycardia seen in early shock.

Cortisol (from the adrenal glands) and growth hormone from the adenohypophysis are released with a concurrent increase in glucagon and decrease in available insulin. This results in a hyperglycemic state accompanying the shock state.

Because of a decrease in circulating free fatty acid and a decrease in lipolysis, protein catabolism becomes the dominant source of energy increasing the acidotic state seen in shock.

CLINICAL PRESENTATION

In early, reversible shock, there may be few if any *significant* changes in the patient. A slight tachycardia, slightly increased or normal blood pressure, or slightly decreased pressure may be seen. The patient is alert, perhaps a little anxious, and asks for something to drink. Respiratory evaluation shows a slightly rapid and deep respiratory pattern without signs of distress.

The skin is warm and dry in this very early shock state. Cyanosis is not present as evidenced by normal nailbed refill.

Towards the end of the early, reversible shock and into the late reversible hypovolemic shock states, the patient evidences definitive signs and symptoms. There is a definite tachycardia accompanied by hypotension, decreased cardiac output, decreased CVP, and decreased PCWP values. The patient's respiratory pattern is hyperpneic, tachypneic, and somewhat labored. The skin is cold and clammy: cold because of compensatory vasoconstriction; clammy secondary to release of catecholamines.

If the patient is still alert, he or she asks for water and appears to be more apprehensive than in the early state of shock.

Refractory shock develops if the cause of shock in the early and late stages of reversible shock is not corrected. This shock stage *may* be reversed with aggressive therapy in a patient who was previously healthy. There is a stagnation of blood in the microcirculation which will begin to coagulate unless rapidly reversed. (Blood will not coagulate as long as it keeps moving.) Acidosis is present. Heart rate is very fast, but a continuing hypotension exists. Frequently, blood pressure can be obtained only by Doppler use. The pulse is weak, thready, and rapid with a narrowing pulse pressure. Cyanosis is evident throughout the body and jugular neck veins collapse with pressure and are slow in refilling. The patient may be semi-conscious but moves restlessly. Urine output is less than 25–30 cc/hour. Disseminated intravascular coagulation may occur.

In irreversible shock, tissue perfusion is negligible due to clotting in the microcirculation since vasodilatation of the capillaries occurred at the end of the previous state of shock as compensatory mechanisms failed. Heart contraction is weak as the increased PCWP indicates a failing left ventricle and an increased CVP indicates a failing right heart. Acidosis counters the effect of the catecholamines and further vasodilatation occurs. Respirations are rapid but drop very soon unless the shock can be reversed. The patient is comatose and without movement. The patient's skin is ashen, gray, and cold. There is a frank cyanosis of nailbeds, conjunctiva, and oral mucosa. The patient is anuric. The clammy skin is due to electrolyte and water loss through the pores of the skin. Body temperature decreases; this is accompanied by a decrease in respirations and increasing rales. Eventually, the patient straight lines as the heart stops contracting.

TREATMENT OF HYPOVOLEMIC SHOCK

The treatment of first priority is to obtain and maintain a patent airway. After this is assured, attention can be directed towards replacing lost vascular volume. The treatment modalities are controversial: crystalloid or colloid infusion.

Often, whole blood and a crystalloid solution (e.g., Ringer's lactate) are used to provide a balance between infusion of RBCs, electrolytes, and fluid which would affect all three compartments (intravascular, intracellular, and extracellular). Interstitial and intracellular compartments are not replenished by blood. The blood would increase vascular volume, osmotic pressure, and oxygen carrying capacity.

The colloid proponents claim that increasing the colloid osmotic pressure in the vascular tree will "pull" interstitial fluids back into the vascular system. Since the liver produces new plasma proteins, a plasma albumin deficit is corrected within 24

hours. Many authorities feel there is greater risk of overtransfusion with colloids (which remain in the patent vascular tree) than with crystalloids which can be absorbed into intracellular and interstitial spaces.

Other solutions may be used to restore normal circulating volume. Fresh whole blood is the ideal replacement fluid. Blood and its component parts are discussed in Chapter 38 and will not be detailed in this chapter.

NURSING INTERVENTIONS

Primary action is the procurement and maintenance of a patent airway. Frequent suctioning may be required if the patient cannot cough effectively to remove secretions. Chest physiotherapy and all measures related to adequate bronchial hygiene are especially important to prevent infection in the post shock period of debilitation.

Monitoring hemodynamic parameters of shock usually involves a CVP line or a pulmonary artery catheter and gives guidelines of the effectiveness of treatment. Nursing procedures relating to any CVP or pulmonary artery catheter are applicable to the shock patient.

Positioning of the patient has traditionally been the Trendelenberg position or use of "shock blocks." Recent research indicates that a *supine* position provides adequate circulation of the brain AND away from the brain preventing stagnation, cerebral ischemia, and hypoxic damage. If a concurrent head injury exists, the head of the bed may be in a low Fowler's position. In cases of severe shock, a supine position with legs elevated 20–30° by pillows may increase venous return or mast pants may be used.

Cardiovascular status, in addition to hemodynamic monitoring, is continuously monitored for signs of dysrhythmias. Dysrhythmias due to electrolyte disturbance are common with massive blood transfusions and with inadequate vascular volume.

Vasomotor tone is normally controlled by constriction secondary to sympathetic and catecholamine factors. This severe vasoconstriction worsens the shock state. Vasodilating drugs are often used *IF* blood volume is restored *before* administration of these drugs such as nitroprusside (Nipride®), chlorpromazine (Thorazine®), and phentolamine (Regitine®).

Steroids may increase tissue perfusion by capillary vasodilatation. They may also help cellular uptake of nutrients and oxygen and stabilize lysosome activity improving cell membrane integrity. Dexamethasone (Decadron®) and methylprednisolone sodium succinate (Solu-Medrol®) are the most common steroids used to reverse the effects of extensive hypotension and hypovolemia.

Acid-base disturbances may be severe, and mixed metabolic and respiratory acidosis are common. Respiratory acidosis is corrected by suctioning and adequate ventilation. Metabolic acidosis may be corrected by intravenous sodium bicarbonate. One equivalent per kilogram of body weight is an initial loading dose. Additional doses depend upon the ABG values.

Fluid overload may occur for up to 36 hours post shock. After volume has been restored with crystalloid infusion, large quantities of interstitial and third space fluid is shifted back into the vascular system. This may cause a severe fluid overload, pulmonary edema, or water intoxication. Administration of albumin will increase vascular osmotic pressure and "pull" fluid from the interstitial and intracellular spaces into the vascular system which will dispose of excess fluid through the kidneys.

Renal function is monitored hourly with an in-dwelling Foley catheter. Severe or sustained hypovolemia may result in acute tubular necrosis (ATN). If the kidneys are unable to increase their function in eliminating the accumulated waste products, diuretics may be required. If diuretic therapy is not adequate, peritoneal or hemodialysis may be employed. Diuretic therapy may be with a 20% glucose infusion to produce osmotic diuresis. Furosemide (Lasix®) or ethacrynic acid (Edecrin®) are often used to support kidney function.

Nutritional support is essential since a shock state rapidly depletes glucose storage with a resulting negative nitrogen balance, and protein catabolism increases acidotic states. Hyperalimentation (total parenteral nutrition—TPN) may be instituted to provide adequate nutritional needs. If the shock state was not caused by gastrointestinal or esophageal bleeding, an N/G tube may be inserted and a continuous drip infusion of commercial food substitutes is started. Isocal® and Vivonex® are two often used food substitutes.

Stress ulcers may occur secondary to necrosis of the gastric mucosa during the hypovolemic period leading to ulcer formation. Intravenous cimetidine (Tagamet®) is often used until oral antacids are tolerated or until the danger of stress ulcers has passed.

Emotional support consists of the continuous presence of the nurse. Short brief comments regarding his or her condition and the use of monitoring equipment will help decrease patient anxiety. Explanations to family members about the patient's current status and nursing procedures usually console the family and the patient.

COMPLICATIONS OF HYPOVOLEMIC SHOCK

Sustained tissue hypoxia will lead to tissue necrosis and release of endotoxins into the system. Brain damage secondary to stagnation or prolonged hypoperfusion occurs as glucose is consumed. Coma, seizures, and intracerebral hemorrhage may occur.

Pulmonary embolism, infarction, or ARDS is likely to occur as the hypovolemic state continues.

Electrolyte disarrangement and acid-base alterations are a result of both the shock state and renal failure.

Cardiac dysrhythmia may herald the onset of irreversible shock resulting in death.

— 38

Blood and Component Therapy

Learning Objectives

By the end of this chapter, the nurse will be able to:

1. Define the end objective of blood transfusions.
2. State four reasons for transfusions.
3. Describe the characteristics of:
   a. Whole blood
   b. Packed cells
   c. Fresh frozen plasma
   d. Cryoprecipitates
   e. Platelets
   f. Plasmanate
   g. Salt-poor albumin
   h. Granulocytes
4. List the purpose of each of the above (a–h) for transfusion.
5. Identify the contraindications, if any, of the above (a–h) for transfusion.
6. Define the major types of transfusion reactions.
7. List four nursing interventions in transfusion reactions.

The primary reason for transfusing blood is to increase the oxygen available for preventing tissue hypoxia. Other reasons may include improving the hemoglobin/hematocrit levels in asanguinous bleeds, increasing intravascular volume, and replacing deficient or utilized substances such as protein, platelets, and clotting factors.

Transfusion with Whole Blood

Whole blood is approximately 500 cc of blood cells, serum, platelets, proteins, and other intravascular nutrients and substances. Whole blood is the best substance to transfuse in hemorrhage bleeds since it replaces both volume and elements.

Whole blood may be preserved for up to 21 days under controlled refrigeration at 4°C or 39°F. However, the blood must be preserved with acid-citrate-dextrose (A.C.D.) solution or with citrate-phosphate-dextrose (C.P.D.). C.P.D. preserved blood has a higher pH than A.C.D. blood and therefore is less acid than A.C.D. blood. This may be an important factor in multiple transfusions.

A.C.D. preserved blood has more citrate than that needed to combine with the collected blood. If citrate ions are infused too rapidly, the liver cannot remove them all and the excess combines with ionized calcium in the bloodstream reducing the amount of circulating calcium. This results in hypocalcemia which results in neuromuscular irritability. Signs and symptoms include muscular cramps, hyperreflexia, carpopedal hand position, convulsions, and cardiac arrest. These complications are likely to occur in patients with liver disease. The slow transfusion of blood in these patients may prevent such complications.

During the 21-day storage limit, the blood slowly deteriorates so only approximately 70–80% of the original blood cells remain. The deterioration of RBCs releases potassium into the plasma. The increase in plasma potassium begins in day 1 raising the potassium level to 7 mEq/L and 23 mEq/L by day 21. Old blood should not be transfused into oliguric or anuric patients since the excess potassium cannot be excreted by the kidneys. Elevated potassium levels are characterized by peaked T waves on the EKG, nausea/diarrhea, colic, and vague muscular weakness starting with the extremeties and extending to the trunk, including respiratory muscles. The patient may have paresthesia of hands, feet, tongue, and face. Apprehension and a slow and/or irregular pulse rate is common. If potassium levels reach 10–15 mEq/L, cardiac arrest and death will occur due to a flaccidness and dilatation of the heart.

Cold blood is rapidly warmed as it mixes with circulating blood at *normal* infusion rates. Rapid replacement of cold blood predisposes the patient to a cardiac arrest. With massive, rapid transfusions the blood can move through a heating coil (Figure 38-1) and reach body temperature, thus reducing cardiac arrest.

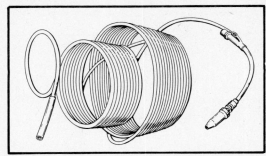

Figure 38-1. Heating coil for blood transfusion.

Serum hepatitis is always a risk since no *highly* reliable tests to identify the hepatitis antigen has been found.

RED BLOOD CELLS (PACKED RBCS)

Packed RBCs provide the advantage of less blood volume (200–250 cc) to infuse, decreasing the chance of fluid overload, and raises the Hgb 1.3 gm%/unit (twice that of whole blood). Over a period of 6 hours a 3–4% increase in Hct will be achieved. In old packed cells, there is a decrease in pH and in 2,3-DPG. The decrease in 2,3-DPG binds hemoglobin and oxygen tightly, lowering the available oxygen in the tissues. The raising of Hgb and Hct may not significantly affect tissue hypoxia.

Packed RBCs are used in severe anemias without blood loss, in patients with CHF, and cautiously in patients with underlying cardiac disease or with renal failure.

Blood transfusion reactions are not common with packed RBCs but are due to platelet or WBC antigens. Usually, there is not a significant change in the clinical picture with the rare reactions that do occur.

FRESH FROZEN PLASMA (FFP)

Plasma is indicated when there is little or no actual blood loss, for example, in burns and crush injuries. In an emergency, FFP may be used as a volume expander in hypovolemic bleeds until fresh whole blood is available.

PLASMA

This is the fluid portion of blood after centrifuging to remove the RBCs. The plasma may be commercially prepared as a liquid, frozen, or dried. Each unit of FFP is about 200–250 cc/unit and has a 1-year shelf life.

Due to freezing the plasma, all clotting factors are preserved especially V and VII, except for platelets. The plasma takes about 20 minutes to thaw and is then ready for use.

CRYOPRECIPITATES

Cryoimmunoglobulins are serum proteins that precipitate at temperatures below 20°C. Cryoglobulins must be obtained and processed at temperatures above 20°C and ideally before refrigeration which may cause cryoproteins to be caught in the blood clots. Many authorities feel that cryoprecipitates are antigen-antibody protein compounds.

Cryoprecipitates usually consist of 20–30 cc/unit of blood and must be infused *immediately* after thawing. Cryoprecipitates contain factors VIII, XIII, and fibrinogen. It is not uncommon to infuse as many as 30 bags of cryoprecipitates at one time using a special transfusion administration set.

The administration of cryoprecipitates is indicated in DIC, hemophilia A, and von Willebrand's disease.

PLATELETS

Less than 40,000–50,000 platelets/mm^3 is considered inadequate for hemostasis. Prolonged bleeding time is a better index for the need of platelet transfusion than an actual platelet count. There is an expected increase of 10,000/unit (platelet)/m^2, and 4–6 platelet pacts are given through a special administration set. A postplatelet transfusion bleeding time is the most accurate index of response to therapy.

In septic and/or febrile patients, platelet infusion should be doubled to effect an increase in platelet count.

In thrombocytopenia, splenomegaly, and DIC, platelet transfusions are useful until more definitive therapy can be insti-

tuted. Alloimmunity may require cross-matching to have any value for platelet transfusion. Platelets can be safely kept at room temperatures for up to 3 days and are inactivated if refrigerated.

VOLUME EXPANDERS

Albumin, plasma protein fractions (Plasmanate®), and, in some institutions, Dextran-40 and Dextran-70 are commonly used for volume expanders.

Salt-Poor Albumin

This is a concentrate of human serum albumin packaged in 50 cc ampules with a total protein of 12.5 gm in 50–100 cc amounts. It is not low in sodium content nor does it supply any clotting factors. Its sole value is its blood volume expansion increasing colloid osmotic pressure for up to 24 hours (time may be as low as 4 hours).

Plasmanate (Plasma Protein Fractions)

This is a commercially prepared hypertonic solution of alpha and beta globulins, human albumin, sodium, and chloride. Because it is hypertonic, it "pulls" fluid from the extracellular and intracellular fluid spaces into the vascular system.

Blood volume may be expanded for up to 48 hours with a maximum administration of 2,000 ml/day at a rate not greater than 8 ml/min.

It is *contraindicated* in dehydrated patients and patients with clotting dyscrasias and/or congestive heart failure. It is *indicated* in burn cases, hypovolemic shock, hypoproteinemia, and rarely in cases of cerebral edema. [Since it is hyperosmolar, it will "pull" edema (if present) from the ECF and ICF fluid of the brain. However, other solutions such as mannitol or 10–20% glucose achieve an osmotic diuresis and may be preferred.]

Dextran

This is commercially available in two forms: Dextran-70 (Macrodex®) or Dextran-40 L.M.W.D. (low molecular weight dextran).

Dextran-70 is a 6% solution in 0.9 normal saline or D$_5$W composed of both small and large molecules. It has colloid effects similar to plasma. Once infused, 40% of the smaller molecules is excreted or degraded within 24 hours and 70–90% of the larger molecules are excreted in the same time period. Dextran-70 has a half-life of 24 hours and is essentially degraded completely in 72 hours.

Dextran-40 (L.M.W.D.) is a 10% solution in 0.9 normal saline or D_5W. This 10% solution has 2 to 2½ times the colloid osmotic pressure of normal plasma. This rapidly expands the intravascular volume. With a 500 ml infusion of L.M.W.D., intravascular volume is increased by about 1,000 milliliters. This gradually drops over the next 12–24 hours.

Dextran's greatest value lies in its expansion properties in addition to its lowering of blood viscosity. The lower blood viscosity is due to a lower Hct and reduction of platelet and RBC aggregations improving tissue perfusion. L.M.W.D. may help prevent a vascular thrombus occlusion of a vessel or graft.

Major complications of Dextran use are allergic reactions, imparied coagulation (due to interference with platelet aggregation), and difficulty in future type and crossmatching attempts for whole blood infusions. The allergic reaction may range from urticaria to anaphylaxis, which may occur immediately or after more than 30 minutes. Nausea, vomiting, and hypotension may occur.

Dextran therapy is CONTRAINDICATED in oliguric patients, CHF patients, and patients with blood clotting dyscrasias.

GRANULOCYTES

Centers performing leukopheresis have the ability to filter out granulocytes. Each unit is about 200–300 cc and the recipient must be compatible with the donor. An infusion of granulocytes improves phagocytosis from the marginal cells, not increasing the already circulating WBC pool. The marginal cells are those being released from the bone marrow.

It is common for the patient to have fever and chills during granulocyte infusion. Steroids and antihistamines given before the infusion will help control the fever, whereas meperidine hydrochloride (Demerol®) will control the chills.

Reactions to Blood and Component Therapy

In spite of meticulous procedures for blood and component therapy, reactions do occur. There are four major reactions.

1. Circulatory overload occurs when too much fluid or too rapid an infusion is administered to patients with underlying cardiac, renal, liver, pulmonary, or hematologic disease. With proper monitoring and assessment, circulatory overload should not occur. If it does occur, prompt and appropriate intervention will remove sufficient fluid to restore the normal fluid status.

2. Bacterial reaction to transfusion therapy is the most common reaction and is characterized by the development of a fever in a previously afebrile patient. If the patient is febrile, a rising temperature may indicate a reaction.

3. Allergic reactions may occur with almost any product transfused. A slight reaction may be manifested by a mild urticaria. A severe allergic reaction is indicated by anaphylaxis which may or may not be reversible.

4. Hemolytic reactions usually occur within the first 30 minutes of the transfusion. It results in actual hemolysis of the RBCs and the transfusion must be stopped.

SIGNS AND SYMPTOMS OF A REACTION

The signs and symptoms will differ with the type of reaction, length of transfusion, the substance being infused, and the intensity of the reaction.

Common signs and symptoms may include chills, fever, hives, hypotension, cardiac "palpitations," tachycardia, flushing of the skin, headache, loss of consciousness, nausea/vomiting, shortness of breath, back pain, and hemoglobinuria. In some instances, warmth along the vein carrying the infusion may be detected.

NURSING INTERVENTIONS

The nurse must immediately stop the infusion (saving the substance being transfused) and keep the vein open with 0.9 normal saline. Accurate assessment of patient status must be completed quickly and efficiently for a comparison with pretransfusion baseline data. The physician and the blood bank are notified of the reaction and physician orders are instituted. If the reaction is anaphylactic, emergency resuscitative measures are instituted while personnel contact the doctor and laboratory and save the substance being transfused.

Nursing support of the patient and family is best achieved by rapid but efficient and professional conduct in instituting all necessary interventions. Education as to the cause of the reaction may prevent a recurrence, for example, hypersensitivity to Dextran-40 (L.M.W.D.). The patient can avoid future infusion if he or she carries this information in his or her wallet—much like a medic alert card or chain.

— 39

Normal Coagulation and Disseminated Intravascular Coagulation

Learning Objectives

By the end of this chapter, the nurse will be able to:

1. List three essential steps in coagulation.
2. Explain platelet aggregation.
3. List at least five clotting factors and their synonyms.
4. Name and describe the activation of three cascades.
5. Identify the one factor necessary in each cascade for the cascade to continue.
6. Define syneresis.
7. Compare the fibrinolytic and anti-thrombin systems.
8. Define disseminated intravascular coagulation.
9. Explain the pathophysiology of disseminated intravascular coagulation.
10. Explain split fibrin products and list their names.
11. Identify five treatment modalities in disseminated intravascular coagulation.
12. List six nursing assessments used almost continuously in the patient with disseminated intravascular coagulation.

Vasoconstriction and platelet aggregation are two essential steps in hemostasis that were covered in Chapter 37. The third hemostatic mechanism is coagulation.

Normal Coagulation

Normal coagulation is dependent upon the presence of all clotting factors and separate, but interrelated components, all functioning correctly. These components are the extrinsic cascade, the intrinsic cascade, and the common final pathway.

CLOTTING FACTORS

Confusion often occurs with the nomenclature assigned to the specific clotting factors. Consequently, an international committee agreed that all clotting factors would be designated by roman numerals for the inactive clotting factors. It was further agreed that once activated, the clotting factors would be identified by the roman numeral and a subscript "a." Table 39-1 lists the clotting factors and their synonyms. There is no designated factor VI.

Table 39-1. Clotting factors and their synonyms.

Factor	Synonym
I	Fibrinogen
Ia	Fibrin
II	Prothrombin
IIa	Thrombin
III	Thromboplastin
IV	Calcium
V	Acglobulin (labile factor, proaccelerin)
VII	Proconvertin (Autoprothrombin I)
VIIa	Convertin
VIII	Antihemophiliac globulin (AHG)
IX	Christmas factor (Autoprothrombin II) Plasma thromboplastin component (PTC)
IXa	Activated PTC
X	Stuart-Prower factor (Autoprothrombin III)
XI	Plasma thromboplastin antecedent (PTA)
XII	Hageman factor
XIIa	Activated Hageman factor
XIII	Fibrin-stabilizing factor

Most of the clotting factors are found in circulating blood, the blood elements and tissues surrounding, and within the microcirculatory system. Clotting factors I (fibrinogen); factor II (prothrombin); and factors V, VII, IX, and X are synthesized in the liver. Factors XI and XIII may also be synthesized in the liver. Factor VIII is most likely synthesized in some way by macrophages in the spleen. Lymphocytes and the bone marrow may work in conjunction with the macrophages.

There are four clotting factors that are dependent upon vitamin K for synthesis by the liver—namely factors II, VII, IX, and X. Current research indicates that factor XI may also be vitamin K dependent. It is known that at least 30 substances may be connected with the clotting process; however, the 17 listed in Table 39-1 are the most significant.

Cascades

A cascade is similar to a row of dominoes standing on their ends. When the first domino falls, it strikes the next domino starting a chain reaction and continues until all the dominoes have been toppled. This necessitates positioning the dominoes so that each will connect with the next. Within the circulating blood, there is a plethora of clotting factors to continue a cascade once initiated. It is interesting to note that there is at least one specific spot in each of the three cascades (extrinsic, intrinsic, and final common pathway) that requires calcium ions (Ca^{++} factor IV) to continue activation of these cascades. These sites are identified in Figure 39-1 showing the normal coagulation process.

EXTRINSIC CASCADE

This cascade (Figure 39-2) is activated by injury to vessels and tissue which has an end result of releasing thromboplastin into the circulatory system.

A second mechanism for activating clotting factors is the release of phospholipids from platelets and damaged tissue which is thought to increase the rate of blood coagulation through both extrinsic and intrinsic cascades.

INTRINSIC CASCADE

This cascade (Figure 39-3) is initiated when factor XII (the Hageman factor, the surface substance) comes into contact with collagen or the basement membrane of the damaged endothelium of the blood vessels; thus the name "intrinsic" with the necessary factors present in the circulating blood.

COMMON FINAL PATHWAY CASCADE

Both the extrinsic and intrinsic cascades react to completion and, in the presence of

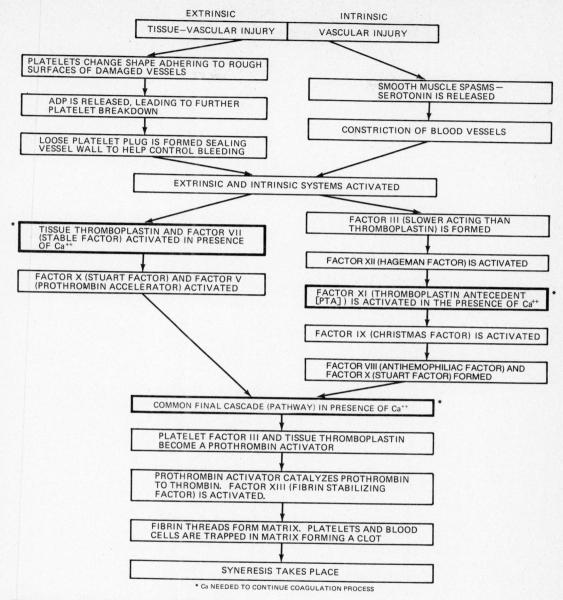

Figure 39-1. Normal coagulation process.

calcium ions, join to form the common final pathway (cascade) shown in Figure 39-4.

Syneresis is the final step in coagulation and the first step in clot stability. Syneresis is the process of particles suspended in a gel beginning to aggregate and form a compact mass—the clot. Clot retraction occurs soon after syneresis is complete. Platelets contain an enzyme, thromboplastin. This enzyme causes the fibrin strands and cells in the clot to be drawn together expressing a clear, serous fluid. Clot retraction is responsible for drawing the edges of damaged vessels together, fostering healing.

Anticoagulation

When the vascular damage has been repaired, the dissolution of the clot begins.

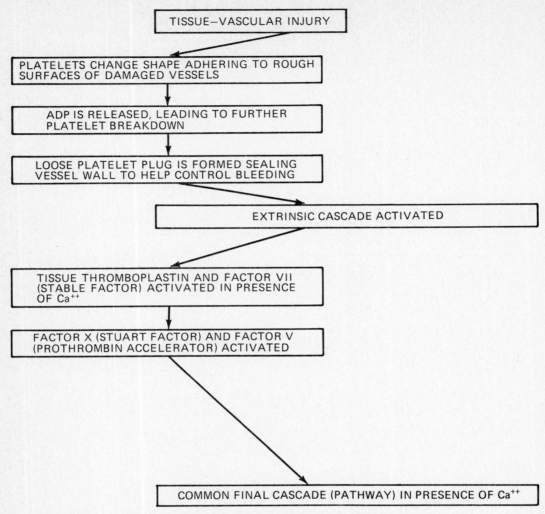

Figure 39-2. Extrinsic cascade segment of overall normal coagulation process.

This is termed fibrinolysis. Until this point, the various cascades have clotted the injured vessels but have not caused massive intravascular clotting because excess thrombin is carried away from the clot site by the circulating blood and antithrombin III is released from mast cells.

There are actually two mechanisms to prevent excessive clotting: the fibrinolytic system and the anti-thrombin system.

THE FIBRINOLYTIC SYSTEM

In this system, plasminogen is converted to plasmin. Plasmin "lyses" the clot and is

present in two forms: free plasmin and bound plasmin.

Free Plasmin

This form of plasmin is normally destroyed by the antiplasmins in the plasma. In some cases, there may be more plasmin than antiplasmin. In these instances, plasmin, other plasma proteins, and many coagulation factors are destroyed. This is pathologic proteolysis.

Bound Plasmin

This bound plasmin is found bound to the fibrin in the clot making the plasmin insolu-

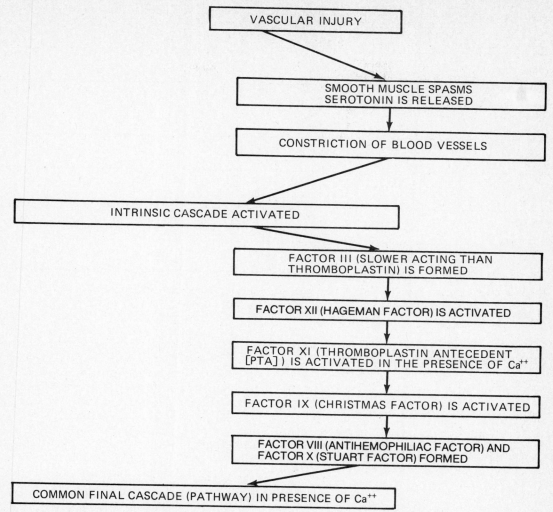

Figure 39-3. Intrinsic cascade segment of overall normal coagulation process.

ble. Bound plasmin phagocytizes the clot and functions in fibrinolysis in a natural physiologic proteolysis.

The fibrinolysis may produce fibrin split products. These are fragments of fibrin and fibrinogen called X, T, D, and E. An elevation of the fibrin split products normally indicates a pathologic process of excess clotting factor consumption.

ANTITHROMBIN SYSTEM

This sytem protects our bodies from excessive intravascular clotting by neutralizing the clotting capability of thrombin. (Antithrombin III is the neutralizing agent.) Heparin is released from most cells. Heparin functions as a serine protease to inhibit all serine proteases in all cascades. These include Xa, Ha, Vt1$_2$, and thrombin. It interrupts the action of thrombin on fibrinogen.

When clot retraction is complete, profibrinolysis is activated by factor XII. This activation results in fibrinolysin (plasmin) which phagocytizes the clot and other clotting factors present in excess of the normal amount. In this way, both intravascular clotting and bleeding are controlled.

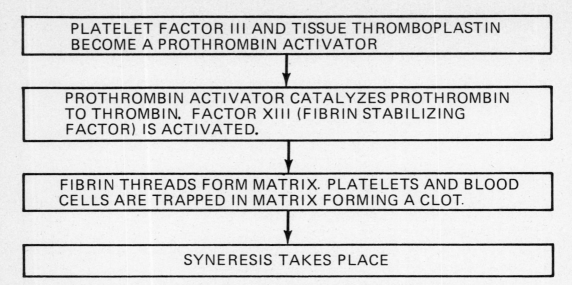

Figure 39-4. Common final pathway (cascade) of the normal coagulation process.

Hemostatic Screening Tests

Specific tests can be performed to evaluate blood clotting activity, to identify abnormalities, and to ascertain patient response to therapy.

PROTHROMBIN TIME (PT)

The PT measures activity level and patency of the extrinsic cascade and the common pathway. Normal values are the same as control (should be 11–16 seconds).

PARTIAL THROMBOPLASTIN TIME (PTT)

The PTT measures activity level and patency of the intrinsic cascade and common final pathway. Normal values are 60–85 seconds.

BLEEDING TIME

This tests the platelet plug formation time. Normal values are less than 4 minutes (Ivy), 1–4 minutes (Duke), and 1–9 minutes (Mielke).

PLATELET COUNT

This is a specific count of platelets seen in a blood smear. Normal values are 150,000–450,000 platelets/mm². Values below 100,000 platelets/mm² are pathognomonic for thrombocytopenia, the cause of which must be determined. Lower platelet count results in excessive bleeding since there is an insufficient number of platelets to clot.

In summary, normal clotting has three stages—namely (1) vascular injury activates thromboplastin activity in *both* the extrinsic and the intrinsic pathways, (2) thromboplastin converts prothrombin to thrombin, and (3) thrombin converts fibrinogen in the plasma at the site of injury to form a fibrin plug.

Disseminated Intravascular Coagulation

The abbreviation DIC will be used in this text. DIC is a state of hypercoagulability in the system which utilized all the clotting factors resulting in hemorrhage.

ETIOLOGY

Many factors may precipitate DIC including multiple trauma, crush injuries, hemorrhagic shock, malignant hypertension, incompatible blood transfusion, any and all cancers, burns, and coronary bypass surgery. The most common causes are obstetrical conditions, for example, amniotic fluid embolism and abruptio placentae.

PATHOPHYSIOLOGY

Regardless of the etiology, specific pathophysiological signs occur in DIC. The common denominator is the release of procoagulants into the circulatory system. Free hemoglobin, cancer tissue fragments, amniotic fluid, and bacterial toxins are some procoagulants that may activate the clotting cascades. Activation of the cascade results in diffuse intravascular fibrin formation. This fibrin is deposited in the microcirculation.

With the clotting of the capillaries, blood is shunted to the arteriovenous anastomoses (refer to Chapter 37, Figure 37-1). This shunting causes the capillary tissue to use anaerobic processes. The microcirculation, with its stagnant blood and production of lactic and pyruvic waste products, causes acidotic blood.

The effects of this produce three procoagulant factors in the capillary blood.

1. Acidosis, which is a strong procoagulant
2. Stagnation of the blood, which increases the concentration of procoagulants
3. The "normal" procoagulants in the blood

This results in massive sequestration of clotted blood in the capillaries (Figure 39-5).

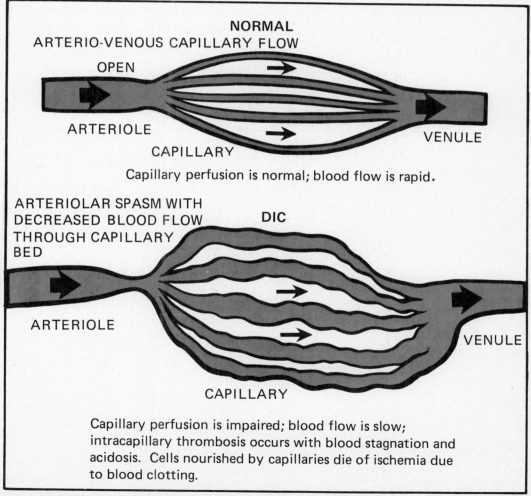

Figure 39-5. Sequestration of clotted blood in the capillaries.

DIC develops rapidly so coagulating factors are depleted in the microcirculation, clotting faster than the clotting factors can be replenished. Without circulating coagulant factors, hemostasis cannot be maintained (Figure 39-6) and the patient begins to bleed.

CLINICAL PRESENTATION

Almost always, patients have arterial hypotension along with shock. This is caused by arterial vasoconstriction of the precapillary sphincter and vasodilatation of the capillaries, forcing the aforementioned arterial-venous anastomoses. Bleeding occurs after injections and/or venipunctures, from incisions, in the mucosa of the mouth, in the respiratory system, in the gastrointestinal system, and in the genitourinary system. It is common for several of these systems to be bleeding simultaneously; rarely is only one system involved.

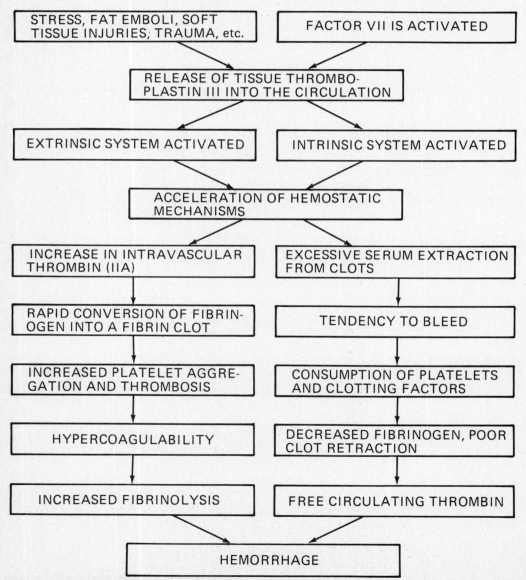

Figure 39-6. DIC alters the coagulation process.

When circulating fibrinogen is completely used up, some circulating thrombin still exists since fibrinogen has not converted it to fibrin. The activation of the clotting process produces thrombin. Thrombin increases clotting which produces more thrombin and fibrin and converts plasminogen to plasmin. Antithrombins (especially antithrombin III) destroys thrombin function. But in DIC, thrombin production exceeds antithrombin III. Thus thrombin promotes uncontrolled coagulation. The initiation of fibrinolysis results in dissolution of clots and degrades fibrin into its fractions which further adds to the bleeding due to their anticoagulation products.

In an attempt to restore hemostasis, the liver produces more fibrinogen or the patient is transfused with blood, plasma, or fibrinogen. This perpetuates the process, making the DIC more severe and intractible.

Pulmonary compromise may require intubation. Following the trend of ABGs and observing for signs and symptoms of hypoxia will show when suctioning and/or mechanical ventilation is needed.

Cardiac status must be monitored for dysrhythmias secondary to acidosis, hypovolemia, hypervolemia, and electrolyte imbalances. Early recognition and treatment of dysrhythmias may prevent progression to more serious dysrhythmias.

Renal problems develop due to fluid overload, fluid depletion, and hypotension. The oliguric or anuric patient cannot eliminate heparin adequately, so the dose must be titrated to match the patients' utilization and excretion of the drug.

Monitor the amount of bleeding and identify the system involved. All drainage should be tested for blood, unless there is a frank, observable bleed.

Watch for signs of thrombus formation. If thrombi develop, the symptoms will vary according to the system involved. The kidneys are most often involved (oliguria or anuria).

Intracranial bleeding may be identified by altered LOC; orientation to person, place, and time; pupil reactions; and extremity movement. These must be checked frequently. Any change will indicate a possible bleed.

Avoid infection. The DIC patient is at high risk for infection primarily due to all the entry ports for bacteria. Development of a fever is an indication to culture blood, urine, sputum, and any other drainage. If the bacteria is identified, appropriate antibiotics are started.

Monitor fluid balance especially if the patient receives multiple blood transfusions and other fluids or has another pre-existing disease.

Skin care to preserve skin integrity is very important. Care must be taken to treat the patient very gently and to maintain good body alignment with adequate support. Sufficient but not excessive pressure is applied to sites of intramuscular injections or venipunctures by laboratory personnel to prevent hematoma formation.

Petechiae are pinpoint flat lesions that appear as reddish purple spots on the skin, buccal mucosa, and conjunctivae. Purpura is characterized by reddish brown spots usually evidencing some fluid presence. Ecchymoses are black and blue bruises.

Psychosocial support is extremely important to decrease the anxiety of the aware patient as he or she is frightened by all the lost blood and the flurry of activity around him or her. Very brief explanations should be given; for example, "I'm giving you some medicine through the vein to help stop your bleeding."

Being honest with the patient's family as well as with the patient will help to decrease anxiety and foster a positive relationship between all parties involved.

TREATMENT OF DIC

The primary treatment of DIC is to treat the underlying disease which is easier said than done in the face of a patient hemorrhaging.

The second treatment is to halt the DIC. This is accomplished by several concurrent actions. It is necessary to replace the clotting factors so the serum is converted back to plasma. At the same time, the effects of thrombin must be stopped. Also at the same time, correction of acidosis, hypotension, hypovolemia, and hypoxia must be attempted since these four conditions act as procoagulants to continue utilization/depletion of clotting factors. Vitamin K (formation of prothrombin) and folic acid (thrombocytopenia) are administered to correct these deficiencies.

The use of heparin remains controversial since it is difficult to assess its effectiveness. Heparin neutralizes free circulating thrombin by combining with antithrombin III which inactivates the thrombin. Heparin functions as an anticoagulant to prevent further thrombus formation in the microcirculatory system. (It does not alter the thrombi already formed.) Heparin *prevents the activation of factor* X. Heparin also inhibits platelet aggregation.

Caution: If used, **heparin should be given intravenously,** *not* subcutaneously. Factors affecting subcutaneous heparin include the absorption rate which is dependent on the amount injected, the depth of injection, body temperature, and cardiovascular status. If a hematoma develops at the injection site, absorption is markedly altered. The amount of heparin needed may be too much for subcutaneous administration. The delay in reaching a therapeutic blood level may be too long with subcutaneous administration. Intravenous heparin overcomes *all* the problems of subcutaneous administration.

After heparin therapy is started, whole blood, fresh frozen plasma, and/or platelet transfusion are administered.

COMPLICATIONS

DIC may become an exsanguinating hemorrhage. Death is not uncommon.

NURSING INTERVENTIONS

Assessment of patients at high risk of DIC include looking for development of petechiae, purpura, and ecchymosis. Oozing of blood from injection sites, I.V. lines, and invasive monitoring lines all may indicate the onset of DIC.

40

Pathologic Hematologic Conditions

Learning Objectives

By the end of this chapter, the nurse will be able to:

1. Identify problems of patients with reduced erythrocytes.
2. Explain the proper position of the patient placed on a hypothermia blanket to treat an uncontrolled fever.
3. Explain why piloerection is to be avoided in using hypothermia blankets.
4. Identify complications that may be related to specific complaints related to leukopenia.
5. List six nursing interventions for the leukopenic patient.
6. Explain the pathophysiology involved in patients with decreased platelets.
7. List five nursing interventions for the patient with decreased platelets.
8. List four complications of bone marrow suppression.
9. List one nursing intervention for each complication of bone marrow suppression.
10. Explain the pathophysiology of Hodgkin's disease.
11. Explain the classification and staging of Hodgkin's disease.
12. Identify the causative factor in Hemophilia A, B, C, von Willebrand's disease, and sickle cell anemia.
13. List the treatment modalities of the aforementioned diseases.
14. Explain nursing interventions appropriate for the patient with Hodgkin's disease.
15. Define the pathophysiology of multiple myeloma.
16. List the clinical presentations of multiple myeloma.
17. Identify treatment and nursing interventions for patients with multiple myeloma.

Pathologic states to be considered in this chapter include decreased erythrocytes, decreased leukocytes, decreased thrombocytes, problems associated with bone marrow suppression, hemophilia, von Willebrand's disorder, sickle cell disease, lymphomas, and multiple myeloma.

Decreased Erythrocytes (Anemia)

A reduction in the number or quality of erythrocytes or excessive destruction of RBCs produces an anemia. Anemia is considered present if the Hgb is less than 10 gm/dl.

ETIOLOGY

Anemia may be the result of intrinsic or extrinsic factors. Intrinsic factors are due to alterations of the cell membrane, the hemoglobin content of the erythrocyte, and/or the enzymes basic to the cell formation. Extrinsic causes of decreased erythrocytes may be due to acquired hemolytic factors including drugs, systemic disease and such, or directly caused by a bleed or frank hemorrhage.

PATHOPHYSIOLOGY

Many body systems are affected by anemia. The respiratory, cardiovascular, and neurologic systems are the most adversely affected by the anemia.

The respiratory rate is increased to increase oxygenation of the RBCs to prevent tissue hypoxia. Increased 2,3-DPG in the RBCs combines with hemoglobin, which decreases its affinity for oxygen. This shifts the oxyhemoglobin dissociation curve to the right facilitating oxygen release to the tissues in an effort to prevent tissue hypoxia. Acid-base imbalances occur frequently.

The cardiovascular system responds to decreased oxygen levels by increasing cardiac output and the cardiac rate. This decreases the time it takes to circulate blood through the body. There is a redistribution of blood from nonessential tissues to areas requiring more oxygen (brain and heart). The neurologic response to decreased levels of oxygen is a hyperpnea and a vasodilatation to allow more blood to circulate through the brain to oxygenate the brain tissue.

CLINICAL PRESENTATION

General symptoms of anemia include fatigue, lassitude, tachypnea, tachycardia, orthostatic hypotension, angina, and sometimes a murmur. Alteration or decrease in LOC ranging from confusion to coma may occur. Symptoms will vary depending upon the type of anemia and the speed with which the decrease in erthrocytes occurs.

TREATMENT

Treating the underlying condition may resolve the anemia. In some instances blood transfusion or blood fractions may be employed.

NURSING INTERVENTIONS

Planning nursing care to provide periods of rest for the patient helps preserve patient stamina for recovery.

Monitoring the patient's respiratory status to ensure adequate ventilation will allow rapid intervention to prevent hypoxemia and tissue hypoxia.

Cardiovascular monitoring is essential since hypoxemia, oxygen saturation of the RBCs, and acid-base abnormalities occur in states of decreased RBCs.

Decreased Leukocytes

Leukopenia results in a greater possibility of infection and complications of infection for the patient.

ETIOLOGY

There are multiple causes of decreased WBCs (leukopenia). All infections including bacterial, viral, rickettsial, protozoal, and overwhelming infection may cause leukopenia. Drugs can induce a leukopenia as can malignant states and several systemic diseases.

PATHOPHYSIOLOGY

Leukopenia may result in a decrease in neutrophils or lymphocytes or both, theoretically. In clinical practice, mild to moderate leukopenia is mainly due to a reduction in neutrophils. Severe leukopenia results in reduction of both neutrophils and lymphocytes.

Neutropenia lowers resistance to infection allowing bacterial invasion of mucous membrane. In severe neutropenia, microorganisms invade the bloodstream, resulting in sepsis.

CLINICAL PRESENTATION

Classic signs of infection include redness, heat (localized), and pus formation which are NOT usually present in leukopenia.

Fever is the classic symptom with sudden high onset, chills, sweating, headache, and muscle pains. Nausea and vomiting may occur.

TREATMENT

A fever pattern should be identified before treatment, *except* when fever is threatening vital function such as the brain (confusion to coma).

After a temperature pattern is identified, treatment may include acetaminophen (Tylenol®) and/or a hypothermia blanket. Aspirin is avoided since it alters platelet aggregation and results in bleeding.

Cultures should be obtained to identify the invading organism and determine specific antibiotic therapy. If one's temperature is too high to wait for culture reports, broad-spectrum antibiotics are used intravenously.

NURSING INTERVENTIONS

Intramuscular injections are contraindicated since each injection could allow bacterial entrance to the body. A central line should be considered to decrease the number of venipunctures and to provide an I.V. route for administration of antibiotics or WBCs. Most antibiotics can be given through the same central line if there is good flushing of the tubing after each drug

is administered in case of incompatibility which would cause precipitation.

If the patient is placed on a hypothermia blanket, the blanket should come only to the shoulders. The head should NEVER be on the blanket. To cool blood going to the head, gloves can be filled with ice and placed against the neck. This effectively cools the blood of the carotid arteries. It is important to prevent shivering, usually accompanied by piloerection. Shivering increases body metabolism generating more heat. This may cause an increased ICP, resulting in an intracranial bleed.

Oral infections, especially *Candida albicans*, occur often with patients who are leukopenic. Inspection of the mouth should be included in mouth care and use of medication if *Candida albicans* is present.

Skin care and meticulous handwashing may prevent other opportunistic bacteria from gaining entrance to the body and starting a secondary infection. Applying lotions to the skin to prevent dryness and cracking also soothes the patient and makes him or her more comfortable. While administering skin care is the opportune time to inspect the patient for areas of redness or blistering which may become decubiti or cellulitis without prompt treatment.

COMPLICATIONS

Impending complications or complication in its early stage tend to be associated with certain complaints. A complaint of a sore throat or chest pain may indicate pneumonia. Complaints of frequency or burning on voiding may indicate a urinary infection. Complaints of being cold and asking for more blankets in a warm environment may indicate a systemic infection. Complaints of rectal pain or pain with defecation may indicate an irritated rectal mucosa or a perianal abcess.

With rectal complaints, the nurse must perform meticulous and frequent perianal care to help prevent the irritated mucosa from becoming further irritated and deteriorated. This precludes the use of rectal thermometers, medications, or enemas. Immediate thorough perianal cleaning is done after each bowel movement.

Decreased Platelet Function

Platelet aggregation is the first primary step towards coagulation. If platelets are decreased or absent, hemorrhage may occur.

HEMORRHAGE

This is the major problem for patients with a decreased platelet level. The most common sites of bleeding occur in the gums, nose, GI tract, bladder, and brain.

TREATMENT

Treatment consists of halting the current bleed while treating the underlying cause. Intravenous replacement of lost volume is an immediate priority. This may include whole blood, packed RBCs, FFP, platelets, plasmanate, and a colloid or crystalloid fluid.

Epistaxis may be life-threatening and so this hemorrhage must be stopped quickly. With the patient in a high-Fowler's position, a nose clip, ice, or packing may be employed to stop the hemorrhage.

NURSING INTERVENTIONS

Once the hemorrhage is controlled, patient education is a major goal.

Mouth care is important since one of the prime sites of bleeding is the gums. A very soft bristle brush (or baby toothbrush) and use of cotton swabs or Water Pics® will clean the gums. Mouth washes should be mild or diluted with water before use.

Maintaining skin integrity is often a major problem. Educating the patient to use an electric razor, instead of a straight razor, to use gloves when washing dishes, to avoid aspirin or aspirin-containing drugs, and to avoid physical games which may result in bruising (backyard football, etc.) will help the patient avoid severe bleeds.

While in the critical care unit, medication should be given I.V. to reduce hematomas. If medication must be given I.M. or S.Q., pressure must be applied to the puncture site for a period of time necessary for blood to clot to prevent hematomas. The same is true for venipuncture sites. As small a needle as possible is used for both injections and venipunctures.

Patients on oxygen therapy must be evaluated often. Nasal prongs may irritate the nasal mucosa. Endotracheal tubes and N/G tubes will also irritate the nasal and oropharyngeal mucosa. Mouth care with glycerine swabs will soothe the buccal cavity mucosa and vaseline may make nasal prongs more tolerable. Some patients, especially mouth breathers, prefer a mask instead of prongs.

Women should be taught to count the pads used during menstruation since this may cause a significant bleed leading to hemorrhage.

Evaluate the patient's sensorium. Changes *may* be the first sign of intracranial bleeding. If the patient is semi-comatose and combative, the use of restraints may need to be considered. However, they might cause bleeding into the tissues at the points of restraint.

Complications of Suppressed Bone Marrow

Bone marrow suppression usually results from radiation and/or chemotherapy.

The complications of bone marrow suppression include a decrease in production of RBCs causing anemia, a decrease in platelets causing bleeding, and a decrease in leukocyte production causing infections.

The radiation and chemotherapy used to suppress the bone marrow also have effects on body systems.

Nausea and vomiting are two very common symptoms and are very difficult to handle. Antiemetics and/or sedation may help relieve the nausea sufficiently for the patient to eat a small bland diet. Soda crackers with coke syrup may relieve the nausea. For some patients, warm or cold ginger ale or lemon/lime soda may help. Experiment to find what will help each patient. Nutritional needs must be assessed to ascertain a positive nitrogen balance. If fluids are necessary, hyperalimentation may be instituted in the absence of neutropenia.

Mouth sores may decrease the patient's appetite simply because it hurts to eat. If the mouth develops sores, it is usually due to *Candida albicans* or stomatitis. Many mouth washes and medications may relieve the *Candida albicans*, whereas a change in diet to eliminate spicy, sour, or acid food may make the patient more comfortable.

Alopecia (loss of hair) is often most emotionally devastating for the patient. Reassurance that the hair loss is temporary and will grow back is not often a help to the patient. Along with reassurance, the nurse can offer toupees, wigs, scarves, and so on to cover the head as the hair grows back.

Hyperuricemia is caused by cell breakdown taking place faster than the kidneys can excrete the by-product, uric acid. If the patient's overall condition and, in particular cardiac status, can tolerate the fluid, fluid should be forced up to 3 liters/day to help prevent renal calculi, along with a diet which will result in an alkaline urine. Allopurinol (Zyloprim®) is a commonly used preventive medication. A skin rash indicates an allergy and the medication should be stopped.

Hemophilia and von Willebrand's Disease

Hemophilia is the name given to three inherited disorders that have bleeding in common. This bleeding is due to a lack of or deficiency in a plasma clotting factor. Von Willebrand's disease is included in this section since it also lacks a clotting factor.

Hemophilia A (the most common) is also known as "classic hemophilia." These people have normal amounts of factor VIII but the factor is *structurally abnormal* and therefore functions differently than normal factor VIII in the intrinsic clotting cascade.

Hemophilia B is also known as Christmas disease (or PTC). It has a factor IX deficiency. It occurs about one-fifth as often as hemophilia A.

Hemophilia C is caused by a deficiency of factor XI. It is transmitted as an autosomal trait so it appears equally between females and males. Some authorities feel hemophilia C occurs more often than hemophilia A. It is simply undiagnosed.

Von Willebrand's disease is an actual lack of factor VIII. The lack of this factor may be total or there may be a reduced amount of *structurally normal factor.*

ETIOLOGY

Hemophilia A and B are sex-linked recessive disorders. They affect men mainly, but rarely a woman has these diseases. It is more common that the female is a "carrier" and transmits these diseases to the male. Hemophilia C is an autosomal trait. All three hemophilias are genetically determined.

PATHOPHYSIOLOGY

Bleeding in hemophilia A occurs in the intrinsic cascade, therefore most hemophilia As bleed into joints, muscles, subcutaneous tissue, and the kidneys (the areas of the body which do not have tissue thromboplastin). The disease is present at birth, but not suspected (if not circumcised) until 3 or 4 months of age. This is the time teeth erupt and the infant may begin crawling and bruising easily whenever he or she falls.

Hemophilia B affects clotting factor IX which is in the intrinsic cascade, so symptoms and treatment are the same for both hemophilia A and B.

Hemophilia C has a deficiency in clotting factor XI and is a much milder bleeding disorder.

Von Willebrand's disease is an autosomal dominant mode of inheritance, so it should occur equally among men and women. However, it occurs more often in women than men. Von Willebrand's disease may have another factor (VWF) that is difficult to separate from factor VIII. Von Willebrand's disease has an effect upon platelet aggregation.

CLINICAL PRESENTATION

Hemarthroses (hemorrhages into joints) are the most common symptoms of both hemophilia A and B. Hemarthroses usually occur after exercise or some form of physical exertion. Spontaneous bleeds may occur in severe hemophiliacs. Hemorrhage may occur in muscle mass forming a hematoma which is extremely painful. These hematomas (masses) press against nerves resulting in transient motor and/or sensory loss. Gastrointestinal bleeding is the next most common symptom. Often there is no evidence of ulceration to account for the bleed. Epistaxis is common.

Joint deformity with eventual crippling may occur. Hematuria is often present in hemophiliacs and may continue for weeks without a known cause.

Hemorrhage into the CNS is rare in hemophiliacs but is extremely severe when it does occur. It is not uncommon for these patients to die subsequent to the hemorrhage (often caused by some trauma).

Hemophiliacs seem to fluctuate in the frequency and severity of the bleed during the year. Hemophiliacs tend to bleed less with age. The reasons for these two variables are unknown at this time. All of these symptoms except hemarthroses occur in von Willebrand's disease also.

DIAGNOSIS

A familial tendency to excessive bleeding is known and the family frequently reports the diagnosis to the physician as "the bleeding disease." The clinical condition can be verified by laboratory tests. The PTT is prolonged. Factor assays reveal decreased factor VIII in hemophilia A and it is variable (from normal to decreased) in von Willebrand's disease. Factor IX is decreased in hemophilia B. Platelet aggregation is normal in hemophilias and decreased in von Willebrand's disease.

TREATMENT

The objective of therapy, which cannot cure the disease, is to prevent crippling deformities and prolong life expectancy. Stopping the bleed and increasing plasma levels of deficient factors during the bleed will help prevent the degenerative stages (destruction of the joints).

In hemophilia A, cryoprecipitated antihemolytic factor, AHF, is administered to raise the factor to 25% of normal which will allow coagulation. Surgery requires increasing the AHF to 50% of normal. If AHF is not available, fresh frozen plasma or plasma fraction, rich in AHF, may be administered.

In hemophilia B, administration of fresh frozen plasma or factor IX will increase the blood level of factor IX.

In von Willebrand's disease, the infusion of cryoprecipitates or blood fractions that are rich in factor VIII (and subsequently VWF) will shorten bleeding time. Prior to surgery or in bleeding states, I.V. infusion of cryoprecipitates or fresh frozen plasma is needed to raise factor VIII level to 50% of the normal.

A patient with hemophilia or von Willebrand's disease needs the care of a hematologist for surgical procedures and dental extraction.

NURSING INTERVENTIONS

During hemophiliac bleeds, administration of the deficient clotting factor or plasma is ordered. AHF is effective from 48 to 72 hours. This means repeat transfusions may be required to stop the bleed.

Apply cold compresses to the injured area, raise the injured area if possible, and cleanse the wound, if one is present. Thrombin-soaked fibrin or sponge may be utilized in some institutions. Restrict activity for 48 hours after the bleeding is controlled to prevent recurrence. Control pain with analgesics such as acetaminophen (Tylenol®), propoxyphene hydrochloride (Darvon®/, Dolene®, Proxagesic®), codeine, or meperidine hydrochloride (Demerol®). Avoid intramuscular injections to prevent a hematoma at the injection site. Aspirin is contraindicated because it affects platelet aggregation. If the patient bleeds into a joint, immediately elevate the joint and immobilize it in slight flexion. Watch for signs of further bleeding such as increased pain and swelling, fever, or possibly shock-like symptoms. Monitor the patient's PTT.

In von Willebrand's disease, monitor the patient's bleeding time for 24–48 hours after surgery and observe for signs of new bleeding. During a new bleed, elevate the injured part and apply cold compresses and gentle pressure to the bleeding site.

Education of the causative factors and treatment of minor injuries is indicated, as well as conditions in which the patient should contact his or her doctor or go to the emergency room for treatment.

Educate the patient and parents (if the patient is a child) in how to control minor trauma and warn against using aspirin or aspirin-containing drugs. Refer the parents to a genetic counseling service.

Psychosocial support should be instituted with referrals to the National Hemophilia Society, local hemophiliac groups, genetic evaluation, psychotherapy for better acceptance of the disease, and an association with other patients managing successfully.

Sickle Cell Disease

Sickle cell disease is also referred to as sickle cell anemia because of the pathophysiology.

ETIOLOGY

This congenital hemolytic anemia occurs most often in blacks and arises from a defective hemoglobin molecule referred to as hemoglobin S.

There is homozygous and heterozygous inheritance. Homozygous inheritance eventually results in the disease since the amino acid valine substitutes for glutamic acid in the B hemoglobin chain.

Heterozygous inheritance results in the person having the sickle cell trait. The trait patient is often asymptomatic.

PATHOPHYSIOLOGY

With abnormal hemoglobin S, the RBCs become insoluble when hypoxia occurs. Because of this, RBCs become rigid, rough, and elongated. The hemoglobin (Figure 40-1) becomes shaped like a crescent or sickle (and thus its name).

Sickling causes hemolysis and the altered cells tend to collect in the capillaries and small vessels. This impairs normal circulation and results in pain, swelling, and tissue infarctions, causing anoxia. This increases blood viscosity causing further impairment of circulating blood. Blockages extend on the capillaries and small vessels leading to further sickling obstruction. A vicious cycle has started.

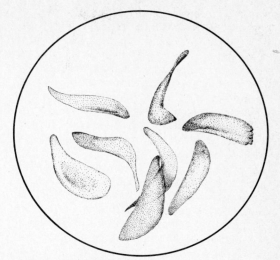

Figure 40-1. Sickle-shaped RBCs.

CLINICAL PRESENTATION

Several types of crises occur but common at some time to all are a tachycardia, cardiomegaly, murmurs, pulmonary infarctions, chronic fatigue, dyspnea (with or without exertion), hepatomegaly, jaundice or pallor, aching bones, chest pain, ischemic leg ulcers, and increased susceptibility to infection. Infection, stress, dehydration, and hypoxic states (strenuous exercise, etc.) may induce a crisis.

The most common crisis is the *painful crisis*. This is a vaso-occlusive or infarctive crisis. It does not usually develop for the first 5 years, but it sporadically appears after that. It is a result of RBCs obstructing blood vessels by rigid, tangled sickle cells. This causes tissue anoxia and possible necrosis. It causes severe thoracic, abdominal, muscular, and bone pain. Jaundice may occur along with dark urine and a low grade fever. After the crisis resolves, infection may occur in from 4 days to several weeks secondary to occlusion and necrosis of the blood vessel.

Autosplenectomy occurs with long-standing disease. Autosplenectomy is the process of splenic damage and scarring, so the spleen shrinks and is no longer palpable. After autosplenectomy, the patient is very susceptible to *Diplococcus pneumonia* which is rapidly fatal without immediate aggressive treatment. Lethargy, sleepiness, fever, and/or apathy occur as signs and symptoms of infection.

Aplastic (megaloblastic) crisis is a result of bone marrow suppression and is often associated with a viral infection. Signs and symptoms include fever, markedly decreased bone marrow activity, pallor, lethargy, dyspnea, possible coma, and RBC hemolysis.

Acute sequestration develops in some children from 8 months to 2 years old. There is a sudden, massive entrapment of RBCs in the liver and spleen. Symptoms of this rare crisis are lethargy and pallor. If not treated, it progresses to hypovolemic shock and death. This is the leading cause of death in sickle cell children under 1 year old.

A hemolytic crisis is rare and usually confined to those who have a glucose-6-phosphate dehydrogenase (G6PD) deficiency. This crisis usually occurs as an infectious response to complications of sickle cell disease rather than to the disease itself.

DIAGNOSIS

A family history and the clinical picture point towards sickle cell disease. A blood smear (Figure 40-2) shows sickle celled RBCs rather than normal RBCs.

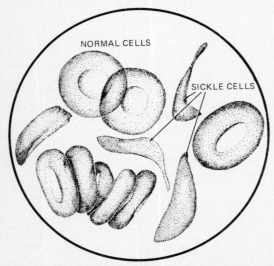

NORMAL CELLS

SICKLE CELLS

Figure 40-2. Comparison between normal and sickle RBCs.

Hemoglobin electrophoresis showing hemoglobin S is pathognomonic.

TREATMENT

Treatment is palliative since no cure and no reversible treatment has been established for this disease. Usually home care will suffice, but in a crisis state, hospitalization is needed.

Treatment of aplastic crisis includes transfusion of packed RBCs, oxygen, and supportive therapies. In sequestration crisis, treatment includes whole blood transfusion, oxygen, and large amounts of oral or I.V. fluids.

NURSING INTERVENTIONS

Supportive care during exacerbations will help avoid such crisis and provide a more normal life. During the crisis, apply *warm* compresses to painful areas and cover the child with a blanket. NEVER use a cold compress which results in vasoconstriction and prolongs the crisis. Encourage bedrest and administer analgesics, antipyretics, and antibiotics as ordered. Patient and family education will help avoid some crises. Such education would include not drinking large amounts of cold fluids, not swimming in cold water, and avoiding clothing that restricts circulation and any activity that would produce hypoxia, such as flying in small (unpressurized) aircraft. A large fluid intake will prevent dehydration and decrease blood viscosity reducing the chance of another crisis. Stress the importance of childhood immunizations and prompt treatment for infections. Emotional, social, and mental development is normal if the parents are not overprotective.

Sickle cell disease makes women poor obstetrical risks, but if pregnancy occurs, such women may benefit from folic acid supplement. Surgery is dangerous only if hypoxia occurs. Usually, one unit of RBCs is given to help prevent hypoxia.

Lymphomas

There are two basic classifications of lymphomas—namely, Hodgkin's disease and non-Hodgkin's lymphoma.

PATHOPHYSIOLOGY

A lymphoma is a proliferation of cells of the lymphoid series which becomes a solid tumor.

Hodgkin's Disease

Hodgkin's disease accounts for one-half of the malignant lymphomas.

DIAGNOSIS

The presence of Reed-Sternberg cells in a biopsy is pathognomonic for Hodgkin's disease. Reed-Sternberg cells are multinucleated with a large nucleolus in the nucleus. It is common to see Reed-Sternberg cells as mirror images of each other.

CLASSIFICATION

It is important to classify and stage Hodgkin's disease to determine prognosis and treatment.

Four major histiocyte (cell morphology) patterns are defined.

1. Lymphocyte predominance
2. Nodular sclerosis
3. Mixed cellularity
4. Lymphocyte depletion

This histiocyte classification is recorded as A, B, C, and D. A is the first and indicates the best prognosis.

STAGING

Staging is designated by a roman numeral. Stage I indicates involvement of the lymph node chain or two contiguous chains on the same side and above the diaphragm. Stage II is the involvement of two noncontiguous lymph node chains above the diaphragm and still on the same side of the body. There may be involvement of one extralymphatic organ also. Stage III involves lymph node or chains above *and* below the diaphragm but contained within the lymphatic system. Stage IV is involvement in the various organs of the body (brain, liver, spleen, etc.), indicating a widespread disease.

An example of classification and staging is IIIB. This patient would have involvement on both sides of the diaphragm, but it would be confined to the lymphatic tissues with mixed cellularity.

CLINICAL PRESENTATION

The presentation symptoms may range from no systemic symptoms (stage IA) to severe cachexia (stage IV).

Typically, a patient in stage IA may not show identifiable lymphadenopathy. But Reed-Sternberg cells appear in the bone marrow aspiration and lymph nodes may be slightly enlarged.

The patients in a B stage have fever, night sweats, and loss of weight. The patients in C and D stages will have palpable lymph nodes throughout the body and nodular infiltration of the liver, spleen, and bones. Other symptoms include progressive anemia (as the bone marrow is infiltrated), edema of the face and neck, possible jaundice due to infiltration of the liver, cachexia, and pain.

TREATMENT

Generally, people with IA, IIA, and IIIB are good candidates for extensive radiation therapy. Patients with IIIB (depending upon the physician), IVA, and IVB are treated with chemotherapy.

Stages IB and IIB generally receive both radiation and chemotherapy. Some patients regardless of staging may receive both chemotherapy and radiation.

An exploratory laparotomy allows visualization and biopsy of retroperitoneal lymph nodes. A splenectomy is usually done for definitive pathologic evidence of disease. A laparotomy also allows radiopaque clips to be placed in the abdomen to become guides for future radiation therapy.

NURSING INTERVENTIONS

Monitoring, supportive, and educational factors are the objectives of nursing interventions.

Monitoring the patient for reactions to treatment is essential. Hyperkalemia can be the result of cytotoxic drugs of the chemotherapy and it may cause cardiac dysrhythmias. Hypercalcemia may develop as the carcinogen cells infiltrate the marrow of various bones. The disease causes bone destruction which occurs faster than the kidneys can excrete the end product, calcium. So a hypercalcemic state exists and it, also, may cause cardiac dysrhythmias.

Supportive care may include administering analgesics, antiemetics, and drugs to reduce fever. With regard to in-patients, bathing (tepid water) should be with a lotion or mild soaps without removing the radiation markings.

Observe the patient closely for side effects and complications. "Normal" side effects include anorexia, nausea, vomiting, diarrhea/constipation, and of course, continual changes in the hematologic picture.

COMPLICATIONS

In addition to the "normal" side effects, intestinal obstruction and desquamation of radiated skin may occur. Fatigue of the patient necessitates pacing nursing procedures to allow the patient some rest periods.

It would be helpful to educate the patient and family, with the help of a dietitian, to decide upon small, palatable meals to avoid a negative nitrogen balance. Refer the patient to the local American Cancer Society for future support.

Non-Hodgkin's Disease

These lymphomas are due to an uncontrolled proliferation of lymphatic cells. They include Burkitt's tumor, reticulum cells (sarcoma), and lymphosarcoma.

ETIOLOGY

The cause is unknown but suspected to be viral with racial/ethnic connection since Caucasians and Jewish descendents have this disease more than other groups. It is 2–3 times more frequent in males than in females. The incidence rises with increasing age and is most predominant at or after 50 years old.

DIAGNOSIS

In an exploratory laparotomy, lymph nodes, bone marrow, liver, and any suspicious tissue are taken for biopsy. Other tests used to differentiate Hodgkin's disease from non-Hodgkin's lymphoma include liver and spleen scan, CT scan of the abdomen, IVP, and chest and bone x-rays.

STAGING

Staging follows the same general classification of Hodgkin's disease differing in that these lymphomas may involve an organ; it it not restricted even in stages I, II, and III, to simply lymph node or lymphatic tissue.

CLINICAL PRESENTATION

This is essentially the same as in Hodgkin's disease.

TREATMENT

Radiation is used in stages I and II. In stage III both radiation and chemotherapy are used. Chemotherapy is used in stage IV.

NURSING INTERVENTIONS

These are essentially the same as for patients with Hodgkin's disease.

COMPLICATIONS

These are essentially those described earlier for Hodgkin's disease.

Multiple Myeloma

As indicated by its name, this condition has widely disseminated tumors of immature plasma cells. These tumors occur as neoplasms of red bone marrow initially, but gradually spread producing osteolytic lesions throughout the skeleton.

ETIOLOGY

No causative factors are known at this time. However, the disease mainly attacks men 50 to 70 years old.

DIAGNOSIS

A triad of symptoms are pathognomonic for multiple myeloma, namely, lytic bone lesions (or diffuse osteoporosis), plasma cells in a bone marrow study, and gammaglobulin abnormalities.

Other laboratory tests may show slight abnormalities. The CBC differential will have 40–50% lymphocytes, but rarely more than 3% plasma cells. An elevated red cell rate (ESR) is usual. Urine may show a positive Bence Jones protein (albumin in the urine) and hypercalciuria. Bence Jones protein, if positive, confirms the disease.

Bone marrow studies show an abnormal number of plasma cells in the marrow. Serum electrophoresis will reveal an abnormal globulin spike indicating an abnormal electrophoresis but also an immunological abnormality. X-rays show osteoporosis.

PATHOPHYSIOLOGY

Immature plasma cells infiltrate the flat bones initially (vertebrae, skull, ribs, and pelvis) and continue their infiltration until all bones are involved. This massive bone involvement often results in collapse of the vertebrae causing pressure on spinal nerves and varied symptomology depending upon which vertebrae collapse. The plasma cells are sometimes known as M proteins and they produce abnormal immunoglobulins. This results in a reduced body protection against antigens. As the multiple myelomas progress, they infiltrate body organs: liver, spleen, lymph nodes, lungs, adrenal glands, kidneys, and the G.I. tract. With this infiltration, the kidneys cannot excrete uric acid and calcium to prevent hyperuricemia and hypercalcemia leading to renal obstruction followed by renal failure.

A positive Bence Jones urine is a reliable but not conclusive test since it rarely, if ever, is found in other conditions and very often found in multiple myelomas.

CLINICAL PRESENTATION

From looking at the pathophysiology, one would safely identify bone pain—usually severe and constant back pain, arthritic aching, swelling, tenderness, and the symptoms of collapsed vertebrae.

Other signs and symptoms include fever, malaise, parathesias, and pathologic fractures (fractures occurring without physiologic stress or trauma).

As the disease advances, vertebral compression may become acute. There is an associated anemia, thoracic deformities (a ballooning effect), and loss of body heighth secondary to multiple vertebral compressions.

Renal compromise or failure occurs due to the protein (Bence Jones) causing a pyelonephritis caused by damage to the tubules.

Infections occur since bone marrow infiltration by plasma cells decrease the normal blood elements.

Severe, recurrent, inexplicable infections occur with a resultant neuropathy. An example is a URI (such as pneumonia) with permanent weakness to the respiratory muscles.

TREATMENT

Prognosis is poor since symptoms do not occur until wide-spread dissemination has occurred. After diagnosis without treatment, survival is 2–3 months once symptoms occur. Long-term treatment using a combination of selective radiation and alternating cyclic chemotherapy with steroids provides 90% remission for up to 2 years. Three percent may survive up to 5 years.

NURSING INTERVENTIONS

Most nursing interventions are aimed at reducing or postponing the complications of multiple myeloma.

Force fluids up to 3,000–4,000 cc/24 hours to prevent renal infection, hyperuricemia, and hypercalcemia. This helps avoid precipitation of uric acid, calcium, and Bence Jones protein. Maintain *accurate* I and 0 records.

Diet changes may need alteration to lower intake of protein and calcium.

Encourage ambulation with a walker with the nurse at the patient's side. If the pain is severe, analgesics may be given 20–30 minutes before walking. Ambulation decreases the chances of URI and avoids the increasing demineralization of bone. Aspirin is often more helpful than narcotics in relieving bone pain. Allopurinol (Zyloprim®) is given for hyperuricemia. Steroids may be used with cytotoxic drugs when chemotherapy is administered. Assess closely for infection since steroids mask them.

If the patient requires a laminectomy, try to get the patient out of bed after 24 hours, if possible. Check for bleeding, hypesthesias, and paresthesia. Return the patient to bed and place him or her in the ordered position, log rolling when turning.

A great deal of emotional support for the patient and family is needed. The family may be very anxious and two things will help the patient and family: (1) Anxiety is reduced if all procedures, especially painful ones, are explained prior to the test and (2) the family is allowed to help as much as they and the patient are able to tolerate during his or her routine care.

41

Anemias and Leukemias

Learning Objectives

By the end of this chapter, the nurse will be able to:

1. Define anemia and explain its pathophysiology.
2. Identify the three types of decreased erythrocyte production.
3. List at least two symptoms of anemia in every body system.
4. Identify the major complications of anemia.
5. Explain the treatments and nursing interventions for patients with anemia.
6. List the four major types of leukemia.
7. Explain the pathophysiology of acute and chronic lymphoblastic leukemia.
8. Explain the pathophysiology of acute and chronic granulocytic leukemia.
9. List four suspected etiologies of leukemia.
10. Briefly explain the clinical presentation of acute lymphoblastic leukemia, lymphocytic leukemia, and granulocytic leukemia.
11. List the complications of each aforementioned leukemia.
12. Explain the complications of chemotherapy.
13. Explain the complications of radiation therapy.
14. Identify nursing interventions in both chemotherapy and radiation therapy.

Anemias are frequently treated in critical care units as a primary symptom of an underlying disease.

Classification of Anemia

Anemias are classified according to pathology, morphology, and etiology. The etiology most usually includes the pathology and the morphology.

ETIOLOGY

There are three major groups or classifica-

tions each having two or more subgroups.

1. Blood loss includes acute posthemorrhage anemia and chronic posthemorrhage anemia.

2. Impaired red cell formation includes the disturbances of bone marrow function as a result of some essential element for erythropoiesis. This would include iron deficiency, activated vitamin D or folate, defective enzymes (pyruvate kinase and G6PD), protein malnutrition,

and scurvy. Impaired red blood cell formation includes causes not due to an essential nutrient deficiency. These include infection, renal failure, drugs, extracorporeal circulation, collagen disease, myxedema, hypopituitarism, and bone marrow infiltration (leukemia, lymphoma, multiple myeloma).

3. Increased red cell destruction, commonly referred to as hemolytic anemias, may be corpuscular defects or abnormal hemolytic mechanisms (extracorpuscular).

PATHOPHYSIOLOGY

The basic factor, regardless of cause, is insufficient oxygen-carrying capacity of the blood. This may be due to reduced numbers of RBCs or abnormal structure of RBCs. This results in tissue hypoxia with specific compensatory mechanisms. These mechanisms usually include tachycardia to circulate the blood more rapidly (causing increased workload on the heart). Vasoconstriction of nonessential vasculature (extremities, gut, and such) shifts the blood to more essential organs (the brain and heart). An increased production of erythropoietin is caused by the hypoxic kidneys. Within 3–5 days, there is an increase in circulating RBCs, but not necessarily normal RBCs, depending upon the cause of the anemia. Hypoxia shifts the oxyhemoglobin curve to the right to release as much oxygen to the tissues as possible. Increased 2,3-DPG also shifts the oxyhemoglobin curve to the right aiding in oxygen release at the tissue level.

CLINICAL PRESENTATION

The signs and symptoms depend upon the cause of the anemia. A common triad of symptoms are pallor, easy fatigability, and generalized muscular weakness. Pallor is best judged by the conjunctiva of the lower eyelid. It is also judged in the nailbeds, the skin, and mucous membrane of the mouth. With a severe bleed, the skin is dead white (in a Caucasian). In acute anemia, there may be an ashen tint to the skin. In advanced pernicious anemia, the skin may have a lemon-yellow tint.

Cardiovascular symptoms may include dyspnea on exertion, "palpitations," angina (due to myocardial ischemia), heart murmur (most often soft midsystolic murmurs), and systolic bruits over the carotid arteries. In severe anemia, a high output state may develop and is characterized by an increase in jugular venous pressure (JVD), peripheral vasodilatation, warm and flushed skin, and a high pulse pressure with a collapsing pulse. Congestive heart failure may occur in patients who have borderline cardiac disease. But severe anemia may cause CHF in patients with no prior evidence of cardiac disease. Edema may occur as a result of capillary permeability. EKG changes occurring with severe anemia (< 6 gm/dl) are abnormal QRS complexes, depressed S-T segments, and a flattening or inversion of T waves. These changes disappear with correction of the anemia.

Renal symptoms include a slight proteinuria and decreased ability to concentrate urine. In patients with renal dysfunction, nitrogen is retained, increasing the BUN.

Central nervous system involvement is common in severe anemia. Symptoms include faintness, headache, tinnitus, roaring or banging in the ears, seeing "spots," drowsiness, lack of concentration and decreased LOC. If alert, the patient may complain of paresthesias of the hands and feet.

Gastrointestinal symptoms include anorexia, nausea, and constipation. Weight loss is *not* a common symptom of uncomplicated anemia. Hematochezia may occur.

Reproductive symptoms in women may include amenorrhea or menorrhagia. Loss of libido is the predominant male symptom.

The skeletal system symptoms are predominantly joint and bone pain. The sternum seems especially tender and may be the site for a bone marrow study (instead of the posterior iliac crest).

RED CELL INDICES

The hemoglobin and hematocrit are decreased (as is the RBC count). Mean cell volume (MCV), mean corpuscular hemoglobin (MCH), and mean cell hemoglobin concentration (MCHC) are the commonly used RBC indices.

Mean cell volume (MCV) represents the *average volume* of RBCs. MCH is the *average weight* of Hgb contained within each RBC. MCHC represents the *average concentration* of Hgb contained in each RBC. Red cell indices are useful in diagnosing specific types of anemia. Red cell indices may also indicate or contraindicate a bone marrow test.

COMPLICATIONS OF ANEMIA

Correct diagnosis of etiology of the anemia is essential for proper treatment and is often difficult. Tissue hypoxia may place compensatory mechanisms on the body inducing further physical stress and possible death. The mechanisms most often include the cardiovascular, neurologic, and renal systems. Anemia may result in susceptibility to infection and/or hemorrhage, both of which may be fatal.

NURSING INTERVENTIONS

Since many anemias are due to an irreversible etiology, they must be considered chronic and often progressive. Nursing support is of paramount importance psychologically.

Nursing care consists of evaluation, assessment, intervention, and evaluation of treatment in each body system: pulmonary, cardiovascular, neurologic, renal, G.I., and integumentary. Actual procedures depend upon the type of anemia and the aggressiveness of the therapy. Nursing procedures will be modified according to the underlying cause and the relevant nursing standards of critical care nursing.

Leukemias

Leukemia may be defined as a malignant neoplasm affecting the entire reticuloendothelial system including the bone marrow, lymph system, and spleen.

Leukemias are not often a cause for admission to a critical care unit unless there is a life-threatening situation (infection or bleeding) during remission or unless very aggressive and extensive treatment is planned.

Basically, there are four classifications of leukemia—two acute and two chronic forms. Although each type differs in its clinical presentation and progression, some generalizations regarding all leukemias can be determined.

CELL DIVISION

Neoplasm may be defined as a mass of uncontrolled progressive proliferation of cells ignoring normal hemostatic mechanisms. Some cells, such as neurons, are not usually capable of mitosis (division) at the time of birth. The mass of neurons increases mainly by elongation rather than by mitosis. Other cells, such as bone, divide continuously until adulthood (or maximum normal growth is obtained). During adulthood, some cells do not normally divide but will become capable of mitosis under specific conditions. (If the liver is damaged and a portion is removed, the remaining cells assume the earlier characteristics of mitosis and will replace the lost tissue.) Some cells maintain the ability to divide (epithelial cells, RBCs, WBCs), whereas others do not maintain this function (neurons) and are not replaced after injury or death.

For mitosis to occur, specific cells must "receive" specific RNA and DNA during the maturation stages. The differentiation may be one of four types:

1. Hypertrophy is an increase in the size of the cells NOT the number of cells. For example, hypertrophy occurs in muscle tissue with exercise and in the uterus during a pregnancy.

2. Hyperplasia is an increase in the number of normal cells in a normal arrangement of the affected tissue. Hyperplasia may be compensatory or pathological. A compensatory hyperplasia occurs when one kidney is removed and the other enlarges to maintain functional activity. Pathological hyperplasia is often due to hormonal excesses such as hyperthyroidism secondary to excessive amounts of TSH.

3. Metaplasia is the replacement of one type of fully differentiated cells by another type of fully differentiated cells not normally occurring in the area of replacement. Mucus-secreting columnar epithelium in the gallbladder may be replaced by stratified squamous epithelium when gallstones are present. This is an adaptive, protective metaplasia secondary to irritation from the gallstones.

4. Dysplasia is an alteration in the size, shape, and organization of differentiated cells. In normal stratified squamous epithelium, mitosis occurs in the basement membrane and matures as the cell reaches the surface layer. Dysplastic stratified squamous epithelium has mitosis occurring in all levels, so at the surface there is a disorganized, varied maturation of cells. Dysplasia often occurs in the respiratory system in smokers. Most often the dysplasia will disappear when the irritant is removed. However, some dysplasias become neoplasms. Neoplasms may be benign or malignant. Neoplasms of the hematopoietic tissue are leukemias. Abnormal proliferation of cells produced by the red bone marrow is called granulocytic, myelocytic, or myelogenous leukemia. Abnormal proliferation in the lymphoid tissue is lymphocytic, lymphatic, or lymphogenous leukemia. Abnormal proliferation of immature lymphocyte precursors is termed lymphoblastic leukemia.

COMMONALITIES OF LEUKEMIA

In acute leukemias, the bone marrow produces leukemic cells almost totally, to the exclusion of normal cell production.

Historically 100% fatal, some leukemias now appear to be cured, whereas others appear to be in a remission state.

Leukemic cells have morphological abnormalities. These abnormalities are both metabolic and maturational changes. In some cases, cell differentiation is completely halted. Future leukemic cells will continue both the metabolic changes and differentiation of the leukemic cell.

Hormonal effects appear to have both stimulator and inhibitor factors influencing leukemic development. Research continues in this area.

Leukemic cells appear to prefer metastasizing through the lymph system.

Leukemic cells are so undifferentiated that on occasion, a specific type of leukemia cannot be determined, especially in acute leukemias. These leukemias are grouped as "blast" type leukemias. In chronic leukemia, the leukemic cells have matured beyond the blast stage and are thus more capable of identification and differentiation.

ETIOLOGY

For most forms of leukemia, a specific carcinogen cannot be identified, and more than one carcinogenic agent may be involved in each type of leukemia.

Suspected etiologic factors include viruses and viral components, chromosomal abnormalities, ionizing radiation (even in small doses), a congenital factor, hormonal and immunological factors, and ingestion of carcinogenic additives in foods.

COMMON COMPLICATIONS OF LEUKEMIA

Most, if not all, leukemias may include organ enlargement as the organ is infiltrated by leukemic cells, such as hepatomegaly, splenomegaly, and lymphadenopathy. Bleeding occurs when the leukemic cells invade the bone marrow, prohibiting normal function (platelets not produced and a cytopenia develops). The kidneys fail to function at their proper (healthy) level due to leukemic cell invasion.

Neurological invasion causes a variety of problems including stroke, intracerebral hemorrhage, and vision problems if the infiltrate impinges upon the optic nerve system. Meningeal infiltration results in increased ICP, headache, papilledema, meningismus, and vomiting. Spinal cord compression leading to paraplegia may occur. Meningeal infiltration (meningeal leukemia) has commonly occurred in children. With more effective treatment prolonging life, it is seen more and more in adults.

Normal erythropoieses cannot be maintained as the bone is invaded. Lack of normal cell production and release results in bleeding, anemia, hemorrhage, fever, and infection (due to neutropenia or leukopenia).

Leukemic cells invade surrounding tissues utilizing the metabolic elements in the tissues. The proliferation of certain leukemic cells is so rapid that the body is depleted of vital nutrients and marked weight loss occurs. The rapidness of leukemic growth may lead to death. Utilization of the body metabolytes leads to electrolyte disturbances, especially calcium. Demineralization of bones occurs in response to granulocytic infiltration of the bone. This produces a hypercalcemic state. Hyperuricemia occurs for two reasons: the increased metabolism of cells from too rapid a proliferation using the body's nutrients, and an accumulation of cellular waste products and dead cells from effective therapy. The hyperuricemia may affect renal function leading to renal failure.

Chronic Lymphocytic Leukemia (CLL)

This leukemia proliferates in lymphoid tissue, blood, and bone marrow causing an increase of abnormal B-lymphocytes. Humoral immunity (antibodies-immunoglobulins) is affected adversely and infections occur.

CLINICAL PRESENTATION

Chronic lymphocytic leukemia (CLL) may start insidiously with no symptoms until the patient sees a physician for another reason, for example, a routine physical or easy fatigue, exertional dyspnea, and weakness. Swollen lymph glands, especially the cervical ones, and the development of lacrimal and salivary gland dysfunction are often the reasons for seeking medical treatment. Cough, hoarseness, or dyspnea may indicate mediastinal node involvement. Intra-abdominal lymph node involvement produces abdominal and gastrointestinal complaints. Generalized skin involvement may include pruritus, macular/papular lesions, herpes zoster, or hyperpigmentation. CLL occurs 2½ times more often in males than in females and the average age at onset is between 50 and 70 years old.

There is lymph node swelling and splenomegaly in the majority of patients.

DIAGNOSIS

Laboratory data are frequently diagnostic. Thrombocytopenia causes gums to bleed, easy bruising, and petechiae. If severe, gastrointestinal bleeding may occur. There is an increase in total leukocyte count and an absolute increase in the number of small lymphocytes. Leukocyte count often ranges from 200,000–400,000/mm^3. It is *rarely* under 15,000/mm^3.

Bone marrow studies differ according to the stage of the disease. In early CLL, at least 20% of the marrow is infiltrated. Throughout the course of CLL, 40% of the bone marrow is infiltrated. In the last stages of CLL, the bone marrow appears packed with small lymphocytes.

TREATMENT

CLL patients seem to live well with this disease, so concomitant illnesses are treated. Infection appears quite commonly.

Splenectomy is used, especially with hemolytic anemia and thrombocytopenia. The results are unpredictable and, if good, are of short duration.

Adrenocorticoid steroids are beneficial if hemorrhage or hemolytic anemia develops.

Radiation and chemotherapy are unpredictable in patient response, with some having a sustained remission and others having no response to therapy.

NURSING INTERVENTIONS

Primary nursing care must be designed to relieve the patient's symptoms and prevent infection.

Maintaining skin integrity to prevent opportunistic microorganisms from gaining entry is essential. Cleaning with mild soap and frequent soaking in the tub is often ordered. Assess for signs of infection—chills, fever, erythema, or swelling of any body part. Frequent gentle massages with body lotion will both help the skin's integrity and comfort the patient.

Observing for complications secondary to thrombocytopenia such as melena, bleeding gums, easy bruising, and anemia is necessary. Dizziness, weakness, and palpitations may also occur.

Patient should be educated to avoid aspirin and aspirin-containing products. Explanation of chemotherapy and/or radiation and their expected side effects are important to stress along with ideas of coping with the side effects. Exploring dietary changes to provide high protein food and high calorie beverages will increase the patient's stamina and sense of well-being.

The patient and his or her family need to be educated to identify symptomatology that should be reported to one's physician. Emotional support for the patient and family will help decrease stress and fear.

Chronic Granulocytic Leukemia (CGL)

Chronic granulocytic leukemia (CGL) is also referred to as chronic myelogenous leukemia (CML). This form of leukemia is found in all races and in both sexes primarily in middle age. It is characterized by excessive production of granulocytes to the exclusion of other cell production, both WBCs and RBCs. Neoplastic granulocytes are found in significant numbers in circulating blood. The more mature cells outnumber the immature cells in peripheral blood, although all stages of maturity are seen in the red bone marrow.

CLINICAL PRESENTATION

Frequently, CGL is found during routine examinations. If not, the patient usually sees a physician 8–9 months after symptoms have started.

The most common initial symptom is pain or discomfort in the left upper quadrant or upper abdomen. Sometimes the patient finds a mass while bathing or showering. There is often a weight loss, fever, and night sweats. Aching in the back and extremities or a pleuritic type of pain in the left upper quadrant of the abdomen and lower portion of the left chest may be the first symptoms for some patients. For others, skin lesions or the occurrence of hemorrhage are first signs.

DIAGNOSIS

The primary finding in CGL on physical examination is splenomegaly. Approximately 90% of the patients have the Philadelphia chromosome (an abnormality of chromosome 22), which appears only in CGL. The cause of the abnormality is unknown. Laboratory tests reveal leukocytosis with leukocytes ranging from 50,000/mm^3 to 250,000/mm^3. Occasionally, a leukopenia (leukocytes < 5,000/mm^3) and neutropenia (neutrophils < 1,500/mm^3) occur in the presence of a high leukocyte count due to an increase in circulating myeloblasts. Serum uric acid may be > 8 mg. Bone marrow is hypercellular with an infiltration of myeloid elements. In an acute state, there is a marked prevalence of myeloblasts.

TREATMENT

Vigorous treatment with chemotherapy is needed in the acute stage. In remissions, the chronic state may be maintained with low doses of chemotherapy.

Ancillary treatment includes splenic radiation, leukopheresis, and allopurinol to prevent hyperuricemia. Splenectomy is controversial.

NURSING INTERVENTIONS

In the face of a chronic state and persistent anemia, nursing care is planned to avoid exhaustion.

Small frequent meals will decrease abdominal discomfort. It is important to prevent constipation with the use of a stool softener as needed. Patient and family education in ways to live with CGL includes advice such as using a soft toothbrush to prevent gum bleeding, using an electric razor instead of a regular razor which might cause bleeding, etc. To prevent hypoxia and atelectasis, stress the need to cough and do deep-breathing exercises on a regular basis.

After the onset of the acute stage, CGL is rapidly fatal regardless of treatment. In this instance, emotional and psychological support with palliative treatment is indicated until death occurs.

Acute Lymphoblastic Leukemia (ALL)

Although acute lymphoblastic leukemia (ALL) is the most severe of the acute leukemias, remission can be achieved in 90% of the children and 40–65% of the affected adults. Remission may last an average of 5 years in children and 1–2 years in adults. Acute leukemia occurs in males more than females, in Caucasians (especially those of the Jewish descent), and in children more than adults. Statistically, acute leukemias occur more often in urban and industrial areas.

As immature cells are released into the circulating blood, they infiltrate other tissues and organs. Invading lymphocytes cause decreased organ function or hemorrhage.

CLINICAL PRESENTATION

Signs may occur insidiously or in a sudden acute onset.

Sudden onset may include a high fever, thrombocytopenia, abnormal bleeding, easy bruising, petechiae, epistaxis, gingival bleeding, purpura, and excessively heavy and lengthy menstrual periods.

Insidiously, signs and symptoms include general symptoms such as low-grade fever, lassitude, weakness, pallor, chills, and recurrent infection.

ALL may cause dyspnea, anemia, tachycardia, palpitations, and abdominal or bone pain.

DIAGNOSIS

Blood counts reveal a thrombocytopenia and neutropenia. Bone marrow study reveals a proliferation of immature WBCs. Lumbar puncture may indicate meningeal involvement indicating that leukemic cells have crossed the blood-brain barrier, thus avoiding the effects of systemic chemotherapy.

TREATMENT

The aim of therapy is to induce remission and restore normal bone marrow functions. Remission may last for up to 5 years in children and 1 year in adults. Vencristine sulfate, prednisone, or both with intrathecal injection of methotrexate or cytarabine is the most common chemotherapy. Bone marrow transplants are being tried.

NURSING INTERVENTIONS

Attempt to maintain the patient's comfort while trying to minimize the side effects of chemotherapy. Maintain patency of veins for future therapy use. Assess patient for signs of meningeal leukemia which includes alteration in LOC, confusion, and headache. Attempt to prevent hyperuricemia by forcing fluids to 2,000 cc daily and administer medication as ordered. Urine pH should be kept above 7.5. Acetazolamide (Diamox®), $NaHCO_3$, and allopurinol (Zyloprim®) are often used. Observe for early signs of cardiotoxicity such as dysrhythmias and CHF.

Protect the patient from infection, if possible. Reverse isolation may be used, but its efficacy in preventing infection is controversial. Avoid Foley catheters and intramuscular or subcutaneous injections. All three of these provide entry ports for microorganisms. Protect the patient's skin by keeping the skin clean and dry, especially the perianal region. Mild lotions or cream may help guard against dry and cracking skin.

Palliative treatment for side effects of the chemotherapy will help make treatment more tolerable. Psychological support of the patient and family is imperative.

Patient and family education of the disease—its terminology, treatment, and side effects—is important. Included in this education are indicators of infection and signs of abnormal bleeding and how to control it. Factors involved in good nutrition and foods that are tolerable in the face of anorexia and nausea must be explored. The objective is high-calorie, high-protein beverages and food. Weight gain from steroid use must be explained and the diet altered as necessary. The dietitian may help the patient and family to plan an appropriate diet.

Physical therapy can help the patient with a reasonable rehabilitation program to use in periods of remission.

COMPLICATIONS

These are usually the sequelae of chemotherapy. They include increasing the chance of an intracerebral bleed, especially with decreased platelets and they often are fatal. Thromboembolic problems may occur with very high WBC levels.

Recurrence inevitably occurs in adults (unless the patient dies from other causes, e.g., a multiple-trauma vehicular accident and such). The reproductive organs and the CNS often harbor leukemic cells which ultimately become active, ending remission and starting an acute phase of the disease.

Acute Granuloblastic Leukemia (AGL)

This form of acute leukemia is also known as acute myeloblastic leukemia (AML). In AGL, there is a hyperplasia of the bone marrow and spleen secondary to uncontrolled formation and release of myeloblasts (precursors to the granulocytes). Remission is much more difficult to achieve than in ALL (acute lymphocytic leukemia).

CLINICAL PRESENTATION

If AGL is going to develop, it usually does so in children and young adults (ages 20–25). After age 25, AGL does not differ greatly from non-lymphoblastic leukemia and must be treated accordingly. Adults (ages 20–25) have a high occurrence of meningeal leukemia without prophylatic therapy.

Signs and symptoms of AGL include the symptoms for both acute and insidious development of acute lymphoblastic leukemia (ALL).

TREATMENT

The objective of treatment is to induce remission by the use of system chemotherapy to restore normal bone marrow function. It is common to use a combination of drugs.

NURSING INTERVENTIONS

Meticulous nursing care encompasses all procedures and areas covered under nursing interventions in ALL, discussed earlier in this chapter.

Hematologic Bibliography

Borg N, Mikas DL, Stark J, Williams SM (eds): Core Curriculum for Critical Care Nursing, 2nd ed. American Association of Critical-Care Nurses. Philadelphia: W. B. Saunders, pp. 346–392, 1981

Brown BA: Hematology: Principles and Procedures. Philadelphia: Lea & Febiger, pp. 23–74, 1973

*Chapman RG, Saiki JH, Nosanchuk JS: Hematologic problems. In Freidman HH (ed): Problem-Oriented Medical Diagnosis, 2nd ed. Boston, MA: Little, Brown and Co., pp. 182–212, 1979

*deGruchy GC, Penington D, Rush B, Castaldi P (eds): Clinical Haematology in Medical Practice, 4th ed. Osney Mead, Oxford, England: Blackwell Scientific Publications, 1978

*Guyton AC: Textbook of Medical Physiology, 6th ed. Philadelphia: W. B. Saunders, pp. 56–102, 1981

*Hematology, hemostasis, immunohematology, and immune responses. In Diagnostics (patient preparation, interpretation, sources of error, post-test care). Nursing 82 books, The nurse's reference library. Springhouse, PA: Intermed Communications, Inc., 1982

Hudak CM, Lohr TS, Gallo BM (eds): Disseminated intravascular coagulation syndrome. In Critical Care Nursing, 3rd ed. Philadelphia: J. B. Lippincott, pp. 409–419, 1982

Kinney MR, Dear CB, Packa DR, Voorman DMN (eds): Hematopoietic disorders. *In* AACN's Clinical Reference for Critical Care Nursing. New York: McGraw-Hill, pp. 579–596, 1981

Leavell BS, Thorup OA: Fundamentals of Clinical Hematology, 2nd ed. Philadelphia: W. B. Saunders, 1968

Muir BL: Infectious agents; and Host-microbe interactions; and Mechanisms of inducible host resistance. *In* Pathophysiology: An Introduction to the Mechanisms of Disease. New York: John Wiley and Sons, pp. 493–566, 1980

Wallner SF: Hematology and oncology. *In* Reller LB, Sahn SA, Schrier RW (eds): Clinical Internal Medicine. Boston, MA: Little, Brown and Co., pp. 241–268, 1979

VII

The Gastrointestinal System

42

Anatomy of the Gastrointestinal System and the Accessory Digestive Organs

---

Learning Objectives

By the end of this chapter, the nurse will be able to:

1. Identify the major components of the gastrointestinal system.
2. Describe and explain the function of the esophagus and the two esophageal sphincters.
3. List and explain the three cellular layers common to digestive organs.
4. List the three divisions of the stomach and two openings of the stomach.
5. Identify and explain the two flexures and three sphincters of the colon.
6. Identify three major arteries of the gastrointestinal tract system and list the structures vascularized by each.
7. Explain the portal vein system.
8. Describe both the intrinsic and extrinsic innervation of the intestines.
9. Identify the main pancreatic duct and the location of the ampulla of Vater.
10. List the regulatory factors of pancreatic secretions.
11. List the components of the biliary system.
12. Identify the component parts of the common bile duct.
13. Describe the innervation and vascularization of the gallbladder.
14. Describe the gross structure of the liver.
15. Describe the hepatic lobule.
16. Explain the blood supply of the liver.

The gastrointestinal tract is sometimes referred to as the alimentary tract. It begins with the mouth and terminates with the anus (Figure 42-1). Structures of the tract include, in descending order, the mouth, esophagus, stomach, small intestine, large intestine, rectum, and anus. The salivary glands, liver, gallbladder, and pancreas are known as accessory digestive organs.

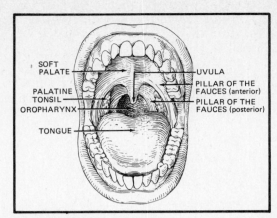

Figure 42-2. The oral cavity.

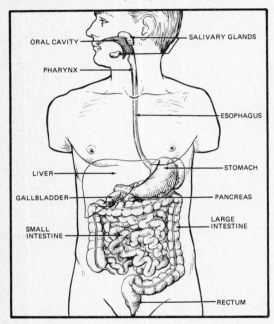

Figure 42-1. The digestive system.

The Mouth

The mouth is commonly referred to as the oral cavity and less commonly as the buccal cavity.

THE ORAL CAVITY

The oral cavity or mouth is composed of all that we can see and feel including lips, cheeks, teeth, gums, tongue, and palate (Figure 42-2), plus the salivary glands.

THE TONGUE

The tongue is a mass of striated and skeletal muscles that is covered by a mucous membrane. (This mucous membrane covers the interior of the entire alimentary tract

lumen.) The surface of the tongue and its side edges are covered with rough elevations called papillae (Figure 42-3). The papillae contain the taste buds. On the undersurface of the tongue in the midline is a fold of mucous membrane called the frenulum (or frenum). The frenulum attaches the tongue to the floor of the mouth.

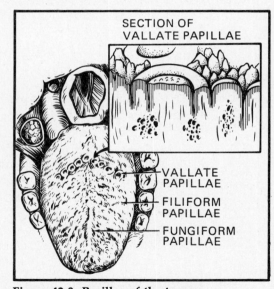

Figure 42-3. Papillae of the tongue.

THE PHARYNX

The pharynx connects the mouth to the esophagus. The pharyngeal walls are composed of longitudinal and circular striated muscle fibers that surround the fibrous tissues helping deglutition (swallowing). The pharynx is divided into three sections.

1. The nasopharynx extends from the nasal cavity to the soft palate. There are swallowing receptors surrounding the opening of the pharynx to stimulate deglutition.

2. The oropharyngeal walls are pulled towards each other from the soft palate to the hyoid bone. This produces a small passage that only well masticated food can enter.

3. The laryngeal pharynx extends from the hyoid bone to the esophagus per se which provides for the epiglottis to cover the trachea during deglutition.

The Esophagus

The esophagus is a 10 to 12 inch long tube located posterior to the trachea and is capable of altering its own lumen size. The first one-third of the esophagus is striated muscle; the last two-thirds, smooth muscle. When food is pushed from the pharynx through the hypopharyngeal sphincter into the esophagus, the pressure of the pushing continues throughout the length of the esophagus and is known as peristaltic waves controlled by vagal response. These peristaltic waves move the food bolus down the esophagus, through the gastroesophageal sphincter, and into the stomach.

The anterior esophageal wall is contiguous with the fibroelastic membrane of the posterior trachea. The superior end of the esophageal tube is opened and closed by the hypopharyngeal sphincter. The distal end of the esophageal tube is opened and closed by the gastroesophageal sphincter. Closure of this sphincter prevents a reflux of food into the esophagus. For food to enter the esophagus, the hypopharyngeal sphincter must open. For food to enter the stomach, the gastroesophageal sphincter must open.

The esophagus itself is contained in both the thoracic and abdominal cavities. The opening in the diaphragm that allows passage of the esophagus is the esophageal hiatus. As soon as the esophagus passes through this opening, it almost immediately enters the stomach. If this opening becomes enlarged, the stomach usually bulges into the opening. This is the common hiatal hernia.

Three cellular layers comprise the wall of the esophagus. The innermost layer of cells is the mucosal layer made up of squamous epithelium. The middle layer is muscle arranged circularly around the lumen. The outermost layer of cells is longitudinal muscle fibers.

The Stomach

The stomach is generally described as having three sections: the fundus, the body, and the pylorus (Figure 42-4). The upper lateral border of the stomach is called the lesser curvature, and the lower lateral border is called the greater curvature (simply because the greater curvature is longer than the lesser curvature). The length of the stomach is about 10–12 inches and the width, 4–6 inches at the widest point.

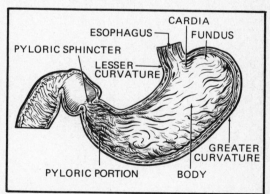

Figure 42-4. Divisions and curvatures of the stomach.

THE FUNDUS

This is the first portion of the stomach that food enters and is classified as a separate entity by the anatomists but not by physiologists since it functions in the same manner as and with the body of the stomach.

LOCATION

The stomach is located in the epigastric, umbilical, and left hypochondriac regions of the abdomen.

OPENINGS OF THE STOMACH

The esophagus has thickened, circular muscles at the distal end just as it passes into the stomach. These thickened, circular muscles form the cardiac sphincter. Relaxation of the cardiac sphincter results in opening of the esophageal lumen. Contraction of the cardiac sphincter results in closing of the esophageal lumen.

The pyloric sphincter has the same anatomical structure and the same physiologic function as the cardiac sphincter. The pyloric sphincter controls the opening at the distal end of the stomach into the duodenum.

LAYERS

The stomach wall is composed of three muscular layers. The outer layer consists of longitudinal muscle fibers. The middle layer consists of circular fibers. The inner layer consists of transverse fibers (Figure 42-5).

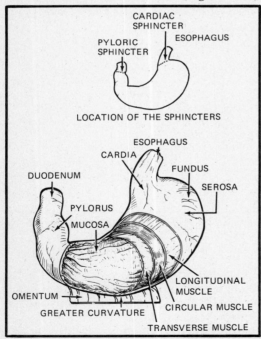

Figure 42-5. Layers of the stomach wall.

The gastric mucosa lines the interior of the stomach. Visceral peritoneum covers the exterior of the stomach and consists of

tissue which "hangs" in a double layer from the greater curvature of the stomach down to cover the anterior side of abdominal viscera. This is the greater omentum (Figure 42-6).

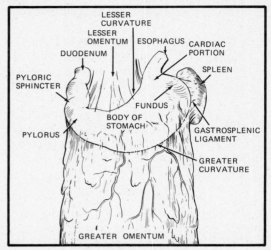

Figure 42-6. The greater omentum.

When not filled, the stomach interior has an appearance of shriveled skin (like on one's fingertips from washing too many dishes at one time). These wrinkled ridges are called rugae and allow for distension.

The interior mucosa of the stomach has a layer called the submucosa. The layer is composed of blood and lymph vessels and connective and fibrous tissue.

GASTRIC GLANDS

There are a tremendous number of gastric glands in the mucosa (Figure 42-7). The gastric gland is narrow at the neck, wider and deeper at the body, and a blind sac at the fundus. The opening of the gland is the foveola (gastric pit). Three types of cells comprise the gastric gland and will be covered in Chapter 43.

Intestine

The intestines are divided into two divisions having significant structural and functional differences. The two divisions are the small and large intestines. They are named as such because the diameter of the small intestine lumen is approximately

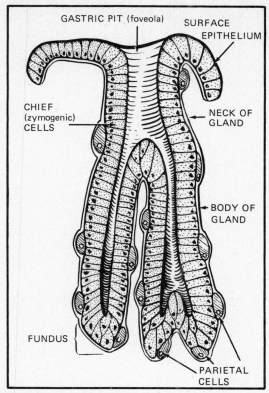

Figure 42-7. Single gastric gland.

1–1½ inches and the diameter of the large intestine lumen is approximately 2–2½ inches.

Small Intestine

The small intestine forms a tubular structure (Figure 42-8) that extends from the pyloric sphincter to the cecum. The 18–20 foot tube is divided into three segments. The first several inches is the duodenum, arising at the pyloric sphincter. It is about 10 inches long, C-shaped, and ends at the ileocecal valve. The middle segment of the small intestine is the jejunum, extending from the ileocecal valve about 8 feet. The third and final segment of the small intestine is the ileum, about 12 feet long. There is no distinct change from the jejunum to the ileum.

LAYERS OF THE SMALL INTESTINE WALL

The small intestinal wall has the same layering as does the stomach. This structural format is similar for the entire digestive tract. (Smooth muscle is involuntary muscle.)

VILLI

Villi (pl., singular is villus) are the distinguishing characteristics of the small intestine (Figure 42-8). These are fingerlike projections into the lumen providing an extensive surface area. An extraordinary number of villi project from the mucosa into the lumen of the small intestine. Each villus contains microvilli to actively absorb nutrients from the intestinal tract. Each villus contains a lymph vessel and a dense capillary bed to aid in the absorption process. This lymph vessel is called a "lacteal."

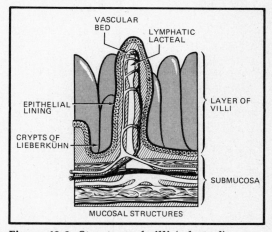

Figure 42-8. Structure of villi (a lacteal).

GLANDS OF THE SMALL INTESTINE

Specialized glands exist in the small intestine. The intestinal lumen is lined with simple, cuboidal, and columnar epithelial cells interspersed with goblet cells. The many goblet cells secrete mucus to protect the mucosa. The goblet cells decrease in numbers markedly towards the end of the ileum.

Crypts of Lieberkühn (Figure 42-9) are tubular glands found between the villi in the submucosa of the duodenum.

Absorptive and secreting cells have been identified but not differentiated in function. It is known that the crypts of Lieberkühn are extremely mitotic and replace villus

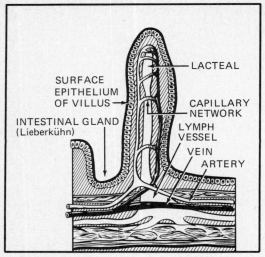

Figure 42-9. Crypts of Lieberkühn.

cells. The entire intestinal epithelial surface is replaced every 32 hours.

Crypts of Lieberkühn are small pits found on the entire intestinal surface except in the area of Brunner's glands. The crypts of Lieberkühn secrete a watery fluid immediately absorbed by the villi. This supplies a carrier substance for absorption by villi as chyme contacts them. This secretion is controlled principally by local nervous reflexes.

Brunner's glands are mucus-secreting glands that are concentrated in the first portion of the duodenum, between the pylorus and the papilla of Vater. The function of Brunner's glands is inhibited by the sympathetic nervous system. Lack of sufficient mucus may be related to the development site of peptic ulcers. Brunner's glands are supposed to protect the duodenum from digestion by the gastric juice.

Peyer's patches are lymphoid follicles that lie in the mucosa and submucosa of the ileum. They participate in antibody syn-·thesis and the body's immune responses.

Large Intestine

The large intestine is also referred to as the colon. It is a 5–6 foot long tube. It extends from the ileum to the anus. It is significantly different from the small intestine in that no villi are in the colon, the diameter is

2½ inches (larger than the small intestine), and it has many sacculations (saclike segmentations) that are called haustra.

There are three segments of the colon: the cecum, colon, and rectum. The colon is further subdivided into four sections: the ascending, transverse, descending, and sigmoid colons.

THE CECUM

This is a blind end sac (Figure 42-10) into which the ileum empties its contents. The vermiform appendix is attached to the base of the cecum. The appendix has no known use and must be surgically removed if it becomes infected to prevent peritonitis.

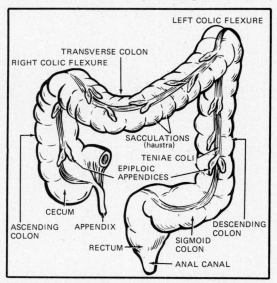

Figure 42-10. The large intestine (anterior view).

THE COLON

Immediately above the cecum is the ascending colon which passes upward to become the transverse colon at the right colic flexure. It then crosses the abdomen and becomes the descending colon at the left colic flexure. At the iliac crest, the descending colon arches backward to form the sigmoid colon (Figure 42-10). The sigmoid colon is the portion of the colon that crosses from the left side to the midline to become the rectum (Figure 42-10), which follows the curvature of the lower sacrum and coccyx.

THE RECTUM AND ANUS

The rectum is about 7 inches long and the distal 1–2 inches are the anal canal (Figure 42-11). Mucous membrane lines the rectum and is arranged in vertical rows called rectal columns. Each rectal column contains an artery and a vein. These veins frequently enlarge to form hemorrhoids. Two sphincters control the anus (the exterior opening of the rectum). The internal sphincter is composed of involuntary smooth muscle. The external sphincter is voluntary striated muscle.

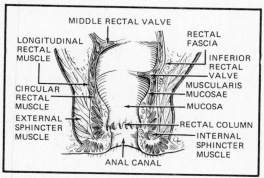

Figure 42-11. Section of the rectum.

LAYERS OF THE COLON WALL

Epithelial cells form the mucosa of the colon, which is actively involved with absorption of water and some electrolytes.

The muscle layers here are different than those in the small intestine. The circular layer becomes somewhat spherical (Figure 42-10) and the longitudinal layer fibers are evenly dispersed in three strips around the colon. These strips are called teniae coli. This results in sacculation since the teniae coli are shorter than the circular muscles. The resulting pouches are the haustra.

Blood Supply of the Gastrointestinal Tract

ARTERIAL VASCULARIZATION

The celiac artery, the superior mesenteric, and the inferior mesentric arteries all branch from the abdominal aorta. Table 42-1 shows the arterial vascularization of the gastrointestinal tract.

VENOUS BLOOD RETURN

The venous circulation of the gastrointestinal system is unique in that the venous blood enters the portal vein system (shown in Table 42-2). *ALL* blood from the gastrointestinal tract enters the portal vein system, which empties into the liver sinusoids. This makes the portal system extremely important for filtering microorganisms and for synthesis of many enzymes, clotting factors, and such needed by the body. Generally, the vein corresponding by name to the artery drains the same areas supplied by the artery.

The portal vein drains into the liver sinusoids. These sinusoids join branches of the hepatic artery to form the hepatic vein. In turn, the hepatic vein drains into the inferior vena cava.

Innervation of the Gastrointestinal System

Compared with the other body systems, the gastrointestinal tract is unique in that it has its own separate intrinsic nervous system. The gastrointestinal tract can be and *is* influenced by the autonomic nervous system.

The intrinsic nervous system has two layers of neurons connected by specific fibers. The outer layer of neurons is called the *myenteric plexus* or *Auerbach's plexus*. It is located between the longitudinal and circular muscle layers. The inner layer of neurons is called the *submucosal plexus* or *Meissner's plexus* and is located in the submucosa.

Generally the myenteric plexus controls movement of the gastrointestinal tract and the submucosal (Meissner's plexus) controls the secretions of the gastrointestinal tract and sensory function through impulses received by stretch receptors in both the gastrointestinal wall and gastrointestinal epithelium.

When the myenteric plexus is stimulated, it results in increasing motor tone of

Table 42-1.   Arterial vascularization of the gastrointestinal tract.

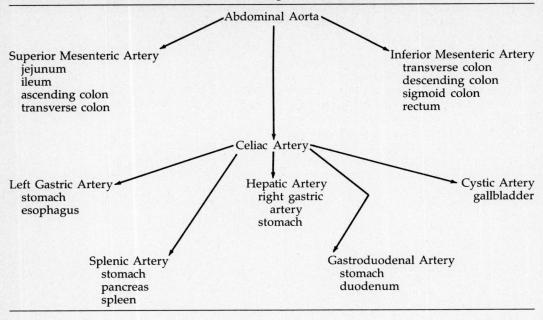

Abdominal Aorta

Superior Mesenteric Artery
  jejunum
  ileum
  ascending colon
  transverse colon

Inferior Mesenteric Artery
  transverse colon
  descending colon
  sigmoid colon
  rectum

Celiac Artery

Left Gastric Artery
  stomach
  esophagus

Hepatic Artery
  right gastric
  artery
  stomach

Cystic Artery
  gallbladder

Splenic Artery
  stomach
  pancreas
  spleen

Gastroduodenal Artery
  stomach
  duodenum

Table 42-2. Venous return of the gastrointestinal tract.

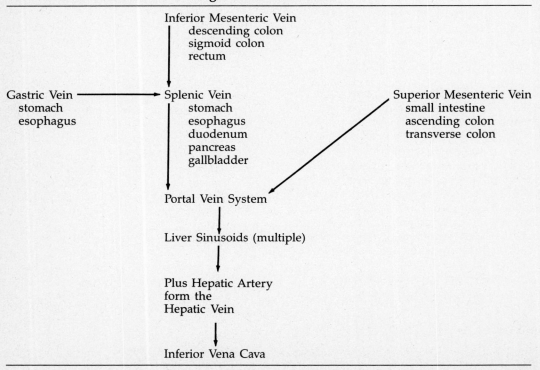

Inferior Mesenteric Vein
  descending colon
  sigmoid colon
  rectum

Gastric Vein
  stomach
  esophagus

Splenic Vein
  stomach
  esophagus
  duodenum
  pancreas
  gallbladder

Superior Mesenteric Vein
  small intestine
  ascending colon
  transverse colon

Portal Vein System

Liver Sinusoids (multiple)

Plus Hepatic Artery
form the
Hepatic Vein

Inferior Vena Cava

the gastrointestinal wall and increasing intensity, rate, and speed of peristaltic waves. Increase in Meissner's plexus activity results in increasing secretions.

Three other plexuses have a minor role in gastrointestinal function. The subserosal plexus is just beneath the outer covering of the gut. Deep myenteric plexuses are located within the actual circular muscle. The mucous plexuses are found throughout the gut and innervated villi and glandular cells.

The autonomic nervous system can alter the effects of the gastrointestinal system at specific points or from the mouth to the stomach and then from the distal end of the colon to the anus. Parasympathetic supply for the gut is from the cranial nerve X (vagus) and sacral nerves. A few cranial parasympathetic fibers innervate the mouth and pharynx. Extensive parasympathetic innervation exists in the esophagus, stomach, pancreas, and first half of the large intestine. The sacral parasympathetic fibers innervate the distal half of the large intestine, especially the sigmoidal, rectal, and anal portions.

The sympathetic nervous system fibers flow along blood vessels of the entire gut. Its neurotransmitter, norepinephrine, inhibits gastrointestinal tract activity. This causes opposite effects than the parasympathetic neurotransmitter, acetylcholine. If strong enough, the sympathetic system can virtually halt activity of the gastrointestinal tract.

The Accessory Digestive Organs

There are four accessory organs that are an aid to the digestive system. They are the salivary glands, the pancreas, the gallbladder, and the liver.

The Salivary Glands

There are three salivary glands, namely the parotid, the submandibular, and the sublingual (Figure 42-12). Each of the salivary glands are paired. The parotid glands are located beneath the skin and anterior and inferior to the external ear. The parotid duct is in the subcutaneous tissue of the cheeks. The submaxillary (submandibular) glands

are under the floor of the mouth near the jaw joint and curve to allow the duct to open at the side of the frenulum under the tongue. The sublingual glands are under the mucous membrane on either side and under the tongue and open by a series of small ducts along the side of the frenulum near the opening of the submandibular gland.

Hormones have no influence on the salivary glands. Salivary secretion is controlled by nerves. Nervous stimuli of the glands occur from the thought, sight, and smell of food.

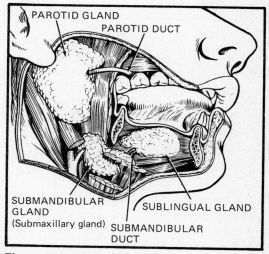

Figure 42-12. Salivary glands.

The Pancreas

The pancreas is a fish-shaped, lobulated gland lying behind the stomach (Figure 42-13). The gland is composed of three segments. The head and neck of the pancreas lie in the C-shaped curve of the duodenum. The body lies behind the duodenum and the tail is a thin, narrow part of the pancreas under the spleen.

The pancreas is both an endocrine and and exocrine organ. The endocrine portion was covered in Chapter 34. The exocrine portion is related to the gastrointestinal system and produces three enzymes whose release is controlled by two hormones produced in the small intestine.

The main pancreatic duct is the duct of

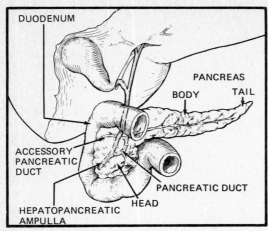

Figure 42-13. The pancreas.

Wirsung which runs the whole length of the pancreas from left to right and joins the common bile duct.

The exocrine part of the pancreas is composed of acinar cells, which are little sacs called alveoli. (Remember the endocrine tissue is the islets of Langerhans.) These cells are arranged around a small central lumen into which the cells drain the exocrine enzymes which they have synthesized. The central lumens drain into multiple ducts which eventually drain into the main pancreatic duct. The ampulla of Vater (Figure 42-14) is the short segment just before the common bile duct enters the duodenum.

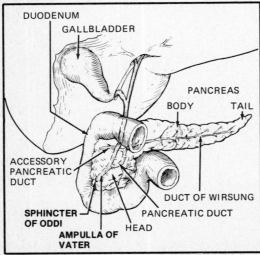

Figure 42-14. The ampulla of Vater and sphincter of Oddi.

Pancreatic secretion is controlled by two factors. In some phases of digestion, the vagus nerve (parasympathetic) stimulates secretion of enzymes. In one phase, the food entering the duodenum stimulates pancreatic secretion by the hormones released in the duodenum.

The Gallbladder

Together, the gallbladder and the liver are known as the biliary system.

STRUCTURE

The gallbladder (Figure 42-15) is a saclike storage structure for bile. It is located on the undersurface of the liver and is held in place by areolar tissue, peritoneum, and blood vessels.

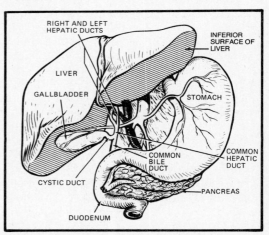

Figure 42-15. Location of the gallbladder.

DIVISIONS OF THE GALLBLADDER

There are four specific portions of the gallbladder (Figure 42-16). The fundus is the distal portion of the body of the gallbladder, which is a blind sac. The body of the gallbladder connects the fundus and the infundibulum. The infundibulum connects the body to the neck. The neck of the gallbladder joins the body of the gallbladder to the cystic duct. Finally, the cystic duct of the gallbladder merges with the liver's duct system (Figure 42-17) to form the common bile duct, which empties into the duodenum when stimulated.

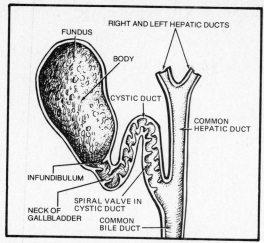

Figure 42-16. Divisions of the gallbladder.

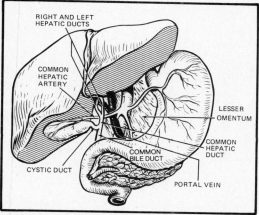

Figure 42-17. Gallbladder and liver duct system.

FUNCTION OF THE GALLBLADDER

The gallbladder stores and concentrates bile. Upon stimulation it provides the passage for bile to leave the liver and enter the duodenum. It also stores up to 50 ml of concentrated bile. The function of the gallbladder in relation to digestion is covered in Chapter 43.

The Liver

The liver is the single largest organ in the body and weighs 3–4 pounds. It is located in the right upper quadrant of the abdomen, lying up against the right inferior diaphragm.

GROSS STRUCTURE

The liver is divided into a right and left lobe by the falciform ligament (Figure 42-18). The falciform ligament also attaches the liver to the abdominal wall and to the diaphragm. The right lobe of the liver is larger than the left. On the inferior liver surface is the quadrate lobe and on the posterior liver surface is the caudate lobe. Both the quadrate and caudate lobes are small.

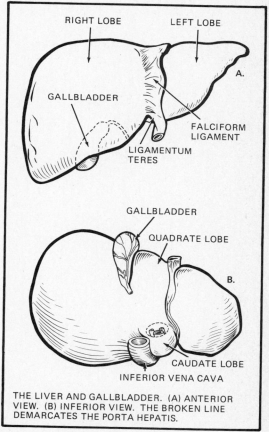

THE LIVER AND GALLBLADDER. (A) ANTERIOR VIEW. (B) INFERIOR VIEW. THE BROKEN LINE DEMARCATES THE PORTA HEPATIS.

Figure 42-18. Divisions of the liver.

FUNCTIONAL UNIT

The hepatic lobule is the functioning unit of the liver (Figure 42-19). It is cylindrical with epithelial cell columns and branches spreading out to the periphery of the lobule. In the surrounding connective tissue, each lobule has a hepatic artery, a portal

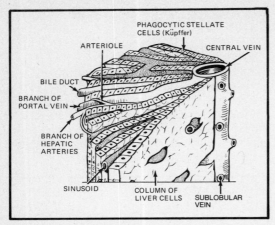

Figure 42-19. A liver lobule.

vein, and a bile duct known collectively as the "portal triad." Between columns of epithelial cells are intralobular cavities called sinusoids. Each sinusoid is lined with Küpffer cells, which are phagocytic cells.

BLOOD SUPPLY TO HEPATIC LOBULES

Each sinusoid receives blood from both the hepatic artery and the hepatic vein. The blood is "cleaned" by the phagocytic Küpffer cells. Products removed from the blood include amino acids, nutrients, sugars, and bacterial debris. Blood leaves the sinusoid by entering the central lobule vein. It then enters the hepatic veins and follows the normal venous circuit. Approximately 1,500 ml of blood enters the liver each minute, making the liver one of the most vascular organs in the body.

43

Physiology of the Gastrointestinal System

Ingested foods cannot be digested by the body in the ingested form. To be assimilated and utilized, the food must be mechanically and chemically altered.

The Mouth

The first step in digesting foods is to alter the food mechanically. The teeth shred, grind, tear, and pulverize foods to make the food small enough to swallow. Each lump of food swallowed is termed a (food) bolus. While the teeth are making the food bolus size, the tongue moves the food around in the mouth so that all of it is masticated and mixed with saliva.

The salivary glands' total daily secretion is between 1 and 1½ liters of saliva. Saliva contains two enzymes of major importance: (1) a serous secretion containing *ptyalin* to digest starch and (2) mucus secretion which contains *mucin* for lubrication. Saliva is composed of 99% water and 1% mucin and amylase.

THE TONGUE

The tongue has several important functions (for anatomical structure, see Chapter 42). It is necessary for speech. It mixes saliva with food being chewed and it pushes the food to the back of the mouth for swallowing. Once started, the reflex act of swallowing becomes involuntary and the tongue pushes the food into the pharynx.

THE PHARYNX

The pharynx connects the mouth and the esophagus and is divided into three sections.

1. The nasopharynx extends from the nasal cavity to the soft palate. Swallowing receptors surround the opening of the pharynx. As the food bolus is pushed towards the back of the mouth by the tongue, these receptors stimulate the pharyngeal walls at the opening of the pharynx. The soft palate rises to block the nasopharyngeal opening, preventing food from entering the nose.

2. The oropharyngeal walls are pulled towards each other from the soft palate to

the hyoid bone. This produces a small passage that only well masticated food can enter. The size of the passage prevents large food masses from entering without additional mastication.

3. The laryngeal pharynx extends from the hyoid bone to the esophagus per se. Muscles attached to the hyoid bone pull the laryngeal pharynx up during deglutition to allow the epiglottis to cover the opening of the trachea, preventing aspiration of food (Figure 43-1).

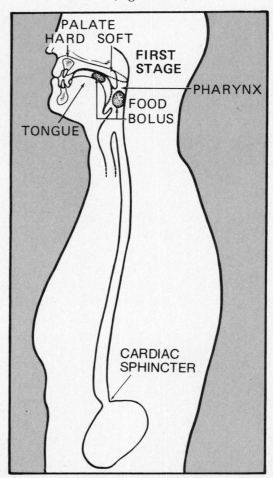

Figure 43-1. First stage of deglutition (swallowing).

The Esophagus

When food is pushed from the pharynx, it must pass through the hypopharyngeal sphincter. When the hypopharyngeal sphincter is relaxed, it is closed due to a passive elastic tension. When the skeletal muscles contract, the spincter opens and a bolus of food may enter the esophagus (Figure 43-2). The sphincter is also open during vomiting to allow the food to be regurgitated. The bolus of food produces a pressure as it enters the esophagus. Gravity plus the pressure, known as a peristaltic wave, advances the bolus down the esophagus.

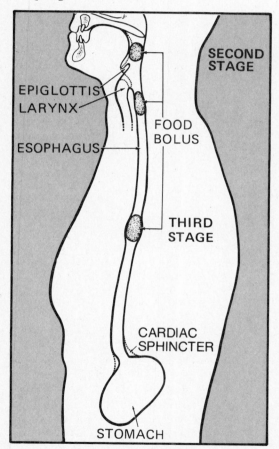

Figure 43-2. The last two stages of swallowing.

The gastroesophageal sphincter, also known as the cardiac sphincter, functions in the same way as the hypopharyngeal sphincter. The gastroesophageal sphincter is between the esophagus and the stomach. It opens to allow the bolus of food to enter and closes to prevent a reflux of food and

acid. If the sphincter cannot close, a condition known as achalasia exists. Achalasia is damage of the myenteric level of nerves that innervate the sphincter and prevent it from closing.

The thoracic segment of the esophagus is under a subatmospheric pressure of -5 mm Hg to -10 mm Hg. The abdominal esophagus is under a pressure of $+5$ to $+10$ mm Hg, so reflux is not uncommon. No enzymes are secreted in the esophagus.

The Stomach

The proximal portion of the stomach, the cardia, receives the bolus of food from the esophagus. This stimulates gastric glands to secrete lipase, pepsin, the intrinsic factor, mucus, hydrochloric acid, and gastrone (inhibits secretion of the acids)—all collectively known as gastric juice. The mucosa of the stomach contains a few gastric glands at the fundus, a great many glands in the body, and fewer glands at the antral (pyloric) portion of the body.

Gastric glands are tubular. The narrow neck of each gland opens into the stomach. Chief cells in the gastric gland's neck have two functions: to secrete mucus and to regenerate cells for both the glands themselves and for the intestinal surface epithelial tissue. Argentaffin cells are present in the tissues of the gastric glands. These cells contain granules which are thought to be the origin of serotonin.

Zymogenic (chief) cells found in the body of a gastric gland secrete pepsin. The fundus (blind end of the gland) has parietal (or oxyntic) cells which secrete hydrochloric acid, water, and the intrinsic factor. The intrinsic factor from the parietal cell is a mucoprotein that is essential for absorption of B_{12}. Once released from the parietal cells, the intrinsic factor adheres to epithelial cells in the ileum. If the ileum is surgically resected, exogenous B_{12} must be taken for life. Hydrochloric acid converts inactive pepsin to active pepsin. The gastric gland's surface epithelial cells secrete mucus and mucopolysaccharides.

The stomach distends to hold a large quantity of food. This distension helps to control the rate at which food enters the duodenum. The stomach also churns the food boluses until a semi-liquid mass exists. This semi-liquid mass is called chyme. The stomach can hold close to 1 liter of food without a change in muscle tone. This is due to the plasticity of the smooth muscles (which is the ability of smooth muscle to extend greatly in length). Laplace's law is evidenced by a large increase in distension of the muscle resulting in very little pressure increase. The stretching of the stomach wall also stimulates the vagal response. The vagal response inhibits muscle activity in the body of the stomach.

The pyloric or antral portion of the stomach has increased depth, size, and muscle and secretes mucus and pepsinogen.

GASTRIC MOBILITY

The rugae allow for a great distension of the stomach without increasing pressure (Laplace's law) which may be termed a receptive relaxation phenomenon. This may allow for stomach contents to approach 6–7 liters before peristaltic contractions are initiated.

Factors affecting gastric motility include quantity of contents, pH of contents, degree of mixing and peristalsis that has occurred, and the capacity of the duodenum to accept chyme from the stomach.

Usually, the fundus of the stomach is stimulated to initiate oscillations which are mild "mixing waves" when about 1 liter of food is in the stomach, but there may be considerably more food present. When the food (bolus) is digested to the chyme state, it is ready for passage into the duodenum.

However, mixing waves alone are unable to achieve this. If no other influences are functional, malabsorption states will occur. To help the conversion of food boluses to chyme, the mixing waves help the hormones and acids mix with the food. Peristaltic contractions occur in the body of the stomach further altering mechanically the food bolus and altering chemically the disintegrating food by complete mixing with the gastric juices. As the peristaltic contractions move towards the antral (pyloric) portion of the stomach, they become very strong in order to force the chyme into the

duodenum. A pH of 1–3 is obtained by the hormone gastrin stimulating the release of hydrochloric acid into the chyme and also stimulating peristaltic contractions which will occur at a rate of about three per minute.

If the duodenum cannot accept more chyme or the chyme is inadequately emulsified or too acidic or hypertonic, the *enterogastric reflex* (which causes lower gastrin and acid secretion) will delay the progression of chyme. This reflex is under vagal influence.

Chyme must be of the proper consistency and acidity and the duodenum must be receptive for the strong antral peristaltic contractions to force the chyme through the pyloric valve. The small size of the pyloric sphincter opening results in little chyme entering the duodenum. Most of the chyme is squirted back towards the body of the stomach as the pyloric valve relaxes and closes. This is an important action in the mixing of the chyme.

GASTRIC EMPTYING

The stomach empties at a rate proportional to the volume of its contents. Other factors affect the opening and closing of the pyloric sphincter to allow gastric emptying.

Chemical composition of the chyme *in the duodenum* determines the rate and quantity of additional chyme entering the duodenum.

The duodenum contains osmoreceptors, chemoreceptors, and baroreceptors which influence duodenal activity. If the chyme has a high fat content upon entering the duodenum, a release of cholecystokinin (CCK) occurs, inhibiting further release of chyme. High fat content is the factor most known for inhibiting gastric emptying.

Other factors such as emotional depression, sadness, and pain (both physical and psychological) inhibit emptying of the stomach. An inadequate fluid intake will retard emptying of the stomach because a large quantity of liquid is necessary to turn fat, protein, and carbohydrates (CHO) into chyme.

Normally, about 2 liters of gastric juices (primarily hydrochloric acid) are secreted per day. The pH is 1–3. This acidity and its resultant irritation affect gastric emptying. The amount of protein present and the osmolality of the stomach contents affect gastric emptying, either inhibiting or accelerating it, depending upon other factors. Acid kills bacteria, breaks down proteins, and initiates some enzyme activity. Chief cells in the stomach secrete the inactive proteolytic enzyme pepsinogen. This is converted to pepsin by hydrochloric acid. Pepsin aids in splitting amino acid bonds.

The mucous cells of the stomach secrete both mucus and water to lubricate the stomach lining and liquify the stomach contents.

The stomach may be emptied rapidly by vomiting which may be due to a markedly distended stomach or duodenum, intense pain, increased ICP, or rotation such as occurs in seasickness. Extreme emotion of anger and sham rage may cause vomiting. Stimulation of the gag reflex may produce vomiting by its stimulation of the vomiting center located in the medulla oblongata (all vomiting requires stimulation of the vomiting center).

CONTROL OF GASTRIC SECRETIONS

Control of gastric secretions may be through autonomic nervous system functions, by hormonal alterations, and/or through baroreceptors.

The control of the gastric secretions, specifically hydrochloric acid, may be broken down into three phases: namely, the cephalic, the gastric, and the intestinal phase. These three phases follow the path of food and then chyme through the alimentary tract. When the stomach is at rest, normal secretions occur at a rate of about 0.5 ml/minute. This is known as the basal rate. With food in the stomach, secretions increase to about 3.0 ml/minute.

The Cephalic Phase

The parasympathetic nervous system via the vagus nerve controls this first phase of regulation of gastric secretion. The sight, smell, taste, or thought of food is sufficient to stimulate the release of hydrochloric acid in preparation for the expected arrival of food boluses. In addition to pleasant thoughts of food, hunger, and hypoglycemia, anger will stimulate secretion of hydrochloric acid.

Vagal control is decreased by certain drugs (especially the anticholinergic drugs), hyperglycemia, and duodenal distension.

The Gastric Phase

This second phase of control over gastric secretion begins when food actually enters the stomach. The predominant regulator in this phase is hormonal. Gastrin is the major hormone and is stimulated by antral distension, secretion of pepsinogen, and an alkaline pH in the stomach. As hydrochloric acid is released in response to gastrin, the stomach contents eventually become acid. When the number of hydrogen ions (acidity) is adequately high, gastrin secretion decreases.

The Intestinal Phase

This phase begins as the name implies— when chyme enters the duodenum. Chyme entering the duodenum is more acid than that in the body of the stomach because as polypeptide fragments move from the body of the stomach to the antrum, they stimulate acid secretion by an unknown mechanism.

When the chyme has a pH below 2.5, there is a slowing of chyme being accepted into the duodenum. In the gastric (second) phase, the chyme becomes more alkaline so that the chyme will move into the duodenum in the intestinal phase.

Fat in the duodenum stimulates the secretion of cholecystokinin (CCK), which directly decreases gastric mobility. Of the food classifications leaving the stomach, carbohydrates (CHO) are the most rapid, followed by protein and then fat.

The Small Intestine

The major function of the small intestine is to absorb nutrients from the chyme. The chyme that enters the duodenum, however, is not sufficiently broken down to allow for nutrient absorption.

Let us digress from following the movement of chyme through the small intestine to explore additional duodenal factors which will make the chyme suitable for nutrient absorption. These additional factors are the digestive role of the pancreas and the biliary system (liver and gallbladder).

The Pancreas

The pancreas' exocrine glands are the acinar glands. The secretions of the acinar glands are enzymes, water, and salts. The pancreatic (acinar) juice is composed of three major types of enzymes: amylytic, lipolytic, and proteolytic. At least 10% of the pancreatic enzymes must be present to prevent malabsorption states.

The amylytic enzyme is predominantly α-amylase (alpha-amylase) first encountered in the saliva. The α-amylase is responsible for hydrolysis of carbohydrates (CHO). The end products of hydrolysis of CHO are glucose and maltose (a disaccharide of two glucose molecules). The difference between salivary and pancreatic amylase is that the latter is able to digest raw starches as well as cooked starches.

The lipolytic enzymes are pancreatic lipase and phospholipase A, which are important in early stages of the digestion of fats. Lipase breaks down triglycerides to free fatty acids and monoglycerides. Bile salts are essential for this function. Phospholipase A hydrolyzes lecithin (a complex lipid) to lysolecithin.

Proteolytic enzymes are actually proenzymes, that is, these proenzymes must be altered to become biochemically active. The three most important proteolytic proenzymes are trypsinogen, chymotrypsinogen, and procarboxypeptidase.

Trypsin is involved in the activation of all three proenzymes to enzymes. Trypsin breaks amino acid bonds of protein chains, forming small polypeptides and single amino acids.

Two other important pancreatic enzymes are nuclease and deoxyribonuclease. These enzymes degrade nucleotides within DNA and RNA molecules.

REGULATION OF PANCREATIC SECRETIONS

In addition to the acinar glands producing enzymes, the cells lining the glands secrete bicarbonate-rich pancreatic juice. Total production is approximately 2 liters per day.

The cells lining the acinar glands contain large amounts of carbonic anhydrase. The alkaline secretions (HCO_3^-) of the duct cells (cells lining the acinar glands) mix with the amylytic, lipolytic, and proteolytic enzymes prior to reaching the major pancreatic duct, the duct of Wirsung.

Secretions of the pancreas are controlled by humoral and neural factors. There are three phases of secretion: the cephalic, gastric, and intestinal phases. The cephalic phase is activated by the same factors as in the cephalic state of the stomach and is mainly controlled by the vagus nerve. The pancreatic juice secreted in this phase is rich in enzymes with minimal amounts of HCO_3^-.

The gastric and intestinal phases are interrelated and controlled by two hormones (secretin and cholecystokinin); which one is in control at any given moment depends upon the composition of the chyme in the duodenum. When the chyme is predominantly undigested proteins and fats, the pancreatic juice will be enzyme-rich. When the chyme is mainly acidic (low pH), the pancreatic juice will be HCO_3^- rich. The secretion of cholecystokinin stimulates the enzyme-rich secretion of pancreatic juices; secretin stimulates the release of HCO_3^- and water-rich pancreatic juice. The pancreatic juices enter the duodenum along with the biliary system secretions at the sphincter of Oddi.

The Biliary System

The biliary system is composed of the liver and gallbladder.

The Liver

The role of the liver in digestion (only one of its many functions) is to synthesize and transport bile pigments and bile salts for fat digestion.

The liver cell, the hepatocyte, synthesizes bile which is then secreted into bile canaliculi (ducts). The bile canaliculi branch and combine, eventually forming the right and left hepatic ducts. Immediately after leaving the liver, the right and left hepatic ducts merge to form the common hepatic duct. The cystic duct of the gallbladder joins the common hepatic duct to form the common bile duct. The common bile duct joins the major pancreatic duct to form the ampulla of Vater just prior to entering the duodenum at the sphincter of Oddi.

The Gallbladder

The gallbladder stores and concentrates bile. The adult gallbladder stores from 30 to 50 milliliters of bile. The major components of bile are bile acids, bile salts (sodium cholate and chenodenoxycholate), and pigments. The pigments are mainly bilirubin, cholesterol, phospholipids, alkaline phosphatase, electrolytes, and water.

Inside the gallbladder, bile salts react with water, leaving a fat-soluble end to mix with cholesterol and/or lecithin. These formed particles are called *micelles*. Gallstones may form when the micelles become supersaturated with cholesterol. If bile salts are absent or diminished in the small intestine, normal fat digestion and absorption cannot occur. This results in fat malabsorption and steatorrhea (fatty stools). Most of the bile salts are re-utilized by reabsorption in the ileum and enter the vascular system to be carried to the liver.

Bile pigments and bilirubin result from the degradation of hemoglobin. Normally, bile pigments do not form stones. However, in some diseases, there is an over concentration of bile pigments resulting in precipitation of bilirubinate stones. Ninety percent of gallstones are composed essentially of cholesterol.

Vagal stimulation increases bile secretions through the sphincter of Oddi. The sphincter of Oddi, in a normal state, remains slightly opened providing for a constant but miniscule amount of bile to enter the small intestine.

During normal digestion, the gallbladder contracts in response to the hormone cholecystokinin, pushing increased amounts of bile through the sphincter of Oddi into the duodenum. The gallbladder does not contract when there is no stimulation by cholecystokinin (e.g., between meals or starvation diets).

Let us return now to the discussion on chyme in the duodenum.

Hormones of the G.I. System

Table 43-1 summarizes the origin, stimulus, activity, and function of the G.I. hormones.

Movements of the Small Intestine

Two types of movement within the small intestine have been identified as mixing contractions and propulsive contractions. Both of these movements continually contribute to the mixing of chyme.

When a portion of the small intestine is distended, baroreceptors stimulate concentric contractions. Each contraction results in a segmentation of the chyme and moves the chyme forward about 1 centimeter. These segmenting contractions normally occur 7–12 times per minute. This helps to mix secretions of the small intestine with the chyme particles.

Propulsive contractions are called peristaltic contractions. Peristaltic contractions may and should be regularly spaced. However, they may be irregularly spaced, isolated, or weak and irregularly spaced. The peristaltic waves (contractions) push the chyme slowly toward the colon. These waves are short and found predominantly in the first portions of the duodenum and jejunum.

Distension of the small intestine activates the nerves to continue the contraction sequence, known as the *myenteric reflex*. As the chyme nears the large intestine, contractions in the ileum increase. As chyme reaches the end of the ileum and is ready to enter the colon, a *gastroileal reflex* is stimulated. The *gastroileal reflex* regulates the movement of chyme from the small intestine into the large intestine. Between the ileum and the cecum is the ileocecal valve, which is normally closed. The tissue immediately before the ileocecal valve is highly

Table 43-1. Gastrointestinal hormones and their functions.

Hormone	Origin	Stimulus	Activity	Function
Gastrin	Antral cells of the stomach	Distension of the stomach due to food present	Increases HCl and pepsin.	Promotes antral activity. Stimulates parietal cells and chief cells.
Secretin	Duodenal cells	Chyme in the duodenum	Increases H_2O secretion.	Stimulates pancreatic and hepatic HCO_3^-. Augments action of cholecystokinin.
Cholecystokinin (CCK)	Duodenal cells	Chyme in the duodenum	Increases gallbladder contraction; decreases stomach tone.	Stimulates pancreas secretion of lipase, amylase, trypsin.
Intestinal peptide (VIP)	Small intestine mucosa	Chyme in the duodenum	Increases H_2O secretion.	Stimulates pancreatic and hepatic HCO_3^-. Augments action of cholecystokinin.
Gastric inhibitory hormone	Small intestine	Blood glucose level	—	Releases insulin.
Polypeptide (G.I.P.)	Small intestine	—		Inhibits gastric secretion.
Vasoactive hormone	—	—	—	Stimulates intestinal juice.

muscular, forming the ileocecal sphincter, and the flaps of the ileocecal valve (Figure 43-3) extend into the cecum. The sphincter is normally contracted except after a meal when it relaxes and allows chyme to move from the ileum into the cecum. Chyme is prevented from returning to the ileum during colonic contraction due to the valve leaflets being floated out to close the ileocecal valve (in much the same ways as the heart valves).

Absorption Mechanisms in the Small Intestine

There are five basic mechanisms for absorption in the small intestine: hydrolysis, non-ionic movement, passive diffusion, facilitated diffusion, and active transport.

HYDROLYSIS

Hydrolysis is the chemical action of uniting compounds with water to split the com-

pounds into more simple compounds. Enzymes and hormones act as catalysts in the process of hydrolysis. Catalysts speed up the process of hydrolysis. (Catalysts speed

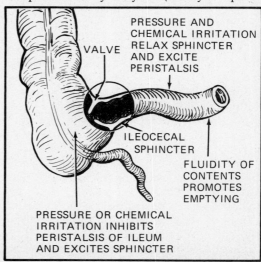

Figure 43-3. The gastroilial reflex.

up a chemical reaction without entering into the reaction.)

NON-IONIC MOVEMENT

Non-ionic transport allows substances to move freely in and out of cells with no energy or carrier substances needed. Such molecules include drugs and unconjugated bile salts.

PASSIVE DIFFUSION

In passive diffusion there is free movement of molecules based on a concentration gradient. Free fatty acids and water are molecules that move by passive diffusion.

FACILITATED DIFFUSION

Facilitated diffusion may be defined as a process by which a carrier picks up an ion, crosses the cell membrane, liberates the ion inside the cell, and then returns outside to pick up another molecule (ion). This diffusion does not require energy and ions cannot move alone against an electrochemical gradient. Fructose is an example of a substance using facilitated diffusion.

ACTIVE TRANSPORT

For nutrients to be absorbed by active transport, energy (ATP) is required. Ions and molecules such as Na^+, K^+, and proteins and glucose require active transport.

Table 43-2 identifies which substances are absorbed in each section of the small intestine.

Carbohydrate Digestion

"Carbohydrates enter the duodenum in the form of starch, polysaccharides (complex sugars), disaccharides, and monosaccharides. The starch and polysaccharides are hydrolyzed under the influence of amylase (from the pancreas and salivary glands) to form maltose (a disaccharide). Maltose thus formed, plus directly ingested disaccharides such as sucrose (cane sugar), lactose (milk sugar), and maltose (malt sugar), are hydrolyzed by intestinal enzymes into simple sugars or monosaccharides which are then absorbed into the bloodstream via the intestinal mucosa."[1]

Approximately 350 grams of carbohydrates are absorbed daily (60% starch, 30% sucrose, and 10% lactose).

[1] A Programmed Approach to Anatomy and Physiology: The Digestive System. Bowie, MD: Robert J. Brady Co., p. 49, 1972

Table 43-2. Absorption in the small intestine.

Substance	Duodenum	Jejunum	Ileum
Proteins	+ +	+ +	+
CHO	+ +	+ +	+
Fat	+ +	+ +	+
Folic Acid	+	+	+
Ascorbic Acid	+	+	+
B_{12}	−	−	+ (requires intrinsic factor and is activated by kidneys)
Calcium	+ + (requires vitamin D and 1,25-dehydroxycholecalciferol)		
Iron	+	+	+
Fat soluble vitamins ADEK	+	+	+ (requires bile salts)
Na^+	+ +	+	+
K^+	+	+	+
Cl^-	+ +	+	+
HCO_3^-	+	+	+
Mg_2SO_4	+	+	+
H_2O	+ +	+	+

The three basic sugars are fructose, glucose, and galactose. Each of these basic sugars has 4 Kcal/gram. Glucose and galactose are actively transported across the small intestine wall into the blood. Fructose is transported by facilitated diffusion.

Protein Digestion

"Proteins which are ingested into the digestive tract are first acted upon by enzymes called proteases. The principal proteases are pepsin (in the gastric secretion) and trypsin (in the pancreatic secretion). These enzymes catalyze the hydrolysis of the very large protein molecules into intermediate compounds (proteoses and peptones) and subsequently into amino acids. In the digestive sequence, protein is broken down into proteoses and peptones in the stomach. These simpler compounds are next broken down into polypeptides and thence into amino acids in the small intestine."[2]

There are approximately 70–90 grams of protein absorbed daily, yielding 4 Kcal/gram.

Of the amino acids, there are eight which are essential. These eight are listed in Table 43-3.

Table 43-3. Eight essential amino acids.

isoleucine
leucine
lysine
methionine
phenylalanine
threonine
tryptophan
valine

Fat Digestion

"Before fats can be digested they must be emulsified, i.e., dispersed as very small droplets. This function is performed in the small intestine by bile which is secreted by the liver and stored in the gallbladder. The emulsification of ingested fat globules provides a greater contact area between the fat molecules and pancreatic lipase, which is the principal fat-digestive enzyme. The end products of fat digestion are glycerides, fatty acids, and glycerol. Some fatty acids and glycerol may be absorbed into the blood via the blood vessels found in the villi of the intestinal mucosa. However, most fatty acids and glycerides are absorbed into the lymphatic system via the lacteals of the same structures."[3]

There are approximately 60–100 grams of fat absorbed daily, providing 9 Kcal/gram.

The Large Intestine

The large intestine has five distinct parts: the ascending colon, the transverse colon, the descending colon, the sigmoid colon, and the rectum.

The large intestine, or colon, is mainly responsible for the absorption of water and some electrolytes and the elimination of waste products. As the chyme moves up the first portion of the ascending colon analward, it is fluid. The chyme is semifluid by the time it enters the transverse colon and becomes mush in this portion of the colon. Intestinal contents are semimush as they enter the descending colon and solid by the time they leave the descending colon and enter the sigmoid colon.

COLONIC MOTILITY

The colon moves its contents slowly through the colon system to allow for fluid absorption so that 800–900 ml of chyme liquid is absorbed along with nutrients. Thus, of the 1,000 ml of chyme (liquid) entering the colon, only 150–250 ml of fluid will be evacuated in the stool per day.

MIXING MOVEMENTS IN THE COLON

Segmentation of chyme in the large intestine is caused by contraction of the inner

---

[2]A Programmed Approach to Anatomy and Physiology: The Digestive System. Bowie, MD: Robert J. Brady Co., p. 50, 1972

[3]A Programmed Approach to Anatomy and Physiology: The Digestive System. Bowie, MD: Robert J. Brady Co., p. 52, 1972

muscle layer, usually resulting in a movement of perhaps as much as 2–2½ cm. There is a slow progress analward with segmentation in the colon. Random contraction results in a lack of coordination resulting in the slow movement of contents through the large intestine.

Mixing movements may also be called haustrations. As the circular segmenting contraction occurs, the teniae coli (the three longitudinal muscles) also contract. This provides for more surface contact of the contents to the lumen wall for absorption.

PROPULSIVE MOVEMENTS IN THE COLON

These are the result of the haustral contractions, which are weak peristaltic contractions. These are insufficient to provide for the necessary expulsion of waste products. A mass movement occurs due to an irritation or distension, usually in the transverse colon. Immediately, rapid contraction (spike potentials) of about 20 cm of the colon *distal* to the irritation or distension occurs. These contractions, as a unit, force the entire mass of fecal material forward. A series of mass movements usually occur for up to 30 minutes and may then occur again in ½–1 full day. Most mass movements occur shortly after breakfast and result in movement of the fecal material initiating the defecation response.

Mass movements can cause increased colonic motility as a result of intense stimulation of the parasympathetic nervous system, irritation secondary to conditions such as ulcerative colitis, osmotic overload, or simply distension, use of drugs such as morphine sulfate and/or magnesium sulfate, and an increase of bile salts. Hypermotility results in diarrhea and may cause severe fluid loss and electrolyte imbalance.

Mass movements are inhibited by all of the anticholinergic drugs and by diets deficient in bulk. This may result in constipation due to extra length of time in the large intestine allowing more fluid absorption.

DEFECATION

The majority of the time, the rectum is empty. However, when mass movements of the sigmoid colon move feces into the rectum, the urge to defecate is stimulated. The stimulus is distension of the rectal wall resulting in the stimulation of the myenteric plexus. These nerves cause peristaltic waves in the rectum and the internal anal sphincter relaxes (receptive relaxation) and then the external anal sphincter relaxes so defecation will occur.

At times, relaxation of the sphincters is not sufficient to provide for defecation. In these instances, a Valsalva maneuver assists in the process of defecation.

44

Gastrointestinal Hemorrhage and Esophageal Varices

Learning Objectives

By the end of this chapter, the nurse will be able to:

1. Define
   a. Hematemesis
   b. Melena
   c. Hematochezia
   d. Endoscopy
   e. Topical thrombin
   f. Portacaval shunt
2. Differentiate between gastric and duodenal ulcers.
3. List four common etiologies in gastrointestinal bleeds.
4. Identify presenting signs of gastric ulcers and duodenal ulcers.
5. List five complications of gastrointestinal bleeds.
6. Describe the treatment for gastrointestinal bleeds.
7. Explain the pathophysiology of esophageal varices.
8. Identify the etiologies of esophageal varices.
9. Describe the clinical signs of esophageal bleed.
10. Differentiate between the treatments of esophageal bleed:
    a. Continuous intravenous vasopressin
    b. Selective angiographic vasopressin
    c. Use of Sengstaken-Blakemore or Linton tubes
    d. Portacaval shunts

Hematemesis is gross vomiting of blood. The blood may be fresh, indicated by a bright red color. The blood may be old, having the appearance of coffee grounds with a black color. The black color is the result of hydrochloric acid acting on the blood. If the blood is excreted in the stool, fresh blood will be dark red. Old blood turns feces black (called melena). Hematochezia is the passage of fresh blood through the rectum.

Gastrointestinal Hemorrhage

Upper gastrointestinal hemorrhage is considered to be a bleed from any site proximal to the cecum. Peptic ulcer disease refers to gastric, duodenal, and stomach ulcerations. Stomach ulcerations apply to those at the gastrojejunostomy junction.

PATHOPHYSIOLOGY

Gastrointestinal bleeding occurs when irritation of the mucosa results in erosion through the mucosa and submucosa. All ulcer bleeding is arterial with three exceptions: (1) A tear cuts across all vessels in its path including veins and capillaries. (2) Malignant tumors may erode into all surrounding tissues and vessels. (3) In patients with esophagitis, erosions move through the papillae which contain arterioles, venules, and the capillary bed.

Arteries are eroded into from the side, which results in two bleeding ends because of arterioarterial anastomoses. In *acute* ulcers, adjacent arteries are normal. Therefore, bleeding is consistent and dangerous. Bleeding most commonly occurs from single or multiple erosions in the stomach and/or duodenum but may occur further down the small intestinal tract. An acute bleed occurs if an artery is at the ulcer base.

Some ulcers may become cancerous. These are usually gastric or specifically peptic ulcers that occur after the age of 50. These are more likely to bleed and the bleeding is more severe than when duodenal ulcers are present.

Duodenal ulcers do not often become cancerous, are usually seen in 30- to 40-year-olds, and account for 80% of the ulcers.

ETIOLOGY

Many varied precipitating causes exist that result in an acute G.I. bleed. Ulcers are the result of an excess of hydrochloric acid. Most of the causes may be classified into specific categories which are (1) stress, (2) drugs, (3) hormonal factors, (4) disease processes, and (5) possible hereditary influence.

Stress includes multiple trauma, head injuries, and burns. People with type A personalities are more prone to peptic ulcer disease than people with type B personalities.

Drugs have a major role in the development of ulcers and resultant bleeding. Drugs have many effects upon the G.I. mucosa. Catecholamines and vasopressors decrease blood supply to the G.I. mucosa. Some drugs stimulate hydrochloric acid release, resulting in ulceration in the susceptible patient. Such stimulants include caffeine, nicotine, and pharmaceutical drugs such as reserpine. Some drugs alter the mucosal and submucosal membrane; the most common drug is alcohol. Aspirin, bile salts, and salicylate-containing drugs are other examples. A decrease in the renewal of the mucosal cells is caused mainly by drugs such as the corticosteroids and phenylbutazone (Butazolidin®).

Hormones cause ulceration by sympathetic stimuli and pituitary gland activity. The sympathetic stimuli result in hypersecretion of hydrochloric acid and pepsin. Catecholamines from the adrenal cortex stimulate gastric secretion.

Multiple systemic disease may result in ulcer formation in the susceptible person.

Duodenal ulcers may have an inherited factor because duodenal ulcers tend to occur in people with type O blood. It is theorized that type O blood people do not secrete blood group antigens that are mucopolysaccharides which may protect the mucosa.

CLINICAL PRESENTATION

Heartburn and indigestion usually signal the start of a gastric ulcer attack. Left epigastric pain occurs after a large meal has distended the gastric wall. A feeling of fullness, weight loss, and recurrent episodes of massive G.I. bleeding are typical.

Duodenal ulcers are characterized by heartburn, mid-epigastric pain, weight gain, and an unusual sensation of hot water bubbling in the back of the throat. Attacks normally occur 2 hours after meals (when the stomach is empty) and after drinking orange juice, coffee, alcohol, or taking aspirin. Eating some food relieves the gastric pain (and thus the weight gain).

Both gastric and duodenal ulcers may extend into the pancreas causing severe back pain, or the ulcers may be asymptomatic.

Acute G.I. bleeding will include symptoms of hemodynamic alterations. These changes include a fall in cardiac output, increased pulse rate, hypotension, diaphoresis, thirst, and oliguria. Restlessness is commonly present.

If G.I. bleeding occurs slowly, pallor, fatigue, and faintness may be the presenting complaints.

DIAGNOSIS

The differential diagnosis between a gastric ulcer and a duodenal ulcer is imperative. A gastric ulcer must be proven benign through biopsy and cytology before massive antacid therapy is initiated.

Endoscopy is the primary diagnostic test for upper G.I. hemorrhage because it is highly accurate (85–95%) and has a low morbidity rate. Endoscopy may be performed as soon as ice saline lavage controls the bleeding and lavage-return is pinkish or clear.

If bleeding cannot be cleared for endoscopy, selective angiography may identify the site of bleeding. Once a lesion has been identified, treatment with vasopressin (Pitressin®) infusion will often control the bleed. The left gastric artery is infused for most mucosal lesions.

An upper G.I. series may be done *after* an endoscopy. It should *not* be done prior to the endoscopy since barium will adhere to the mucosa for several hours and interfere with further examinations.

COMPLICATIONS

If the G.I. bleed started precipitously and is of fresh, bright red blood, the major complication is hypovolemic shock. Replacement transfusions may cause reactions and/or D.I.C. The stress of a shock syndrome may result in myocardial infarction, ulcer perforation, peritonitis, and/or sepsis. Septic shock and death may follow these complications.

TREATMENT

An acute G.I. bleed is a life-threatening emergency and the first objective of therapy is to prevent and/or treat shock.

The estimated blood loss is an index to the severity of the bleed. Maintaining circulating blood volume is the first parameter to be stablilzed. Large-bore intravenous needles will provide a route for fluid expanders and blood transfusions to maintain circulating blood volume.

An Ewald or large size nasogastric tube is inserted to provide access for ice saline lavage. Plain ice water is *NOT* used since it removes electrolytes. The accurate amount of fluid in lavage is subtracted from the total amount of aspiration which determines the true amount of blood loss. When ice saline lavage is unsuccessful in stopping the bleeding, ice saline containing levarterenol bitartrate (Levophed®), which acts as a vasoconstrictor, may be added to the normal saline. The normal dilution is 2 ampuls of levarterenol bitartrate per 1,000 ml of normal saline. Levarterenol bitartrate is now known as norepinephrine injection.

With continued bleeding, the administration of topical thrombin into the stomach may be tried. Thrombin clots the blood at the site of bleeding (by acting with fibrinogen). CAUTION: Topical thrombin is used *only* on bleeding surfaces. It is NEVER injected into blood vessels where it would cause intravascular clotting.

If the source of the bleed cannot be identified and abdominal angiography locates the bleed, vasopressin (Pitressin®) may be used. Vasopressin is usually infused in the left gastric artery for most gastric mucosal ulcerations. After 20 minutes of infusing vasopressin at a rate of 0.2 units/minute, an arteriogram should be repeated to confirm control of the bleeding. If bleeding is controlled, the infusion is continued for 24 hours and then gradually decreased.

NURSING INTERVENTIONS

In addition to the nursing interventions for hypovolemic shock (Chapter 37), fluid and electrolyte balance and adequate nutrition are key objectives of nursing treatment.

Administer medications as ordered, watching for cimetidine (Tagamet®) and anticholinergic side effects. These could include dizziness, rash, mild diarrhea, leukopenia, blurred vision, headache, and urinary retention.

If intra-arterial infusion of vasopressin is used, the patient must be monitored closely for bradycardia, hypotension, water intoxication, and post-vasopressin diuresis. Renal status is measured by urinary output, which should be measured at least hourly.

Tachydysrhythmias are a constant potential complication requiring monitoring and intervention as indicated.

The patency of the N/G tube should be maintained to monitor a recurrence of the bleed.

Emotional support of the patient and family will help reduce stress on the patient and family. This may facilitate patient and family cooperation. As the bleeding is brought under control, reassurance will decrease patient fear.

Esophageal Varices

Esophageal varices are frequently associated with hepatic failure and cirrhosis of the liver. Only esophageal varices will be considered here. Hepatic failure and cirrhosis of the liver will be considered in Chapter 45.

PATHOPHYSIOLOGY

A dysfunctioning liver increases portal vein pressure (portal hypertension) due to the inability of the liver to adequately metabolize, synthesize, or detoxify blood flowing through it. In portal vein hypertension, occlusion of the portal or hepatic vein, or liver parenchymal disease increases collateral blood flow, especially to the stomach and esophagus. Portal hypertension causes a backup of blood shunting into the small plexuses and veins at the esophagogastric junction. This results in hypertrophy of the veins at the distal end of the esophagus resulting in fragile vessel walls which are easily eroded by acid or mechanically traumatized, and thus bleed.

Most commonly, a patient with esophageal varices has a past history of liver disease with or without ascites, splenomegaly, anemia, and/or encephalopathy.

ETIOLOGY

The most common cause of esophageal varices is cirrhosis of the liver resulting in portal hypertension. Varices may also be the result of circulatory abnormalities in the splenic vein or superior vena cava causing a portal hypertension.

DIAGNOSIS

Physical examination may reveal jaundice, ascites, splenomegaly, and anemia if cirrhosis of the liver is a causative factor. Laboratory blood studies show increased SGOT, SGPT, LDH, PT, BUN, and alkaline phosphatase.

A history of weight loss, abuse of alcohol, previous bleeds, poor diet habits, and an emotional crisis are common. Frequently, some physical exertion (e.g., coughing) precipitates a bleed.

CLINICAL PRESENTATION

A sudden, painless hemorrhage occurs. Large quantities of blood are lost by hematemesis. Signs of shock are common. All signs of an acute gastrointestinal bleed may be present.

COMPLICATIONS

The complications are frequently irreversible. They include myocardial infarction, congestive heart failure, and renal failure. Almost always signs of hepatic coma or hepatorenal syndrome are present and indicate impending death.

TREATMENT

No completely satisfactory treatment exists. Three objectives of therapy are to control bleeding, treat shock, and stabilize the patient for a portacaval shunt or other therapy. Control of bleeding may be attempted in five ways.

1. Continuous *slow* intravenous vasopressin in minidoses may be tried.

2. Tamponade of the bleeding vessels may be achieved with the Sengstaken-Blakemore (SB) tube or Linton tube (Figure 44-1). Disadvantages of the SB or Linton tube are aspiration and/or asphyxiation by occlusion of the trachea and rebleed with tube removal. This asphyxiation could occur from accumulated pharyngeal secretions or from an SB or Linton tube that slips and occludes the trachea.

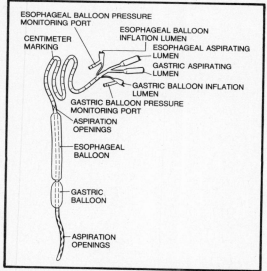

ESOPHAGEAL BALLOON PRESSURE MONITORING PORT
ESOPHAGEAL BALLOON INFLATION LUMEN
CENTIMETER MARKING
ESOPHAGEAL ASPIRATING LUMEN
GASTRIC ASPIRATING LUMEN
GASTRIC BALLOON INFLATION LUMEN
GASTRIC BALLOON PRESSURE MONITORING PORT
ASPIRATION OPENINGS
ESOPHAGEAL BALLOON
GASTRIC BALLOON
ASPIRATION OPENINGS

Figure 44-1. Sengstaken-Blakemore tube.

3. Intra-arterial vasopressin through angiography of the superior mesenteric artery may be attempted. Shock is treated according to normal protocols of fluid and blood replacement, maintenance of electrolyte balance, and vitamin K to reverse the prolonged PT.

4. Portacaval shunts are performed on both an emergency and elective basis to decrease portal hypertension. The results, however, have not appreciably altered the 50% morbidity and mortality rates.

5. Until the 1950s, sclerotherapy was a popular therapy to control bleeding. It is now regaining acceptance but, controlled studies have not been done. Sclerotherapy consists of using an endoscope to inject a substance into a dilated bleeding vessel causing the vessel to sclerose (or harden).

NURSING INTERVENTIONS

A primary objective of nursing interventions is to control the bleeding to prevent or reverse hypovolemic shock (nursing interventions, Chapter 37).

Monitoring electrolyte balance, fluid balance, and nutritional needs will provide for early intervention if a problem appears imminent.

Nursing management of a patient with a Sengstaken-Blakemore or Linton tube to provide tamponade is CONTINUOUS observation for signs of asphyxiation or aspiration. Suctioning pharyngeal secretions is required often. If suctioning does not improve the patient's respiratory status, check for breath sounds in the lungs. If no sounds are heard, most often the SB or Linton tube has slipped and is occluding the trachea. The nurse must *IMMEDIATELY* cut across all the tubes (three) and remove the SB or Linton immediately! For this emergency, scissors are often taped to the head of the bed or wall at the head of the bed.

To prevent ammonia encephalopathy, cathartics such as citrate of magnesia, sorbitol, etc. are administered through the appropriate port of the SB or Linton tube.

If antibiotics are necessary, nonabsorbable ones such as neomycin sulfate are used. This prevents breakdown by intestinal bacteria.

For patients who are receiving intra-arterial vasopressin (Pitressin®), cardiac monitoring and frequent neurological assessments are performed because this drug is a very potent vasoconstrictor. Amyl nitrate, an antagonist vasodilator, should be at the bedside so that it is readily accessible if indications of angina pectoris, myocardial infarction, or encephalopathy occur. Regardless of medical and nursing care, the mortality rate is about 50%.

— 45 —

Cirrhosis of the Liver, Hepatic Failure, and Pancreatitis

Learning Objectives

By the end of this chapter, the nurse will be able to:

1. List three specific forms (etiologies) of cirrhosis of the liver.
2. Identify four complications of cirrhosis of the liver.
3. Enumerate the dietary restrictions in cirrhosis of the liver.
4. Describe the pathophysiology of hepatic failure.
5. List five causes of hepatic failure.
6. Identify six common signs and symptoms of hepatic failure.
7. List four complications of hepatic failure.
8. Describe the three basic interventions in treating hepatic failure.
9. Define acute pancreatitis.
10. Explain the pathophysiology of acute pancreatitis.
11. List six etiologies of acute pancreatitis.
12. Define
    a. Grey Turner's sign
    b. Cullen's sign
    c. Chvostek's sign
    d. Trousseau's sign
13. List a minimum of four presenting signs and symptoms of pancreatitis.
14. List the complications of acute pancreatitis.
15. Identify six nursing interventions in the treatment of acute pancreatitis.

Multiple functions of the liver include the metabolism of CHO, protein, and fat; storage of fat-soluble vitamins, vitamin B$_{12}$, copper, and iron; synthesis of many blood clotting factors, amino acids, albumin, and globulins; deamination of amino acids for glucose; a role in glycolysis and gluconeogenesis; detoxification of many toxic substances; and phagocytosis of many microorganisms.

Cirrhosis of the Liver

Liver functions can be maintained until 50–75% of the hepatocytes (livers cells) are damaged and/or necrotic. Cirrhosis of the liver is the end-stage of many types of liver injury.

PATHOPHYSIOLOGY

There are three specific but artificial categories of cirrhosis which early in the disease have a common pathophysiology. They are (1) Laennec's type cirrhosis, (2) biliary cirrhosis, and (3) postnecrotic cirrhosis. Alternately liver cells are inflamed and/or obstructed causing damage to the cell which occurs first around the central vein. Inflammation recedes and the hepatic lobule regenerates. This cycle is repeated until, at some point, the hepatic lobule is irreversibly damaged. Fibrotic tissue gradually replaces the hepatic tissue as the tissue becomes necrotic.

Areas of necrosis that have become fibrotic alter the shape and contour of the liver decreasing blood flow and lymph flow. This continues until liver function is inadequate in the face of body needs and until hepatic insufficiency, or cirrhosis, is established.

(1) Laennec's type cirrhosis is the most common form and is synonymous with alcoholic, portal, nutritional, and fatty cirrhosis. A dietary deficiency, especially of protein, results in fibrotic scar tissue forming around first the central area of the lobule then the portal area. The fibrotic scar tissue forms nodules and increases fat contents of inflamed cells. Hepatomegaly occurs with this inflammation and recedes to leave a small, nodular, hard-feeling liver.

(2) Biliary cirrhosis is synonymous with obstructive and cholangitic cirrhosis. The scarring that results from inflammation forms around ducts and lobules. Biliary cirrhosis occurs from bile duct disease suppressing the flow of bile, or occluding it in cases of biliary atresia. There is some indication that biliary cirrhosis may have an autoimmune basis.

(3) Postnecrotic or posthepatic cirrhosis occurs following hepatitis or administration of some anesthetics such as halothane.

Other types of cirrhosis include pigment cirrhosis (due to hemochromatosis, etc.), cardiac cirrhosis (caused by right heart failure), and idiopathic cirrhosis (cause unknown).

ETIOLOGY

Laennec's cirrhosis is the result of sustained alcohol abuse and poor nutrition, especially a lack of protein.

Biliary cirrhosis is caused by bile duct disease or obstruction (by stones normally) of the bile ducts.

Postnecrotic cirrhosis is actually a misnomer since cirrhosis occurs due to necrotic tissue. Posthepatic cirrhosis is a more factual nomenclature and occurs after a hepatic infection.

CLINICAL PRESENTATION

Signs and symptoms are similar for all three main classifications of cirrhosis. Vague complaints which occur early are gastrointestinal in origin: nausea, vomiting, anorexia, indigestion, constipation, or diarrhea.

Later signs and symptoms occur due to portal hypertension and hepatic insufficiency. These symptoms include the entire body.

Respiratory changes result in hypoxia secondary to decreased thoracic expansion caused by abdominal ascites.

Central nervous system changes occur because the cirrhotic liver cannot remove ammonia. Ammonia may increase to levels that are toxic to the brain. Consequently, as ammonia levels increase, brain function decreases. Mentation is depressed. Lethargy, slurred speech, asterixis (an uncontrolled, continuous flapping of the hands that indicates the onset of hepatic encephalopathy), paranoia, and hallucinations occur.

Hematologic system symptoms include easy bruising, nose bleeds, anemia, and a prolonged PT time.

The integumentary system (skin) is usually very dry without good skin turgor. Abnormal pigmentation (liver spots, brown spots), spider angiomas, palmar erythema, and jaundice may occur.

The hepatic system symptoms include edema of the lower extremities, ascites, hepatomegaly, jaundice, hepatorenal syndrome, and hepatic encephalopathy. With these symptoms, prognosis is poor.

Other symptoms include a musty smell of the breath (factor hepaticus), muscle atrophy, distended abdominal veins (if ascites is present), and pain in the RUQ, increased by sitting up and/or leaning forward.

Endocrine functions cause some symptoms. These include altered hair distribution with loss of hair on the chest and underarms. There is a testicular hypertrophy, gynecomastia, and menstrual irregularities.

Cardiovascular dysrhythmias are secondary to electrolyte imbalances which may be intractable to treatment.

The renal system may involve the development of the hepatorenal syndrome. The mechanisms are not well understood, however, the liver's inability to detoxify toxins places a very heavy strain upon the kidneys. The kidneys cannot process and excrete many of these toxins, so renal failure develops. This accounts also for the severe, often continuous, pruritis that renal and liver patients develop.

Infections are common and the result of two factors, malnutrition and leukopenia secondary to splenomegaly. Bacteria in the portal blood bypasses the liver so Küpffer cells cannot remove them. Sepsis may result. However, the multiplicity of problems in all body systems adds to the development of infections and sepsis.

DIAGNOSIS

A liver biopsy is the definitive test since cytology studies will detect the inflammation and fibrous characteristics of cirrhosis. Multiple laboratory tests are abnormal. Table 45-1 lists the main laboratory tests.

COMPLICATIONS

The complications of cirrhosis of the liver are the end-stage symptoms of cirrhosis. These include portal hypertension, ascites, esophageal varices, and hepatic encephalopathy (coma). Coma frequently is a sign of impending death.

Table 45-1. Laboratory tests for cirrhosis.

Decreased Levels	Increased Levels
WBC	globulin
hemoglobin	total bilirubin
hematocrit	alkaline phosphatase
albumin	transaminase
serum sodium	lactic dehydrogenase
serum potassium	thymol turbidity
serum chloride	anemia
serum magnesium	neutropenia
cholinesterase	thrombocytopenia
vitamin A	galactose tolerance
vitamin B$_{12}$	urine bilirubin
vitamin C	fecal urobilinogen
vitamin K	urine urobilinogen
folic acid	
iron	

TREATMENT

The primary goal in the treatment of cirrhosis is to maximize liver function. Additional goals include treating the underlying cause and preventing/treating complications.

Dietary enhancement may help restore some liver function. Small meals may be tolerated more than the regular three large meals a day. The diet should be high in protein (0.5 gm/lb/day) to allow regeneration and high in carbohydrate to provide an easy source of energy, sparing the protein as a source of energy. Fat restriction is controversial. Alcohol is prohibited in any form. If hepatic encephalopathy develops, protein intake is markedly restricted. Sodium and fluid intake is also restricted. Multiple vitamins are given since the liver cannot store vitamins A, D, E, and K.

If deterioration is impending or evidenced, paracentesis, administration of salt-poor albumin, ligation of esophageal varices, splenectomy, portacaval shunt, splenorenal shunt, or esophagogastric resection may be attempted.

NURSING INTERVENTIONS

Monitor the neurological status for behavior changes, increasing lethargy, and neuromuscular dysfunction such as asterixis (which is pathognomonic for impending hepatic encephalopathy).

Check the skin, gums, emesis, and stools often for bleeding. Apply pressure at I.M. sites. Notify a physician of the development of bleeding dyscrasias or an increase in bleeding.

Monitor fluid retention by weighing the patient daily and measuring abdominal girth (mark abdomen where measured to ensure all measurements are at the same spot). Check for dependent edema and maintain accurate I & O records.

If paracentesis is performed, note the amount of fluid removed and closely monitor the patient for signs of shock.

Prevent skin breakdown, which is not uncommon, due to edema and pruritus. Bathe the patient with moisturizing lotion, not soap. Turn the patient regularly and ensure rest to prevent an energy drain on the patient.

Educate the patient and family of the importance of proper diet, avoidance of alcohol, moderate exercise, and avoidance of any drugs (including OTC), especially aspirin, unless the physician approves of the use of specific drugs.

Hepatic Failure

When damage and destruction of the hepatocytes become so extensive that the liver cannot perform its normal functions, hepatic failure has occurred.

PATHOPHYSIOLOGY

The pathophysiology of *early* hepatic failure is usually the development of one of the forms of cirrhosis of the liver.

Damaged or destroyed hepatocytes result in decreased liver function which causes more damage to remaining hepatocytes and the cycle is established.

Advanced liver failure, regardless of etiology, occurs when the liver's compensatory mechanisms fail. At this stage, the serum ammonia levels rise. Theorists maintain that ammonia (NH_3), which would normally be converted to urea, remains in the circulation and binds with a carrier forming ammonium ion (NH_4^+). Due to acid/base imbalances, diarrhea, and endocrine dysfunction, the ammonium ion dissociates to form ammonia and a hydrogen ion. Chemically, this reaction is

$$NH_4^+ \rightarrow NH_3 + H^+$$

ammonium ion → ammonia molecule + hydrogen ion

The increase in hydrogen ions causes an acidosis with elevated ammonia levels.

In this advanced state of hepatic failure, the liver is unable to degrade amino acids or synthesize its normal blood clotting factors, so clotting dyscrasias occur. Equally important as the increased ammonia and acidosis is the liver's inability to regulate glucose levels, store glycogen, or form gluconeogenesis. The resulting hypoglycemia may be as deleterious to the brain as the increasing ammonia levels and acidosis leading to a hepatic precoma or frank hepatic encephalopathy.

ETIOLOGY

Multiple causes exist that precipitate liver failure. Most often a chronic liver disease (cirrhosis) exists and an additional stressor precipitates the hepatic failure.

These stressors include, but are not limited to, alcohol ingestion, G.I. bleeding, a dietary intake of large amounts of protein, sedative drugs, and portacaval shunt surgery. Acute liver failure may result from hepatitis (viral or toxic), biliary obstruction, cancers, other acute infections, multiple drugs and anesthetics, and dehydration from rapid diuresis or paracentesis causing a shock state with or without electrolyte imbalances.

CLINICAL PRESENTATION

Early signs and symptoms are the same as cirrhosis of the liver. Moderate signs are altered mental status, incontinence, and tremors (if the patient is alert and can cooperate with testing assessment). A useful test in determining the stage of liver failure is to have the patient sign his or her name daily. As liver failure becomes irreversible, the patient has an increasingly hard time until at precoma stage the writing has become illegible. Advanced signs indicative of impending death include those shown in Figure 45-1 and in coma without response to noxious stimuli.

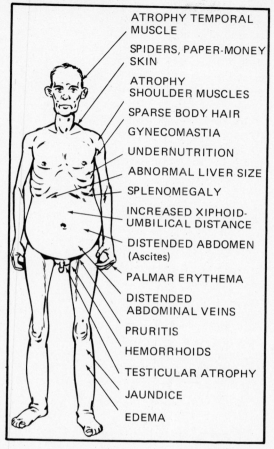

ATROPHY TEMPORAL MUSCLE

SPIDERS, PAPER-MONEY SKIN

ATROPHY SHOULDER MUSCLES

SPARSE BODY HAIR

GYNECOMASTIA

UNDERNUTRITION

ABNORMAL LIVER SIZE

SPLENOMEGALY

INCREASED XIPHOID-UMBILICAL DISTANCE

DISTENDED ABDOMEN (Ascites)

PALMAR ERYTHEMA

DISTENDED ABDOMINAL VEINS

PRURITIS

HEMORRHOIDS

TESTICULAR ATROPHY

JAUNDICE

EDEMA

Figure 45-1. Advanced signs of hepatic failure.

DIAGNOSIS

Diagnosis of hepatic failure is established by a previous history of cirrhosis of the liver, most commonly due to alcoholic cirrhosis. In addition, liver function studies will be abnormal and encephalopathy is present which is progressive in spite of treatment.

COMPLICATIONS

All complications of hepatic coma are life-threatening. They include DIC, hepatorenal syndrome, sepsis and septic shock, and intracranial hemorrhage. These complications most often are intractable to treatment.

TREATMENT

The objective of treatment is to stop the progression of hepatic encephalopathy by decreasing serum ammonia levels.

Neomycin sulfate and kanamycin sulfate (Kantrex®) prevent intestinal bacteria from converting amino acids into ammonia. Sorbitol-induced catharsis produces an osmotic diarrhea which further empties the intestines to help reduce conversion of products to ammonia.

Dietary protein is decreased or eliminated to prevent its degradation into amino acids and ammonia. Hyperalimentation with $D_{10}W$ or $D_{50}W$, essential amino acids, vitamins, and minerals is the preferred diet. Lactulose keeps ammonia in the intestines and lactulose breaks down to form lactic acid which makes the intestines too acidic for bacterial function.

Electrolytes, especially potassium, may be needed to counter alkalosis.

Hemodialysis sometimes improves hepatic encephalopathy *temporarily*, as does exchange transfusions.

Treatment of hepatic encephalopathy is essentially supportive rather than curative.

NURSING INTERVENTIONS

Frequent assessment of the patient's neurological status is an index of the patient's response to therapy.

Monitor intake and output, fluid status, and electrolyte status. Signs of anemia, infection, alkalosis (increasing serum HCO_3^-), melena, or hematemesis should be reported to the physician to provide an opportunity to prevent complications.

Administer medications as ordered avoiding sedatives and hepatotoxic drugs. Monitor for side effects (even with reduced dosage). The unconscious patient's eyes must be protected with eyedrops if the corneal reflexes are absent.

Emotional support of the patient (if alert) and the family with realistic responses to the patient's condition is appropriate and essential since the expected outcome is very poor.

Acute Pancreatitis

Acute pancreatitis is an inflammatory disease of the pancreas gland resulting in enzymatic autodigestion of the pancreas.

PATHOPHYSIOLOGY

The *theorized* pathophysiology of acute pancreatitis is that an obstruction causes widespread edema of the pancreas. Precipitating factors which seem associated to this condition are abuse of alcohol and biliary tract disease.

Edema of the pancreas, secondary to obstruction of outflow, increases pressure within the pancreatic duct system since pancreatic juices are continuously produced. The increased pressure eventually results in the rupturing of ducts releasing their enzymes into the pancreatic cells.

Trypsin is an important proenzyme catalyst. Trypsin probably activates pancreatic enzymes phospholipase A, elastase, and kallikrein. The functions of these enzymes are speculative. Trypsin causes edema, necrosis, and hemorrhage in the pancreas. Elastase is thought to contribute to the hemorrhage by attacking the walls of small blood vessels. Phospholipase A is thought to have a role in coagulation, and fat necrosis and somehow damages the acinar cell membrane. Kallikrein may be the cause of vasomotor changes, edema, and increased permeability of the vascular tree. Kallikrein also probably causes the pain of pancreatitis.

ETIOLOGY

Alcoholism and biliary tract disease are the most common causes of pancreatitis. Blunt, penetrating, or surgical trauma may precipitate an acute pancreatitis as can cancer of the pancreas. Peptic ulcer disease, certain drugs (steroids, isoniazid, and sulfonamides), and mumps are more uncommon causes. More rarely, stenosis or obstruction of the sphincter of Oddi, spasms of the ampulla of Vater, hyperparathyroidism, and a hereditary factor may be identified as the precipitating event.

CLINICAL PRESENTATION

Epigastric pain radiating to the back and unrelieved by vomiting is almost always present, even in mild cases.

Severe cases may have excruciating pain, continuous vomiting, abdominal rigidity, low-grade fever, tachycardia, or hypoventilation with mottled skin and cold extremities. The patient appears critically ill and if the pancreatitis is of a fulminating type, massive hemorrhage, total destruction of the pancreas, diabetes mellitus, diabetic acidosis, shock, coma, and death is the pattern of the illness.

DIAGNOSIS

Grey Turner's sign (ecchymoses in the thigh and groin), Cullen's sign (ecchymoses around the umbilicus), Chvostek's sign (tapping cheek causes facial muscle spasm), and Trousseau's sign (spasmodic contraction of muscle when supplying nerve has pressure applied to it) are present.

Amylase levels (up to or over 500 units) differentiate pancreatitis from peptic ulcer perforation, appendicitis, cholecystitis, and/or bowel infarction/obstruction. EKG changes mimic a myocardial infarction with S-T segment depression and T wave changes. Table 45-2 identifies specific laboratory tests.

Table 45-2. Laboratory test to diagnose pancreatitis.

Markedly elevated serum amylase levels—often over 500 units. Characteristically, amylase levels return to normal 48 hours after onset of pancreatitis.

Supportive laboratory values include:
1. increased serum lipase levels
2. low serum calcium (hypocalcemia)
3. WBC counts ranging from 8,000–20,000/mm^3, with increased PMNs
4. elevated glucose levels as high as 500–900 mg/100 ml
5. hematocrit sometimes exceeding 50% concentrations

COMPLICATIONS

Progressive pancreatic necrosis and involvement of surrounding tissues causing necrosis usually result in a rapid deterioration of the patient. This progression is characterized by sustained tachycardia, pulse, fever, white count, and a fall in serum calcium levels.

Late complications include hemorrhage, abcess formation, pseudocyst, and intestinal obstructions. If hemorrhage occurs, hypovolemic shock, renal failure (secondary to hypovolemia), septic shock, and myocardial infarction (secondary to myocardial depressant factor release from the pancreas) are possible complications. If an abcess forms, it may produce a fistula, especially if the abcess is surgically drained.

TREATMENT

The objective of therapy is first to achieve and to maintain adequate circulatory fluid volume. If the diagnosis is acute necrotizing pancreatitis, hypovolemic shock is common. Although volume replacement is essential, electrolytes and protein (free amino acids) must be included in fluid therapy. A commonly used fluid replacement is at least 50 gm of albumin and 2–4 liters of Ringer's lactate per day for the first few days (up to three), then substitution of the colloids by crystalloids with the rate equal to the daily loss. Electrolytes must be added as needed to prevent complications from imbalances.

Pain relief is achieved through the use of meperidine hydrochloride (Demerol®), not morphine sulfate. Demerol *may* cause sphincter of Oddi spasm; morphine sulfate almost always does. Diazepam (Valium®) may decrease restlessness. Broad-spectrum antibiotics are used for infections. Hyperglycemia > 300–350 mg/100 ml requires insulin therapy and hypocalcemia must be corrected to prevent tetany (warning

signs—muscle cramps, carpopedal spasm, and convulsions).

NURSING INTERVENTIONS

In the acute cases, pancreatitis is life-threatening and requires both vigorous treatment and vigorous nursing care.

Monitoring the patient's status is more accurate with a pulmonary artery catheter than with a central venous pressure (CVP) line. If a CVP line is used, it should not exceed 10 cm H_2O. If it exceeds this, volume expanders are NOT needed.

All vital signs are checked at least hourly: These include T, P, R, B/P, urine output, and amount of intake. Urine is tested for glucose and acetone. If they are present, serum glucose should be checked for hyperglycemia.

Respiratory status is monitored by ABGs and hourly auscultation of lungs for rales, rhonchi, wheezing, and diminished breath sounds.

Cardiac monitoring is essential to detect dysrhythmias which are frequent with shock and/or electrolyte imbalances.

An N/G tube is inserted and connected to suction to prevent a buildup of acid secretions in the stomach. Mouth and nose care should be given hourly, especially if anticholinergic drugs are administered. CAUTION: Atropine and its derivatives are contraindicated in narrow angle glaucoma.

Medicate the patient as ordered. (Demerol® is preferred for pain.) Observe for side effects of all medications, especially antibiotics.

Emotional support is very important because the pain is severe, the N/G tube is uncomfortable, and the monitoring equipment increases apprehension.

Gastrointestinal Bibliography

Borg N, Mikas DL, Stark J, Williams SM (eds): Core Curriculum for Critical Care Nursing, 2nd ed. American Association of Critical-Care Nurses. Philadelphia: W. B. Saunders, pp. 399–438, 1981

*Gastrointestinal disorders and hepatobiliary disorders. *In* Diseases (causes and diagnosis, current therapy, nursing management, and patient education). Nursing 82 books, The nurse's reference library. Springhouse, PA: Intermed Communications, Inc., pp. 648–747, 1982

*Guyton AC: Textbook of Medical Physiology, 6th ed. Philadelphia: W. B. Saunders, pp. 784–835, 1981

Jeejeebhoy KN (ed): Gastrointestinal Diseases: Focus on Clinical Diagnosis. Garden City, NY: Medical Examination Publishing Co., Inc., 1980

Mallory A, Sunder JM: Gastroenterology. *In* Reller LB, Sahn SA, Schrier RW (eds): Clinical Internal Medicine. Boston, MA: Little, Brown and Co., pp. 195–236, 1979

Mehta SJ, Friedman HH: Gastrointestinal problems. *In* Friedman HH (ed): Problem-Oriented Medical Diagnosis, 2nd ed. Boston, MA: Little, Brown and Co., pp. 144–180, 1979

Palmer ED: Practical Points in Gastroenterology, 3rd ed. Garden City, NY: Medical Examination Publishing Co., Inc., 1980

Perrillo RP: Liver disease. *In* Freitag JJ, Miller LW (eds): Manual of Medical Therapeutics, 23rd ed. Boston, MA: Little, Brown and Co., pp. 239–251, 1980

*A Programmed Approach to Anatomy and Physiology of the Digestive System. Bowie, MD: Robert J. Brady Co., 1972

*Proteins, protein metabolites, and pigments, and carbohydrates. *In* Diagnostics (patient preparation, interpretation, sources of error, post-test care). Nursing 82 books, The nurse's reference library. Springhouse, PA: Intermed Communications, Inc., pp. 217–259, 1982

Stenson WF: Gastrointestinal diseases. *In* Freitag JJ, Miller LW (eds): Manual of Medical Therapeutaics, 23rd ed. Boston, MA: Little, Brown and Co., pp. 261–278, 1980

Thal ER, McClelland RN, Shires GT: Abdominal trauma. *In* Shires GT (ed): Care of the Trauma Patient, 2nd ed. New York: McGraw-Hill, pp. 290–342, 1979

*Toskes PP: The Digestive System: Disease, Diagnosis, Treatment. Bowie, MD: Robert J. Brady Co., 1975

Zukerman BR: Gastrointestinal bleeding. *In* Freitag JJ, Miller LW (eds): Manual of Medical Therapeutics, 23rd ed. Boston, MA: Little, Brown and Co., pp. 253–260, 1980

VIII

Shock States

46

Anaphylactic and Septic Shock

Learning Objectives

By the end of this chapter, the nurse will be able to:

1. Define anaphylactic shock.
2. Explain the pathophysiology of anaphylaxis.
3. List the two most common etiologies of anaphylaxis.
4. Describe the clinical presentation of anaphylaxis.
5. Explain the rationale for three treatments in anaphylaxis.
6. Explain the pathophysiology of septic shock.
7. Explain why antibiotic therapy may be an etiology of septic shock.
8. Describe the clinical presentation of the warm stage of septic shock.
9. Describe the clinical presentation of the cold stage of septic shock.
10. List four treatments and interventions for septic shock.

Anaphylactic Shock

Anaphylaxis is an acute, generalized, and violent antigen-antibody reaction which may be rapidly fatal even with prompt emergency treatment.

PATHOPHYSIOLOGY

Upon first exposure to an antigen, antibodies (of the immunoglobulin IgE) are formed and attach to mast cells in tissues and basophils in the vascular system. (Chapter 36 reviews antibody-antigen formation and reactions.) Once antibodies have been formed, a second exposure to the antigen results in an immune reaction (releasing histamine) which may vary from mild to fatal. In its severe form, the reaction is called anaphylactic shock.

The reaction of anaphylactic shock is primarily a histamine reaction setting off a chain of multiple chemical reactions which causes further reactions. The more reactions that occur, the more severe the anaphylaxis and the greater the mortality.

The release of histamine results in vasodilatation of the capillaries (causing hypotension) and a markedly increased cellular permeability. The increase in intracellular fluid alters the cell shape leaving spaces between the previously compact cells. This promotes movement from the vascular system increasing the colloid osmotic pressure. As more colloids move into interstitial spaces, edema and a decreased circulating volume of blood occurs. This has the effect of decreasing cardiac output.

Histamine occurs in two forms in the body named H_1 and H_2. H_1 causes vasoconstriction of the bronchi and intestines. H_2 increases gastric acid secretion and minor cardiac stimulation. Both H_1 and H_2 are responsible for the vasodilatation.

The release and action of histamines result in the release of other amines into the bloodstream. Bradykinin, serotonin, slow-reacting substances, a chemotactic factor attracting eosinophils, prostaglandins, and acetylcholine all play a role in the physiologic development of anaphylaxis. These chemicals may also activate the complement system. These amines increase arteriolar and venous dilatation, capillary permeability, and abnormal shift of fluid from the vascular tree into the interstitial compartment. This shift decreases circulating blood volume but does not decrease total blood in the body. With blood remaining in the microcirculation, decreased systolic and diastolic pressure occurs. These substances and H_1 and H_2 cause an intense bronchiolar constriction which leads to a general hypoxemia.

ETIOLOGY

Drug reactions, especially antibiotics, are the major allergens in anaphylaxis. Other drugs, iodine-based contrast dye, and blood transfusions are also involved in anaphylaxis.

If possible, broad-spectrum antibiotics should not be used before identification of the invading organism. Broad-spectrum antibiotics alter the normal flora, allowing opportunistic bacteria to gain access within the body.

Aside from medications injected or ingested, bites and stings from insects are the major causes of anaphylaxis. Of these, the sting of bees and yellow jackets are the most common, but wasps and hornets may also cause anaphylaxis.

CLINICAL PRESENTATION

The major symptoms resulting from release of histamine and other chemicals are anxiety, severe dyspnea (may have cyanosis), and angioedema. Angioedema is edema in membranous tissues and is most easily seen in the eyes and mouth. It also occurs in the tongue, hands, feet, and genitalia.

There is a diffuse erythema occurring more in the upper body parts than in the lower. Occasionally, abdominal cramps, vomiting, and/or diarrhea may occur. Unconsciousness occurs early in severe anaphylaxis.

As fluid shifts from the capillaries into the interstitial tissue, edema of the uvula and larynx occurs. This edema may produce an acute respiratory obstruction. Laryngeal edema is accompanied by the patient having impaired phonation and a barking or high-pitched cough. If the patient is alert, he or she will show signs of increased anxiety and complain of air hunger.

Cardiovascular effects of anaphylaxis are the same as those associated with other types of shock—mainly hypotension, tachycardia, and changes in the EKG similar to those that occur in myocardial injury. Temporary changes in the S-T segment and the T wave suggest coronary ischemia. However, the serum enzymes are normal.

The changes in ventilation (causing hypoxia) and decreased circulating blood may result in convulsions and unconsciousness. Circulatory failure and laryngeal edema are the usual causes of death in anaphylaxis.

COMPLICATIONS

Myocardial infarction secondary to decreased cardiac output and venous return results in a decreased blood pressure. With decreased cardiac output, increased tissue hypoxia occurs. Increased tissue hypoxia results in increased tissue anoxia and destruction. Hypoventilation occurs due to the decreased venous return of blood to the heart and increases tissue hypoxia.

Pulmonary status, already compromised by bronchiolar constriction, may be further damaged due to overadministration of intravenous fluids which are used to compensate for the decreased vascular volume.

Chemical reactions causing further imbalances may lead to central nervous system convulsions and coma.

If the pulmonary, cardiac, and/or vascular system is refactory to treatment, anaphylaxis is fatal.

TREATMENT

The primary objective of treatment is to dilate the bronchioles which is accomplished by the administration of epinephrine either subcutaneously or intramuscularly. Antihistamines may help control local edema and itching but they cannot alter the circulatory failure and bronchoconstriction to a significant degree. Having administered epinephrine, support of the respiratory system is indicated by mask, intubation, or tracheostomy with the use of a ventilator.

The second goal of therapy is to improve the patient's circulatory status. Promoting the movement of fluid from the interstitial compartment back into the vascular compartment is usually achieved through the use of intravenous fluids. Vasopressors may be used to cause constriction of the blood vessels. However, this can make tissue anoxia more severe and use of them is controversial. The third-space loss of fluid is believed to be caused by leakage through the injured capillary walls. Glucocorticoids help to decrease cellular damage, reduce the severity of anaphylaxis, and prevent inflammation of the damaged tissues. Hydrocortisone given intravenously is the usual drug used. Steroids stabilize the membrane of the basophils reducing the chemical reactions in anaphylaxis.

In addition to maintaining respiratory status, using epinephrine, and administrating glucocorticoids (both those formed by the body in response to stress and synthetic forms), intravenous fluid will increase the circulating blood volume. Intravenous fluids may have electrolytes added to control acid-base imbalances.

NURSING INTERVENTIONS

Assessment of the symptoms in all body systems is extremely important. Research has shown that laryngeal edema and hypo-tension are major factors causing death.

Anaphylaxis may occur in susceptible patients immediately or as much as an hour after injection of an antigen (drug, blood). Respiratory assessment includes identifying signs of stridor, the use of axillary muscles for breathing, and/or cyanosis; auscultating lung fields for rales, rhonchi, or wheezes; and measuring arterial blood gases. Mechanical ventilation should be on stand-by if not already in use. Normal nursing interventions for patients on respirators are applicable for these patients.

Monitoring the patient's cardiac and circulatory status is best achieved by using a pulmonary artery catheter. Death can occur within minutes if there is circulatory failure or pulmonary edema. These parameters must be observed continuously until the patient is stable and then at very frequent intervals (at least every 15 minutes for four times, then every 30 minutes for four times, and then every 1–2 hours).

Antihistamines are not usually helpful in altering circulatory failure and bronchoconstriction. The use of antihistamines does not affect the release of histamine but they do occupy receptor sites, thus preventing the attachment of histamine. Administration of these drugs requires close observation due to their central nervous system depression effect. If epinephrine is used intravenously, monitoring for hypertension and cardiac dysrhythmias is essential. Also, the nurse must maintain a patent line since epinephrine causes tissue necrosis if extravasation occurs.

Renal status is monitored by Foley catheter to prevent fluid overload as the extracellular fluid moves back into the vascular system with appropriate drugs.

In severe anaphylaxis, the patient is frequently comatose, and establishing the monitoring and support systems may leave little, if any, time for psychosocial support. As the patient's condition stabilizes and his or her level of consciousness returns to normal, emotional support is essential. Explaining to the patient what has happened, what all the monitoring equipment is being used for, and that these monitors will be removed as his or her condition improves will help to alleviate the patient's fear.

Septic Shock

Synonyms for septic shock are bacterial shock, toxic shock, bacteremic shock, and endotoxic shock. Gram negative bacterial shock is the most common. Gram positive bacterial shock also occurs.

PATHOPHYSIOLOGY

Most authorities agree that there are two basic stages of septic shock with varying pathophysiology and symptomatology. A warm phase in early septic shock gives rise to a cold phase in the late stage of septic shock.

Warm Phase

Endotoxins are a part of the cell membrane of bacteria. As these bacteria are destroyed by the body's immune system, the endotoxins are released into the vascular system. This begins a series of interactions between body cells and the body's immune system. Endotoxins precipitate a systemic inflammatory response which includes activation of the complement cascade and release of histamine. This results in systemic vasodilation and increased capillary permeability. Capillary pores are enlarged so protein and plasma fluids shift into the interstitial tissues of the microcirculation.

Cold Phase

The cold phase indicates that multiple body systems are compromised by the many chemical reactions initiated by the endotoxins. The lungs, liver, and heart are the major systems involved.

Lungs become less compliant due to extravasation of fluid from the vascular system into the alveoli. Microembolization of platelets and WBCs furthers the release of vasoactive substances which in turn increases lung resistance. Often the patient will develop ARDS at this point.

The liver is unable to filter and detoxify the endotoxins because of microembolization in the liver itself and because the blood entering the liver is more viscous than normal, often sludging in the hepatic microcirculation.

The heart is affected by several actions. Initially, cardiac output is increased, responding to decreased volume and pressure. Tachycardia results. In cold phase septic shock, a myocardial toxic factor (MTF) is released from the prolonged constriction of the splanchnic organs. MTF has a negative inotropic effect. MTF blocks the action of calcium ions essential for cardiac contraction.

The bottom line in septic shock is that tissue hypoxia occurs as a result of increased capillary permeability and vasoactive chemicals trying to neutralize endotoxins.

ETIOLOGY

Patients at a high risk to develop septic shock include the very young, the very old, the debilitated, and those with chronic disease. Other development of septic shock occurs most frequently when there is an infection present in the urinary tract, the respiratory tract, postsurgery, in burns, and in skin and soft tissue infections. The shock may be secondary to meningitis, cellulitis, or decubitus ulcers. Any factor that compromises the body's immune system may result in septic shock. Any and all invasive procedures (pacemaker insertion, blood transfusion, hyperalimentation) may result in septic shock.

CLINICAL PRESENTATION

There may be a wide range of symptoms indicating septic shock or there may be only a drop in blood pressure or slight alteration in mentation. The more rapidly septic shock is diagnosed, the greater the chances for recovery.

In the warm phase there is generally a vasodilation as evidenced by warm skin, a flushed face, and a temperature greater than 102°F. A moderate tachycardia, < 120 per minute, is accompanied by increased cardiac output and increased stroke volume. Pulse pressure is within normal range and many patients have a pulse rate less than 72 per minute. The patient is normally alert in the early warm phase. As the phase progresses from warm to cold there is a decreased venous return, decreased cardiac output, and decreased systolic B/P.

In the cold phase, there is extreme vasoconstriction due to an increase in epinephrine and norepinephrine. This extreme hyperactivity causes a release of histamine, serotonin, bradykinin, kallikrein II, and angiotensin II from the cells. These vasoactive substances are indicative of a deteriorating state. The skin is cold, pale, and clammy. Subnormal body temperature is evidence that the body is unable to maintain metabolic heat production. There is a greater decrease in venous return, cardiac output, and stroke volume than in the warm stage. The patient may be oliguric or anuric due to a decreased glomerular filtration rate. The patient's mental status deteriorates from an alert stage to confusion, incoherence, possible bizzare behavior, and coma.

Cell hypoxia causes a metabolic acidosis as the cell uses anaerobic mechanisms to maintain metabolic function.

Fresh whole blood may be transfused if indicated and some hospitals use an infusion of glucose, potassium, and insulin (GKI). These substances are needed intracellularly to continue metabolic function. Administration of GKI is still controversial.

Sympathomimetic drugs (Dopamine® and Dobutamine®) are sometimes used to counter the vasodilation causing a lowered peripheral resistance.

The use of steroids, although controversial, is gaining acceptance when they are used with additional intravenous fluids and antimicrobial drug therapy.

NURSING INTERVENTIONS

The primary nursing intervention is to assess and maintain a patient ventilatory status. This requires monitoring the patient to identify signs of hypoxia, increased work of breathing, cyanosis, hyperventilation, or tetany. (Staring into space without focusing often is a clue to the development of alkalosis.) If the patient is on a respirator, the routine patient care is carried out including auscultation of lung fields.

Monitoring the cardiovascular system, preferably with a pulmonary artery catheter, is essential because septic shock may rapidly (in minutes) change from early to late shock with no chance of resuscitating the patient. The MTF will cause marked cardiac dysrhythmias leading to asystole.

Renal status is measured by an indwelling Foley catheter on an hourly or less basis. The urine excreted will help to monitor the intravenous fluids to prevent fluid overload as well as to warn of impending renal failure.

Neurologic status is assessed over a period of time to establish a base-line level of mentation. If the neurologic status deteriorates, there will be signs of apprehension, behavioral changes, and decreasing alertness.

Emotional support of the patient is vital since one of the first symptoms is extreme anxiety. An explanation of treatment modalities, monitoring equipment, and nursing procedures will help decrease the patient's anxiety. The same information should be provided to the patient's family to solicit their assistance in meeting the patient's emotional needs.

Shock Bibliography

*Bordicks KJ: Patterns of Shock: Implications for Nursing Care, 2nd ed. New York: Macmillan, 1980

Borg N, Mikas DL, Stark J, Williams SM (eds): Core Curriculum for Critical Care Nursing, 2nd ed. American Association of Critical-Care Nurses. Philadelphia: W. B. Saunders, pp. 154–165, 1981

Hardy JD (ed): Critical Surgical Illness, 2nd ed. Philadelphia: W. B. Saunders, pp. 25–41, 290–325, 508–525, 591–596, 1980

*Meislin HW (ed): Priorities in Multiple Trauma. Germantown, MD: Aspen Systems Corp., 1980

*Perry AG, Potter PA (eds): Shock: Comprehensive Nursing Management. St. Louis, MO: C. V. Mosby, 1983

Trunkey DD: The effects of hormones and toxic factors in shock. In Current Concepts, A Scope Publication. Kalamazoo, MI: The Upjohn Co., 1979

*Walt AJ, Wilson RF (eds): Management of Trauma: Pitfalls and Practice. Philadelphia: Lea and Febiger, pp. 56–75, 136–147, 463–581, 1975

IX

Psychosocial Aspects of Critical Illness

— 47

Psychosocial Ramifications of Critical Illness

Learning Objectives

By the end of this chapter, the nurse will be able to:

1. List Maslow's hierarchy of needs.
2. Define
   a. Self-concept
   b. Self-esteem
   c. Body image
   d. Perception
   e. Need
   f. Distress
3. List nursing interventions for the patient experiencing:
   a. Fear and anxiety
   b. Powerlessness
   c. Loneliness
   d. Pain
   e. Sensory overload
   f. Sensory deprivation
4. Define the two types of crises that exist.
5. Describe the four stages in a crisis.
6. Define suicide.
7. List nursing interventions for the suicidal patient.
8. Define death.
9. List the five psychological stages of death and dying described by Elizabeth Kübler-Ross.
10. List nursing interventions for the dying patient.

It has been shown through research that critical patient's and their families are more stressed than patients and families in non-critical care areas of the hospital. Analo-gously and as one might expect, research has shown that critical care nurses "burnout" from stress more rapidly than other nurse health care providers.

Nursing Stress

Over the past few years research into the areas of nursing stress and burnout has identified the causes of stress and ways of effectively coping with burnout. The reader is referred to any one of the many excellent available books, articles, slide presentations, lectures, seminars, and workshops for an in-depth review of these topics.

Aspects of the Critical Care Nurse

Research has shown that critical care nurses as a group are more aggressive than other nurses, are more comfortable with the extensive use of monitoring equipment than other nurses, and enjoy the challenge of the critically ill and multiple trauma patient. On the average, critical care nurses are younger than nurses in non-critical care areas. Perhaps age is a factor in nursing burnout. This is based on the fact that younger, less experienced critical care nurses may not be aware of their *own* needs which must be met in some form to prevent burnout.

Common Nurse-Patient Needs

A need is any physical or emotional factor *not* being met which causes anxiety in the nurse and/or patient and which should be met. Maslow (perhaps the best authority in this area) has arranged the needs common to all persons.

Maslow's hierarchy of needs builds from the basic physiological survival needs (air, food, shelter, etc.) to safety and security needs to love and belonging to self-esteem and to self-actualization. One probably can never achieve self-actualization. It is probably a dynamic life process. Once one achieves the desired, "final" objective, a new "final" objective appears. Thus, self-actualization needs are probably dynamic.

If one uses Maslow's hierarchy of needs, then the greatest need throughout one's life is to feel adequate as a person (self-actualization). Adequacy has three major components. Any one of these three being negative prohibits the person (patient, nurse, or relative) from feeling completely adequate.

These three components are self-concept, self-esteem, and body image.

1. Self-concept is the total of tangible (brown hair) and intangible (trustworthiness) factors that *intellectually* identifies one's existence, both consciously and subconsciously.

2. Self-esteem is the emotional *feeling* one has about one's self. Rationally or irrationally, one feels at varying times like a success or failure at a task, at life, in relationships, and eventually with himself or herself. A positive self-esteem fosters a positive self-concept and adequacy as a person.

3. Body image is the final component that makes one feel adequate or inadequate. Body image is one's *belief* about one's self, rational or irrational. Body image changes throughout life and often is expressed by one's appearance and the activities in which one engages.

Positive thinking (self-concept), positive feeling (self-esteem), and positive belief (body image) of one's self fosters a feeling of adequacy. Alterations, both positive and negative, in any one of these three concepts alters the remaining two.

Coping with Stress

On one hand, if one's beliefs are negative, one's body image, self-esteem, and self-concept are negative. Thus, frustrating limitations of one's ability to cope in a given situation (i.e., critical crisis) are present.

On the other hand, if one's beliefs are positive, one's body image, self-esteem, and self-concept will provide a source of coping adequately in a given situation (i.e., critical crisis). Coping adequately helps perpetuate future coping successfully. Failing to cope with a situation tends to make future coping more difficult or even impossible.

Attempts to cope with a situation in a critical care area are influenced by the patient's strengths, potentials, and limitations. Most of these three factors have evolved over a period of time and have a social component.

A strength is some inner characteristic

one believes about one's self. It may be an ability to perform some task or it may be an attribute such as dependability.

Potentials are present in everyone and encompass all those abilities, objectives, and goals that one *could* achieve if so desired.

Limitations are the imagined and the real factors which prevent one from performing certain tasks and achieving specified goals. The strengths, potentials, and limitations of each individual affects one's self-concept, self-esteem, and body image.

Stress for Patients

Hans Selye may be considered the first "stress expert." He defines the absence of stress as eustress and explains that eustress may become distress at any given time for any given person.

Illness, especially critical illness, certainly presents distress for patients (unless they are in a coma) and their families. Some of the stresses experienced include fear, anxiety, powerlessness, loneliness, pain, sensory overload, sensory deprivation, and fear of dying.

Not all patients will perceive all these factors as stressors. Perception will differ with each patient and family depending on the interpretation of the stimulus. Perception involves all the body's senses: touch, sound, smell, sight, and taste. A stimulus of any sense will result in an *awareness* of the stimulus unless a person is in a deep coma.

Dealing with Patient Stress

In helping a patient deal with his or her stress, the critical care nurse sometimes becomes frustrated and gives up. The best nursing interventions are simple acts. (Some of these are identified with each stressor.)

The critical care nurse is in the habit of identifying a problem, determining an appropriate action, and evaluating the response to the action taken. That is, the critical care nurse is often expecting a "quick fix." The psychosocial needs for the patient coping with his or her stressors include time for adjustment, sorting things out,

and so on. Psychology and psychiatry are long-term treatment modalities that may be started in critical care areas but rarely, if ever, completed there.

Patient Fear and Anxiety

Fear is a tangible reaction to a specific known danger (fear of dying, fear of a respirator) whereas anxiety is based on an unknown factor. When anxiety becomes severe or panic, specific physical symptoms may be observed. Tachypnea, tachycardia, pupil dilatation, and apprehension/restlessness are present. Anorexia, nausea, vomiting, and diarrhea may occur.

The nursing intervention is to communicate with (not to) the patient that he or she believes the patient is anxious or frightened and identify ways to decrease the patient's fear. Helping the patient ventilate his or her feelings often identifies specific problem areas. This in itself may diminish the fear to a tolerable level.

Communication with the patient is both verbal and nonverbal. The nurses' verbal expressions should be reinforced by nonverbal communication. The nurse should also be observing the patient's nonverbal communication for insight into the problem and possible solutions. Misconceptions of procedures, injuries, and machines may be the stressors and appropriate, honest explanations may reduce the patient's fear to a tolerable level.

Care of the patient by the same nurse as much as feasible provides a basis for interpersonal rapport. This then allows the nurse to identify coping defenses the patient uses effectively. The nurse then incorporates these mechanisms when talking with the patient. Administration of pain medication and/or tranquilizers as ordered and as needed will further assist the patient to cope with the situation.

Powerlessness and Loneliness

POWERLESSNESS

Feelings of powerlessness affect everyone at sometime in one's life. Powerlessness is a feeling that the situation one is in is *completely* out of one's control. The sense of powerlessness is extremely uncomfortable (distress) for most persons. It is one of the first emotions critically ill alert patients experience. The feeling of powerlessness is intensified if the patient is intubated, if extensive casting and traction is used, or if the patient is in Crutchfield tongs as a result of fractured cervical vertebrae.

Nursing interventions in the critical care unit are most effective if they are simple, but sincere.

Simple explanations (as often as necessary) for the reason the patient is in critical care, the use and need of the specialized equipment, and the termination of the use of the equipment provide some basic knowledge. This knowledge gives the patient a sense of some power because he or she understands what is taking place.

Using knowledge that an endotracheal tube will be removed at some specific point will establish a goal for the patient and nurse to work towards. The nurse may need to help the patient re-define some small goals which are realistic, for example, breathing without machine assistance for 5 minutes, then 10 minutes, and so on, rather than establishing a goal of extubation by next week. The long-range goal may indeed be realistic, but using short-term goals will help the patient feel he or she does have some power.

Giving patients choices in relation to type of bath, treatments, dressing changes, the chance to sit in chairs, type of drink (if allowed) and such are small, simplistic actions which usually enable the patients to feel that they do have some power, are less threatened, and able to cope with the critical care situation more effectively.

Throughout this process the nurse must be empathetic and supportive of the realistic goals the patient sets.

LONELINESS

This is a state of stress in which one feels uncomfortably alone. Staff members are constantly around and families visit for short periods, but the person feels isolated and disconnected from his or her "normal self and life-style."

Nursing interventions again are most valuable if they are simplistic, but meaningful. Attempts to relieve this loneliness are helpful ONLY when the patient is willing "to give up" his or her aloneness state. In these instances, allowing a family member to come in, feed the patient, and help with other care as appropriate may be indicated. Such care could include wiping the patient's face with a cool washcloth, moistening teeth, tongue, and gums with glycerol swabs, rubbing the patient's back, and many other such simple, but effective actions.

Patients may give up their aloneness if a family picture or other significant object is nearby (within the limits of critical care space and monitoring equipment).

If the nurse is empathetic, he or she may establish a rapport with the patient and participate in the patient's ventilating of feelings and fears. It is important that the patient's misconceptions be clarified and that the patient be reassured that dreaming and redreaming of the critical illness events is a NORMAL body response. The mind, through dreaming, begins to resolve the crisis. Many critically ill persons fight drifting off into even a light sleep because of such dreams. If the patient does not bring this up and if the nurse has established a modicum of rapport, talking about the illness and the normalcy of dreaming about it may often be the single act that allows the patient and nurse to reach each other. But the patient cannot be *forced* into a relationship that will relieve the aloneness.

Pain

Pain may be defined as an extremely unpleasant stimulus which recalls vividly from the brain similar noxious stimuli of the past. Pain tolerance is an individual experience which may be used to elicit a specific response from family members and/or the nurse.

Appropriate nursing interventions may be immediate medication I.V. (after a heart attack) followed by other comforting measures. On the other hand, appropriate nursing interventions may be to withhold pain medication and try other relief measures first.

Holding the patient's hand and talking softly, repositioning the patient, or applying a cool washcloth to the forehead may decrease the patient's awareness of pain. Very successful pain relief has been achieved through diversion, humor, relaxation techniques, self-hypnosis, and meditation. When these measures fail, medication may be the only solution. But, if given, then when one-half to two-thirds of the effective time of relief has passed, these same nursing interventions may be tried again. And the amount and frequency of pain medication requested may be reduced.

Sensory Overload

Sensory overload may be defined as a state of stress in which multiple stimuli from the environment are perceived by the patient as continuous and unbearable. The patient may withdraw psychologically and/or exhibit bizarre behavior commonly referred to as "ICU-itis" or "CCU-itis." This sensory overload incapacitates the patient and retards healing as precious energy is consumed in the process of the senses being overloaded with stimuli.

Nursing interventions that seem to alter the sensory overload are again those simple acts which provide comfort to the patient. Dimming lights for specific rest periods, decreasing the volume of cardiac monitors, and answering phones and call lights promptly are examples.

Nurses reporting at the change of shift should be away from the patient's bedside and talk quietly to prevent one patient from hearing about another patient but thinking the case is his or her own. Nurses can (and should) ask the intern or resident staff to discuss the cases with their attending physicians at the unit desk instead of at the bedside.

Mouth care administered frequently will help decrease mouth odor, help eliminate a bad taste in one's mouth, and help prevent the breakdown of buccal membranes and cracking of the lips.

Hospital "smells" are a continuous noxious stimulus to most patients. The use of room deodorizers and prompt removal of soiled linens and such will help decrease the "smells."

Touch is an enigma. It is a definite contributor to sensory overload but is also a therapeutic intervention in sensory deprivation. The difference is the type of touch. In sensory overload, tactile sensations are frequent, often painful, occasionally invasive, and seemingly continuous.

Nursing intervention requires some preplanning to decrease the tactile overload. Simple actions again are often the most useful. The nurse can plan to bathe a patient, change a dressing, replace the linens, and reposition the patient as a single act occurring over time. For example, bathe the patient's front, and change dressings. Allow the patient to rest an hour. Reposition the patient on one side; bathe the upper side and the patient's back; if more dressings are present, change them and then change the empty half of the bed's linens pushing the soiled linens against the lower side of the patient. Allow the patient to rest for an hour; then reposition the patient on his or her other side on the clean linens. Finish washing any remaining areas, give a soothing back rub, and complete the linen change. Allow the patient to rest. Changing dressings or I.V. sites is often painful. Performing these procedures separately and interspersed with a positive touch (e.g., back rub) helps decrease sensory overload due to touch. Pain medications may be administered before starting patient care to diminish tactile stimulation. Grouping multiple activities together and spreading them over a period of time benefits the patient but may frustrate the nurse who wants the bath and bed change completed before the first visitors of the day arrive.

Sensory Deprivation

Sensory deprivation occurs most often when doctors and nurses forget that a patient lies under all those tubes and machines. Patients experience a lack of sensory stimuli that are pleasant, meaningful, and comforting. If sensory deprivation is severe or prolonged, patients may become angry, confused, restless, or withdrawn. (The same patient symptoms may occur with sensory overload so the nurse must examine the environment to determine which state is present.)

Nursing interventions are most appropriate if simple and meaningful. Verbal and tactile communications are the most consistently used and useful interventions. Gentle hand holding while quietly talking *with* the patient (not *to* the patient) is invaluable. Direct and consistent eye contact enhances the verbal and touching communication.

Family visits and familiar cherished objects, including pictures, may be supplied *if* feasible. Bedside radios (in call lights or wherever in the area) may be turned to the patient's station of choice to provide some pleasant stimulus.

If at all possible, arranging for an uninterrupted 2 or 3 hours of sleep at night will enable the patient to cope more effectively than almost anything else.

A "locked in" syndrome or "tunnel vision" may occur with both sensory overload and sensory deprivation. In this syndrome, the patient usually lies perfectly still, moving only his or her eyes, if anything. The overwhelming characteristics of critical care areas and sudden critical illness of the patient result in the patient's unwillingness or inability to move or talk.

The Family and Growth and Development

The family is composed of persons forming a unique group. Traditionally, a father, mother, and some children are the nuclear family. Grandparents, aunts, uncles, and so on form the extended family. In our current society, mobility has often separated the nuclear family from the larger supporting family.

The parents assume responsibility for the socialization of their children. Thus, standards, values, and prejudices are a social growth and a reflection of parental values.

Both social and physical growth are defined by Erickson's eight stages of growth and development. The patient's successes and failures in each stage he or she has passed will influence the patient's reaction to a critical care experience. If the nurse is unfamiliar with Erickson's stages, he or she will find excellent books and articles in nursing journals, social science and psychology journals, as well as in some pediatric texts.

Nursing interventions to assist the patient to cope with his or her illness depend in part upon these stages. The nurse may be able to help the patient develop some positive coping skills which will enhance the patient's self-esteem and probably make nursing communications, and thus care, easier.

Interpersonal Communications

Basic to life itself is communication. No one can fail to communicate unless one is truly a mountain hermit. The rest of us communicate with everyone we meet. Communication occurs through body language, facial expression, verbal expressions, and even the manner in which we move. For more in-depth study of the fascinating concept of non-verbal communication, one may wish to read one of the body language books available.

The topics of perception, strength, limitations, potentials, family, growth and development, and interpersonal communication have only been touched upon in this text because the concepts are basic to nursing. Many resources are available on any and all of these topics for a more detailed study if desired.

Human Sexuality

Human sexuality is a component of one's self-concept and is always in a dynamic state of evolving from birth and changing throughout one's life. One's concept of his or her sexuality is often perceived as threatened by critical illness.

Nursing interventions most effective in diminishing this perceived threat are to maintain and to protect the patient's modesty and dignity as much as possible at all times.

Crisis

A crisis exists when one perceives that so many negative stimuli have arisen that one can no longer cope with the situation. This point varies with each person at any given time. Certainly becoming ill and admitted to a critical care area is stressful and to some is a crisis. The family as well as the patient may experience a crisis.

Two types of crises exist. One is situational crisis where a major change in a common circumstance results in an inability to cope with reality. Death is an example of a situational crisis.

The second type of crisis is maturational. Maturing from infancy to old age requires one to develop specific skills (Erickson's eight stages). If the skills are not acquired, it becomes difficult to cope with additional stressors.

According to Fink there appear to be four stages of a crisis.[1] The first stage is shock or disbelief. Anxiety and helplessness are usual signs in this stage of crisis.

The second stage of crisis appears to be denial. If confronted with the reality of a crisis, the individual usually expresses anger and resists changing his or her thought.

The third stage of crisis appears to be acceptance of the crisis which causes depression. The depression may be associated with extreme anxiety through mourning to bitterness. If the depression is severe enough, thoughts or expressions of suicide may be present.

The fourth stage of crisis is adaptation and change. Reality is accepted and a gradual awareness of one's resources and abilities become apparent.

The objective of nursing intervention in crisis is to help the patient cope with the crisis. Some patients cannot cope with the stress or change, and they break down because of the traumatic changes. Some patients will struggle through the crisis and be unchanged. Some patients come through a crisis having grown and become stronger with an enhanced self-esteem.

Nursing interventions include the nurse sharing his or her perception of the crisis

with the patient to validate it. The nurse may help by correcting misconceptions of the patient and help him or her identify reality. Planning ways to cope with crises is helpful. Explain the situation and plan the next step or expected step with the patient.

Short and simple interventions are more helpful than "the hour counseling session." Encouraging ventilation of feelings and supporting the patient and family as much as one can *within* the limits of reality help to resolve the crisis.

Addiction

An addiction exists any time an individual depends upon a substance to feel complete (adequate). An addict admitted to a critical care area may at first still be under the influence of the addicting substance. In these cases, the addict's perceptions are unrealistic. Addicts usually manifest three behaviors while in critical care areas: (1) Addicts fear not having the desperately needed substance and being unable to cope with that situation. (2) An addict *may* be concerned with how those around him or her will react to his or her addiction. This threatens an already decreased self-concept and self-esteem. (3) While withdrawing from an addictive substance, addicts tend to be hyperactive to all stimuli and *crave sweet foods*.

Nursing interventions with addicts must be straightforward and honest. The patient may try to prevent others from approaching too closely. Negative, abusive, and maladaptive behavior occurs often. The nurse must intervene in a calm, direct manner and state what is expected of the patient and what behavior will not be tolerated. Providing clear, concise explanations of machines and treatments is essential. Establishing rapport will be difficult if not impossible. Care for the addict as a *patient* and not an addict will help avoid power struggles.

Suicide

Suicide is a self-destructive action by an individual when overwhelmed and feeling helpless about a situation. One is unable to cope with a situation by less drastic coping mechanisms.

[1] Borg N, Mikas DL, Stark J, Williams SM (eds): Core Curriculum for Critical Care Nursing, 2nd ed. American Association of Critical-Care Nurses. Philadelphia: W. B. Saunders, p. 455, 1981

Many emotions are experienced by the suicidal patient including shame, guild, despair, and hopelessness. Depression is exhibited by actions (or words) that show life is not worth living anymore. Suicide may be considered to be a logical response to the overwhelming situation.

Nursing intervention is usually more effective if the nurse knows why a suicide was attempted. Equally important is how the nurse feels about suicide. A suicidal crisis is normally short-lived (hours to days).

Nursing intervention starts by accepting the attempt at suicide from the patient's perception. Communication, both verbal and non-verbal, may help the suicidal patient see a situation more realistically. Supporting the patient and the patient's family will help develop a non-threatening atmosphere. Talking with the patient and his or her family about receiving psychiatric care is important.

Death and Dying

Death is the psychobiological cessation of all cellular activity throughout the body. Dying is the process of specific cells and cell systems stopping all of their functions until all body systems have ceased to function. Then death has occurred.

Elizabeth Kübler-Ross has identified five *psychological* stages of the dying process. The stages are not necessarily followed in sequence and because of the stresses of dying, stages may be skipped or returned to any number of times. The five stages are (1) denial, (2) anger, (3) bargaining, (4) depression, and (5) acceptance.[2]

---

[2]Dealing with Death and Dying. Jenkintown, PA: Nursing 77 Books, Intermed Communications, 1976

Denial is an important coping mechanism. It allows the patient some inner control to block out overwhelming threats. The patient may then cope with small aspects of a crisis.

Nursing interventions can strongly support the patient and the family during the dying process *IF* the nurse is comfortable with his or her own feelings about death.

The survivors go through the same five stages during the dying of their loved ones. The nurses may not see all these stages in them.

Nurses intervene by responding to the dying patient only after *active* listening to the patient's perception of the situation. Accepting the patient and family as they are helps the nurse to establish rapport and provide support. Nursing interventions that discourage false beliefs and encourage the acceptance of reality are beneficial.

A major nursing intervention is to provide comfort measures for the dying patient. These measures include frequent mouth care, a position of comfort, medication for pain as needed, and allowing the extended family to visit if the patient seems to benefit from this. The dying patient may feel cold to the touch, but the patient is usually hot internally and should not be covered with heavy blankets, just loose sheets.

As death approaches, the patient will look towards light so leave the shades open and lights on. Have family members stand close to the head of the patient since he or she cannot see far away.

All experienced critical care nurses know of patients who have died easily and of patients who have had a very hard time dying. Critical care nurses become involved with some patients more than others and go through the dying grief patterns with the patient. Nurses may cry with the patient and/or family without loss of professionalism.

Psychosocial Bibliography

Borg N, Mikas DL, Stark J, Williams SM (eds): Core Curriculum for Critical Care Nursing, 2nd ed. American Association of Critical-Care Nurses. Philadelphia: W. B. Saunders, pp. 439–471, 1981

*Hudak CM, Lohr TS, Gallo BM (eds): Critical Care Nursing, 3rd ed. Philadelphia: J. B. Lippincott, pp. 17–49, 1982

*Kinney MR, Dear CB, Packa DR, Voorman DMN (eds): AACN'S Clinical Reference for Critical Care Nursing. New York: McGraw-Hill, pp. 323–358, 1981

*Roberts SL: Behavioral Concepts and the Critically Ill Patient. Englewood Cliffs, NJ: Prentice-Hall, 1976

X

Assessment of Body Systems

— 48 ——————————

Assessment Skills

Learning Objectives

By the end of this chapter, the nurse will be able to:

1. List the four skills used in assessment.
2. Identify at least four specifics one checks by inspection.
3. Describe techniques for light and deep palpation.
4. Explain testing for rebound tenderness.
5. Identify at least four specifics one checks by palpation.
6. Identify at least four specifics one checks by percussion.
7. Describe the percussion procedure including positioning of the plexor and pleximeter.
8. List four of the five sounds produced by percussion.
9. Identify at least four specifics one checks by auscultation.
10. List at least five extraneous factors which influence auscultation.

There are four assessment skills which must be developed to accurately and effectively assess a body system. These skills in order are inspection, palpation, percussion, and auscultation, except when assessing the gastrointestinal system. In that case, the order is inspection, auscultation, palpation, and percussion. Auscultation is performed before palpation and percussion to avoid altering abdominal sounds.

Inspection

Inspection is purposeful observation to first obtain a general, overall picture of the patient. It is followed by specific inspection of each body system. Inspection is not only accomplished with the use of one's eyes, but also with other body senses (touch, smell, and hearing) in assessing each body system of the patient. Inspection also utilizes varied instruments such as an otoscope, ophthalmoscope, and speculum as one moves from the general inspection to the specific. Inspection may reveal diaphoresis, use of accessory muscles for breathing, inequality of limb movement, pupillary response to light, and much more general but important information.

Palpation

Palpation is usually the second step in a systematic assessment. Since some people do not like being touched, explaining what you are doing and why will decrease patient resistance. It is also nice to warm your cold hands before starting palpation.

Palpation includes the use of your fingers (front and back), the palms of your hands, and the dorsal surface of your hands. Using the dorsal surface of your hands and fingers (Figure 48-1) provides an accurate way to detect increases in temperature of the body or specific area. (Palmar surfaces are not as sensitive as dorsal surfaces.)

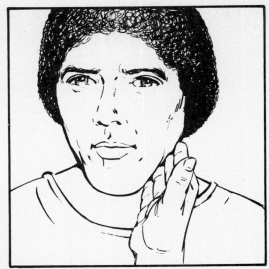

Figure 48-2. Palpation with pads of fingers (lymph nodes, masses, etc.).

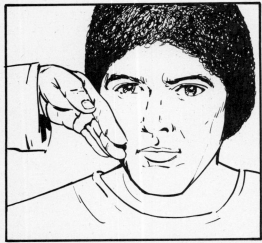

Figure 48-1. Dorsal surface of fingers palpating temperature.

Palpation with the pads of your fingers (Figure 48-2) can identify lymph glands and growths along with the size, position, and motility of each. Effective palpation requires rather short fingernails to avoid patient discomfort in both superficial and deep palpation.

The ball (or palm) of your hand is used to detect fremitus (Figure 48-3). The thumb and index fingers (Figure 48-4) are used to palpate muscle and skin turgor, tissue consistency, and joint movement.

Palpation may be light or deep. Light palpation (Figure 48-5) is done first, followed by deep palpation (Figure 48-6). Light palpation of the abdomen identifies areas of tenderness, abnormal collection of fluid in an area, masses, and/or changes in organs (for example, a nodular liver or splenomegaly). Light palpation involves pressing the

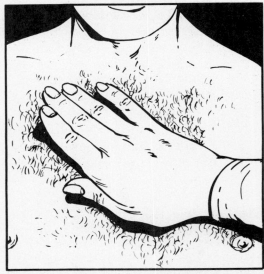

Figure 48-3. Ball of hand palpation for fremitus (vibration).

fingertips gently in a circular movement while pressing down about 2 centimeters. Palpate sensitive and painful areas last.

For deep palpation of the abdomen, either press fingers to a depth of 5 centimeters or place one hand over the other hand's fingers. Keeping the lower fingers on the body, use the upper hand to press downward. This is used to feel for masses and the

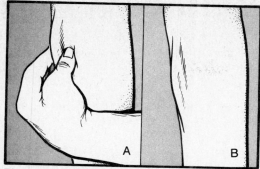

Figure 48-4. Finger testing of skin turgor. Gentle pinching of the skin (A); tenting, a response associated with dehydration (B).

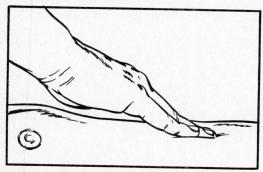

Figure 48-5. Light palpation.

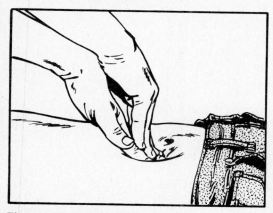

Figure 48-6. Deep palpation.

location of abdominal organs especially in obese patients.

In both light and deep palpation, the examiner's fingers maintain contact with the patient's skin as each quadrant of the abdomen is explored.

Palpation for rebound tenderness requires slow but gentle, deep pressure over

the area of tenderness (if possible). A SUDDEN release of pressure may cause pain. If it does, a test for referred rebound tenderness is to perform the same procedure on the nonaffected side. With a sudden release of pressure, referred pain occurring on the affected side is a conclusive test for true rebound tenderness. A great deal of practice is needed to enable the nurse to use this technique to acquire accurate information.

Percussion

Percussion is used for two reasons. One purpose is to determine the size and density of underlying structures. The other is to stretch certain tendons to obtain a deep tendon reflex.

Percussion requires extensive practice to enable the nurse to both perform and interpret results accurately.

PERFORMING PERCUSSION

Hyperextend the middle finger of the left hand and place the distal phalanx and joint firmly on the skin surface. The finger used in this position is known as the *pleximeter* finger (Figure 48-7). Be certain to keep the remainder of the left hand *off* the patient's skin to avoid dampening the vibrations.

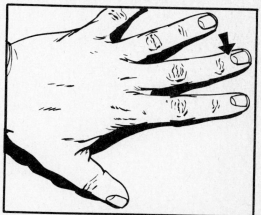

Figure 48-7. The pleximeter finger (noted by arrow).

Place your right arm close to the skin surface with your wrist and hand cocked upward. The middle finger of the right hand is relaxed and partially flexed (Figure 48-8). With a relaxed wrist motion, strike the pleximeter finger quickly and sharply. The right middle finger doing the striking is called the *plexor*.

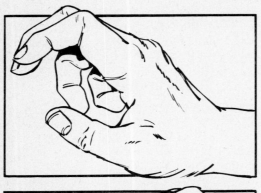

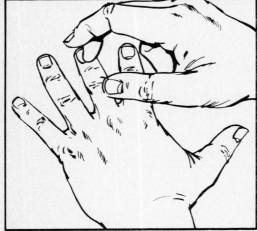

Figure 48-8. Plexor finger function.

A left-handed nurse may simply reverse hands or learn to percuss with both hands. Use the tip of the plexor finger (not the pad) and keep the plexor fingernail short to avoid damage to the pleximeter finger. Aim the plexor to strike the pleximeter finger at the point that is exerting the most contact with the skin. This should be the base of the terminal phalanx of the distal interphalangeal joint. Movement for percussion is at the wrist. Other than the two fingers, the elbow, entire arm, and shoulder are NOT involved in percussion. The pattern for percussion should be one or two blows in a spot and then one or two blows in the parallel spot for comparison of sounds.

SOUNDS OF PERCUSSION

With much practice and experience the nurse will be able to identify five sounds and differentiate four of them by intensity, pitch, and duration. Table 48-1 identifies the sounds according to these characteristics.

You can practice these sounds by percussing your own or a friend's thigh (flatness), liver (dullness), normal lung (resonance), emphysematous lung (hyperresonance), and puffed out cheek or gastric air bubble (tympany). Naturally, the more one practices, the more readily the sounds can be differentiated.

Another form of percussion is the fist percussion. This is commonly used to test for tenderness over the kidneys, at the costovertebral angle, and over the liver and the

Table 48-1. Characteristics of percussion sounds.

	Relative Intensity	Relative Pitch	Relative Duration	Example Location
Flatness	Soft	High	Short	Thigh
Dullness	Medium	Medium	Medium	Liver
Resonance	Loud	Low	Long	Normal lung
Hyperresonance	Very loud	Lower	Longer	Emphysematous lung
Tympany	Loud	*	*	Gastric air bubble or puffed out cheek

*Distinguished mainly by its musical timbre.
Note: Reproduced from Bates B: Guide to Physical Examination. Philadelphia: J.B. Lippincott, p. 87, 1974. Reprinted with permission of J.B. Lippincott.

gallbladder. The nurse puts one hand flat against the back of the patient over the appropriate site. With the other hand made into a fist, the nurse strikes the hand on the patient's back in the appropriate region.

Auscultation

This is the most difficult assessment skill to perfect. It involves listening to various sounds made by the body's organs. These are primarily the lungs, heart, blood vessels, stomach, and intestines. The stethoscope is the utensil used for auscultation. The diaphragm of a stethoscope transmits high-pitched sounds. The bell of a stethoscope transmits low-pitched sounds.

QUALITY OF A STETHOSCOPE

The stethoscope itself must be in perfect working condition. The bell and diaphragm allow air leaks if there is any damage to them. The tubing of the stethoscope should be between 12 and 15 inches long, have a ⅛ inch lumen, and be free of cracks or leaks at points of attachment. The ear tips are inserted facing forward and should be sized to fit the ear canal snugly to block out noise but not cause distress from too tight a fit.

TIPS FOR USING A STETHOSCOPE

Close all doors to shut out noise. Turn off radios and/or TVs. Ask the patient not to talk until directed. Clothing, bedsheets, and jewelry moving around or touching the tubing may distort sounds.

Moving the stethoscope over hair may sound like rales. Warm the stethoscope before placing it against the patient's body to prevent shivering (piloerection), which causes rales-type sounds or distorts other sounds.

Extensive practice to learn normal sounds will enable the nurse to differentiate between normal and abnormal sounds. Further practice will enable the nurse to distinguish not only the abnormal sounds but to associate them with specific disease entities.

Auscultation is used to listen for bruits, heart sounds, lung sounds, abdominal sounds, and such.

These skills make the critical care nurse an invaluable member of the health care team because of his or her input from continuous patient assessment and early identification of new difficulties and also responses to treatment modalities.

— 49

Assessment of the Patient with a Respiratory Dysfunction

Learning Objectives

By the end of this chapter, the nurse will be able to:

1. Define the normal shape of the thorax and abnormal shapes of the thorax. Indicate their significance and include the barrel chest, the pectus excavatum, and the pectus carinatum.
2. Describe deformities of the chest wall caused by kyphosis, scoliosis, and kyphoscoliosis.
3. Briefly describe normal chest excursion.
4. Identify five respiratory patterns and the characteristics of each.
5. Explain why cyanosis is an unreliable parameter of inspection of the respiratory system.
6. Identify three reasons for percussing the chest field.
7. Explain palpation to detect fremitus.
8. Describe the progression of percussion of the posterior chest wall starting with the top of the shoulders.
9. List three main groups of lung sounds.
10. List four normal breath sounds including the inspiratory to expiratory ratio.
11. Define abnormal lung sounds and list three adventitious lung sounds.
12. Differentiate between a pleural rub and a pericardial rub.
13. Explain the use of egophony in assessing pulmonary status.
14. Explain the use of pectoriloquy in assessing respiratory status.
15. Explain the use of bronchophony in assessing pulmonary status.

Prior to instituting assessment of any system certain general factors relative to the system being assessed should also be known. An up-to-date personal patient history with the current chief complaint and a family history may add important data to the health care practitioner.

Physical Landmarks

Specific anatomic landmarks are used to communicate exact locations of abnormal sounds to all members of the health care team. Each lung serves as a comparison for the other lung so percussion, palpation, and auscultation abnormalities in one lung can be compared to the other lung. For this reason, identification of the site by anatomical location is most accurate.

ANTERIOR CHEST LANDMARKS

These include the suprasternal notch, the supraclavicular area, the clavicular area, the mid-clavicular area, the infraclavicular area, the mammary area, and the hypochondriac area (Figure 49-1).

POSTERIOR CHEST LANDMARKS

These include the seventh cervical vertebra, the suprascapular area, the scapulae, the inferior scapular tips, the interscapular area, and the mid-vertebral column (Figure 49-2).

APPROXIMATION OF LANDMARKS

These are approximations and are not definitive. The suprasternal notch is immediately superior to the sternum. The angle of Louis is aligned with the second rib anteriorly and the fifth thoracic vertebra posteriorly. The xiphisternal articulation is aligned with thoracic vertebrae nine to eleven. These approximate landmarks will help guide the nurse in assessment and assist in accurate descriptions of the location of any abnormalities noted.

AXILLARY DIVISIONS OF THE CHEST

Occasionally assessment of the respiratory system will involve the axillary region. It is however more commonly used in cardiac assessment. Figure 49-3 identifies the three divisions of the axilla.

General Inspection

Prior to assessing any body system, general observations provide much information. The general skin color and appearance are

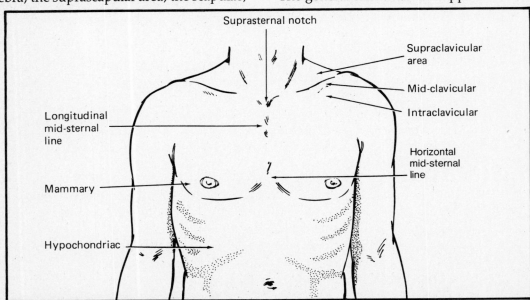

Figure 49-1. Landmarks of the anterior chest.

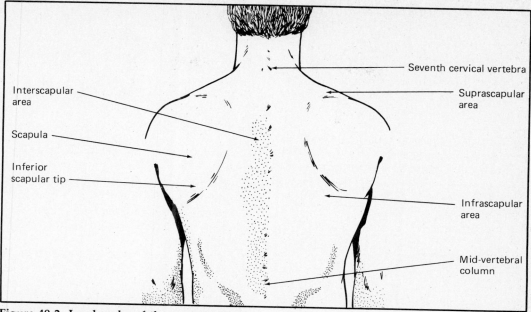

Figure 49-2. Landmarks of the posterior chest.

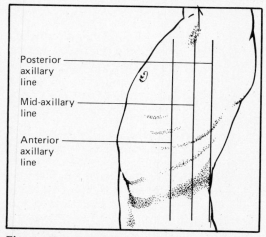

Figure 49-3. Landmarks of the axillary chest.

important. For example, a person may be emaciated or obese with or without difficulty in breathing. There may be signs of fatigue, nervousness, or decreased energy level. Specific illness, past and present, and familial histories are usually available in the admission notes on the patient.

Inspection

Inspection of the respiratory system includes general appearance, size and shape of the chest, appearance of the bony thoracic cage, color, respiratory pattern/rate, the need for use of accessory muscles on inspiration or lack there of, and effort (if any) on exhalation.

Inspection of the chest begins with the skin which is usually lighter in color than the exposed areas of skin (unless tanned from the use of a sunlamp or sunbathing). The skin should appear smooth and not nodular, flakey, or scaling.

The shape of the thorax should be observed from the position of the ribs in relation to the angle of Louis anteriorly and the C-7 vertebral spinous process posteriorly. The shape of the normal adult chest should be larger in the lateral diameter than in the anteroposterior diameter (Figure 49-4A). The ratio may range from 1:2 to 5:7. The thorax should appear symmetrical.

ABNORMALITIES IN THE SHAPE OF THE CHEST

The barrel chest has a lateral increase in size to equal the anteroposterior size (Figure 49-4B). This is normally associated with emphysema.

The pectus excavatum (Figure 49-4C) is a funnel-shaped chest. The lower portion of the sternum is depressed. This may cause compression on the heart and vessels producing a murmur.

The pectus carinatum (Figure 49-4D) is commonly called a pigeon chest. In this instance the sternum is displaced anteriorly. The displacement produces grooves on the chest which accentuate the deformity.

Kyphosis, scoliosis, and kyphoscoliosis are abnormal configurations of the posterior chest wall. Kyphosis is an abnormal con-

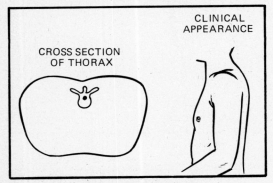

Figure 49-4a. Normal adult thorax.

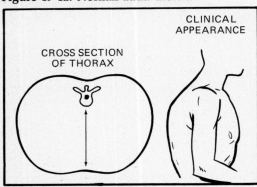

Figure 49-4b. Barrel chest.

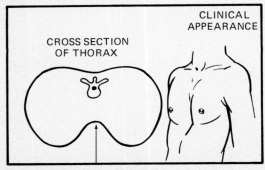

Figure 49-4c. Funnel chest.

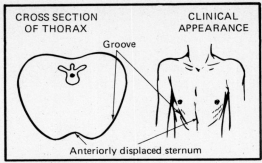

Figure 49-4d. Pigeon chest.

vexity in the thoracic spine causing a "hunchback." Scoliosis is an abnormal S curvature of the thoracic spine and is frequently seen with kyphosis producing a kyphoscoliosis.

Deformities in the configuration of the thorax may make it difficult to assess the respiratory system completely.

Observation of the respiratory pattern is made during the general observation. If the pattern is abnormal, describe it and count respirations for a full minute to obtain an accurate rate and pattern. Respiratory patterns were explained and diagrammed in the respiratory section of this text (Chapter 1) and will not be repeated here.

CYANOSIS

This is an unreliable parameter because of many extraneous factors. Cyanosis does not occur without a drop of at least 5 gm of Hgb per 100 ml of blood. Usually, cyanosis is first seen in the conjunctiva, buccal membranes, under the tongue, and under the knee. Defects in hemoglobin or hemoglobin binding capacity, cardiac output, skin thickness, perfusion of tissues, and inadequate respiration are just a few of the extraneous features relating to cyanosis. This finding must of course be identified as the result of a specific problem to be treated successfully. Note: A cherry red color instead of the bluish tint of cyanosis indicates carbon monoxide poisoning.

CLUBBING OF THE FINGERS

This is most often a cardiac related problem and not usually of pulmonary origin. For this reason, it is covered in Chapter 50.

Palpation

The skin of the chest wall is lightly palpated to reveal any lumps and/or tender areas not seen on simple inspection. The skin should be warm, dry, and smooth to the touch.

CHEST EXCURSION

Palpation of the chest determines if each lung expands to the same degree at each tested spot. The technique is the same for anterior and posterior testing. Place your hands with thumbs together and fingers spread widely over the center of the patient's chest (anterior—sternum; posterior—vertebral spinous processes). Have the patient take a deep breath. If normal, the fingers and thumbs will move apart to an equal degree. Note any deviation. Each lobe of the lung (or its equivalent area) should be tested in the same manner.

TACTILE FREMITUS

Fremitus is the vibration felt through the chest wall while the patient is speaking. Some degree of fremitus is normal. To test for this, palpate using the palm of your hand, comparing the observations from each side of the chest. Palpate anterior and posterior portions of the chest. Figure 49-5 shows the progression sequence for palpating the posterior chest wall. Fremitus is usually decreased or absent over the sternum.

Increased fremitus is usually associated with conditions that enhance sound transmission. Such conditions include pneumonia, lung tumors, and fibrosis.

Decreased fremitus most often occurs in conditions that do not enhance sound transmissions. Such conditions include pleural fluid and air.

It is normal for fremitus to be most intense directly over the sound and to decrease as the examining hand moves towards the periphery.

POSITION OF THE TRACHEA

Palpation of the trachea in a normal state is midline. If deviated, the trachea moves **towards** the side of atelectasis, a pneumonec-

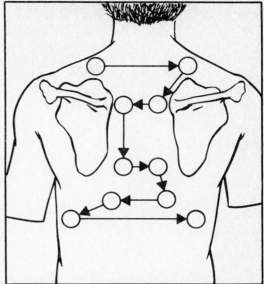

Figure 49-5. Palpation of the posterior chest (starting at the upper left shoulder and proceeding downward).

tomy, a unilateral fibrosis, and during the inspiratory phase of flail chest.

The trachea moves **away** from a side of a tension pneumothorax, a pleural effusion, and during the expiratory phase of a flail chest.

SUBCUTANEOUS EMPHYSEMA

This is also referred to as subcutaneous crepitus. It is caused by air escaping into tissue under the skin. Etiologies include tracheal leak, pneumothorax, or a leak from the mediastinum. Fractured ribs are a common precipitating factor. Gentle pressing (light palpation) on the skin feels like the sound of a crackling bowl of Rice Krispies®.

PALPATION OF THE DIAPHRAGM

An estimation of the level of the diaphragm on **each** side of the chest can be made using the ulnar side of the extended hand. Hold the extended hand parallel to and touching the posterior chest. With the patient repeatedly saying "99", move your hand downward until fremitus is no longer felt. This marks the diaphragmatic level, which is usually higher on the right than on the left side of the chest.

Percussion

Bony structures and soft tissue such as the heart, liver, and diaphragm have greater density (due to increased cell mass) than the air-filled pulmonary system.

When percussing the lung-filled portions of the chest, the characteristic sound is a resonant sound, which is of low intensity and pitch and of long duration in the healthy lung. In overinflation of the lungs a hyperresonant sound is heard (refer to Chapter 48 for review of the characteristics of each sound). A dull sound is transmitted with percussion of the liver, heart, and bones due to the increased cell mass of these structures. Percussion follows a specific pattern comparing one lung to the other beginning at the apex of each lung (Figure 49-6).

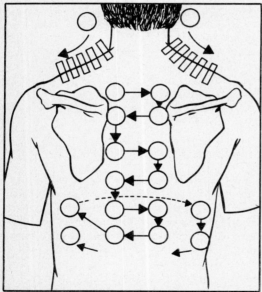

Figure 49-6. Percussion of the lungs (starting at the top of the shoulders and proceeding downward).

LEVEL OF THE DIAPHRAGM

Percuss the posterior chest wall in a series of progressive downward steps. A level of dullness is reached during quiet respiration which represents the level of the diaphragm. Figure 49-7 shows the location and sequence of percussion with the sound changing from resonant to dull at the level of the diaphragm. Excursion of the diaphragm is determined by measuring the levels of dullness on full expiration and full inspiration. The distance is normally 5–6 centimeters.

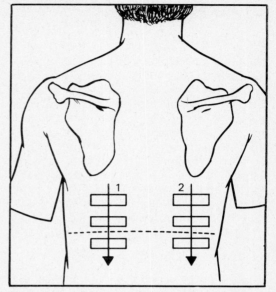

Figure 49-7. Percussion determining diaphragmatic excursion.

Auscultation

Auscultation is an ongoing assessment to determine the normal sounds and alterations of the pulmonary system, for example, resolution of pneumonia, development of edema, the position (or change in position) of endotracheal tubes and such. Each sound has four characteristics important in auscultation. These are the pitch, the intensity, the quality, and duration. Frequency (or pitch) of sound is related to wave cycles per second. A high-pitched sound (high-frequency) has more wave sounds per second than a low-frequency sound. The greater the amplitude or intensity, the louder the sound. The lesser the amplitude or intensity, the softer the sound. Quality of the sound is denoted by descriptive terminology; such words as breezy, tubular, harsh, fine, bubbling, and creaking are frequently used words. Duration (or longevity) compares the inspiratory or expiratory phase in the respiratory cycle. Figure 49-8 presents a graphic illustration of the normal breath sound characteristics.

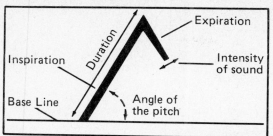

Figure 49-8. Schematic drawing of normal breath.

Breath Sounds

There are three main classifications of lung sounds: normal sounds, adventitious sounds, and abnormal voice sounds.

NORMAL BREATH SOUNDS

There are four normal breath sounds: tracheal, bronchial, bronchovesicular, and vesicular. Figure 49-9 depicts the tracheal breath sounds.

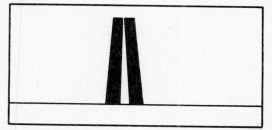

Figure 49-9. Tracheal breath sounds.

Tracheal Sounds

These sounds have a high pitch, are loud, and have the quality of being tubular and harsh. The duration of inspiration (I) is equal to that of expiration (E) with a slight pause between the two phases. Tracheal sounds are normally heard only over the trachea. The ratio of I:E is 1:1.

Bronchial Sounds

Bronchial sounds (Figure 49-10) are heard over the manubrium and along the sternal borders. They are high pitched, high intensity, loud, tubular, and harsh quality sounds. Expiration is twice as long as inspi-

ration with a very brief pause between them. The ratio of I:E is 2:3.

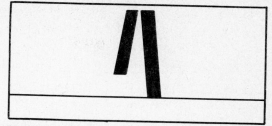

Figure 49-10. Bronchial breath sounds.

Bronchovesicular Sounds

Bronchovesicular sounds (Figure 49-11) are normally heard over the upper third of the sternum and interscapular area. These sounds are of moderate amplitude, medium to high pitch, and similar to that of blowing, muffled sounds. The ratio of I:E is 1:1.

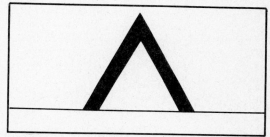

Figure 49-11. Bronchovesicular breath sounds.

Vesicular Sounds

Vesicular sounds (Figure 49-12) are made by the noise of alveoli opening on inspiration and a glottic hiss (air moving through the larynx) during expiration. These are best heard in the periphery of the lung. Vesicular sounds are of low amplitude, medium to low pitch, and similar to that of breezy, swishing, or rustling sounds. Inspiration is three times as long as expiration, but there is no separation between the sounds. The ratio of I:E is 3:1.

Figure 49-13 shows the location of the four types of breath sounds for auscultation.

ADVENTITIOUS BREATH SOUNDS

There are four adventitious breath sounds: rales, rhonchi, wheezing, and a pleural friction rub.

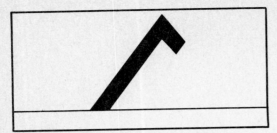

Figure 49-12. Vesicular breath sounds.

Rales

Rales are caused by the passage of air through secretions present in alveoli and tubular air passageways.

Rales can be subdivided into fine, medium, and coarse rales. Fine rales (Figure 49-14A) are sometimes called crepitant rales. They are heard at the end of inspiration. Fine rales are the vibrations of the separation of alveolar walls which have lightly adhered to each other because of the presence of pus and fluids in the alveoli. Fine rales are auscultated in the periphery of the chest. Fine rales sounds may be produced by rubbing a strand of hair between your thumb and finger.

Medium or subcrepitant rales (Figure 49-14B) are caused by fluid or mucus-filled bronchial walls that are separated by inspiration. The sound has a low pitch, high amplitude, and a wet, moist quality occurring in early to mid-inspiration.

Coarse or bubbling rales (Figure 49-14C) are heard in the larger airways that contain fluid or mucus secretions. The sound is of low pitch and has a loud bubbling quality. It is most frequently heard during expiration but can also be heard during inspiration.

Rhonchi

Rhonchi may be either musical (sibilant) or sonorous. Sibilant rhonchi have a high pitch and possess a musical quality. Sonorous rhonchi are low pitched and sound like someone snoring. Rhonchi (Figure 49-15) are continuous sounds secondary to air passage through edematous, spasmodic airways or through tubules filled with mucus. Even though they are continuous sounds, they are most frequently heard during expiration. Characteristics are variable depending upon the extent of pulmonary abnormalities.

Wheezing

Wheezing results from air passing through airways which have a decreased lumen due

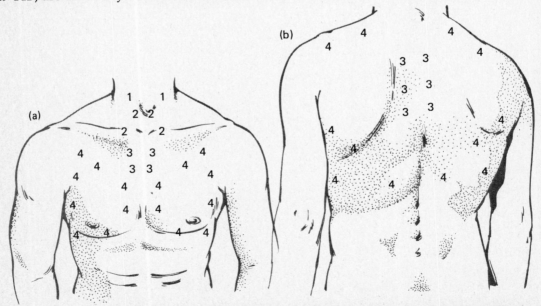

Figure 49-13. Locations of breath sounds: (a) anterior chest; (b) posterior chest. (1) denotes tracheal sounds, (2) bronchial sounds, (3) bronchovesicular sounds, and (4) vesicular sounds.

A

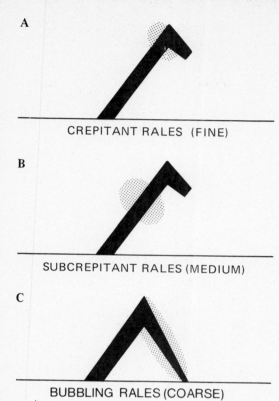

CREPITANT RALES (FINE)

B

SUBCREPITANT RALES (MEDIUM)

C

BUBBLING RALES (COARSE)

Figure 49-14. Schematic drawing of rales.

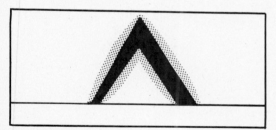

Figure 49-15. Rhonchi.

to smooth muscle contraction, edema, or secretions (Figure 49-16). Wheezing is commonly heard during expiration but may be heard during inspiration.

Pleural Friction Rub

This is a scratchy sound due to inflamed pleura rubbing against each other without the normal lubricating substance (Figure 49-17). A pleural rub sounds like rubbing

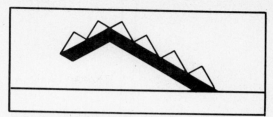

Figure 49-16. Wheezing.

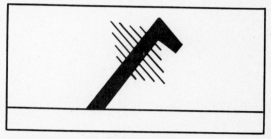

Figure 49-17. Pleural friction rub.

leather together. It is heard during inspiration and expiration. (A pericardial rub sounds like rubbing sandpaper.)

VOICE SOUNDS

Three sounds, bronchophony, egophony, and whispered pectoriloquy are heard in patients with pulmonary consolidations and occasionally in patients with pleural effusion (which compresses the lung parenchyma).

Bronchophony

An increase in the intensity and clarity of spoken words or syllables heard with a stethoscope indicates the presence of bronchophony (an abnormal sound).

Egophony

With the patient saying "ee", auscultation of both lung fields from superior to inferior lobes reveals the "ee" sound changing to an "ay" sound. Again, this indicates lobe consolidation.

Whispered Pectoriloquy

While having the patient whisper a word repeatedly, the transmission of this sound through the stethoscope is unusually clear throughout most lung lobes.

50

Assessment of the Patient with Cardiovascular Dysfunction

Learning Objectives

By the end of this chapter, the nurse will be able to:

1. Identify the use of percussion in assessing the cardiovascular status.
2. Identify at least four sounds of auscultation and the significance of each.
3. Describe the procedure for inspecting neck veins.
4. List factors of inspection for the arms, legs, and chest.
5. Define clubbing and its associated early and late changes.
6. List the pulses normally palpated.
7. Define pulsus alternans, pulsus paradoxus, and pulsus bisiferens.
8. Explain what S_1 represents.
9. Explain what S_2 represents.
10. Describe a physiological split S_1.
11. Describe a pathologic split S_2.
12. Explain the meaning of S_3 and S_4.
13. Define murmur.
14. Differentiate between systolic and diastolic murmurs.

The same four skills are used in the assessment of the cardiovascular system that were used in assessing the respiratory system. The same anatomical landmarks used in examining the respiratory system are used with the cardiovascular system. The assessment begins with the patient's history.

Inspection

Observe the overall physical appearance of the patient. Check the skin and mucous membranes for hydration, skin turgor, perfusion, petechiae, and angiomas.

The heart lies within an angle in the chest

with the right border of the heart (primarily the right atrium) located at the right side of the sternum between the third and fifth intercostal spaces. The apex of the heart is formed primarily by the left ventricle. During ventricular contraction, the apex rotates close to the chest wall. This positional change often produces a palpable and/or visible thrust known as the "point of maximal intensity" (PMI). The PMI is well localized, is about 2–3 cm in diameter or smaller, and can be seen briefly in the fifth intercostal space. The PMI is less observable in either an obese or muscular person due to the density of the chest. Sometimes having the person hold his or her breath at end-expiration enables visualization of the PMI.

The precordium is inspected for the PMI, heaves, lifts, any shape or contour that may affect cardiac function, the breathing pattern, and pulses.

INSPECTING NECK VEINS

Place the patient in a 45° angle supine. Shine a light tangentially (obliquely) to illuminate neck veins. The internal jugular is more reliable than the external jugular. If the neck vein is distended, measure the distance from the manubrium to the top of the distended neck vein. Add 4 cm to this measurement and this is a guide for central venous pressure. The normal value is 4–15 cm H_2O.

Check for a hepatojugular reflex (HJR). With the patient in the same 45° angle position used to determine the CVP, compress the upper right abdomen for 30–45 seconds. If HJR is present, the jugular veins will become more pronounced and the level of filling seen in the neck veins will rise.

INSPECTION OF THE EXTREMITIES

When inspecting the extremities, compare one arm to the other and one leg to the other. Look for ulcerations, edema, color changes, and distribution of hair. Feel for temperature changes in the four extremities and check all peripheral pulses.

Clubbing of the fingernail beds is evi-

dence of long-standing hypoperfusion and hypoxia. Figure 50-1 shows the normal angle between the fingernail and the nail bed which is usually around 160°. In early clubbing, the nail base is springy and is at a 180° angle. In late clubbing, the nail base is visibly swollen and the angle between the nail and the nail base exceeds 180°.

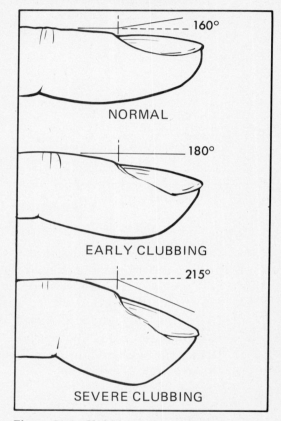

Figure 50-1. Clubbing of the fingernails.

Palpation

Palpate for the PMI where it was seen using the palmar surface of the fingers. If the PMI was not seen, palpate in the intersection of the mid-clavicular and mid-sternal lines. After palpating for the PMI, the rest of the precordial region is palpated to determine the presence or absence of thrills, thrust, heaves, retractions, bulges, and lifts. The precordial region is palpated as shown in Figure 50-2. The apical, mid-precordial, parasternal, pulmonic, aortic, sternoclavicular, and epigastric areas are usually palpated in this order.

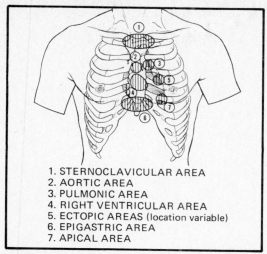

1. STERNOCLAVICULAR AREA
2. AORTIC AREA
3. PULMONIC AREA
4. RIGHT VENTRICULAR AREA
5. ECTOPIC AREAS (location variable)
6. EPIGASTRIC AREA
7. APICAL AREA

Figure 50-2. Precordial regions palpated to determine abnormalities.

Thrills are palpable murmurs. "Thrills should be identified as systolic or diastolic by their relationship with the PMI. Thrills are generally associated with pathological states. A thrust is an outward chest movement of increased amplitude; a heave is an outward movement of prolonged duration with or without increased amplitude. Retraction is an inward movement. The word *lift* (sic) describes outward movement of sternal or peristernal area."[1]

When palpating pulses, the rate, pattern, and intensity are assessed and recorded. With the exception of the carotid arteries, all pulses should be palpated in opposing positions at the same time for comparison. Figure 50-3 identifies the major pulses for palpation.

The carotid arteries are palpated individually to prevent occlusion of the arteries perfusing the brain. When palpating the carotid artery, one must be careful not to rub the area. This may cause reflex slowing of the heart. This is especially important in the elderly and the patient with a known

[1]Burns KR, Johnson PJ: Health Assessment in Clinical Practice. Englewood Cliffs, NJ: Prentice-Hall, p. 171, 1980

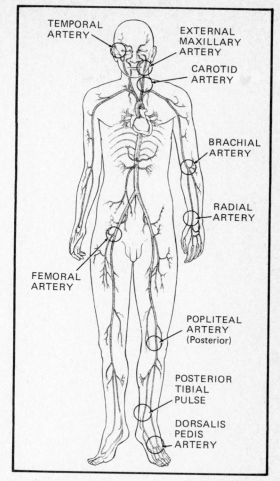

Figure 50-3. Major pulses to be palpated.

cardiac pathology. NOTE: If one cannot palpate the carotid artery, attempt to palpate the superficial temporal artery which is a bifurcation of the external carotid artery.

The pattern of rhythm of the pulse is recorded as regular, irregular, irregularly regular, or irregularly irregular. A regular pulse occurs in a methodical sequence. An irregular pulse has no descriptive pattern. An irregularly regular pulse has a describable pattern such as 1, 2, 3, 4, skip, 1, 2, 3, 4, skip. An irregularly irregular pulse has no pattern, such as, 1, 2, skip, 1, 2, 3, 4, skip, 1, skip, and so forth.

TYPES OF PULSE

The normal pulse is regular in rhythm and consistent in intensity. A full or increased pulse may be regular in rhythm but has a consistently increased intensity. Bounding pulses are variable in rate and very forceful in maximal intensity. A weak pulse has minimal pulsation. Palpable pulses that are rapid, weak, and of variable intensity are termed *thready*. In **pulsus alternans,** the pulse is alternately weak and strong. In **pulsus paradoxus** the pulsation is decreased during respiratory inspiration and increased during expiration. Changes in intrathoracic pressure are responsible for the changes in pulse intensity of pulsus paradoxus. **Pulsus magnus** is a strong, bounding, and rapid pulse. **Pulsus parvus** is a small, weak pulse. **Pulsus bisiferens** is a pulse characterized by two impulses palpated during one systole.

ALLEN'S TEST

The Allen's test confirms adequate peripheral circulation in the ulnar and radial arteries. This test should be performed on all patients prior to hemodynamic monitoring through a peripheral artery.

Have the patient rest his or her arm on the overbed table. Put a rolled washcloth under his or her wrist for support and then have the patient make a clenched fist. Using the first two fingers of each of your hands, occlude the ulnar artery with one hand and the radial artery with the other hand. After occluding both arteries for about 30 seconds, have the patient unclench his or her fist and hold the patient's hand in a relaxed position. At this point, the palm of the patient's hand should appear blanched. NOTE: Do not allow the patient to hyperextend his or her fingers since this may cause a false blanching. Now remove the fingers occluding the patient's ulnar artery. If the artery is patent, the patient's hand will flush indicating a rush of oxygenated blood into the hand.

Repeat the Allen's test on the patient's other wrist and document your findings for both the patient's left and right wrists.

Percussion

With the advent of the stethoscope, percussion is used less often. Percussion's main use is to identify the external borders of the heart to determine the presence of a cardiomegaly. However, x-rays and other diagnostic tests provide more reliable data.

Auscultation

Auscultating heart sounds is the major task in assessing cardiovascular status. It is also the most difficult skill for most nurses to accomplish. The key factors noted in auscultation are the pitch, intensity, duration, and quality of the heart sounds. It is necessary for one to recognize that the anatomical locations of the heart valves and the points of maximal sound transmission are *not the same*. Figure 50-4 shows the anatomical location of the heart valves and Figure 50-5 shows the areas for auscultation.

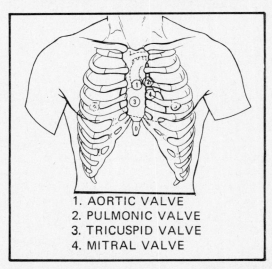

1. AORTIC VALVE
2. PULMONIC VALVE
3. TRICUSPID VALVE
4. MITRAL VALVE

Figure 50-4. Anatomical location of heart valves.

NORMAL HEART SOUNDS

Contraction of the heart produces two primary sounds. S_1 is the first heart sound and is usually described as lub. The S_1 sound is associated with the turbulent blood flow against the mitral and tricuspid valves following their closure. S_1 is followed by a quiet period called systole.

The second primary sound is S_2. It is described as dub. It is associated with turbulent blood flow against the closed aortic and pulmonic valves. S_2 is followed by another quiet period, diastole. At the base of the heart, S_1 is the lighter sound and S_2, the

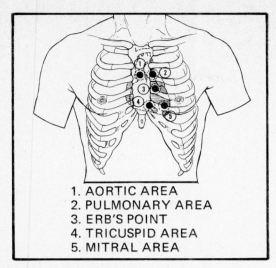

1. AORTIC AREA
2. PULMONARY AREA
3. ERB'S POINT
4. TRICUSPID AREA
5. MITRAL AREA

Figure 50-5. Areas for auscultation.

heavier, louder sound. Figure 50-6 shows the relationship schematically.

The heart may produce two more sounds which are called S_3 and S_4. S_3 occurs in 0.12–0.14 seconds after S_2. S_3 is thought to be due to increased pressure required to complete ventricular filling. S_3 is common in young people and those who have a slow

ventricular rate (like joggers). S_3 disappears around the age of 20 and its presence after the age of 30 is indicative of a cardiac myopathy. S_3 occurs late in diastole or in early, rapid ventricular filling and is heard best over the pulmonic valve area with the bell of the stethoscope. The cadence (Figure 50-7) with an S_3 sounds like Ken-**Tuc**-Ky with the emphasis on *Tuc.* An S_3 sound may be a warning sign of impending congestive heart failure.

S_4 occurs in diastole either just before S_1 or within S_1. It is thought that last ventricular filling, tensing of atrioventricular valve structures, and atrial muscular contraction cause S_4. S_4 is normally differentiated from S_1 only in young children. S_4 is heard just before S_1 and is best heard in the pulmonic valve area with the bell of the stethoscope. The cadence (Figure 50-8) of S_4 sounds like **Ten**-nes-see with the emphasis on the *Ten.* S_4 sounds are related to atrial contraction and often occur in myocardial infarction. Discriminating S_3 and S_4 from a split S_1 or S_2 sound is very difficult and requires a great deal of experience. Figure 50-9 graphically illustrates the relationship of heart sounds to the cardiac cycle.

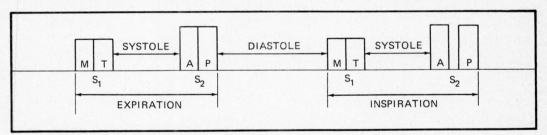

Figure 50-6. The relationship between S_1 and S_2.

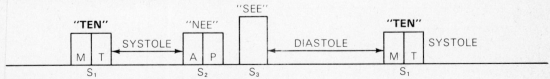

Figure 50-7. A schematic representation of S_3.

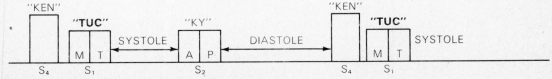

Figure 50-8. A schematic representation of S_4.

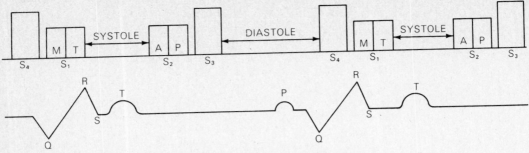

Figure 50-9. The relationship of heart sounds to the cardiac cycle.

Splitting of the Heart Sounds

SPLITTING OF HEART SOUND S_1

S_1 splitting is due to asynchronous closure of the mitral and tricuspid valves. Changes in the conduction time and blood volume are the causes for altering the timing of the closing of the valves. These factors result in a separate sound for closure of each AV valve. One *actually* hears a second sound.

A distinction among S_3, S_4, and a split S_1 is that these are heard best with the bell of the stethoscope and the normal S_1 is heard best with the diaphragm of the stethoscope.

Splitting of the first sound is often heard in hyperthyroidism, anemia, tachycardia, and mitral stenosis. In a split S_1 the sound may be normal, is best heard at the apex or PMI of the heart, and sounds like **T-lub-dub**. Figure 50-10 depicts the relationship of a split S_1.

PHYSIOLOGIC SPLITTING OF S_2

S_2 split usually occurs during inspiration because increased blood flow to the right side of the heart prolongs right ventricular systole delaying pulmonic valve closure. The physiologic splitting of S_2 is best heard in the pulmonic valve area with the diaphragm of the stethoscope and sounds like Lub-**dub**. The splitting sound appears during inspiration and disappears with expiration. Figure 50-11 shows a schematic representation of the normal physiological splitting of S_2.

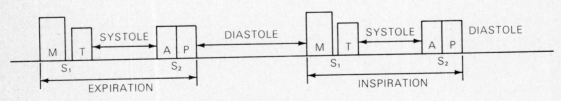

Figure 50-10. Representation of split S_1 sounds.

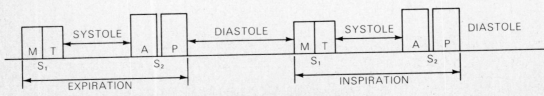

Figure 50-11. Representation of normal physiologic S_2 splitting.

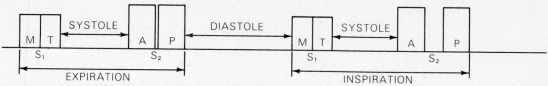

Figure 50-12. Representation of fixed S₂ splitting.

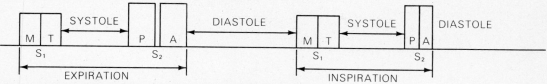

Figure 50-13. Representation of paradoxical S₂ splitting.

FIXED SPLITTING OF S_2

A fixed splitting of S_2 is abnormal and is constant in both inspiration and expiration. It is this constancy which differentiates pathological splitting from physiological splitting. A fixed split S_2 is best heard in the pulmonic valve area as Lub-**T-lub.** Figure 50-12 is the schematic relationship of the fixed splitting of S_2.

Paradoxical splitting is the result of pulmonic valve closure preceding aortic valve closure. Paradoxical splitting is most often caused by left bundle branch block and severe aortic stenosis. In paradoxical splitting, the splitting appears on expiration and disappears on inspiration. Figure 50-13 is a schematic representation of paradoxical splitting.

Extracardiac Sounds

Extra heart sonds may be heard in early, mid, or late systole.

EARLY SYSTOLIC EJECTION CLICKS

Early clicks occur shortly after S_1. Aortic ejection clicks are heard at both the base and apex of the heart. Aortic clicks normally occur with dilatation of the aorta, hypertension, and aortic valve disease.

Pulmonary ejection clicks are best heard in the pulmonic area of the heart. These clicks may be heard when there is pulmonary artery dilatation, pulmonary hypertension, and/or pulmonic stenosis.

MID-LATE SYSTOLIC CLICKS

Most mid and late systolic clicks are probably related to a ballooning of the mitral valve or some other mitral valve deformity. These clicks are often associated with late systolic murmurs.

PERICARDIAL FRICTION RUB

This rub is produced by inflammation of the pericardial sack. There may be three short components associated with the friction rub. These components are atrial systole, ventricular systole, and ventricular diastole. If all three sounds are present, the diagnosis is almost certain. However, often only the first two components are present. If just one sound is present, it is easy to confuse the friction rub with a murmur. The rub is most often heard at the third intercostal space (ICS) at the left sternal border (LSB), but this is variable. A friction rub does not commonly radiate in any area. The intensity is variable and may increase if one has the patient lean forward and exhale. A friction rub sounds scratchy and close to the ear, perhaps because it is a high-pitched sound.

VENOUS HUM

A venous hum is most common in children. It is a benign sound caused by turbulence of blood in the jugular veins. It is a continuous murmur which is loudest in diastole and softest in systole with no silent interval. The hum radiates to the first and second

ICS from the medial one-third of the right clavicle. The sound ranges from soft to moderate and can be completely obliterated by pressure on the jugular vein. The sound is humming, roaring, and of low pitch.

MEDIASTINAL CRUNCH

These crunches develop when there is air in the mediastinum. Movement of the heart produces pressure on these small air pockets. The mediastinal crunch sound is either random or it occurs during ventricular systole. A mediastinal crunch may be associated with crepitation in the neck secondary to subcutaneous emphysema. These sounds are associated with cardiac surgery. However, they can occur in an accident victim. In these cases, the sounds are an ominous sign indicating probable rupture of the trachea or tracheobronchial tree.

SYSTOLIC SNAP

This is the sound heard when the mitral valve opens. It is generally heard in patients with mitral stenosis.

Murmurs

High frequency, high intensity sounds are called heart sounds. Low frequency, low intensity sounds are called heart murmurs.

Murmurs are graded on a scale of one (I) to six (VI). They are usually reported as a fraction such as III/VI with the numerator identifying the severity of the murmur and the denominator identifying the scale used.

In general, if a murmur occurs with a pulse beat, consider it to be a systolic murmur. If the murmur does not occur with a pulse beat, consider it to be a diastolic murmur. Table 50-1 reviews systolic murmurs and their characteristics. Table 50-2 reviews diastolic murmurs and their characteristics.

Table 50-1. Systolic murmurs.*

Pathology	Timing	Location	Referred Sound	Quality	Pitch	Intensity	Schematic Pattern
I Variant VSD	Early systolic murmur	Lower left sternal border	Precardium	Harsh	High	Moderately loud	S_1 ∼∼∼∼ S_2 Constant
II Aortic stenosis	Midsystolic murmur (ejection)	First or second right intercostal space	Apex and neck (carotid arteries), heard over complete thorax; may be accompanied by thrill.	Harsh	Mid scale to high	May be difficult to hear (faint) or easily heard with stethoscope (loud)	S_1 WWW∼ ∼WWW S_2 Decrescendo/ Crescendo
a. Aortic valvular calcification							
b. Dilatation of aortic root							
c. Coarctation of the aorta							
d. Idiopathic hypertropic subaortic stenosis							
III Pulmonic stenosis		Third left intercostal space	Toward left shoulder	Harsh	Mid scale to high		
IV Tetralogy of Fallot	Midsystolic murmur (ejection)	Left sternal border, 3rd and 4th interspace	Toward left shoulder, neck, or apex	Harsh	Mid scale to high depending on severity	Moderately loud to loud	S_1 WWWW∼ ∼WWWS_2 Decrescendo/ Crescendo

Table 50-1. Continued.*

Pathology	Timing	Location	Referred Sound	Quality	Pitch	Intensity	Schematic Pattern
V Click-murmur syndrome	Late systolic murmur (ejection)	Apex	Toward left axilla	Blowing	Mid scale to high depending on severity	Moderately loud	S_1 ⑂Wwww- -wwwW⑊ S_2 Decrescendo/Crescendo
a. Mitral-valve prolapse	Late systolic murmur (ejection)	Lower left sternal border (mitral area)	Toward left axilla	Blowing	Mid scale to high depending on severity	Moderately loud	S_1 ～～～ S_2 Constant
b. Multiple systolic clicks	Late systolic murmur (ejection)	Lower left sternal border (mitral area)	Toward left axilla	Blowing	Mid scale to high depending on severity	Moderately loud	S_1 ⑂Wwww- -wwwW⑊ S_2 Decrescendo/Crescendo
VI Mitral regurgitation (insufficiency)	Pansystolic (holosystolic) regurgitation murmurs	Lower left sternal border (mitral area)	Toward left axilla	Blowing	High	Loud	S_1 ～～～ S_2 Constant
VII Tricuspid regurgitation (insufficiency)	Pansystolic (holosystolic) regurgitation murmurs	Lower left sternal border (tricuspid area)	Toward apex	Blowing	High	Moderately loud	S_1 ～～～ S_2 Constant
VIII Ventricular septal defect (VSD) or (IVSD)	Pansystolic (holosystolic) regurgitation murmurs	Lower left sternal border over defect	Precordium	Harsh	High	Loud—depending on size	S_1 ～～～ S_2 Constant

*Adapted from Cardiovascular system. *In* Assessment (patient history, anatomy and physiology, physical examination, nursing diagnosis). Nursing 82 books, The nurse's reference library. Springhouse, PA: Intermed Communications, Inc., pp. 348-349, 1982

Table 50-2. Diastolic murmurs.*

Pathology	Timing	Location	Referred Sound	Quality	Pitch	Intensity	Schematic Pattern
I Aortic regurgitation (insufficiency)	Early diastolic	Second right ICS† and LSB†	Toward sternum	Blowing	High	Moderately loud	S_1 S_2 ⋙ S_1 Decrescendo
II Pulmonic regurgitation (insufficiency)	Early diastolic	Second or third ICS	Toward sternum	Blowing	High	Moderately loud	
III Patent ductus arteriosus (PDA)	Early diastolic	Second left ICS	Toward neck (carotid arteries)	Harsh	Mid scale to high	Moderately loud to loud	S_1 ∼∼∼ S_2 Continuous
IV Mitral stenosis	Mid to late diastolic	Apex	Sound does not radiate	Rumble	Low	Soft—may be heard without difficulty	S_1 S_2 ⋙ S_1 Crescendo
V Tricuspid stenosis	Mid to late diastolic	Lower left border (xiphoid area)	Sound does not radiate	Rumble	Low	Soft—may be heard without difficulty	

*Adapted from Cardiovascular system. *In* Assessment (patient history, anatomy and physiology, physical examination, nursing diagnosis). Nursing 82 books, The nurse's reference library. Springhouse, PA: Intermed Communications, Inc., pp. 348–349, 1982

†ICS = intercostal space; LSB = left sternal border

— 51

Assessment of the Patient with Neurologic Dysfunction

Learning Objectives

By the end of this chapter, the nurse will be able to:

1. Identify significant family and medication histories that have an effect on the nervous system.
2. Identify the procedure to assess six of the twelve cranial nerves.
3. Define Weber's test and the Rinne's test.
4. List three assessment skills used in evaluating the motor system.
5. List three or more factors one should inspect in assessing the motor system.
6. Differentiate between superficial and deep-tendon reflexes.
7. Describe the superficial abdominal reflexes in a normal assessment.
8. Explain the testing of the cremasteric reflex in men.
9. Describe the plantar reflex in relation to the term Babinski.
10. Differentiate between the grasp reflex, the snout reflex, and the glabellar reflex.
11. Briefly describe how to test the following deep-tendon reflexes:
    a. The jaw-jerk
    b. The biceps reflex
    c. The brachioradialis test
    d. The triceps reflex test
    e. The finger flexion test
    f. The patellar reflex test
    g. The achilles (ankle-jerk) test
12. Briefly describe methods for assessing light touch, pain, and temperature sensations.
13. Briefly explain testing deep sensory modalities of vibration and proprioception.
14. Explain assessment of the cortical discriminatory sensations in relation to:
    a. Stereognosis
    b. Topognosia
    c. Graphagnosia (graphesthesia)
15. Differentiate between gait dystaxia, arm dystaxia, and leg dystaxia.
16. Explain the Doll's eyes test.
17. Describe decorticate positioning.
18. Describe decerebrate positioning.
19. List and define six common respiratory patterns associated with neurological dysfunction.

The chances are that a nurse may not perform a complete neurologic examination of a patient. However, all of the aspects of a patient's neurological health are important in establishing a baseline for comparing specific neurologic changes.

A neurological assessment includes a patient history (which is extremely important and usually difficult to obtain); medications being taken; and signs and symptoms of altered function in the cerebrum (changes in LOC), the cerebellum (changes in coordination), the cranial nerves (facial asymmetry), the motor system (abnormal movements), the sensory system (paresthesias), and the reflexes (hypo-hyper pathologies).

Patient History

Significant family history of a systemic disease may have some bearing on the patient's current status. Systemic diseases which affect the patient are important because of their symptomatology and current treatment. Medication history includes psychoactive drugs, anticoagulants (including aspirin), anticonvulsants, and alcohol use and abuse.

Inspection

Inspection of the patient begins as soon as one sees the patient. Is the patient awake or not? Is he or she disheveled, lying quietly in bed, or having abnormal positioning of hands and feet (decerebrate/decorticate posture)? Is the patient restrained, combative but not restrained, or thrashing about in a bizarre manner? Does the patient seem to understand his or her environment or recognize you as a nurse and not as a threat? Does he or she make eye contact with you or mostly gaze away from you? Is the patient's facial expression confused, angry, impatient, alert, or flat? Is the patient's face symmetrical or does one eye and one corner of the mouth droop or are the folds of the face symmetrical? Inspection of the patient's head and face may reveal depressions, lumps, areas of tenderness, swelling, and ecchymoses.

If the patient is able to talk, is his or her speech normal, clear and appropriate, or dysarthric (difficulty in speaking), dysphonic (difficulty in producing sound), dysprosodic (difficulty with syllables and rhythm of speech), or dysphasic (difficulty in understanding or expressing words)? Are all four extremities moved equally? Does the patient's mood seem labile, swinging from one extreme to another?

If the patient is not unconscious, test his or her long-term memory (birthdate, place of birth, etc.) and short-term memory (where he or she is and why). Assess the patient's orientation to person, place, and time. Assess the patient's abstract reasoning by having him or her explain a simple proverb (e.g., a stitch in time saves nine). Does the patient converse with you or does the patient simply utter a stream of words? By this point, one will have assessed the alert patient's level of consciousness and have a baseline for future comparisons.

Palpate the carotid arteries ONE at a time to prevent significant interruption of cerebral perfusion. If palpation reveals a bruit, auscultate the carotids, the eyes, temples, great vessels, and mastoid processes to confirm the presence of a bruit. Inspect the face for symmetry and the presence, absence, or size of palpebral fissures.

Testing Cranial Nerves (Conscious Patient)

If the patient is alert **and** cooperative, the nurse can check all 12 cranial nerves. If the patient is not alert **or** not cooperative, not all of the cranial nerves can be tested. Figure 51-1 shows the origin and function of all 12 cranial nerves.

OLFACTORY NERVE (CN I)

This nerve cannot be tested in the unconscious patient. In the conscious patient, anosmia (loss of sense of smell) is tested by having the alert patient close one nostril and sniff a familiar nonirritating odor such as coffee or cloves. Repeat this with the other nostril.

OPTIC NERVE (CN II)

To test this nerve, test the patient's visual acuity. Test each eye separately. Have the

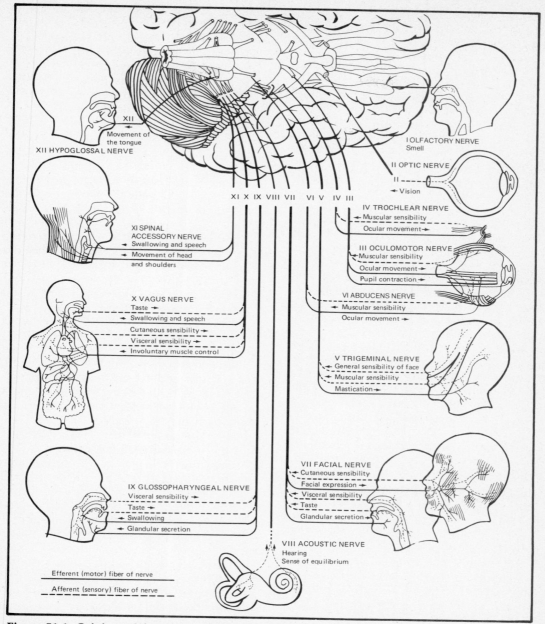

Figure 51-1. Origin and function of the twelve cranial nerves.

patient read something printed on a card at varying distances to obtain a rough estimate of his or her visual acuity. If it is possible to test the visual fields, stand directly in front of the patient and have the patient stare at your nose. Bring an object (finger) from outside the patient's scope of vision towards the patient's nose. Each quadrant is tested in each eye. If the nurse is able to stand directly in front of the patient, the nurse can compare the patient's visual field with his or her own.

OCULOMOTOR (CN III), TROCHLEAR (CN IV), AND ABDUCENS (CN VI)

These three cranial nerves are tested concurrently. Observe the pupil size and shape, comparing right to left. Test light reflexes and pupil dilatation. Direct light reflex is checked by shining a light directly into the eye. The pupil should constrict briskly. Check each eye. The consensual light reflex is tested by shining a light into one eye and checking to see if the *other* pupil is constricted. It should be. Repeat, testing the other eye. Test the accommodation reflex by having the patient stare at your finger as you move the finger directly towards the patient's nose. The eyes should converge and follow the finger towards the nose; the pupils should constrict. Range of ocular movement is tested by having the patient follow your finger through full range of motion. Nystagmus may occur during the test or with the eyes resting. Nystagmus is a jerking back and forth movement of the eye and is abnormal except at the extremes of a lateral gaze. The rate of normal nystagmus is 20 times per minute. Occasionally, nystagmus is rotational. If all of these tests are normal, it may be recorded as **PERRLA** (pupils equal, round, react to light with accommodation).

TRIGEMINAL (CN V)

This nerve has both a motor and a sensory tract. The motor tract is tested by having the patient clench his or her teeth. While the teeth are clenched, palpate the masseter muscles and the temporal muscles. Assess the patient's ability to chew.

The sensory tract innervates the face. It has three branches. To test all three, have the patient close his or her eyes and with a pin touch the patient's forehead, cheeks, and jaws on each side. The patient should be able to discern a dull or sharp pinprick in each area. Test the corneal reflex by *gently* touching the cornea with a wisp of cotton. Blinking and tearing is the normal reflex.

FACIAL (CN VII)

This nerve provides motor activity of the face such as smiling, frowning, raising eye-brows, and opening eyes against resistance. All of these facial activities should be symmetrical and equal in strength. The facial nerve also is responsible for taste. Taste buds are on the anterior two-thirds of the tongue AND on the sides of the tongue. Sugar and salt are the normal substances used to test taste. (Of course, the patient will have to rinse his or her mouth in between the salt and sugar.)

ACOUSTIC (CN VIII)

This nerve has two segments: The cochlear branch is responsible for hearing and the vestibular branch is associated with balance.

In the alert patient, the cochlear nerve may be tested by whispering near each ear of the patient. The patient's ability to hear the sound indicates an intact cochlear branch. If no sound or a diminished sound is heard, more extensive testing is warranted. Both the Weber and Rinne's tests use a tuning fork to test transmission of sound.

In the Weber's test, one places a vibrating tuning fork midline on the patient's anterior skull. With the stem of the tuning fork in place, sound should be heard equally with each ear. If the sound is heard unequally, the ear with the decreased hearing has the impaired cochlear nerve.

Rinne's test consists of placing the stem of a vibrating tuning fork on the mastoid bone. When the sound stops, the tuning fork is held in front of the ear canal. Sound should again be heard because air conduction of sound is greater than bone conduction of sound. If the patient does NOT hear more sound via air conduction, a middle ear disease is suspected. An impaired cochlear nerve function is suspected if the air-to-bone conduction is less in one ear as compared to the other.

Often the vestibular portion of CN VIII indicates dysfunction when patients complain of nausea, vomiting, or sweating. Other signs include the development of vertigo, nystagmus, postural deviation, and hypotension.

Often an ice water Caloric test is done to establish vestibular function. It is essential that the tympanic membrane be intact and that the ear canal not be occluded. The head of the bed is elevated to 30° in order to position the semicircular canals on a vertical plane. The physician irrigates the ear canal with ice cold water (not more than 200 cc).

If the vestibular portion of CN VIII is intact, the patient usually develops nausea, vertigo, and horizontal nystagmus towards the untested ear. Postural deviation and past-pointing occur on the irrigated side. The ice water Calorics should be tested on both ears by the physician.

GLOSSOPHARYNGEAL (CN IX)

Several steps are used to test both the afferent and the efferent arc of CN IX.

In order to test CN IX completely, have the patient identify taste at the back of the tongue. An abnormal response is loss of taste. This frequently occurs with a tumor or injury to the brain stem.

Touch cotton (such as a Q-tip®) to the soft palate. Absent sensation on the affected side of the palate may be caused by neck trauma. Have the patient say "ah." With this syllable, the palate should elevate symmetrically. Use a tongue blade to test the gag reflex. With the gag reflex, the palate and uvula should rise. In addition to testing the glossopharyngeal nerve, this tests the efferent arc of CN X.

The glossopharyngeal nerve also affects the patient's speech and may be tested if the patient's speech seems abnormal. If there is a question, have the patient say these three specific sounds in order: "kuh, kuh, kuh," "la, la, la," and "mi, mi, mi." These three sounds will test the ability of the soft palate, tongue, and lips (in this order) to interact in forming words.

If dysarthria or dysphagia is suspected, ask the patient to swallow water and observe the patient's ability to do so. During the examination, watch to see how well the patient handles salivation.

VAGUS (CN X)

Pressure on the carotid artery normally slows the heart rate and may cause hypertension.

Hoarseness may indicate damage to the vagus nerve. Inspect the soft palate and larynx. Sagging of the soft palate, a gag reflex, or deviation of the uvula (to the normal side) are indications of damage to the vagus nerve secondary to a tumor, injury to the brain stem, or neck trauma.

SPINAL ACCESSORY (CN XI)

This nerve innervates the sternocleidomastoid and the trapezius muscles. Observe these muscles for symmetry, atrophy, or hypertrophy. Test these muscles from each side. The strength should be the same. There are three tests to be performed for these muscles:

1. Have the patient shrug his or her shoulders against the downward pressure you apply on both of the patient's shoulders. The resistance and strength of the trapezius muscles should be symmetrical.

2. Have the patient push his or her head against your hand to assess the strength of both sternocleidomastoid muscles, which should be the same.

3. Have the patient turn his or her head to one side and resist your attempts to turn his or her head back to midline. Palpate the opposite sternocleidomastoid muscle. Repeat on the other side. The size and strength of muscle should be the same on both sides. Abnormal findings would be a lack of muscle contraction, inequality of muscle contractions, and fasciculations.

HYPOGLOSSAL (CN XII)

This nerve is responsible for normal tongue movements required for speaking and swallowing. Have the patient stick out his or her tongue. It should be midline. Observe the asymmetry, deviation to one side, loss of tongue tissue on one or both sides, and fasciculations. An abnormal position from midline will result in the tongue protruding towards the affected side. This may be the result of neck trauma associated with major vessel damage. Also, test the strength of the tongue by having the patient move his or her tongue from side to side, pushing it against the cheeks. Strength should be equal on both sides.

The Motor System

The motor system is normally assessed for gross abnormalities from the first contact with the patient. Motor system screening includes the patient's station and gait.

The Romberg test evaluates the patient's station by having the patient stand with feet close together and with eyes opened and then closed. Involuntary swaying of the trunk with eyes closed is abnormal and known as a positive Romberg test.

Tandem (heel-to-toe) walking with one's eyes open is considered to be abnormal if the trunk sways. Table 51-1 describes abnormal gait.

Have the patient hop in place on each foot alternately. Note imbalance or poor coordination.

Have the patient stand on one foot and perform a shallow knee bend with the angle of the knee at 45°. Repeat, standing on the other foot. Normally there is no difficulty; however, a weakness of the quadriceps makes this maneuver difficult or impossible. To evaluate plantar and dorsiflexion of the ankles, have the patient walk first on his or her toes and then on his or her heels. If there is no motor weakness, the patient can do this easily. With motor weakness, the patient cannot do this.

Screening upper extremity motor function is partially subjective. Have the patient grip your hands and decide if the strength of the grip is symmetrical. Next have the patient stand unsupported with the arms at his or her side. Ask the patient to then raise both arms to shoulder level with palms pronated, then supinated. Deviations from normal include weakness, asymmetry, or abnormal muscular movements. Table 51-2 defines abnormal muscle movement.

Table 51-1. Abnormal gaits.*

Gait	Pattern Observed
Hemiplegic gait	Leg is stiff and extended; movement of foot results from pelvic tilting upward on involved side; the foot is lifted and leg swung at pelvic level; arm remains flexed, adducted, and does not swing.
Spastic (diplegic) gait	Short steps, dragging the ball of the foot across floor; legs are extended.
Steppage gait	Elevating hip and knee excessively high to lift "drop foot" off ground.
Dystrophic gait	Legs far apart, shifting weight from side to side like waddling; abdomen is often protruding and lordosis is common.
Tabetic gait	Legs positioned far apart, lifted high, and forcibly brought down with each step, stamping heel on ground.
Cerebellar gait	Staggering gait with lurching from side to side; often swaying of the trunk occurs.
Parkinsonian gait	Shuffling gait with short steps; the entire trunk is flexed as are the knees, and the head is hunched forward.
Dystonic gait	Jerky dancing movements that appear nondirectional.
Astasia	Uncontrolled falling.

*Burns KR, Johnson PJ: Health Assessment in Clinical Practice. Englewood Cliffs, NJ: Prentice-Hall, p. 329, 1980.

Table 51-2. Abnormal muscle movements.*

1. Fasciculations: irregular contractions of muscle fiber bundles.
2. Myotonus: involuntary persistence of muscle contraction.
3. Choreiform movement: involuntary, intermittent, jerky movements of muscle groups, one at a time.
4. Ballism: flailing movements, usually involving limbs on one side.
5. Tremors: involuntary rhythmic movement due to alternating contractions of the flexor and extensor at a joint.
6. Dystonia: hypertonic trunk musculature resulting in slow, twisting movements of the trunk.
7. Athetosis: slow, twisting movement of the head and distal extremities.
8. Myoclonus: singular or serial, rapid, jerking movement (5–50 times per minute) of a muscle in the extremities, face, oral cavity, or diaphragm (hiccup).

*Burns KR, Johnson PJ: Health Assessment in Clinical Practice. Englewood Cliffs, NJ: Prentice-Hall, pp. 329–330, 1980.

Assessment of Reflexes

There are two types of reflexes: superficial and deep tendon reflexes.

SUPERFICIAL REFLEXES

The primary superficial reflexes tested are the corneal reflex and the gag reflex (refer to cranial nerves V and IX, respectively), the abdominal reflexes, cremasteric reflexes, anal reflexes, and plantar reflexes.

The superficial abdominal reflexes (Figure 51-2) are elicited by stroking the skin lateral to midline with a blunt-edged object (i.e., the handle of a reflex hammer, a tongue depressor, the blunt end of a safety pin). These reflexes are tested in the upper, middle, and lower quadrants bilaterally. The normal response is deviation of the umbilicus toward the stimulus.

The cremasteric reflex is elicited by stroking the inner thigh in a distal direction. The normal result is an elevation or movement of the ipsilateral testicle upward toward the body (Figure 51-3).

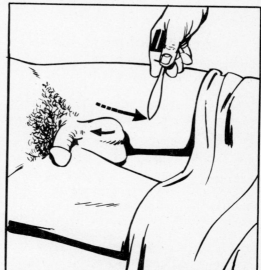

Figure 51-3. Eliciting the cremasteric reflex.

The anal reflex is elicited by pricking the perianal area. The normal response is contraction of the external anal sphincter.

The plantar reflex is obtained by scratching the lateral edge of the sole from heel to

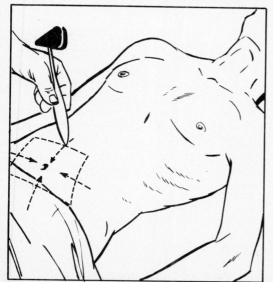

Figure 51-2. Eliciting the abdominal reflex.

toe. The expected result is plantar flexion of all the toes.

DEEP TENDON REFLEXES

The deep tendon reflexes include the pectoralis, biceps, triceps, jaw, and brachioradialis reflexes, the finger flexor reflex, the patellar (knee) reflex, and the achilles (ankle-jerk) reflex. Table 51-3 shows deep tendon reflexes, methods of assessment, and expected responses for the major deep tendon reflexes. Figure 51-4 through Figure 51-10 picture the deep tendon reflexes being elicited.

The jaw jerk is elicited by having the patient open his or her mouth and relax the lower jaw. The center of the chin is tapped with a reflex hammer. Normal response is no reaction. An abnormal response is the snapping shut of the lower jaw.

Deep tendon reflexes are assessed from a 0–5 grade. The reflex grading system either consists of a numeric notation (0–5) or it uses plus signs of which the symbol (#) recorded is the same as the arabic number. Table 51-4 presents both grading systems of the deep tendon reflex. Figure 51-11 shows these reflexes on a stick figure.

Other Pathologic Reflexes

There are several responses usually tested along with the deep tendon reflexes. Not all of these responses are reflexes but are deviations associated with pyramidal tract disease and often with other hyperactive reflex responses.

CLONUS

Clonus is a rhythmic, alternating flexion and extension in response to muscle stretch. The oscillations of clonus may be sustained or intermittent. The rate may vary from 5 to 50 per minute. Ankle clonus is tested by having the patient relax his or her knee and foot, keeping the leg slightly flexed. The foot is then suddenly dorsiflexed by the nurse's hand and **held** in dorsiflexion. The normal response is no response. If clonus is present, the foot will oscillate between flexion and extension and rhythmic clonic contractions of the muscles will be seen. This is normally reported as 4-beat clonus, 6-beat clonus, and so forth.

THE BABINSKI PHENOMENON

This is elicited by stroking the lateral sole from heel to toe and across the ball of the foot to the medial sole with a blunt object. The normal Babinski response is plantar flexion of the toes (Figure 51-12). The abnormal response (positive Babinski sign) is fanning of the toes with dorsiflexion of the great toe (Figure 51-13).

Variations of a positive Babinski are referred to as an equivocal Babinski sign which may indicate a milder or early stage of pyramidal tract disease. A definite positive Babinski sign is considered by most neurologists to be pathognomonic of pyramidal tract disease.

HOFFMANN'S SIGN

Normally Hoffmann's sign is no response to a forced flexion of the distal phalanx of the middle finger. It is elicited with the wrist held horizontal, pronated, and relaxed. A positive Hoffmann's sign (Figure 51-14) is a flexion-adduction of the fingers with opposing flexion-adduction movement of the thumb. A positive Hoffmann's sign is associated with upper motor neuron disease.

Hypo and hyper reflexes are always abnormal states.

The Sensory System

The assessment of the sensory system includes superficial sensation, deep sensation, deep pain, and discrimination. In the male, testicular pain is assessed. The body is evenly assessed with comparison of one side to the other side. The nurse should test patient reliability by attempting to determine if the patient is saying what he or she thinks you want to hear or what is actually perceived.

SUPERFICIAL SENSATIONS

These are the sensations of light touch, pain, and temperature. With the patient relaxed and eyes closed, test superficial sensations.

Table 51-3. Deep tendon reflexes, methods of assessment, and expected responses.*

Reflex Center	Method	Expected Response
Pectoralis (C$_5$ to T$_1$)	Patient's arm semiabducted; place thumb over tendon anterior to axillary crease; tap the thumb.	Contraction of muscle (seen or felt)
Biceps (C$_5$, C$_6$)	Patient's arm flexed and pronated; support elbow, place thumb over tendon in anticubital fossa, and strike thumb.	Muscle contraction usually with flexion of the forearm
Triceps (C$_7$, C$_8$)	Patient's arm flexed at elbow is supported by examiner; strike the triceps aponeurosis (do not mediate).	Contraction +/− extension of forearm
Brachioradialis (C$_5$, C$_6$)	Patient's forearms resting on abdomen, if lying, or tap, if sitting; the radial surface 1–2 inches above the wrist is tapped (do not mediate).	Flexion and supination of forearm
Finger Flexor Reflex	Hold patient's wrist, relaxed and pronated; with fingers flexed and relaxed, tap a tongue blade across fingertips.	Flexion of fingers and terminal phalanx of the thumb are seen and felt
Knee or Patellar Reflex (L$_2$, L$_3$, L$_4$)	Patient's legs semiflexed and dangling, directly strike quadriceps tendon below patella (do not mediate).	Contraction of muscle with extension of leg
Ankle Jerk, Achilles (S$_1$, S$_2$)	Patient's ankle relaxed and foot extended; apply gentle pressure to ball of foot creating dorsiflexion, and strike the Achilles tendon.	Plantar flexion of foot

*Burns KR, Johnson PJ: Health Assessment in Clinical Practice. Englewood Cliffs, NJ: Prentice-Hall, p. 331, 1980.

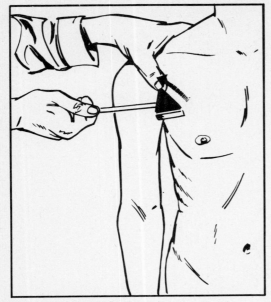

Figure 51-4. Pectoralis reflex.

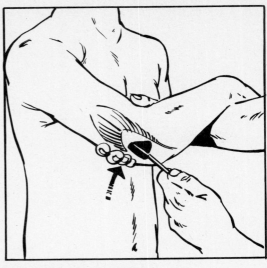

Figure 51-6. Triceps reflex.

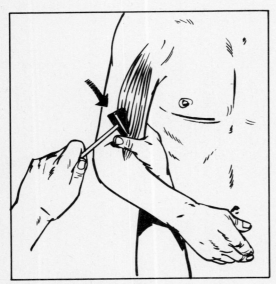

Figure 51-5. Biceps reflex.

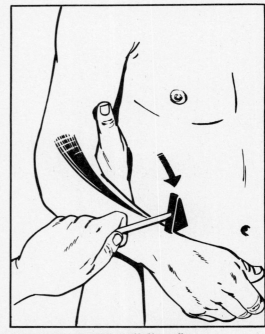

Figure 51-7. Brachioradialis reflex.

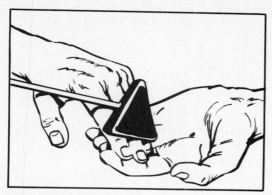

Figure 51-8. Finger flexor reflex.

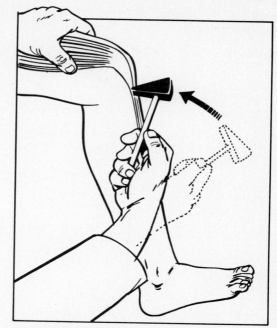

Figure 51-9. Knee-jerk or patellar reflex.

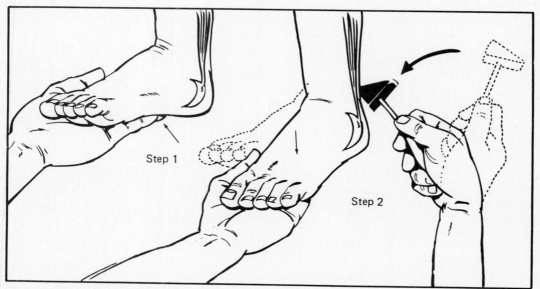

Step 1

Step 2

Figure 51-10. Ankle jerk reflex.

Table 51-4. Grading systems of deep tendon reflexes.*

Grade	Reflex Response
0	(0) absent
1	(+) sluggish or diminished
2	(+ +) active or normal
3	(+ + +) slightly hyperactive or increased response
4	(+ + + +) brisk with intermittent or transient clonus
5	(+ + + + +) very brisk with sustained clonus

*Burns KR, Johnson PJ: Health Assessment in Clinical Practice. Englewood Cliffs, NJ: Prentice-Hall, p. 330, 1980.

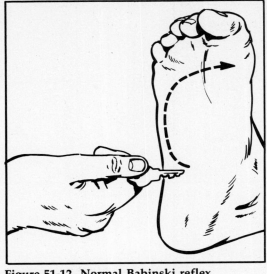

Figure 51-12. Normal Babinski reflex.

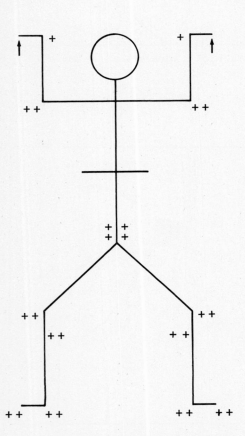

Figure 51-11. Deep reflexes depicted on stick-figure.

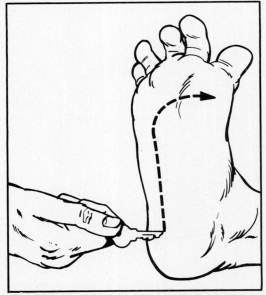

Figure 51-13. Positive (abnormal) Babinski reflex.

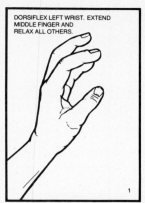
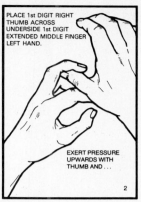
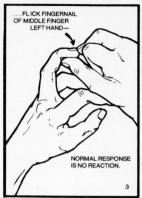
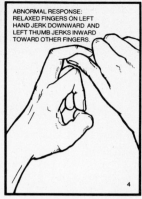

Figure 51-14. Hoffmann's sign.

Light Touch

Use organized but unpatterned testing. For light touch use a wisp of cotton and touch both arms, the trunk, and both legs. Ask the patient to identify when and where he or she is being touched.

Pain

Pain sensation is usually tested with a safety pin. With the patient's eyes closed, ask the patient to tell you when and where he or she is being touched and if the touch is sharp or dull. Decreased pain sensation is called hypalgesia. Loss of sensation is called analgesia. Unpleasant but not painful sensations are called paresthesia.

Temperature

This is not normally tested if the pain sensation is intact. To test temperature sensation, fill two test tubes, one with hot water and one with cold water. To test temperature sensation, follow the same pattern as testing for pain, only this time have the patient identify whether the sensation is hot or cold.

DEEP SENSATION

Deep sensation is first tested by testing vibration sense using a tuning fork.

VIBRATION SENSE

Place the vibrating tuning fork over the patient's sternum so that the patient recognizes the vibrating sensation. Vibration is tested over bony prominences. Because loss of vibration sense usually occurs distal to proximal, test distal areas first. Vibratory sense loss occurs in the lower extremities before the upper extremities. Thus, place the vibrating tuning fork over toe joints, then ankle bone, then the knee, and so on. If the vibratory sense is felt in the toes and in the finger joints, vibratory sense is intact and no further testing is needed. This test is not valid in the very elderly since a normal vibratory loss occurs with age. If the patient feels no vibrations in the toes, then vibratory testing proceeds to the ankle, the knee, the iliac crest of the hip, the lower ribs, and the head. If vibratory sense is lost in the fingertips, then testing of the wrist, elbow, and shoulder is indicated.

PROPRIOCEPTION

Proprioception is the identification of the position of the finger and great toe bilaterally. Hold the distal phalanx of the digit on its lateral surfaces. Do NOT hold the great toe or thumb by its superior and inferior planes since the pressure exerted to move the great toe or thumb will be a clue to the patient as to its position. When holding the distal phalanx by the lateral surfaces, a clue will not be given to the patient. If the position sense is impaired, continue to test proprioception by moving the next proximal joint.

DEEP PAIN

Deep pain is first assessed by noting the degree of pressure required by the examiner's thumb to produce pain on the calf muscle of the patient. Usually a great deal of pressure is required. Next the achilles tendon is pinched between the examiner's thumb knuckle and index finger until the patient indicates pain. Normally even slight pressure is painful.

SENSORY DISCRIMINATION

These tests are used to evaluate cortical sensory function.

STEREOGNOSIS

Stereognosis is the ability to identify familiar objects placed in the patient's hand while his or her eyes are closed. Items used include coins, keys, paper clips, and such.

GRAPHESTHESIA

This is the ability of the patient to recognize numbers or letters drawn on the palm of his or her hand with the patient's eyes closed. Normally these symbols are easily recognized by the patient. The terms graphesthesia is sometimes used synonymously with graphagnosia.

TOPOGNOSIA

Have the patient, with eyes closed, identify which finger the examiner is touching and if the sensation is on the right or left side of the finger. The patient should be able to do this easily.

DIFFUSE CEREBRAL DYSFUNCTION

The next three reflexes are all abnormal if they are present.

Grasp Reflex

In this reflex the patient grasps something placed in his or her hand and is unable to release it on command. Normally a person is able to release the object.

Snout Reflex

This reflex is similar to the newborn infants' rooting reflex. In the snout reflex, the patient involuntarily purses his or her lips when the side of the mouth is touched.

Glabellar Reflex

This reflex consists of the patient repeatedly blinking in response to each tapping on the forehead.

Assessment of the Patient with an Altered State of Consciousness

Altered state of consciousness will be referred to as a coma state in this text since unconsciousness can exist ONLY when both cerebral hemispheres are affected by injury or metabolic conditions. The injury or metabolic disease state may affect the diencephalon, the pons/mid-brain, or the reticular formation. If there is a lesion of the cerebrum, medulla, or spinal cord, it will not cause a coma if the lesion is unilateral. The following five assessments will provide a basis for determining patient response to treatment modalities.

1. **Level of consciousness** is best determined by the amount of force necessary to obtain a patient response. Since there is a lack of agreement on the words used to identify levels of consciousness (lethargy, stupor, obtundation), it is best to describe the force of stimuli needed to obtain a response from the patient and record this. If the patient can be aroused, determine his or her orientation to person, place, and time and describe the patient's behavior, emotional state, and his or her ability to speak clearly. The patient's LOC will have some bearing on the motor system, so motor reactions of the extremities and patient posturing must be identified.

2. **Pupillary response** was discussed previously in this chapter and includes a direct light reflex and a consensual light reflex. Descriptions of the pupil are made in comparison with the other pupil and are measured in millimeters. Response to the direct light response should be described as brisk, sluggish, fixed and dilated, fixed and constricted, or as a hippus reflex.

3. **Motor ability** of the patient in an altered state of consciousness can still be

tested. First observe what motor activity the patient has in response to noxious stimuli or spontaneously. This may identify a hemiplegia. Both hemiparesis and hemiplegia may be tested by lifting both of the patient's arms or both of the patient's legs off of the bed and then releasing them simultaneously. The hemiparetic extremity will fall faster and more limply than the nonhemiparetic extremity.

There may be increased muscular resistance (paratonia) to passive movement which usually occurs when there is decreased frontal lobe function. If paratonia is present or only one sided, there is normally a lesion of the frontal lobe and an increased ICP. Decerebrate rigidity (extensor posturing) has been described in the neurologic section and is associated with lesions of the pons/mesencephalon area. Decorticate rigidity (flexor posture) was also described in the neurologic section and is associated with lesions of the internal capsule.

4. **Cranial nerve testing** was covered in detail earlier in this chapter. Additional testing of cranial nerves V–VII is accomplished by applying pressure to the supraorbital ridge and looking for facial grimacing which will be decreased or absent on the same side as a hemiplegia if present. The ice water Caloric test, also called the oculovestibular reflex, was explained under testing of cranial nerves earlier in this chapter.

The Doll's eyes phenomenon is a synonym for the oculocephalic reflex. This test is done to confirm the patency of cranial nerves III, IV, and VI. To perform this test, hold the patient's eyelids open and briskly but gently turn the patient's head to one side. If the cranial nerves are intact, the patient's eyes will move in contraversive conjugate deviation. NOTE: The Doll's eyes phenomenon CANNOT be performed unless there is proof that a cervical injury is not present.

5. **Vital signs** are checked very frequently since hypothermia increases the metabolic needs of the central nervous system which may already be compromised. Hypothermia may result in cardiac dysrhythmias and has not been proven to prevent secondary effects of the cerebral condition causing a coma. Pulse and blood pressure are routinely checked although they are acknowledged as unreliable parameters in central nervous system disorders.

Respirations are often valuable in identifying cerebral dysfunctions. The most common respiratory patterns associated with a cerebral insult are posthyperventilation apnea, Cheyne-Stokes respiration, central neurogenic hyperventilation, apneustic breathing, ataxic breathing (Biot's), and cluster breathing. These were described and schematically presented in the respiratory section of this test and will therefore not be repeated here.

— 52

Assessment of the Patient with Renal Dysfunction

Learning Objectives

By the end of this chapter, the nurse will be able to:

1. List both family and patient historical facts that are pertinent to the renal system.
2. Explain skin color and pigmentation in the chronic renal failure patient.
3. List three observations to be made regarding edema.
4. Describe the respiratory pattern in altered renal function.
5. Explain the various urine colors and the cause of these.
6. Describe the procedure for percussion of the kidneys.
7. Identify the reason for percussion.
8. List the areas one auscultates for bruits in a renal assessment.
9. List two pathologies that a bruit may support.

As with all of the body system assessments, a personal and familial history is extremely important. It is helpful to know if other family members have a history of kidney disease, high blood pressure, diabetes mellitus, cardiovascular disease, or malignancies.

The patient's history is important to identify any of the familial traits and other precipitating causes of renal disease. The assessment of renal function in this text refers to renal failure and end-stage disease.

Inspection

Generalized inspection of the renal failure patient involves checking the appearance of the skin and its characteristics, eye disorders, muscle characteristics, including tetany and asterixis, the respiratory pattern, state of hydration, and urine characteristics.

SKIN AND ITS CHARACTERISTICS

The renal patient often has an abnormal skin color. Pallor is common due to anemia which is the result of decreased erythropoietin production. This results in a decreased number of RBCs. The decreased number of RBCs results in the skin's grayish tinge. Decreased oxygenation of the blood due to the decreased RBCs may result in hypoxia and an alteration in the LOC. The skin may have bruises and ecchymoses because of its fragility. The skin turgor depends upon the patient's state of hydration. Renal failure causes the glands in the skin to stop functioning. This causes subcutaneous calcium deposition resulting in purpura, which itches intensely.

EYE DISORDERS

Cataracts, papilledema, and dilated, convoluted veins are often seen in moderate-to-severe renal failure.

MUSCLE CHARACTERISTICS

The most common muscle dysfunctions are seen with the uremic syndrome of end-stage disease and may consist of tremors, weakness, and generalized debilitation. Muscle abnormalities include tetany and asterixis.

Tetany is caused by severe hypocalcemia or too rapid a correction of acidosis. This is tested by Chvostek's sign and Trousseau's sign.

Chvostek's sign is positive when tapping the finger over the supramandibular portion of the parotid gland results in an ipsilateral muscle spasm of the upper lip. This test is not always valid.

Trousseau's sign is the development of a carpopedal spasm when a B/P cuff is inflated over the upper arm. If no spasm is present after 3 minutes, the test is negative. In this case, remove the B/P cuff and have the patient hyperventilate (more than 30 breaths a minute). This causes a respiratory alkalosis that can produce carpopedal spasm.

Asterixis

Asterixis is indicative of a deteriorating uremic state with a poor prognosis. Asterixis may be seen as irregular movement of the wrists with a flapping movement of the fingers upon hyperextension of the arm. Asterixis normally occurs within 30 seconds of hyperextension of the arm.

THE RESPIRATORY PATTERN

The respiratory pattern changes from eupnea to a Kussmaul pattern as acidosis develops and becomes severe. Kussmaul respirations were defined and schematically shown in the respiratory section of this text and will not be repeated here.

STATE OF HYDRATION

Evaluate the patient's state of hydration by checking the mucous membranes in his or her mouth and his or her skin turgor. Mild dehydration is present if the buccal mucosa is dry. Severe dehydration is evidenced by parched, cracked lips and sunken eyes. Evaluate the patient's skin turgor by pinching a fold of the patient's skin over a bony area and then releasing it. If the patient is not dehydrated, the skin will immediately return to its normal state. This is most commonly done on the dorsal surface of the hand and the forearm.

To evaluate a patient's state of hydration, the nurse also needs to check the patient's neck veins for distension; dependent edema occurring in the ankle, sacral, and/or scrotal area; or total body edema (anasarca) occurring in the periorbital, abdominal, and pulmonary spaces. These symptoms indicate that the patient is in fluid overload and not dehydrated. Measure and compare the patient's intake and output daily. The normal hourly urine output is 30–100 ml. The normal 24-hour output is 720–2,400 ml. One thousand milliliters equal about 1 kilogram (2.2 pounds). With this information, the nurse can determine if the patient is in a negative fluid balance or a positive fluid balance.

URINE CHARACTERISTICS

Normally, urine is a clear yellow liquid. Abnormalities include grossly bloody urine, cloudy urine (pyuria), or orange urine due to bilirubin (bilirubinuria). The nurse may observe nocturia, polyuria, polydipsia, oliguria, and anuria.

Palpation

Palpation is used to obtain an idea of the size and shape of the kidneys. Palpation may reveal tenderness, and occasionally masses and cysts (although these are often difficult if not impossible to identify).

The right kidney is easier to palpate than the left, but even with bimanual palpation (Figure 52-1), usually only the top of the right kidney can be palpated since it is positioned slightly lower than the left.

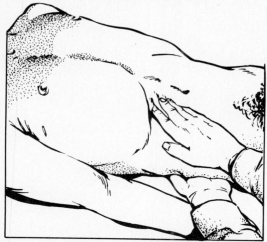

Figure 52-1. Bimanual palpation of the kidney.

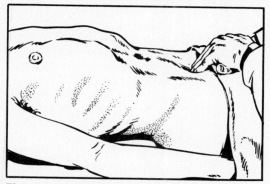

Figure 52-2. Palpation of the urinary bladder.

Palpate the urinary bladder bimanually (Figure 52-2) starting some 2 inches above the symphysis pubis. If empty, the bladder cannot usually be palpated. If the bladder is barely palpable, it is mildly distended. If easily palpable, it is markedly distended and an obstruction or disease state may be responsible. In a man, the prostate should be palpated for obstruction and retention of urine.

Percussion

In order to adequately percuss the kidneys, fist percussion is used rather than finger percussion (the techniques for fist percussion were discussed in Chapter 48). The percussion is performed over the costovertebral angles to elicit tenderness and/or pain. Either of these would indicate infection, calculi, masses (cysts, tumors, abcesses), hydronephrosis, or polycystic disease.

Auscultation

Using the bell of your stethoscope, try to auscultate the renal arteries, especially if the patient has hypertension. Listen for renal artery stenosis, which will be a bruit in the periumbilical area. Also listen for aortic bruits, which are best heard in the flanks or the intercostal region of the anterior abdomen.

Further Assessment

After all the information from inspection, palpation, percussion, and auscultation has been gathered, further studies to determine renal function are specific laboratory and radiologic studies. The nurse can determine more about the patient's conditions if he or she refers to the chart for serial laboratory results and diagnostic test results. This will give the nurse an overall assessment of the patient with renal dysfunction.

53

Assessment of the Patient with Endocrine Dysfunction

Learning Objectives

By the end of this chapter, the nurse will be able to:

1. Explain why history is important in assessing the endocrine system.
2. Identify the major areas of inspection and list the significant findings.
3. Describe palpation of the endocrine system.
4. Describe percussion of the endocrine system.
5. List other diagnostic tests for assessing the endocrine system.

The endocrine system acts as a regulator of all body systems. The endocrine system has eight glands that interact throughout the body to maintain growth and development, body systems function, emotional states, and physical appearance.

Most endocrine diseases present characteristic alterations in facial features and general appearance. Each endocrine disorder produces a striking physical similarity among those afflicted. Because the changes are so obvious and so characteristic of a specific endocrine dysfunction, an experienced endocrinologist can make a diagnosis often at first glance. At the same time, the diagnosis of endocrine diseases is difficult, if not impossible, for the general practitioner and other health care providers who have not had the opportunity to study and to examine patients with specific disorders.

History

Some endocrine diseases are inherited while others have a tendency to be inherited. Subsequently, establishing a family history is very important.

A patient history reveals information about his or her endocrine system. For example, trauma may cause diabetes insipidus, especially if the head is involved. Surgical procedures may have an effect on other body parts. For instance, removing both ovaries causes a premature menopause in a young female.

Diabetes mellitus developing during a pregnancy or after delivery of an infant weighing more than 10 pounds may indicate maturational development of diabetes mellitus in coming years.

The use of drugs including alcohol may produce signs of endocrine dysfunction.

Any and every change from a person's "normal" behavior or habits may indicate the onset of endocrine dysfunction and medical attention should be sought.

Inspection

Inspection is the primary assessment skill used in assessing the endocrine system. Palpation and auscultation are of slight value.

GENERAL APPEARANCE

The physical appearance, which includes the emotional state, is usually seen first and can rule out many suspicions immediately and make one think of a specific disease right away.

In the general assessment, the patient's apparent state of health is noted along with any signs of distress. General body development including height, weight, body build, and body fat are evaluated. The distribution of body fat differs in men and women. In men, fat is normally found over the entire body. In women, fat is predominant in the shoulders, breasts, buttocks, inner thigh, and the symphysis pubis. In overweight persons, fat distribution seems to accumulate in identical areas in both men and women.

Observing the patient's speech may make you suspicious of hyperthyroidism if the patient cannot talk fast enough or of myxedema if the patient slurs his or her words and sounds hoarse.

Skin color is important in determining the presence of hyperpigmentation, which may range from a slight tan to brown. Racial considerations have to be included in assessing the skin color. This is best done by looking at the mucous membranes of the mouth. Hyperpigmented gums are normal for black people; however, in a white person this may indicate Addison's disease. Hypopigmentation also occurs. Vitiligo is a condition in which splotches of skin of a black person lose their color and become white. In Caucasians, hypopigmentation results in albinism—a lack of skin coloring; albinos must stay out of the sun or bright light. Jaundice causes yellowing of the sclerae whereas jaundice due to myxedema does not affect the sclerae.

It is important to observe the patient for symmetry and appropriate proportions of the head, arms, and legs to the body. Dwarfism, giantism, and acromegaly are all dysfunctions which may be easily observed. Acromegaly is identified by an overgrowth of membranous bones and tissues. The forehead and the lower jaw both extend further out from the face than normal. The tongue may be so enlarged that it cannot be contained within the mouth. Hands and feet may become huge and the acromegaly patient may develop a kyphosis due to the vertebrae increasing in width and weight. Further testing would then be done on this patient to rule out tumors and to control the concurrent hyperglycemia.

The distribution of hair is observed over the scalp, face, and body. One also can determine if the hair is thick or thin, smooth or coarse, and dry or oily. The presence of hair on a woman's chest (hirsutism) is indicative of endocrine imbalance and indicates further exploration and/or treatment.

The eyes may reveal a great deal of information if properly inspected. Sunken eyes may be caused by severe dehydration. Visual acuity is tested with a Snellen chart or some other reading test. Testing peripheral visual fields may reveal a marked decrease in visual acuity secondary to glaucoma or to a pituitary tumor. Exophthalmos would indicate immediate testing for hyperthyroidism which is the most common cause for a pituitary tumor.

Inspection of the mouth includes observing the coloration of the mucous membranes as discussed earlier and determining if the membranes are normally moist or dry; dryness indicates dehydration. The tongue is evaluated for hypertrophy or atrophy, unusual color, and tremors. If tremors are present, neurological examination may reveal a concomitant neurological dysfunction.

The neck of the patient is observed as the patient swallows. The observer is looking for movement of the thyroid cartilage or any other detectable masses. A lack of noted movement during swallowing may be pathological so the neck will be palpated.

By this point in the inspection of the patient, the nurse should be able to accurately state the patient's level of consciousness with supporting data. The general behavior of the patient should be noted as normal (as expected) or abnormal with specific detailed data. Medications that the patient may be taking may alter the patient's LOC which should be noted.

Palpation

In palpating the thyroid gland, the nurse may stand facing the patient or behind the patient with the patient's chin lowered slightly. Having the patient lower his or her chin relaxes the neck muscles making palpation easier.

The thyroid gland is palpated for size, shape, symmetry, nodules, and tenderness or painfulness. To correctly palpate the thyroid gland, your index and middle fingers are used to feel the thyroid tissue directly below the cricoid cartilage. Palpation is done during swallowing since this raises the trachea, the larynx, and the thyroid gland, but no other structures. Next palpate the thyroid gland while standing behind the patient and use your thumbs to palpate for the same characteristics as previously noted. Enlarged thyroids may be due to goiters. Any masses or nodules felt require additional diagnostic tests to determine the endocrine dysfunction. Feel over the thyroid arteries for a thrill indicating turbulence of blood in these vessels which warrants further diagnostic studies.

Palpation should be used to determine any masses in the abdomen or enlargement of the kidneys. Tumors of the adrenal gland may displace the kidneys low enough to be palpated. This of course would indicate an abnormality and warrant further testing. Palpation of the abdomen is covered in Chapter 48.

Auscultation

Whether or not thrills were palpated over the thyroid arteries, the thyroid gland should be auscultated to determine the presence of bruits.

Percussion

This is not used in the assessment of the endocrine system.

Other Studies

With inspection being probably the most useful assessment tool in endocrine dysfunctions, other diagnostic studies including laboratory studies and radiologic studies must be included to finalize the diagnosis.

54

Assessment of the Patient with Hematologic Dysfunction

Learning Objectives

By the end of this chapter, the nurse will be able to:

1. Identify pertinent historical data relevant to the hematologic system.
2. List medications that may alter the hematologic system.
3. List five factors to be observed when inspecting the hematologic system.
4. Explain the palpation of the hematologic system.
5. Explain the percussion of the hematologic system.
6. Explain the auscultation of the hematologic system.
7. List three findings of auscultation of the hematologic system.
8. List three findings of inspection of special tests of the hematologic system.

Probably the most valuable skill in assessing the patient with a hematologic dysfunction is the ability to obtain a complete factual history. The familial history is an important record of hematologic disorders such as anemias, malignancies, RBC dyscrasias, bleeding disorders such as hemophilia, or clotting disorders as in polycythemia. Since many of the hematologic disorders are inherited or have the tendency to be inherited, detailed familial and patient histories are required.

History

For the individual patient, current problems and significant hematologic disorders in the past are pertinent. The most impor-

tant factors are types of surgery, allergies, multiple blood transfusions, recurrent infection without an identifiable cause, slow wound healing, exposure to certain chemicals, and whether one works in a radiation area.

Extremely important to the health care provider is a current and accurate history of medications. These would include vitamins, steroids, anticoagulants, allergy medicine, antidysrhythmic drugs, immunosuppressive drugs, cancer drugs, and drugs that contain aspirin.

Inspection

With an accurate family and patient history known, inspection becomes more valuable in looking for specifics.

The skin is inspected for pallor, cyanosis, jaundice, ulcerations or lesions, swelling, and neuromuscular alterations. If lymph nodes are swollen and/or red, detailed palpation should be performed.

The skin is affected by prolonged bleeding. There may be excessive bruising, petechiae, ecchymoses, epistaxis, and retinal hemorrhage; hemorrhage from any orifice may cause the skin to be pale. Because of retinal hemorrhage, there may be a loss of visual acuity and/or blindness may occur.

Hematologic dysfunction may result in the mouth deteriorating with gingival bleeding, ulcerations of the tongue, ulcerations of the buccal mucosa, and dysphagia.

The assessment must include observation of the entire body looking for signs of infection, ulcers anywhere on the body, masses large enough to be identified, and deformities especially of the joints.

Because of hematologic dysfunctions, especially those involved with bleeding into joints, some patients lose the sensations of pain, touch, position, and vibration.

The patient's behavior indicates his or her mood and general mental status. Irritability and other emotional expressions may occur as a result of bleeding or because of an immune disorder.

Palpation

All superficial lymph nodes, even if they are not swollen or red, must be gently palpated to determine tenderness, size, and location. It should also be noted if the lymph nodes are moveable or fixed and if they are hard, soft, or firm. The nurse tests for tenderness of the sternum and adjacent ribs, providing these are not fractured, as in a trauma case.

Bleeding into the joints may cause pain or lack of mobility of those joints because of hemarthrosis. Bones may ache as a result of pressure inside the bone marrow as it expands to meet the replacement needs of formed blood elements. Repeated bleeding into the joints eventually results in decreased mobility of those joints.

Palpation of the spleen is not usually possible unless it is enlarged. If there is splenomegaly, the spleen is usually very tender. Only light palpation is required to detect tenderness and pain. Deep palpation of an enlarged spleen may rupture it.

The liver is palpated to determine hepatomegaly and/or nodules and hardness. Both hepatomegaly and splenomegaly may be caused by cell overproduction as in polycythemia or leukemia or by defective cells being rapidly destroyed (hemolytic anemias).

Percussion

The assessment skill of percussion as described in Chapter 48 is used to determine if the liver or spleen is enlarged. The lungs and heart are also percussed since hematologic disturbances may result in pulmonary emboli and other lung problems. Cardiac problems may also develop secondary to hematologic dysfunction. These problems might include palpitations, angina pectoris, and prosthetic heart valves.

The abdomen is assessed by percussing as explained in Chapter 48. This may reveal abdominal pain, abdominal masses, hematochezic stools, or black stools indicating the presence of melena. By referring to the patient's history, the nurse may learn of ulcers, changes in bowel habits, alcohol abuse, or vitamin K deficiency.

Auscultation

This assessment tool is used to determine murmurs, bruits, rubs, tachycardia/bradycardia, pulmonary edema, abnormal lung sounds, and bowel sounds.

Auscultation of the abdomen may reveal the presence of aneurysms of the aorta and impedance of blood flow at the ileo-femoral bifurcations.

Auscultation of the carotid bruits indicates a probable decreased cerebral perfusion secondary to atherosclerotic disease.

The auscultation of pericardial and pleural rubs was covered in Chapters 49 and 50.

The genitourinary tract is affected by hematologic disorders. This may result in urinary tract infections, bladder dysfunction, hematuria, and menstrual disorders in the female.

All of the nervous system functions are impaired if hematologic disorders occur. This includes all sensory, motor, and mentation functions.

— 55

Assessment of the Patient with Gastrointestinal Dysfunction

Learning Objectives

By the end of this chapter, the nurse will be able to:

1. List the correct order for assessment skills to be used.
2. Identify the four regions of the abdomen.
3. List the factors observed during inspection of the G.I. system.
4. Briefly describe percussion of the abdomen.
5. Differentiate between superficial and deep palpation.
6. Briefly describe palpation of the abdomen.

An assessment of the gastrointestinal (G.I.) system is different from that of other body systems because of the order in which the examination steps are performed. One starts with inspection and then auscultates the abdomen before continuing with percussion and palpation. This is because percussion and palpation may alter the bowel sounds.

History

Pertinent history about the patient's family is important, but in the G.I. system it is not as crucial as in other systems. The *patient's* history is important, both past history and information on the current disorder.

Anatomic Sites

Anatomic landmarks are used in describing the location of pain, masses, tenderness, scars, and other abnormal findings. The abdominal divisions are shown in Figure 55-1 with the major structures located in each section.

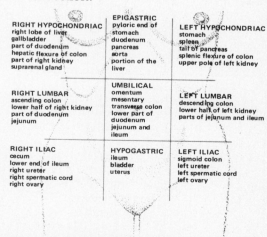

RIGHT HYPOCHONDRIAC	EPIGASTRIC	LEFT HYPOCHONDRIAC
right lobe of liver	pyloric end of stomach	stomach
gallbladder	duodenum	spleen
part of duodenum	pancreas	tail of pancreas
hepatic flexure of colon	aorta	splenic flexure of colon
part of right kidney	portion of the liver	upper pole of left kidney
suprarenal gland		

RIGHT LUMBAR	UMBILICAL	LEFT LUMBAR
ascending colon	omentum	descending colon
lower half of right kidney	mesentary	lower half of left kidney
part of duodenum	transverse colon	parts of jejunum and ileum
jejunum	lower part of duodenum	
	jejunum and ileum	

RIGHT ILIAC	HYPOGASTRIC	LEFT ILIAC
cecum	ileum	sigmoid colon
lower end of ileum	bladder	left ureter
right ureter	uterus	left spermatic cord
right spermatic cord		left ovary
right ovary		

Figure 55-1. Abdominal divisions and major structures in each division.

Inspection

Inspection of the G.I. system begins with the mouth and ends with the rectum. The mouth is inspected for any masses, swelling or bleeding of the gums, and abnormalities of internal structure.

After inspecting the patient's mouth with the patient in a supine position, the shape of the abdomen is noted. Abdominal contours (Figure 55-2) may be flat, scaphoid, rounded, indrawn, or distended.

The umbilicus is inspected for its contour and location on the abdominal wall; if the umbilicus is everted, signs of inflammation or hernia may be present.

The skin over the entire body, including the abdomen, is inspected for scars, varicosities, lesions, rashes, spider angiomata, and striae. Pulsations are usually aortic and are usually seen in the epigastrium.

The presence of any lesions, masses (mobile or fixed), draining wounds,

Figure 55-2. Abdominal contours.

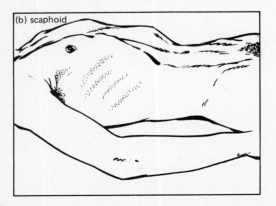
(a) flat

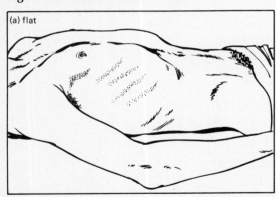
(b) scaphoid

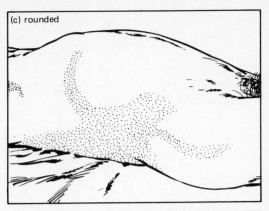
(c) rounded

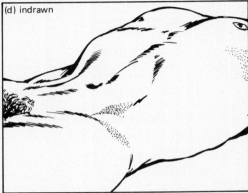
(d) indrawn

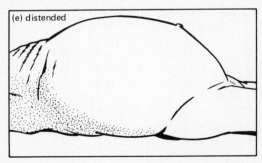
(e) distended

fistulas, ostomies, or asymmetries indicates a need for further examination. Striae may be silvery faded lines from extensive abdominal extension such as occurs in a pregnancy or they may be purple striae which occur with rapid, high-dose steroid use or Cushing's syndrome. An abnormal pubic hair distribution (normal distribution is diamond-shaped in males and triangular in females) may indicate an endocrine disorder. Further testing is warranted.

The abdomen is also inspected for normal peristaltic waves in thin adults.

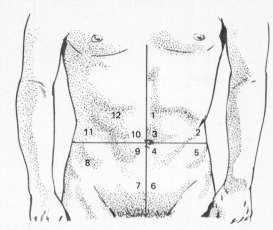

Figure 55-3. Abdominal sites for auscultation.

Auscultation

This is the next assessment tool used in assessing the G.I. system. The auscultation is performed in a clockwise fashion covering the entire abdomen. The abdominal sites for auscultation are shown in Figure 55-3.

All of the numbered sites of Figure 55-3 are auscultated. Each time you move the stethoscope, remove it from the abdomen and then replace it. Dragging the stethoscope across the abdomen frequently causes involuntary muscle spasms which will alter the sounds heard. Normal abdominal sounds are the peristaltic sounds which are high-pitched, gurgling noises occurring five or more times per minute. The diaphragm of the stethoscope transmits these sounds most easily.

Two abnormal types of bowel sounds may be heard upon auscultation. The first type is the absence of sound or extremely weak and infrequent sounds which may indicate bowel immotility associated with peritonitis or paralytic ileus. Auscultation must be performed for 3–5 minutes prior to a determination. The second type of abnormal sound is a frequent, loud, rushing, and high-pitched sound which may indicate mechanical obstruction or hypermotility of the bowel. Auscultation should be noted with relation to hours after eating.

The abdomen should be auscultated for other abnormal sounds such as bruits and peritoneal friction rubs. Bruits may indicate aortic aneurysms or other pathological conditions.

Percussion

Using the mediated method (Figure 55-4), percuss the abdomen to determine density of the area and underlying structures. Nor-

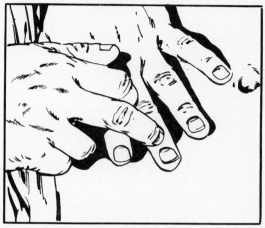

Figure 55-4. Mediated percussion of the abdomen.

mally, the sounds that are produced range from tympany to dullness. Flatness is an abnormal sound. Percussion over the stomach, the epigastric area, or upper midline section normally yields a tympanic sound.

If a dull sound is obtained in percussing the abdomen, it may be necessary to determine the absence or presence of fluid. If the

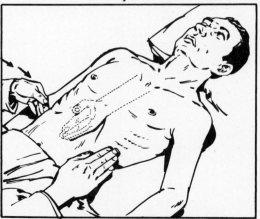

Figure 55-5. Percussion for abdominal fluid wave (ballottement).

patient is alert and can cooperate, have the patient place the outer edge of his or her hand longitudinally along the midline of his or her stomach (Figure 55-5). This is to prevent fat waves from traveling across the abdomen and being interpreted as fluid waves. If the patient cannot assist, have another person place his or her hand mid-abdomen. Place the fingertips of your right hand in the subject's lumbar area at the side. With your left hand, quickly thrust your fingers into the opposite lumbar side region. If fluid is present, the right hand will feel the wave. If ascites is present and severe, fluid waves may be seen as well as percussed.

Percuss the outline of the liver by beginning in the right mid-clavicular line at the mid-sternal level and progress downward. When the upper edge of the liver is reached, a dull sound will be produced. The upper liver is generally located between the fifth and seventh intercostal space. Continue to percuss downward until the lower level of the liver is located. The upper and lower boundaries should be no more than 10 cm apart.

Palpation

Palpation begins with light technique described in Chapter 48. The examiner places his or her hand palm side down with fingers extended just above the abdomen. To actually palpate, the pads of the fingers are placed on the abdomen and light pressure is applied to about 1 cm or the depth of subcutaneous tissue; the fingers are moved in a circular pattern. Palpate one quadrant completely before proceeding to the next quadrant. Light palpation of the abdomen is utilized to determine the characteristics of the skin and subcutaneous tissue and to elicit any areas of tenderness. If the patient has tenderness in a specific area, palpate that area last. Guarding of the abdomen is voluntary or involuntary. Involuntary guarding persists through the entire respiratory cycle. This results in a tense abdominal musculature. Voluntary guarding is used during inspiration, with the muscles relaxing during expiration. Light palpation of the inguinal area often reveals the pres-

ence of small lymph nodes (0.5–1 cm in diameter). These nodes are termed shotty; they most frequently occur after pubescence and remain throughout adulthood.

55-6). The fingers of the free hand press upon the joints of the other hand. The upper hand then applies pressure onto the lower hand. Deep palpation is 4–5 cm in depth or a suitable distance past the subcutaneous tissue. All quadrants of the abdomen are palpated like this to outline underlying contents and structures.

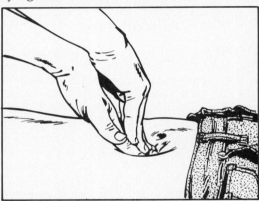

Figure 55-6. Deep palpation by manual method.

The liver is palpated in the right upper quadrant by placing a hand parallel to the rectus muscle and just under the inferior angle of the right costal margin (about 2.5 cm below the percussed lower liver border). Have the patient take a deep breath, allowing the "abdominal hand" to rise with the protruding abdominal wall. During expiration, exert a slow, gentle, downward and forward pressure with the abdominal hand to a depth of 4 or 5 cm. Once the correct depth is reached, the patient is asked to take another breath. The examiner keeps his or her hand on the abdominal wall without moving it. Inspiration aids in the descent of the liver. The fingers must palpate the liver's edge, but the liver must also rise some with the abdominal wall to prevent pain. The liver's edge feels firm and it has a sharp ridge of relatively straight contour.

Although the spleen is not normally palpable, the splenic area is palpated. The same procedure for palpating the liver is used in palpating the spleen. Splenic enlargement is graded as slight (1–4 cm below costal margin), moderate (4–8 cm below costal margin), and great (8 cm or more below costal margin).

Palpation of the kidney is performed by pressing directly upward beneath the costal margin at the mid-clavicular line while the patient takes a deep breath. The downward movement of the diaphragm also displaces downward the inferior margin of the kidney which may be felt at this point. The right kidney is more often felt because it is lower than the left kidney. The kidneys are not normally palpable in the adult unless the adult is very thin; even then, only the lower pole of the kidney is palpable.

Large masses or a distended bladder may be palpable in the abdominal region. Large masses may be found in any quadrant with deep palpation. Manipulation of the mass should be minimal, but it is essential to determine size and characteristics. Palpation of the bladder begins 2.5–5 cm above the pubic area. The palpating fingers gently press down and curve backward towards the hand. If the bladder is distended (which in the adult is over 5 ounces or 150 cc), palpation may start higher on the abdominal surface and work downward until the bladder is encountered. A description of the location, in centimeters from the umbilicus or the pubic area, is recorded.

— 56 —————————————

Assessment of the Psychosocial Needs of the Patient

Learning Objectives

By the end of this chapter, the nurse will be able to:

1. List the assessment skills used in assessing the patient with a psychosocial dysfunction.
2. List eight parameters that may be explored.
3. List two nursing interventions for each of the eight parameters above.

There appears to be a general agreement among all nurses that the psychosocial needs of all patients are important and may have a direct relationship on the outcome of their illness.

A very definite line of demarcation is felt to exist between the nurses in academia and the nurses in critical care clinical practice. The former stress the paramount importance of identifying the patient's psychosocial needs and directing nurses' activities to meeting these needs. The latter acknowledge the psychosocial needs of the critically ill patient but stress that their primary responsibility is to provide the physical care required to keep the patient alive. The clinical practitioner feels that meeting most psychosocial needs of the patient is important but secondary to meeting life-threatening physical needs since a lot of the psychosocial care of the patient will occur after

transfer from the critical care unit to a general floor.

The normal assessment skills of inspection, percussion, palpation, and auscultation cannot be used in treating a patient's psychosocial needs. Inspection is the basic, if not only, assessment skill used.

Inspection

The order in which the patient's psychosocial needs are observed varies from institution to institution and indeed from nurse to nurse. One order based on patient needs may first include pain and then communication patterns, followed by coping methods (strengths and potentials), needs and stress limitations, perception, sleep patterns, body image, and self-esteem. Many more psychosocial phenomena could be listed (refer to Chapter 47), but these are probably the major factors to be considered in a critical care unit.

Pain or the degree of pain that a patient is experiencing may be ignored during a critical phase such as intubation or cardiac arrest. During other settings, the nurses are able to observe the patient and see the degree of pain expressed nonverbally by the patient. Pain may be enhanced by or caused by fear and anxiety. Thus it is appropriate and indeed necessary to ask the patient if he or she is having pain and to have the patient describe the location, intensity, and duration of the pain. If needed, pain medication should ALWAYS be given. However, often the nurse talking to, reassuring, and repositioning the patient may be sufficient to stop the pain or decrease it to a level that can be tolerated or that would require less medication.

Communication patterns cannot be established with the semi-lucid patient. Observing the patient who is moderately alert, the nurse may be able to identify the manner in which the patient most often expresses his or her needs and/or feelings both verbally and nonverbally. By observing the patient, one may also identify specific nurses with whom the patient can communicate and those with whom the patient cannot communicate. In answering the patient's questions, the nurse should explain answers as simply, as concisely, and as truthfully as possible. If a nurse is untruthful with a patient with whom he or she has established good rapport, the rapport would be jeopardized and a communication link that could have been beneficial would have been lost.

Strengths and potentials are observed by the nurse as positive attributes or resources that the patient can use to help in the current situation. The patient may use several coping mechanisms, but close observation by the nurse may identify the *most* successful coping mechanism used by the patient. The nurse can then support the patient in a manner compatible with this coping mechanism. She or he may be able to reinforce the patient's ability to cope by directly talking to the patient regarding things that will make the critical care experience more tolerable.

Needs and stress limitations are those needs that the patient has that MUST be met and the stress that MUST be reduced. Close observation of the patient will often allow the nurse to identify specific needs and stressors. But the most effective manner to identify these needs and stresses is to ask the patient what he or she needs, what is stressful to him or her, and what may the nurse do to help with the most important needs and the worst stressors.

Perception is how the patient views his or her situation and the critical care setting. Perception is one aspect of psychosocial needs of which observation must be verified by the patient. The nurse may question the feelings the patient has and ask for verification of the emotions he or she has seen pertaining to the patient's reaction to and perception of his or her current situation. If the nurse has identified the patient's perception, he or she may be able to question the patient regarding actions that will help the patient cope with his or her situation.

Sleep patterns are almost always interrupted by the patient's admission to critical care units. The patient's sleep is interrupted by many factors including the taking of vital signs, administering medication, noise from monitoring machines, and pain. The nurse may observe the amount of time the patient appears to sleep and attempt to determine if the patient ever achieves REM sleep. Sleep for relatively long periods of time may be achieved by decreasing noises, lights, and the number of times the nurse "must" awaken the patient for some reason. If the patient does not receive sufficient, good quality sleep, the nurse may become aware of a decreased ability of the patient to cope with the situation and the gradual onset of "ICU-itis" or "CCU-itis." The administration of pain medication or a hypnotic substance may be beneficial.

Body image is usually damaged with admission to a critical care unit. If able to talk, the patient may make statements revealing concepts of his or her body image. If the patient has had an extremity or portion thereof amputated as a result of trauma or disease, the body image is definitely altered. The nurse may help the patient to accept this change in body image by LIS-TENING to the patient's comments about himself or herself and any equipment around the patient. The nurse should support the patient emotionally through fostering the patient's use of previously identified coping mechanisms. The nurse should also observe and record the patient's reaction to his or her body image. General support and possibly the use of humor may help the patient to accept a new body image.

Self-esteem may be defined as how a patient feels as a person—adequate or inadequate. The nurse should encourage the patient to ventilate his or her feelings and listen especially for comments related to the patient's perception of himself or herself. The nurse, as time and the patient's condition allows, may help the patient to strengthen a low level of self-esteem through ventilation of the patient's feelings.

Communication and sleep patterns, needs, insights into self-esteem, and body image should be recorded AND reported to the nurses on the general floor when the patient is transferred from critical care.

There are many opportunities to help the patient psychosocially and to prepare the patient and his or her family emotionally for transfer from the unit. However, the primary goal of critical care nursing is the treatment of the immediate, life-threatening event that has occurred. Secondary to this, *good* critical care nurses are continually trying to meet as many of the psychosocial needs of the patient as possible.

Assessment of Body Systems Bibliography

Assessing Your Patient: Nursing Photobook. Springhouse, PA: Intermed Communications, 1980

*Assessment (patient history, anatomy and physiology, physical examination). Nursing 83 Books, The nurse's reference library. Springhouse, PA: Intermed Communications, 1983

*Bates B: A Guide to Physical Examination. Philadelphia: J. B. Lippincott, 1974

Borg N, Mikas DL, Stark J, Williams SM (eds): Core Curriculum for Critical Care Nursing, 2nd ed. American Association of Critical-Care Nurses. Philadelphia: W. B. Saunders, 1981

*Burns KR, Johnson PJ: Health Assessment in Clinical Practice. Englewood Cliffs, NJ: Prentice-Hall, 1980

Chaney PD (ed): Assessing Vital Functions Accurately. Nursing Skillbook, Nursing 77 Books. Springhouse, PA: Intermed Communications, 1977

Coping with Neurologic Disorders: Nursing Photobook. Springhouse, PA: Intermed Communications, 1981

Dealing with Emergencies: Nursing Photobook. Springhouse, PA: Intermed Communications, 1980

Ensuring Intensive Care: Nursing Photobook. Springhouse, PA: Intermed Communications, 1981

Giving Cardiac Care: Nursing Photobook. Springhouse, PA: Intermed Communications, 1980

Jackson J: The Whole Nurse Catalog. New York: Churchill Livingstone, 1980

Performing GI Procedures: Nursing Photobook. Springhouse, PA: Intermed Communications, 1981

Providing Respiratory Care: Nursing Photobook. Springhouse, PA: Intermed Communications, 1980

*Roberts SL: Behavioral Concepts and the Critically Ill Patient. Englewood Cliffs, NJ: Prentice-Hall, 1976

Appendix I

Systems Abbreviations, Formulae, and Tests

In this appendix, select abbreviations, formulae, and tests have been included that the nurse may or should be able to use in applying the nursing process to patient care.

Respiratory

Respiratory Abbreviations
Major:
C—Concentration of gas in blood
F —Fractional concentration in dry gas
P —Pressure or partial pressure
Q—Volume of blood
Q̇—Volume of blood per unit time
R —Respiratory exchange ratio
S —Saturation of hemoglobin with O_2
V̇—Volume of gas
V̇—Volume of gas per unit time

Symbols for Gas Phase:
A—Alveolar
B —Barometric
D—Dead space
E —Expired
I —Inspired
L —Lung
T —Tidal

Note: Abbreviations are *all* capitals

Symbols for Blood Phase:
a —arterial
c —capillary
c —end-capillary
i —ideal
v —venous
v̄ —mixed venous

Note: Abbreviations are *all* lowercase

A patient history will help in calculating various formulae.

HISTORY

A 47-year-old black male has a long history of tuberculosis with cavitary lesions in both upper lobes. He was admitted with hemoptysis. He underwent a right upper lobectomy and a right thoracoplasty. The patient has had a stormy postoperative course including chest tubes for complete collapse of the RML.

Current information is on postoperative day 14. The patient is in ICU, on a Puritan Bennett MA-1 with no spontaneous respirations. Parameters are:

Ventilator
V_T = 1000 cc
IMV = 14/min.
FI_{O_2} = 40%

Lab Values (ABGs)
pH = 7.49
Pa_{CO_2} = 36
Pa_{O_2} = 95
Saturation = 97%

Hgb = 12, Body weight = 210 lbs (95 kg)
PE_{CO_2} = $\dot{V}_E$ into Douglas bag and run through gas
    analyzer = PE_{CO_2} = 19

Using the Given Data

1. **Dead space**

$$V_D = \frac{(PA_{CO_2} - PE_{CO_2})}{PA_{CO_2}} \times \dot{V}_E$$

$$= \frac{(36 - 19) \times 14 \text{ liters per minute (lpm)}}{36}$$

$$= 6.61 \text{ ml}$$

When PA_{CO_2} = 36, PE_{CO_2} = 19, $\dot{V}_E$ = 14 lpm

2. **Physiologic Dead Space (Bohr Equation)**

$$\frac{V_D}{V_T} = \frac{PA_{CO_2} - PE_{CO_2}}{PA_{CO_2}}$$

$$= \frac{36 - 19}{36}$$

$$= 0.47 \text{ ml}$$

When PA_{CO_2} = 36, PE_{CO_2} = 19, $\dot{V}_E$ = 14 lpm

Three Methods of Determining Alveolar Ventilation

1. $\dot{V}_A = V_T - V_D$
            $= 1000 - 470$
            $= 530 \text{ cc}$

When V_T = 1000,
        V_D = 470 (Physiologic dead space from Bohr equation multiplied to remove decimal)

OR

$$\dot{V}_A = (V_T - V_D) \, F$$
$$= (1000 - 470) \, 14$$
$$= 7420 \text{ ml/min.}$$
$$= 7.42 \text{ lpm}$$

When $V_T = 1000$, $V_D = 470$, $F = 14$ (ventilator IMV = 14/min.)

2.
$$\dot{V}_A = \frac{\dot{V}_{E_{CO_2}} \times 0.863}{P_{A_{CO_2}}}$$

$$= \frac{304 \times 0.863}{36}$$

$$= 7.29 \text{ lpm}$$

Where $304 = \dot{V}_{E_{CO_2}}$,
(3.2 ml/kg Body Weight $= 95 \times 3.2 = 304$ ml)
0.863 = respiratory quotient, $P_{A_{CO_2}} = 36$

3.
$$\dot{V}_A = \frac{\dot{V}_{E_{CO_2}}}{F_{A_{CO_2}}\%} \times 100 \times F$$

$$= \frac{19 \text{ ml}}{36\%} \times 100 \times 14$$

$$= \frac{19 \text{ ml}}{3.6\% \times 100} \times 100 \times 14$$

$$= \frac{19 \text{ ml}}{3.6} \times 100 \times 14$$

$$= 5.278 \times 100 \times 14$$

$$= 527.8/\text{breath} \times 14 \text{ (IMV)} = 7,388 \text{ ml/min} = 7.388 \text{ lpm}$$
rounded off $\dot{V}_A = 7.4$ lpm

When MAV = maximum alveolar volume,
from: 1000 V_T (on respirator) $\times$ 14 IMV (on respirator)
thus: $1000 \times 14 = 14,000 = V_{A_{CO_2}} = V_{a_{CO_2}} = V_{E_{CO_2}}$
$$= P_{A_{CO_2}} = F_{A_{CO_2}}$$

Minute Alveolar Ventilation

1. Minute Alveolar Ventilation
$$\dot{V}_E = \dot{V}_D + \dot{V}_A$$
$$\dot{V}_E = \dot{V}_D = 470 \text{ cc (from Bohr equation multiplied to remove decimal)}$$
$$\dot{V}_A = 530 \text{ cc}$$
$$\dot{V}_D = 6.6 \text{ liters}$$
$$\dot{V}_A = 7.4 \text{ liters}$$
$$\dot{V}_E = 14.0 \text{ lpm}$$

Oxygen Formulae

1. O_2 Capacity (combined)
$$= \text{Hgb} \times 1.34 \text{ ml O}_2 \qquad \text{given: Hgb} = 12 \text{ as stated in parameters}$$
$$= 12 \times 1.34 = 16.08 \text{ ml O}_2$$

2. O_2 Content
$$= (Hgb \times 1.34) \times Saturation + (Pa_{O_2} \times 0.003)$$
$$= (12 \times 1.34)0.97 + (95 \times 0.003)$$
$$= 15.6 + 0.29$$
$$= 15.89 \text{ ml}$$

3. Saturation
$$Sa_{O_2} = \frac{O_2 \text{ content}}{O_2 \text{ capacity}} \times 100(\%)$$

$$= \frac{15.89}{16.08}$$

$$= .988 \times 100 = 98.8\%$$

4. O_2 Transport
$$= O_2 \text{ content} \times 10 \times \text{cardiac output}$$
$$= 15.89 \times 10 \times 5.1$$
$$= 810.39 \text{ ml } O_2/L$$

5. $A - aDO_2$
$$PA_{O_2} = 95 \text{ (given)}$$

$$= (P_B - P_{H_2O}) \, FI_{O_2} - \frac{Pa_{CO_2}}{0.8}$$

$$= (760 - 47).40 - \frac{36}{0.8}$$

$$= (713).4 - 45$$
$$= 285 - 45$$
$$= 240$$
$$240 - 95 = 145 \text{ mm Hg}$$

Arterial blood gas interpretation is covered in Chapter 3.

Cardiac Formulae

Oxygen Consumption = Average amount of expelled O_2 into Fick bags in ml/min.

$$\text{Cardiac Output} = \frac{O_2 \text{ Consumption (liters/min.)}}{AVO_2 \text{ Difference (vols.)}}$$

$$\text{Cardiac Index} = \frac{\text{Cardiac Output (C.O.)}}{\text{Body Surface Area (B.S.A.)}}$$

$$\text{Stroke Volume} = \frac{\text{Cardiac Output}}{\text{Heart Rate}}$$

$$\text{Total Pulmonary Resistance} = \frac{\text{PA Mean}}{\text{Cardiac Output}} \text{ (mm Hg/L/min.)}$$

$$\text{Pulmonary Vascular Resistance} = \frac{\text{PA Mean} - \text{LA Mean}}{\text{Cardiac Output}} \text{ (mm Hg/L/min.)}$$

$$\text{Systemic Vascular Resistance} = \frac{\text{Peripheral Arterial Mean}}{\text{Cardiac Output}} \text{ (mm Hg/L/min.)}$$

Sites of Infarction

Using leads I, II, III, aVR, aVL, and aVF, one can determine the type/site of acute infarctions.

Rule: Q wave plus an elevated ST = MI (myocardial infarction).

To determine a site of infarction, use the leads listed next.

Leads

I — aVR = $\underline{R}$eaches out and down; it probes but gives no answers.
II — aVL = $\underline{L}$ateral M.I.
III — aVF = In$\underline{F}$erior M.I.
V_1, V_2, V_3 = pure anterior M.I.
V_2, V_3, V_4 = anterior: anteri_septal M.I.
V_3, V_4 = septal M.I.
V_5, V_6 = apical M.I.

Figure A-1 shows three types of QRS complexes in myocardial infarctions.

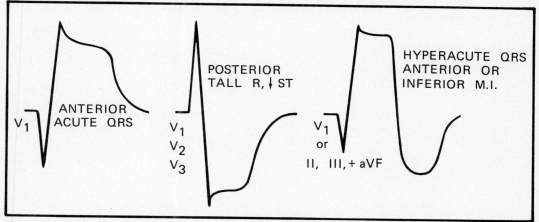

Figure A-1. Typical complexes in specified myocardial infarctions. Hyperacute is most likely to have fatal dysrhythmia.

Notes:

1. Hyperacute QRS complex indicates the patient is likely to develop fatal dysrhythmias.
2. Q wave > 2 mm deep and > 0.04 seconds wide is a significant Q and usually indicates a transmural M.I.
3. Inverted T, a depressed ST, and no Q wave usually indicates a subendocardial M.I.
4. For setting priorities when understaffed or overpopulated: in$\underline{F}$erior M.I.—$\underline{F}$ouls up your night (multiple dysrhythmias, etc.); anterior M.I.—often dies in the night.

Axis Deviation

For strictly CCU-oriented nurses, axis deviation is probably well understood. For non-cardiac critical care nurses, axis deviation is usually a difficult concept to understand. The following Figure A-2 will help these nurses.

Comparing leads I and III or I and aVF, the following identifies the axis deviation by the relationship of the QRS complexes.

A variant form is to use lead III instead of aVF which would equal from 2–7 on the clock circle in Figure A-2 as full range of normal axis, that is, 30°–90° as an approximate normal axis.

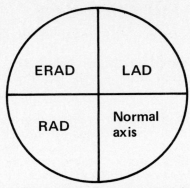

Figure A-2. LAD = Left axis deviation; RAD = Right axis deviation; ERAD = Extreme right axis deviation.

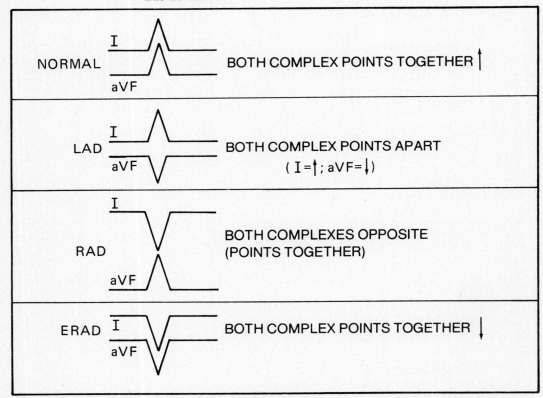

Figure A-3. A method of rapid determination of degree of axis deviation in a 12 lead EKG.

Neurologic Section

1. Normal ICP = 50–200 cm of H_2O or 4–15 mm Hg
   To convert cm of H_2O to mm Hg use formula:

$$\frac{cm\ H_2O}{1.36} = mm\ Hg$$

Obtain ICP from monitor readout to use in formulae a and b.
  a. MAP = SAP
     (mean arterial pressure = systemic arterial pressure)
  b. CPP = MAP − ICP
     (CPP = cerebral perfusion pressure)
  c. CPP = CBF
     (approximates cerebral blood flow)
2. Queckenstedt's Test
   With a spinal needle in place, a manometer is attached and a pressure reading is obtained. Then the neck veins of the patient are gently compressed. An immediate rise in CSF pressure occurs. The pressure is released and the manometer reading falls to the original value. This indicates patent circulation of the cerebrospinal fluid. No change in the manometer reading indicates obstruction of CSF flow.
   Other relevant tests and results are found in the neurologic section and in Chapter 51 on neurologic assessment.

Renal Section

The creatinine clearance test is probably the most reliable laboratory test used to determine renal function. This is due to the fact that creatinine is a constant end-product of creatine use in the body in an irreversible equation. Creatinine varies little in the relation to diet, urine volume, or physical exertion. It is proportional to total muscle mass.

The formula for creatinine clearance is:

$$C = \frac{(U \times V)}{P}$$

where C = clearance rate
  U = urine concentration of creatinine
  V = volume of urine durine test period
  P = plasma concentration of creatinine
  The plasma is drawn half-way through the time span of the test.

Normal results may occur until more than 50% of the total nephrons have been damaged. For men, normal creatinine clearance is 105 ± 20 ml/min./1.73 m^2 of body surface. For women, normal creatinine clearance is 95 ± 20 ml/min./1.73 m^2 of body surface. These approximate values are in normal, healthy 20-year-olds and will decrease about 6 ml/min./decade.

Many other urine tests and diagnostic procedures will be used when the creatinine clearance is abnormal.

Other Sections

Endocrine, hematologic, gastrointestinal, and psychosocial system abnormalities are seen on inspection and in various laboratory tests.

The assessment chapters identify specific observations to make, the systems in which other assessment skills may be used, and the order of use.

In addition to laboratory tests, x-rays, ultrasound, nuclear medicine, angiography, and possible biopsy are extremely important in the aforementioned systems.

Appendix II

Laboratory Values[1]

Laboratory values differ from institution to institution. Those given here will be similar to those in other institutions but not exact. Therefore, it is necessary for a nurse to learn the values of his or her own institution.

Most hospitals maintain a list of specific laboratory values (known as panic values) which are life-threatening and must be reported to the physician immediately. The laboratory technician normally repeats the tests, notifies the lab supervisor, and then reports the results to the nurse on the floor. Information as to who reported the abnormal value, the time of reporting, and the name of the person who received the report is recorded in some fashion.

Panic Values—Chemistry

	Less Than	Greater Than
Serum Calcium	7 mg/dl	12.0 mg/dl
Serum Glucose (Newborn)	30 mg/dl	300 mg/dl
Serum Glucose	50 mg/dl	500 mg/dl
Serum Potassium (Newborn)	2.5 mEq/L	8.0 mEq/L
Serum Potassium	3.0 mEq/L	6.5 mEq/L
Serum Potassium (Hemolyzed Specimen)	3.0 mEq/L	8.0 mEq/L
Serum Sodium	120 mEq/L	160 mEq/L

Panic Values—Hematology

	Less Than	Greater Than
Hemoglobin	5 gm	N/A
Hematocrit	15.0%	N/A
WBC	1,000/cu mm	100,000/cu mm
Platelet Count	30,000/cu mm	1,000,000/cu mm

COAGULATION

P.T.	Greater than 30 seconds
P.T.T.	Greater than 110 seconds
Fibrinogen	Less than 100 mg/dl

[1]Used with permission of Mr. Ron Noble, MT (ASCP), Director of Administrative Services and Chief Technologist for Pathology, Richland Memorial Hospital, Columbia, South Carolina.

Panic Values—Microbiology

Positive Blood Culture
Positive Cerebrospinal Fluid Gram Stains or India Ink Preps
Positive Acid-Fast Smears of Cultures

List of Laboratory Normal Values

Procedures	Normal Values
Acid Phosphatase, Prostatic	0–0.8 IU/L
A/G Ratio	1.0–2.2
Albumin, Serum	3.0–5.5 gm/dl
Alkaline, Phosphatase	30–115 IU/L
Alpha-1 Antitrypsin	
age: 6 weeks–adult	85–213 mg/dl
Alpha-2 Macroglobulin	146–369 mg/dl
Amino Acid Screen, Urine	Negative
Ammonia, Plasma	11–35 micromoles/L
Amylase, Serum	20–110 IU/L
Amylase, Urine	4–37 IU/2 hrs.
Anti-DNase B Titer	
preschool	1:60
school age	1:170
adult	1:85
Antinuclear Antibody (ANA) Titer	Less than 1:20 usually rules out autoimmune disease
Anti-Smooth Muscle Antibody (ASMA)	Negative
Anti-Strep Screen	Negative
Anti-Strep Titer	Less than 4-fold rise in titer
Anti-Thrombin III Assay	80–120%
Bence Jones Protein	Negative
Bilirubin, Direct, Serum	0–0.3 mg/dl
Bilirubin, Fecal	Negative
Bilirubin, Indirect, Serum	
after age 1 month–adult	0.2–8.0 mg/dl
Bilirubin, Micro	0.2–1.2 mg/dl
Bilirubin, Total	0.2–1.2 mg/dl
Bilirubin, Urine	Negative
Bleeding Time	
Ivy (forearm puncture)	0.5–6.0 minutes
Simplate (modified Ivy)	2.3–6.0 minutes
Blood Urea Nitrogen (BUN)	10–26 mg/dl
Calcium, Serum	8.5–10.5 mg/dl
Calcium, Urine	50–150 mg/24 hrs.
Calcium, Urine Screen	Negative
Ceruloplasmin	18–45 mg/dl
Chloride, CSF	118–132 mEq/L
Chloride, Serum	96–106 mEq/L
Chloride, Urine	110–250 mEq/24 hrs.

Cholesterol
  under age 40 years   140–270 mg/dl
  over age 40 years   150–330 mg/dl
Cholesterol, HDL
  low risk   Less than 35 mg/dl
  intermediate risk   35–55 mg/dl
  high risk   Greater than 55 mg/dl
CO_2, serum   24–30 mEq/L
Cold Agglutinins   Negative
Complement, C-3   83–177 mg/dl
Complement, C-4   15–45 mg/dl
Complement, Total Hemolytic   56–150 CH100 units
Complete Blood Count (CBC)
  red blood count: male   4.1–5.5 $\times$ 10⁶/cu mm
                 female   3.9–5.2 $\times$ 10⁶/cu mm
  white blood count   4,500–10,500/cu mm
  hemoglobin: male   13.0–17.5 gm/dl
             female   11.5–16.0 gm/dl
  hematocrit: male   39–53%
            female   36–48%
  MCH   26–34 micromicrograms
  MCHC   31–37%
  MCV   80–100 cubic microns

  Platelet count   150–450 $\times$ 10³/cu mm
Creatine Phosphokinase (CPK)
  male   15–120 IU/L
  female   10–80 IU/L
Creatinine Clearance
  male   105 $\pm$ 20 ml/min.
  female   95 $\pm$ 20 ml/min.
Creatinine, Serum   0.7–1.5 mg/dl
Creatinine, Urine   1000–2000 mg/24 hrs.
C-Reactive Protein, Quantitative   Negative or <0.6 mg/dl
Differential White Count
  polys   40–70%
  bands   0–10%
  eosinophils   0–6%
  basophils   0–2%
  lymphocytes   15–45%
  reactive lymphocytes   0–6%
  monocytes   1–10%
Dilantin®
  therapeutic range   10.0–20.0 mcg/ml
  toxic level   Greater than 30 mcg/ml
Eosinophil Count   0–450/cu mm
Estriol   Varies according to weeks
                             of gestation and from day
                             to day in same patient
Euglobulin Clot Lysis   2–4 hrs.
Fat, Fecal (qualitative)   Small amount of neutral
                             fat is normal

Fat, Fecal (quantitative) — 1–7 grams/24 hrs. as fatty acids

Fibrin Split Products — Up to 10 mcg/ml
Fibrinogen — 180–400 mg/dl
Globulin, Serum — 2.4–3.5 gm/dl
Glucose, CSF — 40–70 mg/dl
Glucose, Serum (fasting)
   under age 50 years — 70–115 mg/dl
   over age 50 years — 85–125 mg/dl
Glucose, Urine — Negative
Ham's Test — No hemolysis
Haptoglobin — 27–139 mg/dl
Hematocrit
   male — 39–53%
   female — 36–48%
Hemoglobin
   male — 13.0–17.5 gm/dl
   female — 11.5–16.0 gm/dl
Hemoglobin F — Less than 2% in adults
Hemosiderin — Negative
Herpes I and II
   Immunofluorescence Titer — Less than 1:100 not significant

5HIAA (Serotonin) — 2–4 mg/24 hrs.
Homocystine — Negative
17-Hydroxycorticosteroids (17-OH)
   male — 3–10 mg/24 hrs.
   female — 2–6 mg/24 hrs.
Immunoglobulin A, Adult (IgA) — 70–312 mg/dl
Immunoglobulin E, Adult (IgE) — 0–104 IU/ml
Immunoglobulin G, Adult (IgG) — 639–1349 mg/dl
Immunoglobulin M, Adult (IgM) — 56–352 mg/dl
Immunoglobulin G, CSF — Less than 12% of total protein

17-Ketogenic Steroids (17-KGS)
   male — 5–23 mg/24 hrs.
   female — 3–15 mg/24 hrs.
Ketones, Urine — Negative
17-Ketosteroids
   male — 8–10 mg/24 hrs.
   female — 4–15 mg/24 hrs.
Lactic Acid, CSF — 0.6–2.2 mEq/L
Lactic Acid, Serum — 0.6–2.2 mEq/L
Lactic Dehydrogenase (LDH) — 60–225 IU/L
L. E. Prep. — Negative
Lee-White Clotting Time — 6–12 mins.
Lipase, Serum — 4–24 IU/dl
Lithium®
   therapeutic range — 0.5–1.5 mEq/L
   toxic level — Greater than 2.0 mEq/L
Magnesium, Serum — 1.5–2.0 mEq/L
Microsomal Antibody Titer — Less than 1:100
Monotest — Negative

Nitroblue Tetrozolium (NBT)	Less than 10% NBT positive neutrophiles
Occult Blood, Fecal	Negative
Occult Blood, Urine	Negative
Orosomucoid	30–135 mg/dl
Osmolality, Serum	270–295 mOsm/kg
Osmolality, Urine	40–1400 mOsm/kg
Osmotic Fragility	
initial hemolysis	0.44 ± 0.02
complete hemolysis	0.32 ± 0.02
Ox-cell Hemolysin Titer	Less than 1:56 titer
pH, Urine	Approximately 6.0
Phenobarbital	
therapeutic range	15.0–25.0 mcg/ml
toxic level	Greater than 25.0 mcg/ml
Phosphorus, Inorganic, Serum (adult)	2.5–4.2 mg/dl
Phosphorus, Urine	400–1300 mg/24 hrs.
Plasma Hemoglobin	Less than 3 mg/dl
Plasminogen	80–120%
Platelet Count	$150–450 \times 10^3$/cu mm
Potassium, Serum	3.5–5.0 mEq/L
Potassium, Urine	30–90 mEq/24 hrs.
Protein, Total, Serum	6.0–8.5 gm/dl
Protein, Total, Urine	25–75 mg/24 hrs.
Pseudocholinesterase	7–14 IU/ml
Rheumatoid Factor (RA)	Negative
Quinidine®	
therapeutic range	2.3–5.0 mcg/ml
toxic level	10 mcg/ml or higher
Red Cell Count	
male	4.1–5.5 million/cu mm
female	3.9–5.2 million/cu mm
Red Cell Indices	
MCH	26–34 micromicrograms
MCHC	31–37%
MCV	80–100 cubic microns
Reducing Substances, Fecal & Urine	Negative
Reticulocyte Count	0.5–1.5% in adults
	2–6% in newborn
Salicylate	
therapeutic range	2–29 mg/dl
Sedimentation Rate	
male	0–15 mm/hr.
female	0–20 mm/hr.
child (1–14 years)	0–15 mm/hr.
Semen Analysis	
pH	Approximately 7.7
volume	1.5–5.0 ml
count	60–150 million/ml
Serological Test for Syphilis	Non-reactive
Serotonin, 5HIAA, Quantitative	2–4 mg/24 hrs.
Serum Iron (adult)	35–140 mcg/dl
Serum Iron Binding Capacity	245–400 mcg/dl

SGOT	0–41 IU/L
SGPT	0–45 IU/L
Sodium, Serum	136–145 mEq/L
Sodium, Urine	40–220 mEq/24 hrs.
Specific Gravity, Urine	1.010–1.030
Sugar Water Test	No hemolysis
Sweat Chloride	
normal	Up to 30 mEq/L
borderline	30–60 mEq/L
positive (presumptive)	Greater than 60 mEq/L
Tegretol® (Carbamazepine)	
therapeutic range	Varies—3–8 mcg/ml effective in most patients
toxic level	Greater than 10 mcg/ml
Theophylline	
therapeutic range	10–20 mcg/ml
toxic level	May occur at levels greater than 15 mcg/ml
Thrombin Clotting Time	8–10 sec.
Tobramycin®	
trough levels	Greater than 2 mcg/ml may indicate tissue accumulation
Total Serum Solids (TSS)	5.5–8.0 gm/dl
Transferrin	204–360 mg/dl
Triglycerides	30–135 mg/dl
Uric Acid, Serum	
male	3.9–9.0 mg/dl
female	2.2–7.7 mg/dl
Valproic Acid®	
therapeutic	50–100 mg/ml
Viscosity, Serum	1.4–1.8 relative viscosity
VMA	0.5–12.0 mg/24 hrs.
White Blood Count (WBC)	4500–10,500/cu mm

Index

Page numbers followed by an **f** refer to figures; those followed by a **t** refer to tables.